PET/MR: Functional and Molecular Imaging of Neurological Diseases and Neurosciences

Jie Lu • Guoguang Zhao
Editors

PET/MR: Functional and Molecular Imaging of Neurological Diseases and Neurosciences

科学技术文献出版社
SCIENTIFIC AND TECHNICAL DOCUMENTATION PRESS

Springer

Editors
Jie Lu
Department of Radiology
and Nuclear Medicine
Xuanwu Hospital
Capital Medical Uniersity
Beijing, China

Guoguang Zhao
Department of Neurosurgery
Xuanwu Hospital
Capital Medical University
Beijing, China

ISBN 978-981-19-9901-7 ISBN 978-981-19-9902-4 (eBook)
https://doi.org/10.1007/978-981-19-9902-4
Jointly published with Scientific and Technical Documentation Press

This Springer imprint is published by the registered company Springer Nature Singapore Pte Ltd.
The registered company address is: 152 Beach Road, #21-01/04 Gateway East, Singapore 189721, Singapore

Preface

Brain disorders seriously endanger the life and health of people in China due to their high morbidity, mortality, and disability rate. Nowadays, research, development, and clinical application of neuroimaging techniques are developing rapidly, aimed at further improving the accuracy of diagnosis of brain disorders. The invention and application of integrated positron emission tomography/magnetic resonance (PET/MR), a product of organic combination of functional brain imaging and molecular imaging techniques, is aimed at fulfilling the exploration of brain disorders and brain science. Based on the theory of brain function and molecular biology and with the help of modern medical imaging techniques, it truly realizes in vivo visualization of different parts of the signaling pathways in the human body.

Basic studies in molecular biology can fully exert their research significance only if they are applied to humans. Integrated PET/MR builds a bridge between basic research in molecular biology and its in vivo clinical application in humans. It can dynamically, objectively, and quantitatively transform the neurotransmitters, immune proteins, and tissue-specific biomarkers into intuitive spatial distribution images, followed by fusing with structural images to achieve accurate identification and delineation of lesions with high sensitivity and specificity. Moreover, integrated PET/MR can be useful to adequately identify the pathological tissues and healthy tissues, locate targets, and outline the boundaries. Using integrated PET/MR in combination with advanced innovative techniques (e.g., analysis methods for brain science, neuromodulation, surgical robots, and image-guided precision neurosurgery) can lead to new ideas for the diagnosis and treatment of neurological diseases such as glioma, brain metastases, epilepsy, and Alzheimer's disease.

This book comprehensively summarizes the latest progress regarding the application of integrated PET/MR in the diagnosis, treatment, and research of brain disorders at Xuanwu Hospital, Capital Medical University. It also introduces the latest achievements in the field of brain science in China and abroad. Each chapter offers perspective and practicability, which will help medical imaging technologists master the essentials of integrated PET/MR diagnosis. The book also has important reference value for scientific research in brain functional and molecular imaging. Therefore, it is especially suitable for practitioners in the fields of neuroimaging, neurology, neurosurgery, and other related major fields of brain science. We believe that the publication of this book will play a vital role in promoting PET/MR in terms of basic research and clinical application.

Those who share the same desire succeed, and those who help each other win! Let us look forward to great achievements of the application of "Integrated PET/MR Brain Functional and Molecular Imaging" in brain disorders and brain science. With PET/MR and related techniques, research ranging from brain disorders to brain science is bound to make great progress!

Beijing, China Guoguang Zhao

Preface

Time flies, and 7 years have passed in the blink of an eye. Looking back on the installation and use of positron emission tomography/magnetic resonance (PET/MR) equipment 7 years ago (July 2015), it seems like only yesterday. I can still vividly remember the feeling when I welcomed the first time-of-flight PET/MR equipment in Southeast Asia. I had no experience and no team at that time, but I confronted the challenge with complete enthusiasm, and concomitantly bore the huge psychological pressure of fearing failure and living up to the expectations of the leaders of our hospital. Relying on my skills in magnetic resonance imaging (MRI), I led a novice team consisting of a newly enrolled graduate student (Bixiao Cui) with a background in nuclear medicine, a nuclear medicine technologist (Jie Ma) with only 2 months of experience in PET/CT, and a nurse (Dongmei Shuai) to start the exploration in PET/MR. The hardships are indescribable. The efforts of countless all-nighters, weekends, and holidays gradually paid off, resulting in my first speech in an international conference, publication of our first PET/MR monograph, and publication of our first article in European Journal of Nuclear Medicine and Molecular Imaging! These 7 years were full of sweat, tears, toil, and pain, as well as the joy of harvest and success! Over the past 7 years, the team has also continued to grow and expand, forming an integrated cross-functional team of members specializing in medicine and engineering, and research groups specializing in various brain disorders including cerebrovascular disease, brain tumor, epilepsy, Alzheimer's disease, and Parkinson's disease. Every member has injected new vitality into the team and contributed to new results. At this point, I would like to thank them sincerely for their hard work, dedication, and persistence and for their company throughout this journey, which has given me the courage to keep going forward.

With the development of PET/MR equipment and its popularization and application in our country, there is an urgent need for interdisciplinary talents who are skilled in PET and MRI in clinical practice. Our previous publications including *Integrated PET/MR: Operation Specifications and Clinical Application*, *Integrated PET/MR Practice Manual*, and *Integrated PET/MR Imaging: Case Atlas* mainly focused on the standardization of clinical operation of the equipment and manifestations of typical clinical cases. Based on previous work, this book summarizes our team's experience in studying brain disorders and brain science as well as the latest research progress in China and abroad. It comprehensively introduces the research progress in PET/MR brain functional and molecular imaging including its clinical application in brain disorders and the status quo of brain science. The book consists of 16 chapters including introduction of the equipment, principles of functional brain imaging, its application in brain disorders, and research in brain science, gradually deepening chapter by chapter. The content related to functional brain imaging includes functional MRI, perfusion imaging, principles of dynamic PET imaging, and data post-processing methods. The related brain disorders include Alzheimer's disease, Parkinson's disease, epilepsy, brain tumor, cerebrovascular disease, brain injury, depression, schizophrenia, multiple sclerosis, migraine, and other major diseases. Therefore, this book has great clinical practicability.

We have received great support and help from many colleagues while writing this book. We would like to express our deep gratitude to Professor Jiehui Jiang from Shanghai University; Professor Lijun Bai from Xi'an Jiaotong University; Professor Su Lui from West China Hospital of Sichuan University; Professor Jiliang Fang from Guang'anmen Hospital, China Academy of Chinese Medical Sciences; Professor Baoci Shan from the Institute of High Energy Physics, Chinese Academy of Sciences; Professor Chuantao Zuo from Huashan Hospital of Fudan University; Professor Yufeng Zang from Hangzhou Normal University; Professor Xiang Li from Vienna General Hospital, Medical University of Vienna; Professor Jun Liu from the Second Xiangya Hospital of Central South University; Professor Yong He from Beijing Normal University; and Professor Junling Xu from Henan Provincial People's Hospital. They participated in the writing of this book in their spare time and provided valuable opinions and suggestions despite their busy work schedules. I would like to express my heartfelt thanks to them! Due to the limited knowledge of the author, inadequacies and omissions are inevitable in the book, and all colleagues are welcome to offer criticism and corrections.

Beijing, China Jie Lu

Contents

About the Editors

Guoguang Zhao, M.D., Ph.D. Prof. Zhao is the President of Xuanwu Hospital, Capital Medical University, National Medical Center for Neurological Disorders, the coordinator of the China International Neurosurgery Institute and the director of the national neurosurgical robot committee. Prof. Zhao has focused on stereotactic neurosurgery and brain functional diseases. He has dedicated himself to the promotion and application of neurosurgical robots in China, where he co-developed China's first neurosurgical robot. To date, Prof. Zhao has published over 50 papers in prestigious journals such as *The Lancet Public Health, Alzheimer's & Dementia, and Science Bulletin*, of which the highest impact factor was 72. Prof. Zhao has presided over projects of the National Key Research & Development Program, and National Natural Science Foundation, and edited or translated five books.

Jie Lu, M.D., Ph.D. Prof. Lu is the Vice President and the Director of Department of Radiology and Nuclear Medicine, Xuanwu Hospital, Capital Medical University, mainly engaged in brain function and molecular imaging research. Her team took the lead in the multi-modal imaging research of brain diseases using PET/MR, developing new individualized technology and innovative scanning sequence for brain function analysis. To break through the difficult problem of individualized application, Prof. Lu independently developed deep learning technology for the diagnosis of brain disease by multi-modal neuroimaging methods and established a full-process automatic platform for image post-processing and diagnosis. To date Prof. Lu has published more than 200 SCI articles as the first or corresponding author, with the representative works published in international authoritative journals such as *Neuron, Nat Commun, Radiology, Brain, Neurology, EJNMMI*. Among them, the most cited article was cited for 495 times, listed in the top 1% ESI highly cited papers. Prof. Lu was the main editor of 6 PET/MR monographs, authorized 7 related patents, chaired or participated in 12 expert consensuses, presided over 18 research projects. Prof. Lu now serves as the editorial board of several international academic journals, such as EJNMMI, Neuroimage, and JMRI.

1 Introduction to Positron Emission Tomography/Magnetic Resonance (PET/MR) Imaging

Bixiao Cui, Kun Guo, and Jie Lu

Molecular imaging is an emerging interdisciplinary field that integrates multiple disciplines including medical imaging, nuclear medicine, clinical medicine, molecular biology, chemistry, physics, and computer science. Molecular imaging can be used to observe molecular and biological functions in the living body. Positron emission tomography/magnetic resonance imaging (PET/MR) combines PET and MRI into a single modality and is currently the most advanced medical imaging available.

1.1 History of PET/MR

During the past few decades, there has been growing interest in multimodal imaging equipment. A large number of studies have shown that the combination of two or more imaging modalities can improve diagnostic performance. Thus, in 1998, the first PET/computed tomography (PET/CT) system was created, which was widely accepted by medical imaging experts, clinicians, and molecular imaging researchers worldwide. PET/CT integrates both PET and CT into a single machine, providing a multimodal imaging approach that has now become a routine diagnostic tool in clinical practice. However, the clinical application of PET/CT has several shortcomings. First, although the information acquired using CT can assist physicians in determining the anatomical location of lesions, it has a lower image resolution for soft tissues than that obtained using MRI. Second, MRI does not emit ionizing radiation, and therefore, it is more suitable for children as well as patients who may need to undergo repeated examinations. PET is a type of functional imaging technique that can detect abnormalities in the metabolism of various human tissues with extremely high sensitivity and accuracy. Therefore, the integration of PET and MRI into a single system enables the acquisition of a full range of data regarding the structure, function, and metabolism of the human body. This information is highly valuable in the diagnosis and treatment of diseases. Due to the complementary characteristics of MRI and PET, researchers began exploring the potential of integrated PET/MR systems.

In 1990, the first structural design patent was issued for inclusion of a PET detector in an MRI scanner. In 1997, researchers placed scintillation crystals within a 0.2 Tesla (T) open MRI system and connected them to photomultiplier tubes (PMTs) housed outside of the magnetic field via 4 m long optical fibers; they used this technology to perform PET/MR on anatomical phantoms. However, progress of the early development of the integrated PET/MR technology was slow due to compatibility-related difficulties, such as the

B. Cui · K. Guo · J. Lu (✉)
Department of Radiology and Nuclear Medicine, Xuanwu Hospital, Capital Medical University, Beijing, China

J. Lu, G. Zhao (eds.), *PET/MR: Functional and Molecular Imaging of Neurological Diseases and Neurosciences*, https://doi.org/10.1007/978-981-19-9902-4_1

feasibility of placing PET detectors within the magnetic field of the MRI scanner and PET image attenuation correction.

To minimize the mutual interference between PET and MRI technologies, one of the key technical requirements was the development of PET detectors and photodiodes that could detect 511 KeV high-energy photons in a strong magnetic field. Previous studies found that the scintillation crystals used in PET/MR needed an electromagnetic compatibility close to that of the human body to be effective. However, the electromagnetic compatibility of traditional scintillation crystals, such as lutetium gadolinium oxyorthosilicate and gadolinium oxyorthosilicate, differs significantly from that of the human body. This difference can affect the homogeneity of the magnetic field of the MRI scanner, producing artifacts that preclude the use of these materials in PET/MR. However, the increased research activity and clinical use of cerium-doped lutetium oxyorthosilicate (LSO) and cerium-doped lutetium yttrium oxyorthosilicate (LYSO) effectively solved the problem of electromagnetic susceptibility. Additionally, the PMTs traditionally used in PET/CT systems were highly susceptible to magnetic fields; however, the magnetic field of the MRI system can alter the trajectory and skew the detection of electrons, indicating that PMTs are not feasible in PET/MR systems.

Avalanche photodiodes (APDs), however, are not affected by magnetic fields and can be coupled with PET scintillation crystals directly or via very short optical fibers. Studies evaluating APD-based PET/MR have been conducted in both small animals and the human brain. Furthermore, ADP-based PET/MR for whole-body imaging has been successfully developed and utilized; the Biograph mMR by Siemens combines LSO crystals and APDs to enable both the detection of gamma (γ) particles in strong magnetic fields and the conversion of scintillation photon signals to electrical signals. However, despite the relative maturity of the APD technology, APDs are limited by their low signal amplification gain (10^2–10^3), slow output signal, and low temporal resolution. In recent years, improved detectors using silicon photoelectric multipliers (SiPMs) have gradually become a technological hotspot in PET/MR research. SiPMs have the same amplification gain and temporal resolution as traditional PMTs, as well as other advantages such as improved consistency, small size, low operating voltage, and compact structure. Xi et al. used SiPMs to construct a monolithic PET detector array and calculated the optimal size of the SiPM array for clinical imaging, which yielded a relatively high detection efficiency. SiPMs are sensitive to temperature, implying that the stability of the signal output depends on the bias voltage and temperature changes. With the continuing advances in temperature control technology, it will soon be possible to resolve the issue of temperature sensitivity in SiPMs.

Rapid progress has been made in the development of integrated PET/MR technology, due to the increasing sophistication of new photoelectric detection technology. In November 2006, the Knoxville Medical Center in Knoxville, Tennessee, USA, used an integrated Siemens PET/MR scanner to perform the world's first simultaneous acquisition of human brain fusion images. In 2011, Phillips unveiled the 3.0T sequential Ingenuity TF PET/MR scanner (Fig. 1.1a), which combined MRI with a redesigned PET component with special magnetic shielding. In the same year, Siemens released the integrated Biograph mMR PET/MR scanner (Fig. 1.1b), which allowed for the fused acquisition of MR and PET images within the same machine, enabling synchronous and concentric MR and PET imaging. At the end of 2014, General Electric launched the world's first integrated PET/MR scanner with time of flight (TOF) function (Fig. 1.1c). The introduction of TOF technology significantly shortened the scan time, reduced the dose of radiopharmaceuticals administered to patients, and significantly enhanced the image contrast. In the same year, Siemens released the second-generation integrated Biograph mMR PET/MR scanner, which was equipped with high-definition PET technology (HD PET) that improved the resolution, contrast, and signal-to-noise ratio of PET images. In addition, the application of its unique BodyCOMPASS

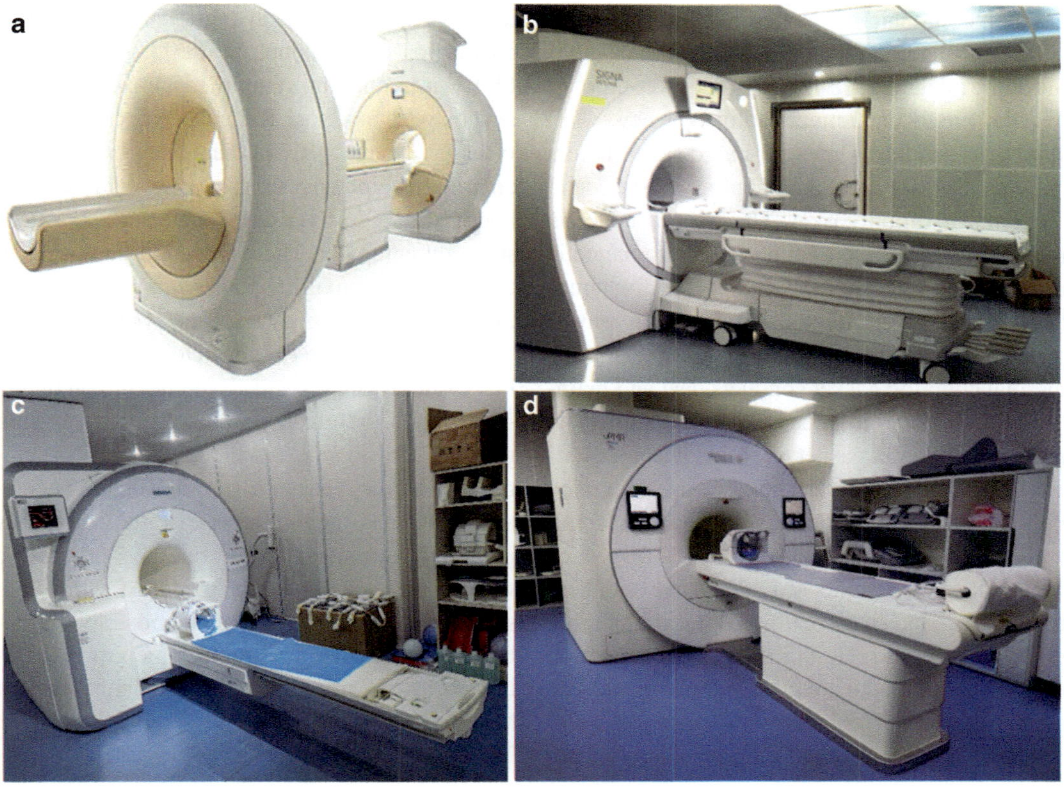

Fig. 1.1 PET/MR scanners: sequential Ingenuity TF PET/MR (**a**); integrated Biograph mMR PET/MR (**b**); integrated Signa TOF PET/MR (**c**); and integrated uPMR 790 PET/MR (**d**)

technology enabled MRI-based PET calibration during functional imaging, so as to ensure data accuracy. In China, research on PET/MR began relatively late compared to other countries. In 2018, United Imaging launched the uPMR 790 PET/MR scanner (Fig. 1.1d), which was fully integrated with artificial intelligence technology. Deep learning methods were implemented to achieve a series of unique innovations in imaging workflow automation, including one-click intelligent localization, bed planning, and attenuation correction, simplifying the workflow while also enhancing the quality of standardized imaging.

1.2 PET/MR Equipment

The integrated PET/MR scanner is a novel multimodal imaging system that merges PET and MRI into a single machine. This configuration enables two different simultaneous acquisition of data by two different modalities within the same space, while also drawing on the independent functions of each equipment. Therefore, PET/MR combines high soft tissue resolution and multiparameter, multi-functional imaging characteristics of MRI, with high sensitivity for radiotracer metabolism and quantitative characteristics of PET into a single system.

1.2.1 Components of the Integrated PET/MR System

The hardware of the integrated PET/MR system is primarily composed of a gantry, examination table, and console. Other components include the corresponding coils, cabinets, and post-processing workstation. The gantry consists of the PET and MRI components, and its basic structure (from inner- to outermost) includes the MRI body coil, PET detector module, MRI gradient coil, main magnetic field coil, and magnetic field shielding coil. The PET detector module of the integrated PET/MR system is composed of the photoconductive radiofrequency (RF) shielding module, lutetium-based scintillators (LBSs), SiPMs, thermal coupling gasket, and aluminum fixation gasket. The photoconductive RF shielding module eliminates electromagnetic interference from the MRI components, whereas the LBSs intercept photons; the SiPMs convert photon signals into electrical signals, and the thermal coupling gasket conducts heat and maintains the detector at a constant temperature. The aluminum fixation gasket fixes the detector module in place. The primary coils of the integrated PET/MR system include the joint head/neck coil, body coil, breast coil, and flexible coils (Fig. 1.2).

The console is composed of a display and keyboard, which includes control buttons for initiating scanning on the display, adjusting the examination table, and communicating with the patient. The equipment cabinet room houses a variety of equipment, including the MRI RF cabinet, PET cabinet, conduction plate cabinet, heat exchanger cabinet, PET water cooling system, helium compressor, and magnet monitor. The MRI RF cabinet provides the system's RF gradient and generates and controls equipment signals. The PET cabinet houses the PET power supply unit and PET reconstruction computer. The conduction plate cabinet contains other auxiliary power supplies. The heat exchanger cabinet is used for the system's air and water cooling, as the PET detector is cooled by the PET water cooling system. The helium compressor controls the magnetic pressure using helium gas, while the magnet monitor allows for observation of the magnetic pressure and liquid helium level. The image post-processing system processes image data transmitted to the post-processing workstation, which requires hardware with a high storage capacity, large memory, and fast computing power, together with supporting post-processing software, and typically uses miniaturized high-performance computers.

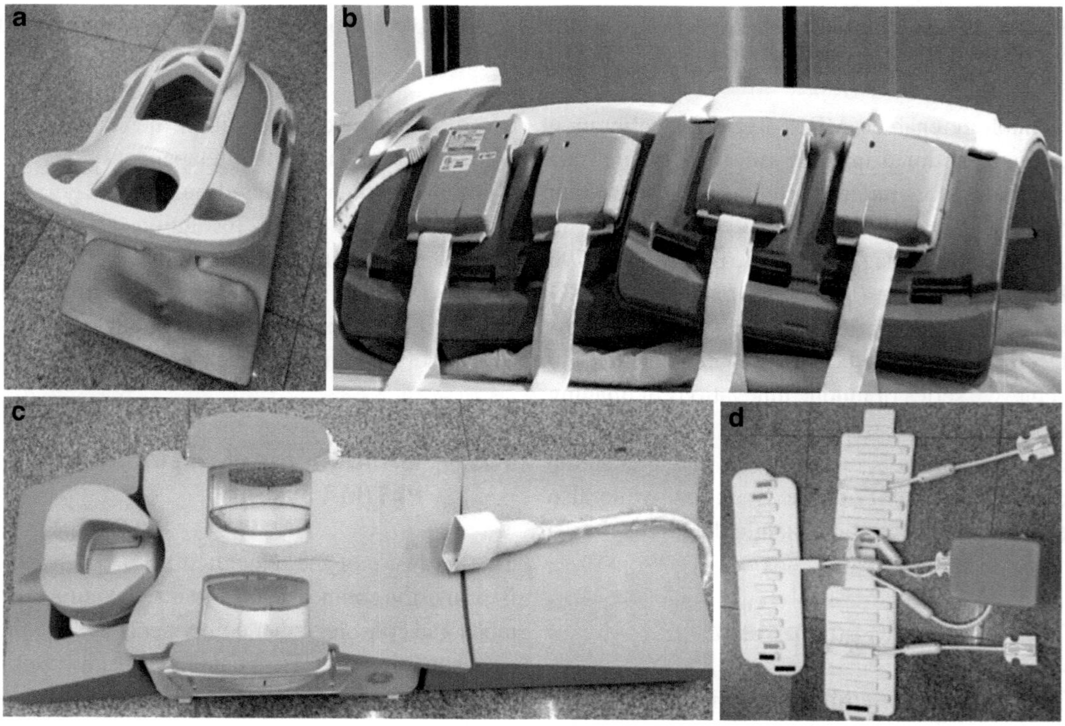

Fig. 1.2 MRI surface coils: joint head/neck coil (**a**); body coil (**b**); breast coil (**c**); and flexible coil (**d**)

1.2.2 Hardware Compatibility

Integrated PET/MR involves integration of a full-ring PET detector into the gradient and RF transmitter coils of the MRI system. While the RF and gradient coils emit RF and gradient pulses, the PET detector receives the γ photons released after positron emission decay, thereby achieving fully iso-field and iso-centric imaging. As the PET detector is embedded in the MRI system, substantial improvements to the RF transmitter and gradient coils are needed. Therefore, the device thickness had to be decreased, to make room for installation of the PET detector while maintaining adequate MRI performance; moreover, the bore diameter is often reduced to 60 cm.

The core challenge in successful deployment of an integrated PET/MR system lies in ensuring compatibility of the PET and MRI hardware. Therefore, the scintillation crystals used for PET imaging must have low magnetic susceptibility. However, traditional scintillation crystals, such as lutetium gadolinium oxyorthosilicate and gadolinium oxyorthosilicate, are highly susceptible to a magnetic field, which can affect the homogeneity of the magnetic field of MRI components, easily creating artifacts. SiPM-based Geiger-mode detectors are small in size, with low operating voltage, a compact structure, and decreased susceptibility to magnetic fields. They have superior energy resolution and temporal resolution when compared to APDs. Therefore, they are the preferred choice for photoelectric conversion detectors in integrated PET/MR systems.

1.2.3 Principles of PET/MR Imaging

1.2.3.1 Principles of PET Imaging

In PET imaging, a molecular substance required for metabolism in the body is labelled with a positron-emitting radionuclide, which releases positrons as it decays. The positrons then interact with free electrons in the body to generate annihilation radiation, emitting two γ photons with the same energy (511 keV) in opposite directions. The PET scanner detects the pair of γ photons within a specific time frame (i.e., the coincidence time window) to confirm the occurrence of an annihilation event between the two detectors, and the event is recorded as one event. Since γ photons have a certain level of penetrating power, PET detects γ photons outside of the body to obtain the tomographic distribution of positron-emitting radionuclides for imaging. The PET detector is ring-shaped, and volume data are obtained by detecting the resulting γ photon pairs from annihilation events in any direction within the detector.

1.2.3.2 Principles of MR Imaging

In MRI, the most commonly used atomic nucleus is the hydrogen proton because of its high magnetic susceptibility and wide distribution in human tissues. Each hydrogen proton within the body acts as a miniscule magnet; however, the chaotic arrangement of protons throughout the body causes their magnetization vectors to negate each other and therefore fail to produce a macroscopic magnetization vector. Upon entering the main magnetic field, however, the magnetic field generated by the spin of protons becomes parallel with the main magnetic field, rotating and swinging around the axis of the main magnetic field—a type of rotation known as precession. When an RF pulse that matches the precession frequency of protons is used to excite the nuclei, the energy of the RF pulse is transferred to the protons at a low level, exciting them to a higher energy level; this phenomenon is known as magnetic resonance. The energy of the RF pulse deflects the macroscopic magnetization vector, which gradually returns to a state of equilibrium when the RF pulse is turned off. The time it takes to return to a state of equilibrium is known as relaxation time. Relaxation is divided into two parts: (1) longitudinal relaxation, which is the gradual return of the longitudinal magnetization vector to its initial maximum value (equilibrium state), while T1 relaxation is the time needed to return to 63% of its initial maximum value; and (2) transverse relaxation, which is a gradual decrease of the transverse magnetization vector until it disappears, while T2 relaxation is the time needed for it to decay to 37% of its maximum value. The number of protons varies between different tissues in the human body, resulting in different T1 and T2 values. To highlight one tissue characteristic, weighted imaging techniques can be utilized to suppress the other characteristics as much as possible.

1.2.3.3 Attenuation Correction Technology

The 511 keV high-energy photons detected during PET cause the Compton effect to occur in the human body, during which high-energy protons are either attenuated or scattered. Attenuation correction algorithms are used to estimate the attenuation and scattering ratio of each line of response. The resultant images only provide information on proton density and relaxation time and do not provide an attenuation profile. MR-based attenuation correction (MRAC) is achieved using tissue segmentation, atlas registration, transmission scan, and emission data reconstruction methods.

The most recent integrated TOF PET/MR scanners can perform sensitivity, radionuclide attenuation, and detector dead time corrections on the PET detector, similar to the capabilities of traditional PET and PET/CT. However, γ-ray attenuation, γ-ray random coincidence, and γ-ray scatter corrections are all based on information obtained during MRI. Due to the limited field of view in MRI, it is necessary to combine the MRI signals with the TOF information from PET with no attenuation correction (NAC) in order to restore the contours of the human body. First, the MRI sequence is used to acquire information on water, gas, soft tissue, adipose tissue, and/or bone in the human body, which is combined with PET-NAC to restore the contours of the body. Next, the MRAC attenuation correction map (MRAC μ-map) is obtained for application to the PET images. Adipose tissues have a relatively small attenuation coefficient, but they exhibit high signal intensities in both T1- and T2-weighted MR images; therefore, information on adipose tissue can be isolated in the process of tissue segmentation. To improve accuracy, the matrix of the MRAC μ-map is similar in size to that of the PET scan. Given the structural complexity of human tissues, the use of human body atlases can enhance the speed and accuracy of tissue segmentation. Furthermore, MRI with zero echo time (ZTE) is crucial for accurate depiction of bone structure. As the density of bone cortex is almost three times the average density of bone, precise MRAC can only be achieved using the cortical bone structure. Traditional methods employ ultrashort echo time (UTE) to acquire the overall bone structure, but this technique is insufficient to obtain the cortical bone structure. ZTE, however, can accurately obtain the anatomical structure of the cortical bone. Additionally, TOF technology can help eliminate the impact of foreign bodies on MRAC, thus improving the accuracy of the resulting PET images.

1.3 PET/MR Scan Protocols

Integrated PET/MR involves simultaneous acquisition of PET and MRI. Prior to scanning, the PET parameters are defined before setting the MRI sequences. The main scan modes in integrated PET/MR include a PET scan and an MRI scan. In accordance with actual clinical needs, simultaneous PET and MRI scanning can first be performed, followed by separate scans with certain special MRI sequences (e.g., contrast-enhanced MRI). This section will mainly introduce PET/MR scans of the brain.

1.3.1 Pre-Scan Preparation

Patients must fast for at least 4 h before the scan, although they can drink sugar-free water during this period, and they must also avoid exercising vigorously or for an extended period of time the day prior to the scan. Diabetic patients should maintain their blood glucose concentration at a recommended level of ≤11.1 mmol/L. Patients should disclose their current medication regimens and be accompanied by a family member on the day of the scan. The attending physician obtains a detailed medical history, verifies the patient's order, and confirms the patient's general information, reason for the examination, and scan protocol. The physician also verifies that the patient has no contraindications to MRI, and informs the patient of the scan procedure, precautions, and expectations.

On the day of scan, the patient's height, weight, and blood glucose are measured, and venous access is established. The injection dose is calculated based on body weight, which is 3.7 MBq/kg for the conventional tracer ^{18}F-fluorodeoxyglucose (^{18}F-FDG), and 0.1 mL/kg body weight (0.1 mmol/kg) for the contrast agent. For patients undergoing static imaging, all audiovisual stimuli are blocked out after the radioactive tracer (e.g., ^{18}F-FDG) is injected, the room lights are dimmed, and the temperature is maintained at approximately 22 °C. The patient is asked to keep their eyes closed for 40–60 min while lying on the examination table, during which they should avoid talking, eating, or chewing. For patients undergoing dynamic imaging, a bolus injection of the radioactive tracer is performed with the patient on the scan table, and the technologist begins image acquisition before the injection. Patients receiving dual radioactive tracers are first injected with the tracer with the shortest half-life. They are scanned, and then asked to rest on the scan table with their eyes closed for ≥10 half-lives, after which they are injected with the tracer with a longer half-life. Patients receiving both a radioactive tracer and a contrast agent are injected via two separate intravenous (IV) catheters, so as to prevent the accumulation of radioactive tracers in the IV catheter from affecting image quality. Patients are required to change into hospital provided clothes for the examination; prior to entering the scan room, the patient and their family member/friend must remove all metallic objects from their bodies. Wheelchairs, stretchers, hospital beds, oxygen tanks, monitoring equipment, and other equipment are all strictly prohibited from entering the examination room. Patients requiring oxygen therapy are given MRI-safe oxygen equipment. Patients with limited mobility should use MRI-safe wheelchairs or beds. Nurses are strictly prohibited from bringing any metallic items into the scan room.

1.3.2 PET/MR Data Acquisition

1.3.2.1 Scanning Coils and Body Positions for Integrated PET/ MR

During integrated PET/MR, the joint head/neck coil is used, and the patient wears earplugs to protect their hearing. The patient is placed in the supine position, entering the scanner head first, with both arms by their sides. The long axis of the body should be parallel to the long axis of the scan table, and the coil should be placed close to the shoulders. The head should remain motionless and centered in the scanner, and can be positioned using a head wedge. Due to the small size of children's heads, support cushions can be used to raise the head, centering it with the coil as much as possible, while asking the patient to retract their lower mandible. The glabella or nasal base is used for centering the patient's position, and the patient must close their eyes when the laser light passes over them. The technologist should also instruct the patient to use the alert button if they experience any significant discomfort. The anatomical scan range includes the entire brain, from the foramen magnum through the top of the skull. Details on the scanning process are shown in Fig. 1.3.

1.3.2.2 PET Scan Parameters

PET imaging of the brain consists of a single scan position, and the scan range includes the entire brain. The midline of the scan position is the center of the brain. Acquisitions can either be considered static or dynamic, as previously described in Sect. 3.1. The scanning mode is set to volume scan, which covers the entire brain. The dynamic scan time begins after the injection of the radioactive tracer with the patient on the scan table, and ends when drug metabolism stabilizes, which generally takes around 60 min. The scan time can be selected based on the characteristics of the tracer used. Static scans generally last 8–10 min, or are performed simultaneously with the MRI scan. The scan parameter settings (based on the GE PET/MR) are as follows: TOF and point spread function (PSF) technology; slice

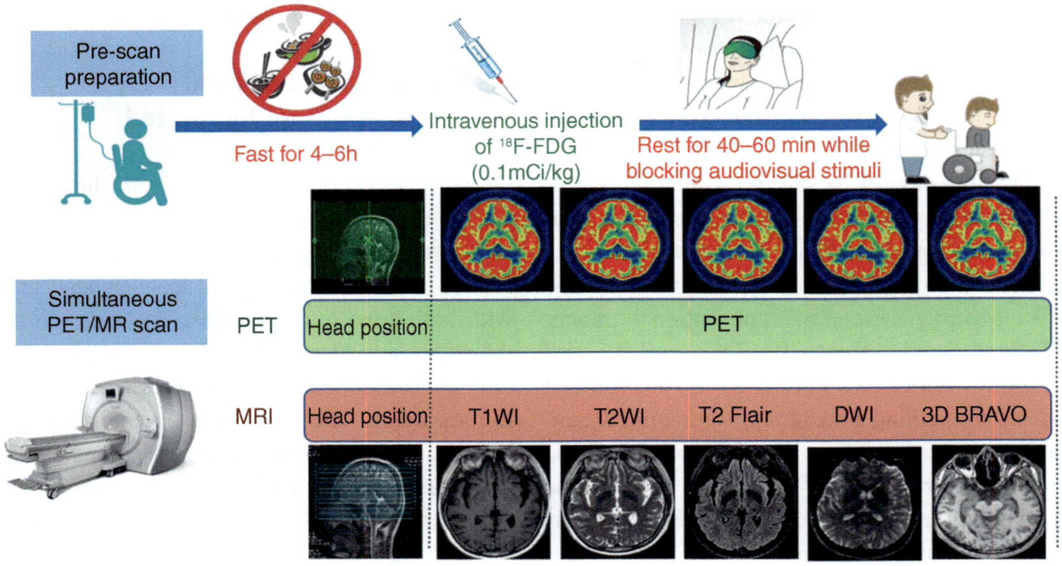

Fig. 1.3 Schematic diagram of the integrated PET/MR scanning procedure

thickness = 2.78 mm; field of view (FOV) = 35 cm; number of iterations = 8; valid subset = 32; matrix size = 192 × 192; full width at half maximum = 3 mm; and MRAC based on the Dixon sequence. The list mode is selected in dynamic scanning for segmenting in chronological order, which is necessary for image reconstruction.

1.3.2.3 MRI Scan Parameters

(1) Conventional MRI sequences: The scan range includes the entire brain, from the foramen magnum through the top of the skull. Conventional scan orientations include the transverse, sagittal, and (when necessary) coronal planes. Transverse scanning is performed parallel to the anteroposterior lines; sagittal scanning is performed parallel to the longitudinal fissure of the brain; and coronal scanning is performed with reference to the sagittal and transverse planes, perpendicular to the longitudinal fissure on the transverse plane and parallel to the brain stem on the sagittal plane. The scan range is determined based on the size of the lesion. Nonenhanced sequences obtained include transverse T2-weighted imaging (T2WI), T1-weighted imaging (T1WI), fluid-attenuated inversion recovery (FLAIR), diffusion-weighted imaging (DWI), sagittal T2WI or T1WI, and coronal T2WI or T1WI; fat-suppressed T1WI can also be performed if necessary, depending on the lesion. The scan parameters (based on the GE PET/MR) are as follows:

- T2WI: transverse scan; repetition time (TR) = 5.758 ms; echo time (TE) = 120 ms; FOV = 23 cm; matrix size = 256 × 256; number of excitations (NEX) = 1; slice thickness = 5.0 mm; interslice gap = 1.0 mm; and scan time = 1 min 9 s. The scan range covers all brain tissue from the skull base through the top of the skull.
- T1WI: transverse scan; TR = 2.529 ms; TE = 11 ms; FOV = 23 cm; matrix size = 256 × 256; NEX = 2; slice thickness = 5.0 mm; interslice gap = 1.0 mm; and scan time = 2 min 47 s. The scan range covers all brain tissue from the skull base through the top of the skull.
- FLAIR: transverse scan; TR = 7.000 ms; TE = 155 ms; FOV = 23 cm; matrix size 256 × 256; NEX = 1; slice thickness = 5.0 mm; interslice gap = 1.0 mm; and scan time = 1 min 52 s. The scan range covers all brain tissue from the skull base through the top of the skull.

- DWI: transverse scan; TR = 2.500 ms; TE = 79.9 ms; FOV = 23 cm; matrix size = 160 × 160; *b*-values = 0 and 1.000 s/mm²; NEX = 2; slice thickness = 5.0 mm; interslice gap = 1.0 mm; and scan time = 1 min 9 s. The scan range covers all brain tissue from the skull base through the top of the skull.

(2) Special MRI sequences: The following special sequences can be utilized, depending on the lesion. Common sequences include the following:

- Three-dimensional T1-weighted imaging (3D-T1WI): sagittal scan; TR = 7.9 ms; TE = 3.2 ms; FOV = 25.6; matrix size = 256 × 256; NEX = 1; slice thickness = 1.0 mm; interslice gap = 0 mm; voxel size = 1.00 × 1.00 × 1.00 mm³; and scan time = 3 min 48 s. The scan range covers all brain tissue from the skull base through the top of the skull.
- Three-dimensional TOF magnetic resonance angiography (MRA): transverse scan; TR = 4 ms; TE = 17.2 ms; FOV = 22 cm; matrix size = 368 × 211; NEX = 1; slice thickness = 1.2 mm; interslice gap = 0 mm; voxel size = 0.85 × 0.6 × 1.2 mm³; and scan time = 2 min. The scan range covers all brain tissue from the skull base through the top of the skull and is centered on the circle of Willis from the top of the corpus callosum to the foramen magnum, or encompasses the target vascular region. This sequence does not have an interslice gap and involves scanning and stitching together 3–4 slices with an overlap of 20–30%. The pre-saturation band is set above the scan area (top of skull). Flow compensation, magnetization transfer, fat suppression, and slice interpolation techniques should be utilized.
- Blood-oxygen-level-dependent functional MRI (BOLD-fMRI): echo planar imaging (EPI) sequence; transverse scan; scan range covers the skull base through the top of the skull, with the topmost slice encompassing the gray matter structure of the entire brain; TR = 2.000 ms; TE = 30 ms; FOV = 22.4 cm; matrix size = 64 × 64; NEX = 1; slice thickness = 3.5 mm; interslice gap = 0.7 mm; voxel size = 3.5 × 3.5 × 3.5 mm³; scan time = 10 min 53 s; and time points ≥ 200. BOLD-fMRI is an imaging technique that reflects the functional activity of local brain tissue through changes in deoxyhemoglobin levels of cerebral blood vessels. Since deoxyhemoglobin is a paramagnetic substance, the decrease in deoxyhemoglobin levels during local brain activity manifests as an increase in T2 signal intensity on fMRI. BOLD signals do not directly reflect the physiological state of neural activity, but are comprehensive effects of secondary physiological responses in the surrounding blood vessels, blood flow, and metabolism elicited by neural activity.
- Diffusion tensor imaging (DTI): EPI sequence; transverse scan; TR = 8461 ms; TE = 75.1 ms; FOV = 22.4 cm; matrix size = 64 × 64; NEX = 1; slice thickness = 3.5 mm; interslice gap = 0 mm; voxel size = 3.5 × 3.5 × 3.5 mm³; scan time = 9 min 56 s; frequency encoded in left/right direction; *b*-values are generally 0 and 1000; number of diffusion gradient directions ≥ 30; and scan range covers the skull base through the top of the skull. DTI is a non-invasive structural imaging method developed based on DWI. It uses the anisotropic diffusion of water molecules in the central nervous system to obtain information on microstructural changes at the molecular level and therefore indirectly infers pathophysiological changes. DTI can be used to acquire the diffusion characteristics of tissues, and its main parameters include mean diffusivity (MD) and fractional anisotropy (FA). The FA value is the ratio of anisotropy of the diffusion process to the overall diffusion, and its value ranges between 0 and 1, with 1 indicating maximum anisotropy in diffusion motion and 0 indicating minimum

anisotropy (i.e., maximum isotropy). FA provides information on the direction of diffusion, which can indicate the cellular arrangement and structural integrity of white matter bundles in the brain. Any pathological process that alters tissue integrity and direction of nerve fiber arrangements can lead to changes in the barriers that restrict the motion of water molecules, thereby causing changes in MD and FA.

- Susceptibility- weighted imaging (SWI): transverse scan; TR = 0.8 ms; TE = 20 ms; FOV = 23 cm; matrix size = 448 × 195; NEX = 1; slice thickness = 2.0 mm; no interslice gap; voxel size = 1.03 × 0.51 × 2 mm^3; scan time = 4 min 21 s; frequency encoded in left/right direction; phase encoded in anterior/posterior direction; and reconstructed images include phase and magnitude maps. SWI primarily shows intracerebral venules, hemorrhages, and even microbleeds, and is a valuable technique for diagnosis of traumatic brain injury, brain tumors, cerebrovascular malformations, cerebrovascular diseases, and certain neurodegenerative diseases. The 3D-SWI sequence involves scanning on the oblique plane and encompasses the entire brain, with adjustments made on the sagittal plane to avoid skull base structures, thereby reducing the impact of susceptibility artifacts from the skull base.
- Arterial spin labelling perfusion-weighted imaging (ASL-PWI): This sequence must be completed before contrast-enhanced scans, as the presence of contrast makes it impossible to perform quantitative analysis of cerebral blood flow. Post-labelling delay (PLD) is selected based on cerebral blood flow velocity, where a shorter PLD (1–1.5 s) is used for a faster blood flow, and longer PLD (1.5–2.5 s) for a slower blood flow. The general parameters are as follows: transverse scan; TR = 5500 ms; TE = 13.78 ms; FOV = 22.4 cm; matrix size = 64 × 64; NEX = 1; slice thickness = 6.0 mm; interslice gap = 0.0 mm; voxel size = 3.5 × 3.5 × 6 mm^3; scan time = 3 min 44 s; and scan range is from the skull base through the top of the skull. ASL uses an inversion recovery pulse sequence to label water protons in the arterial blood at the proximal end of the imaging plane, in order to produce blood flow-dependent image contrast.
- Perfusion-weighted imaging (PWI): EPI sequence; transverse scan; frequency encoded in the left/right direction; TR = 1.600 ms; TE = 35 ms; FOV = 23 cm; matrix size = 128 × 128; NEX = 1; slice thickness = 5.0 mm; interslice gap = 1.0 mm; voxel size = 1.8 × 1.8 × 5 mm^3; total number of scans = 40–50; contrast injection speed is generally >3–3.5 mL/s; scan time = 1 min 41 s; and scan range covers the skull base through the top of the skull. Parameters include cerebral blood flow (CBF), cerebral blood volume (CBV), mean transit time (MTT), and time to peak (TTP).
- Proton magnetic resonance spectroscopy (^{1}H-MRS): This sequence is generally not performed simultaneously with PET, in order to ensure the homogeneity of the local magnetic field. The skull, gas, fat, and major blood vessels should be avoided during positioning. This sequence requires the single-voxel spectroscopy pre-scan water peak suppression rate to be >99% and full width at half maximum <7, or multi-voxel spectroscopy pre-scan water peak suppression rate >96% and full width at half maximum <10. Scan parameters are as follows: axial scan; frequency encoded in the left/right direction; TR = 1.500 ms; TE = 144 ms; FOV = 16 cm; matrix size = 14 × 14; NEX = 2; slice thickness = 15 mm; voxel size = 10 × 10 × 15 mm^3; and scan time = 4 min 28 s. MRS utilizes the chemical shifts of various substances to discern different mole-

cules and their concentrations in a variety of biological tissues. In MRS, the region of interest (ROI) must be placed at the center slice of the lesion, which means that simultaneous iso-centric scanning with PET cannot be performed. The ROI should include the lesion and the surrounding or contralateral normal brain parenchyma, in order to facilitate the comparison between diseased and normal brain tissue. To ensure homogeneity of the local magnetic field, tangential saturation bands must be added if interfering tissues (e.g., skull, gas, fat) are present around the ROI. MRS utilized nuclear magnetic resonance and chemical shifts to achieve the quantitative analysis of specific atomic nuclei and their compounds. Therefore, it is an effective technique for non-invasive *in vivo* assessment of tissue metabolism. The main metabolites detected by ^{1}H-MRS include *N*-acetylaspartate (NAA), choline (Cho), creatine/phosphocreatine (Cr), and lactate (Lac). Of these metabolites, NAA is only found in neurons and is regarded as a neural biomarker; Cho is primarily involved in the synthesis of cell membrane phospholipids and acetylcholine; Cr is an energy metabolite with relatively stable levels and is therefore often used as a reference value to standardize the levels of other metabolites; Lac is a product of anaerobic glycolysis, and an early, sensitive marker of cerebral ischemia.

(3) Special MRI sequences for different neurological diseases:
   - Cerebrovascular diseases: SWI (to reveal cerebral microbleeds); PWI or ASL (to evaluate impairments in whole-brain blood perfusion); or MRA (to detect intracranial arterial diseases).
   - Intracranial space-occupying lesions: contrast-enhanced 3D-T1WI (to better display brain metastases) and ^{1}H-MRS (to help differentiate between malignant and benign tumors).
   - Epilepsy: oblique coronal FLAIR, angled perpendicular to the hippocampus (to show abnormal hippocampal signals).
   - Alzheimer's disease: oblique coronal T1WI, angled perpendicular to the hippocampus (to detect atrophy of the hippocampus).
   - Parkinson's disease: transverse SWI (to detect abnormalities in the red nucleus and substantia nigra).

(4) MRI sequences for brain structure and function research:
   - 3D-T1WI structural imaging (for accurate anatomical segmentation and registration of functional brain imaging).
   - DTI (to evaluate occult white matter changes and abnormalities in white matter tracts).
   - BOLD-fMRI (task-related and resting states, to study the link between brain activation and brain function).

Suggested Readings

Antoch G, Bockisch A. Combined PET/MRI: a new dimension in whole-body oncology imaging? Eur J Nucl Med Mol Imaging. 2009;36(Suppl 1):S113–20.

Bogner W, Hangel G, Esmaeili M, et al. 1D-spectral editing and 2D multispectral in vivo(1)H-MRS and (1)H-MRSI-methods and applications. Anal Biochem. 2017;529:48–64.

Boss A, Bisdas S, Kolb A, et al. Hybrid PET/MRI of intracranial masses: initial experiences and comparison to PET/CT. J Nucl Med. 2010;51(8):1198–205.

Castillo M. History and evolution of brain tumor imaging: insights through radiology. Radiology. 2014;273(2 Suppl):S111–25.

Cattaneo PW, De Gerone M, Gatti F, et al. Development of high precision timing counter based on plastic scintillator with SiPM readout. IEEE Trans Nucl Sci. 2014;61(5):2657–66.

Delso G, Kemp B, Kaushik S, et al. Improving PET/MR brain quantitation with template-enhanced ZTE. Neuroimage. 2018;181:403–13.

Freitag MT, Fenchel M, Bäumer P, et al. Simultaneous carotid PET/MR: feasibility and improvement of magnetic resonance-based attenuation correction. Int J Cardiovasc Imaging. 2016;32(1):61–71.

Hammer BE. NMR-PET scanner apparatus. 1990, WO9101503A1.

Herzog H, Pietrzyk U, Shah NJ, et al. The current state, challenges and perspectives of MR-PET. Neuroimage. 2010;49(3):2072–82.

Judenhofer MS, Wehrl HF, Newport DF, et al. Simultaneous PET-MRI: a new approach for functional and morphological imaging. Nat Med. 2008;14(4):459–65.

Liu F, Jang H, Kijowski R, et al. Deep learning MR Imaging-based attenuation correction for PET/MR imaging. Radiology. 2018;286(2):676–84.

Martinez-Möller A, Nekolla SG. Attenuation correction for PET/MR: problems, novel approaches and practical solutions. Z Med Phys. 2012;22(4):299–310.

Mehranian A, Zaidi H. Joint estimation of activity and attenuation in TOF-PET/MR using constrained Gaussian mixture models. IEEE Trans Med Imaging. 2015;34(9):1808–21.

Merlo Pich E, Jeromin A, Frisoni GB, et al. Imaging as a biomarker in drug discovery for Alzheimer's disease: is MRI a suitable technology? Alzheimers Res Ther. 2014;6(4):51–8.

Miller-Thomas MM, Benzinger TL. Neurologic applications of PET/MR imaging. Magn Reson Imaging Clin N Am. 2017;25(2):297–313.

Okazawa H, Tsujikawa T, Higashino Y, et al. No significant difference found in PET/MRI CBF values reconstructed with CT-atlas-based and ZTE MR attenuation correction. EJNMMI Res. 2019;9(1):26.

Páez D, Orellana P, Gutiérrez C, et al. Current status of nuclear medicine practice in Latin America and the Caribbean. J Nucl Med. 2015;56(10):1629–34.

Pichler BJ, Wehrl HF, Kolb A, et al. Positron emission tomography/magnetic resonance imaging: the next generation of multimodality imaging? Semin Nucl Med. 2008;38(3):199–208.

Roncali E, Cherry SR. Application of silicon photomultipliers to positron emission tomography. Ann Biomed Eng. 2011;39(4):1358–77.

Saeed U, Compagnone J, Aviv RI, et al. Imaging biomarkers in Parkinson's disease and Parkinsonian syndromes: current and emerging concepts. Transl Neurodegener. 2017;6:8.

Sailer AMH, Grutters JP, Wildberger JE, et al. Cost-effectiveness of CTA, MRA and DSA in patients with non-traumatic subarachnoid haemorrhage. Insights Imaging. 2013;4(4):499–507.

Shao Y, Cherry SR, Farahani K, et al. Simultaneous PET and MR imaging. Phys Med Biol. 1997;42(10):1965–70.

Willekens I, Lahoutte T, Buls N, et al. Time-course of contrast enhancement in spleen and liver with Exia 160, Fenestra LC, and VC. Mol Imaging Biol. 2009;11(2):128–35.

Xi D, Xie Q, Zhu J, et al. Optimization of the SiPM pixel size for a monolithic PET detector. Phys Procedia. 2012;37:1497–503.

Yamamoto S, Watabe T, Watabe H, et al. Simultaneous imaging using Si-PM-based PET and MRI for development of an integrated PET/MRI system. Phys Med Biol. 2012;57(2):N1–13.

Research Applications of PET Imaging in Neuroscience

2

Jiehui Jiang

With the recent advances in nuclear medicine imaging equipment and the development of new imaging agents, the applications of positron emission tomography (PET) imaging in the field of neuroscience have grown rapidly. PET imaging allows for the visualization of physiological and pathological changes in the living brain at a molecular level, providing vital and valuable information for the diagnosis and treatment of central nervous system (CNS) diseases. This chapter primarily focuses on the principles of PET imaging, the processing of PET data, and the research applications of PET in neuroscience.

2.1 Principles of PET Imaging

2.1.1 Physical Principles of PET Imaging

PET imaging involves the detection of a radiotracer labelled with a positron-emitting nuclide within the body. When the radionuclide-containing tracer is injected into the body, the radionuclide bound to the tracer accumulates in the target organ(s), from which it emits positrons. Each positron travels approximately 1–3 mm and then collides with a random body tissue. This collision generates annihilation radiation, producing a pair of 511 keV gamma (γ) photons that travel 180° relative to each other. By placing a pair of detectors in the direction of flight for the photon pair, the two photons can be captured simultaneously. The line connecting the two detectors receiving the photon pair is known as the line of response (LOR) and implies that the annihilation event must lie somewhere along this straight line. Therefore, by arranging multiple sets of detectors in a 360° ring, we can obtain one-dimensional information about the lines connecting multiple detector pairs. These signals are then subjected to back-projection and mathematical processing, to obtain a tomographic image of the distribution of the radiotracer.

The positron-emitting radionuclides involved in the process of the generation of annihilation radiation are generally proton-rich nuclides that emit positrons when they decay. The proton in the nucleus decays into a neutron, while also releasing a positron and a neutrino, as shown in Eq. (2.1):

$$P \rightarrow n + \beta^{+} + \upsilon \tag{2.1}$$

where P is the proton, n is a neutron, β^{+} is a positron, and υ is a neutrino. A positron has the same mass as an electron, and the same magnitude of electric charge like an electron, but positive rather than negative. Positron emission (or β^{+} decay) generally occurs in artificial radionuclides.

J. Jiang (✉)
Institute of Biomedical Engineering,
School of Life Sciences, Shanghai University,
Shanghai, China
e-mail: jiangjiehui@shu.edu.cn

J. Lu, G. Zhao (eds.), *PET/MR: Functional and Molecular Imaging of Neurological Diseases and Neurosciences*, https://doi.org/10.1007/978-981-19-9902-4_2

Table 2.1 Physical properties of commonly used positron-emitting radionuclides

Radionuclide	Half-life (min)	Maximum positron energy (MeV)	Maximum range (mm)	Average range (mm)
^{11}C	20.3	0.96	5.0	0.28
^{13}N	10.0	1.19	5.4	0.60
^{15}O	2.0	1.70	8.2	1.10
^{18}F	109.8	0.64	2.4	0.22
^{68}Ga	67.8	1.89	9.1	1.35
^{82}Rb	1.3	3.35	15.6	2.60

The preparation of PET radiotracers requires the generation of radioisotopes by bombarding a target with a proton beam in a cyclotron. Currently, the most commonly used PET radionuclide is ^{18}F, which has a half-life of approximately 110 min. In comparison, other PET radionuclides (^{11}C, ^{13}N, and ^{15}O) have shorter half-lives (20, 10, and 2 min, respectively). Radionuclides commonly used in neuroimaging include ^{11}C, ^{18}F, and ^{15}O.

The physical properties of commonly used positron-emitting radionuclides are shown in Table 2.1.

2.1.2 PET Scanning System

The primary function of the PET scanner, which is composed of the gantry, examination table, electronic cabinet, operator console, analysis workstation, and printing equipment, is to record the annihilation events.

2.1.2.1 Gantry

The gantry is the largest component of the PET scanner and primarily consists of the detector ring, rod source, radiation shielding equipment, event detection system, and coincidence circuitry.

Detector

The detector is the most crucial component of the PET imaging process. It serves to capture incident γ photons and absorb their energy, from which it generates electrical signals that can then be processed by subsequent circuits. The recorded electrical signals provide information for processing, such as the energy deposited in the detectors by the γ photons and the time and position of photon interactions with the scintillation crystals. The PET detector is composed of scintillation crystals, photomultiplier tubes (PMTs), and related electronic circuits. Of these components, the scintillation crystals and PMTs are the core components of the detector, and their arrangement determines its structure. The performance of the PET scanner is dependent on the detector, which plays a decisive role in the scanner's core performance indicators, including spatial resolution, temporal resolution, and sensitivity.

PET detectors are generally constructed using high-density crystals such as bismuth germanium oxide (BGO), lutetium oxyorthosilicate (LSO), or lutetium yttrium oxyorthosilicate (LYSO), which are segmented into smaller elements. Thus, one detector block consists of one crystal block and its coupled PMTs. The most classic arrangement is the 4 × 64 array, in which each detector block is composed of 4 PMTs coupled to 64 crystal elements. Multiple detector blocks are tightly arranged to form a ring, and multiple detector rings are arranged to form a cylinder. The X-Y plane is the PET cross-section, which is parallel to the plane of the detection ring. The Z axis is the long PET axis, which is perpendicular to the plane of the detection ring.

The detectors used in PET scanners can be classified into two major types according to the crystals used: scintillation detectors and semiconductor detectors. Scintillation detectors are the more widely used detectors in PET imaging systems. Nevertheless, semiconductor detectors have gradually been utilized in PET scanners used for small animals, due to their excellent energy resolution and direct photoelectric conversion during detection.

Scintillation Detectors

Scintillation detectors are detectors that use the flash of light (i.e., scintillation) produced when radiation interacts with certain substances to detect ionizing radiation. They are primarily composed of the scintillator, light guide, and PMTs.

1. Scintillator

The scintillator is the core component of the scintillation detector, and its properties have a direct impact on the performance of the detector, particularly its energy, time, and position localization. The scintillator used in early PET systems was thallium-doped sodium iodide (NaI[Tl]). NaI(Tl) has a high light yield and good spatial resolution, but also has poor stopping power and longer luminescence decay, and is prone to deliquescence. As the crystal manufacturing technology advanced, new scintillation crystals were gradually introduced. BGO crystals have a large decay constant, low light yield, and poor energy resolution, but have a high density, strong stopping power, and high sensitivity, and can be used for two-dimensional (2D) PET imaging. LSO and LYSO crystals are currently the preferred choices for scintillators in PET scanners due to their fast response, high light yield, and high density.

Newer halide scintillators, such as cerium-doped lanthanum bromide ($LaBr_3$:Ce), cerium bromide ($CeBr_3$), and cerium-doped lutetium iodide (LuI_3:Ce), have a number of excellent properties, including high light yield, rapid decay, and high energy density. Unfortunately, the raw materials for these halide crystals are costly and difficult to prepare, which has hindered their widespread application in PET imaging. Additionally, cerium-doped gadolinium aluminum gallium garnet ($Gd_3[Al,Ga]_5O_{12}$:Ce, GAGG:Ce), used in a multicomponent garnet scintillator, has excellent light yield, good energy resolution, and no issues with deliquescence or self-radioactivity, exhibiting exceptional comprehensive performance compared to other scintillation crystals. Table 2.2 lists the scintillation crystals most frequently used in PET imaging systems, along with their technical performance indicators.

2. Light guide

Light guides are primarily made of silicone oil or organic glass and are used to fill the gaps between the crystal scintillator and the PMTs. Light guides are meant to minimize the total internal reflection of photons interacting with air, and enhancing the efficiency of the photons entering the PMTs.

3. Photomultiplier tube (PMT)

PMTs are vacuum electron-tube devices that convert weak light signals, those at wavelengths of 200–1200 nm, into electrical signals.

Semiconductor Detectors

Semiconductor detectors use semiconductive materials as the detection medium and work by converting radiant energy into electrical signals. Compared to traditional scintillation detectors, semiconductor detectors bypass the need for multiple energy conversions and have a low signal noise, high energy resolution, and compact device structure. Semiconductor detectors detect radiation based on the generation of electron–hole pairs within the crystals. An electric field is

Table 2.2 Technical performance indicators of common scintillation crystals

Scintillator	Density (g/cm^3)	Light yield (photons/MeV)	Decay time (ns)	Wavelength of luminescence center (nm)	Energy resolution (%)
NaI:T1	3.7	41,000	230	415	9.0 (140 keV)
CsI:T1	4.5	66,000	800	550	14.0 (140 keV)
BGO	7.1	9000	300	480	12.0 (511 keV)
LSO:Ce	7.4	30,000	40	420	9.1 (511 keV)
LYSO:Ce	7.1	32,000	45	420	7.1 (511 keV)
$LaBr_3$	5.3	63,000	16	358	3.3 (511 keV)
LuAP	8.3	10,000	18	365	11.4 (511 keV)
GSO	6.7	12,500	60	440	7.9 (511 keV)
GAGG:Ce	6.6	56,000	90	520	4.9 (662 keV)

applied at both ends of the detector, which causes the electrons and electron holes to drift toward the anode and cathode, respectively. This results in the formation of an output charge, which converts radiation into electrical signals, thus detecting the radiation emitted.

Early semiconductor detectors were primarily composed of silicon (Si) and germanium (Ge). However, both Si and Ge have a relatively narrow band gap, meaning that early detectors needed to operate at liquid nitrogen temperatures in order to suppress the thermal noise produced by the detectors themselves. Furthermore, Si and Ge have lower effective atomic numbers; therefore, their detection efficiencies are too low for detecting γ- or X-rays. In recent years, compound semiconductors, such as cadmium telluride (CdTe) and cadmium zinc telluride (CZT), have been created and utilized in semiconductor detectors. Compared to Si- and Ge-based semiconductor detectors, CdTe- and CZT-based detectors have wider band gaps, allowing them to operate at room temperature. Moreover, they have higher energies and spatial resolutions and can be used to construct detection modules of smaller sizes. Therefore, semiconductor detectors have been regarded as viable alternatives to scintillation detectors.

1. Rod source

A rod source uniformly encapsulates germanium-68 (^{68}Ge) or cesium-137 (^{137}Cs) within a small hollow rod. Depending on the equipment, there are usually 1–3 rod sources with different activities for transmission scans, blank scans, and quality control.

2. Shielding

The internal shielding of the PET scanner consists of two parts: (1) Thick lead plates (or septa) on both sides of the entire detector ring, which serve to shield the detection rays; and (2) 1 mm thick, ring-shaped tungsten plates interposed between individual detector rings, which serve to shield incident photon pairs from the field of view (FOV) of other rings, similar to the function of a collimator.

3. Detection system and coincidence circuitry

The role of an event detection system is to collect incoming electrical signals from the detector, determine if they are valid (511 keV) γ photon signals and transmit information about the position of any valid γ photon signals. The coincidence circuitry receives the photon event signal from the coincidence detection system. Each detector that registers a γ photon generates a timed pulse, which is fed into the coincidence circuitry to identify and select true coincidence events.

Under normal circumstances, a very small window ($\leq$ 15 ns) is set for the coincidence circuits. Timed pulses that are registered simultaneously within this time window are regarded as γ photon pairs generated by the same positron annihilation event and are subsequently recorded by the coincidence circuitry. Based on the positional and temporal information gathered, it is possible to reconstruct a three-dimensional (3D) PET image. Furthermore, annihilation γ photon pairs can only be detected within the FOV of two opposing detectors (180° apart). The technique of using the coincidence between the output pulses from two opposing detectors to determine the position of a scintillation event is known as electronic collimation, which is a major feature of PET imaging. It forgoes the need for heavy lead collimators, improves the sensitivity and uniformity of the point-source response function, avoids the negative effects of lead collimators on resolution and uniformity, and greatly improves detection sensitivity.

Although the coincidence circuitry can detect simultaneous scintillation events, in reality, there is always a time difference between the triggering of the two detectors. This time difference is known as the resolution time and implies that γ photons which arise from different positions but are incident on two opposing detectors within the resolution time are also recorded. Coincidence events which are not generated by annihilation radiation are known as random coincidences. Additionally, γ photons may also randomly undergo Compton scattering during flight, which changes the course of the photons and results in a different LOR to that of the original event. This is known as scattered coincidence.

Random and scattered coincidences create image noise, reducing image resolution and contrast, thereby affecting image quality. Increasing the coincidence count rate to a certain level will lead to a quadratic increase in the count rates for random and scattered coincidences, whereas increasing the degree of activity to a certain extent will, instead, result in poorer image quality. Therefore, we cannot improve the image quality of PET scans simply by increasing radiotracer activity alone.

4. Examination table

The examination table holds the patient during the PET scan. It moves the patient to position the part of the body to be examined within the FOV of the scanner, depending on the requirements of the examination.

5. Electronic cabinet

The electronic cabinet primarily contains the central processing unit, input and output systems, internal and external storage systems, and other components. Its main function is to perform image reconstruction, as well as the processing and storage of image data.

6. Image analysis workstation

The workstation is primarily composed of a computer system with PET-specific software. Its functions include image reconstruction and display, data storage, and data transmission.

7. Printing equipment

The printing equipment consists of image output systems, such as printers and laser cameras. Its main function is to output images, text, or other materials.

2.1.3 PET Image Acquisition

PET image acquisition can be categorized into two types: emission scanning and transmission scanning. Emission scanning can further be divided into the following categories: 2D, 3D, static, dynamic, gated, local, and whole-body acquisition.

2.1.3.1 Emission Scanning

When positron-emitting nuclides enter the human body and decay, they each emit one positron, which travels a very short distance, 1–3 mm, through the nearby body tissue. Once its kinetic energy disappears, the positron collides with an electron to generate annihilation radiation, thus creating two γ photons (both with an energy of 511 keV) that travel in opposite directions. The process by which the PET scanner collects information about these photon pairs to determine the location and quantity of the radiotracer is known as emission scanning.

2D and 3D Acquisition

A 2D acquisition involves the placement of shields (known as septa) between the individual detector rings. During 2D acquisition, the septa block photons from interacting with other detector rings and allow the detection of photon pair signals only within the same ring. Three-dimensional acquisition is a rapid mode in which the septa are removed, and the detectors can detect photon pair signals from other detector rings, expanding the detection range to the entire axial FOV. The intensity of photon pair signals detected in 3D acquisition is 8–12 times higher than that of 2D acquisition, which also significantly enhances sensitivity. However, this also implies that there is a marked increase in scattered and random coincidences in 3D acquisition, leading to a low signal-to-noise ratio and necessitating scatter and random coincidence correction. Three-dimensional acquisition is currently widely used in clinical practice. The schematic diagrams for 2D and 3D acquisition are shown in Fig. 2.1.

Static and Dynamic Acquisition

Static acquisition is the most commonly utilized mode of PET imaging. It involves waiting for a fixed amount of time after the imaging agent is injected into the patient and acquiring the images when the agent has reached equilibrium. Dynamic acquisition refers to a continuous, dynamic mode

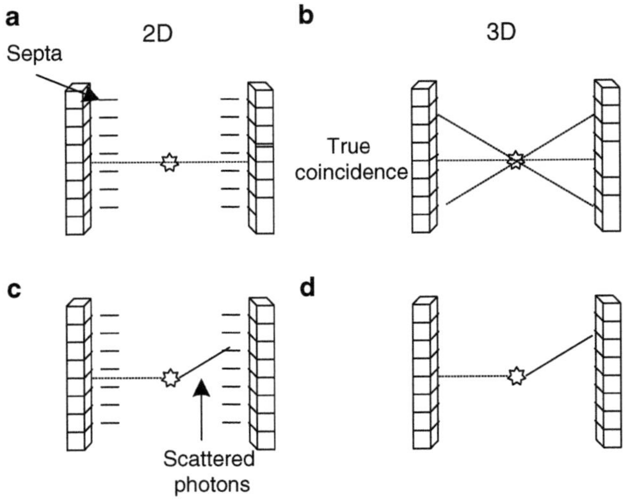

Fig. 2.1 Schematic diagrams of 2D and 3D PET acquisition

of data collection which is performed while actively injecting the imaging agent to obtain a continuous, dynamic image sequence. This enables us to observe the spatial changes of the imaging agent in the body, and to study dynamic changes in vivo.

Gated Acquisition

Gated acquisition includes cardiac and respiratory gated acquisition. As cardiac and respiratory movements are characterized by their cyclic nature, gating can be used to collect information that is synchronized with these cycles, in order to eliminate the effects of cardiac and respiratory motion.

Local and Whole-Body Acquisition

Local acquisition is primarily utilized for the imaging of specific organs (e.g., brain, heart) or certain parts of the body, while whole-body acquisition is mainly used for the diagnosis and evaluation of malignant tumors and associated metastases.

2.1.3.2 Transmission Scanning

Transmission scanning refers to the process in which a rod source is rotated around the body to collect the leftover radiation after the external radioactive source has exited the human body. By combining the results of the transmission and blank scans, we can calculate the attenuation coefficient of the tissues. Hence, transmission scanning can be used to perform attenuation correction on the data from the emission scan.

2.1.4 PET Image Reconstruction

The raw data used in the process of PET image reconstruction includes the one-dimensional projections of the radiation emitted from the patient (i.e., a set of parallel line integrals or ray sums). To convert these data into a usable form, they must first be mathematically transformed (or reformatted) and reconstructed into a set of horizontal images. The primary methods of image reconstruction are analytical, iterative, and deep learning.

2.1.4.1 Analytical Methods

Analytical methods are back-projection methods based on the central slice theorem, with filtered back-projection (FBP) being the most commonly used method. Once the acquisition of PET data is complete, it is confirmed that count values along the LORs between the detectors are directly proportional to the integrals of the radioactivity along these LORs. These line integrals are known as projections, and based on these projection data, we can perform the image reconstruction for each tomographic plane.

In FBP reconstruction, the projection data are convolved under a given projection angle using a filter to obtain the corrected projection data, followed by the back-projection (i.e., reverse to the projection direction) of the corrected projection data to reconstruct the image. In order to improve the computational speed, FBP always converts the raw projection data to the frequency domain for processing. In the frequency domain, the convolution operation is a simple multiplication, which substantially improves the speed of reconstruction. Fourier transform is always applied in FBP processing to convert the image from the spatial to the frequency domain. Once the reconstruction is complete, the inverse Fourier transform is applied to convert the image from the frequency to the spatial domain for ease of image interpretation. The FBP technique primarily includes the following steps:

1. Fourier transform: raw data are converted into frequency domain functions using the Fourier transform
2. Filter: pre-filtering is performed using the ramp filter function
3. Back-projection operation: the image is reconstructed using the back-projection technique
4. Second filter: the appropriate filter function and parameters are selected to filter the reconstructed image and eliminate the high-frequency noise of star artifacts and
5. Inverse Fourier transform: the image is converted from the frequency to the spatial domain for ease of display and interpretation.

2.1.4.2 Iterative Methods

Iterative reconstruction is an algorithm-based method of image processing characterized by convergence. It primarily involves the performance of multiple rounds of iterative algorithm-based comparisons in order to ensure the consistency of the reconstructed data with the actual image data, and is therefore much more computationally expensive. As the computing speeds of microcomputers continue to increase, the application of this reconstruction technique has grown in popularity. The principle behind iterative reconstruction is very simple: at the start of reconstruction, a set of initial cross-sectional estimates is arbitrarily assigned, which is usually a data matrix with all elements set to 1 and using the same size as the original acquisition matrix. Based on these initial estimates, the simulated projection data is calculated and compared to the original projection data, in order to determine the amount of correction needed for each pixel. Using this corrective data, adjustments are made to the matrix values of the initial image data. The adjusted image is then repeatedly subjected to the steps above, and multiple rounds of iterations are performed until a predetermined level of accuracy is attained. A flowchart summarizing iterative reconstruction is shown in Fig. 2.2.

The greatest advantage of iterative reconstruction is the ability to introduce various physical factors and statistical models during the reconstruction process, in order to achieve high-resolution images. One of the more widely used methods is the statistical iterative method, which

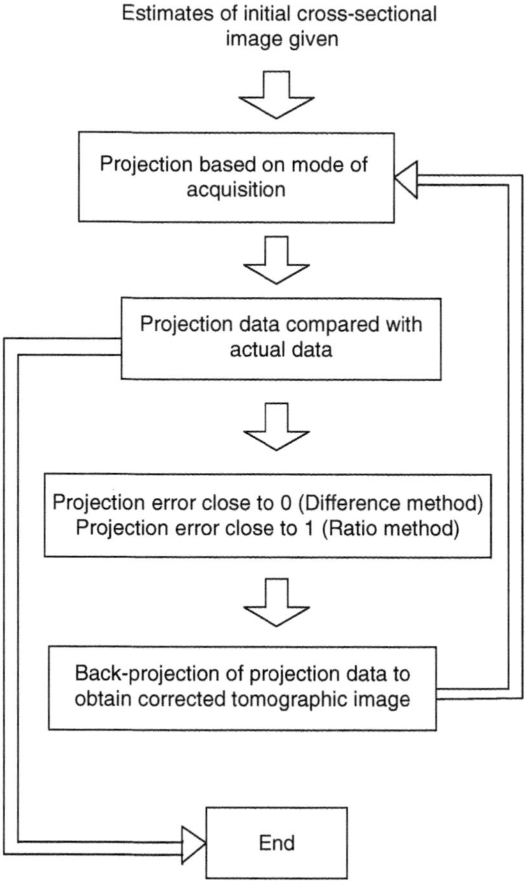

Fig. 2.2 Flowchart of iterative tomographic image reconstruction

regard reconstruction as identifying the distribution of radioactivity under a given set of criteria. Many types of algorithms and mathematical models are utilized in iterative reconstruction, the most common of which include the maximum likelihood estimation and conjugate gradient methods. Iterative methods of reconstruction have a slow convergence and are computationally expensive, and increasing the number of iterations leads to issues such as the "aging" of images or the appearance of high-frequency artifacts. These potential problems can be addressed by introducing fast iterative ordered subsets with an over-relaxation factor into the algorithm, or by introducing stopping rules, performing multi-objective optimization, and adding smoothness constraints, among other techniques, to eliminate high-frequency artifacts. At present, the optimization of iterative reconstruction methods is one of the primary aims of research PET image reconstruction, which has led to the diversified development of this field.

2.1.4.3 Deep Learning Algorithms

Although remarkable progress has been made in the development of PET detectors, most PET systems still employ simple signal processing methods to extract time and position information from detector signals. In quantitative image reconstruction, deep learning can be used to estimate various correction factors, including scatter events, attenuation images, and statistical noise in the reconstructed images. Currently, the majority of deep learning-based PET image reconstruction is focused on the penalized-likelihood reconstruction framework, in which the unknown PET image is estimated as:

$$\hat{x} = \arg\max_{x>0} L\left(y|x\right) - \beta U\left(x\right) \tag{2.2}$$

where $L(y|x)$ is the log-likelihood function, $\beta U(x)$ is the penalty function, and β is the hyperparameter.

In general, deep learning algorithms, such as neural networks, can be applied in the penalty function $\beta U(x)$, or completely replace the latter. Due to the additional constraints of $L(y|x)$, this reconstruction method is more robust to mismatches between the training and test data. In addition, a pre-trained network can be used to represent PET images and perform constrained maximum likelihood estimation:

$$\hat{x} = \max_{x} L\left(y|x\right), \text{s.t.x} = f\left(\alpha\right) \tag{2.3}$$

where $f(\alpha)$ is the pre-trained network and α is an arbitrary input. This method is an extension of the linear representation based on the kernel method. Compared to the kernel method, deep neural networks have a stronger capability for accurate representation and can fully utilize the prior inter-subject information available in the training data. Furthermore, during the process of image reconstruction, the network parameters are fixed, and the network inputs are updated. This makes it possible to add a self-attention generative adversarial network structure and introduce additional constraints on the network input to stabilize the reconstruction process.

To avoid pre-training networks with a large number of training images, some researchers have applied a deep image prior framework when performing PET image reconstruction. In this method, the image reconstruction process is transformed into a network training process through the neural network representation of the PET images. The training labels are the PET sinograms (raw data), and the training objective function is the log-likelihood function of the sinogram data. The network is trained from scratch during the image reconstruction process, without the use of any other training images. This unsupervised learning framework is extended to the process of direct parametric PET image reconstruction.

There are numerous algorithms based on deep learning, such as sparse representation and dictionary learning penalized image reconstruction. However, further investigations are needed on the application of deep learning algorithms in PET image reconstruction.

2.1.5 Data Correction

A number of factors can result in errors in PET imaging, including nonuniformities in detector sensitivity, effects from the rapid decay scattering on the intensity of positron-emitting tracers and the absorption attenuation of the human body, random coincidences due to high count rates, and dead-time losses. If these factors are left uncorrected, they can have a serious impact on PET image quality; therefore, PET data are typically corrected, so as to enhance image quality and eliminate image artifacts. Current methods of data correction include detector normalization, attenuation correction, scatter correction, random coincidence correction, and dead-time correction.

2.1.5.1 Detector Normalization

Detector normalization is also known as detector sensitivity correction. A basic assumption when performing PET image reconstruction is the uniformity of LOR sensitivity. However, due to differences in detector parameters, the actual sensitivities of the detectors are not uniform. Variations in the angle between the LOR and the detector surface can also lead to differences in sensitivity. Moreover, the sensitivity of a detector is related to its geometric dimensions and shape. The process of correcting factors that can lead to differences in detector sensitivity is known as detector normalization. Each LOR should have one normalization factor, which is given below:

$$NOPM_i = \frac{\sum_{i=1}^{M} D_i M}{D_i} \tag{2.4}$$

where D_i ($i = 1, \ldots, M$) is the count response of each detector measured using a uniformly distributed radioactive source, and M is the total number of PET detectors. These normalization factors are stored in the computer as files. When PET measurements are made, the measured values are multiplied by the corresponding normalization factors to implement the correction of detector efficiency.

2.1.5.2 Radionuclide Decay Correction

All radionuclides have a short half-life, and as image acquisition progresses, the radionuclide injected into the human body naturally decays. Thus, decay correction is needed to ensure that the data obtained from the beginning through the end of the acquisition remain unaffected by decay. This type of correction can be calculated according to the decay formula, and the decay correction coefficient is given as:

$$I = \exp\left(t^* In2 / T\right) \tag{2.5}$$

where t is a given moment in time after the onset of acquisition, and T is the half-life of the radionuclide used.

2.1.5.3 Tissue Attenuation Correction

Photons are absorbed when they pass through human tissues, and this absorption is known as radiation tissue attenuation, which can distort the acquired images. Therefore, attenuation correction is needed to prevent image distortion and artifacts. The simplest form of attenuation correction is to assume that the density of human tissues is uniform; the correction is given by Eq. (2.6):

$$I_0 / I = \exp\left(\mu, x\right) \tag{2.6}$$

where I_0 is the radioactivity before attenuation, I is the radioactivity after attenuation, μ is the tissue attenuation coefficient, and x is the attenuation length.

It is worth noting that there are substantial variations in the densities of different tissues, and therefore, the above correction method deviates significantly from actual conditions. To achieve a more accurate attenuation correction, the anatomy within the FOV is usually irradiated with ring-shaped or rotating rod sources to obtain data on the penetrating LORs in every direction, and to calculate the tissue attenuation coefficient for all positions within the FOV.

The two penetrating sources above each have their advantages and disadvantages: Ring-shaped sources have a higher acquisition efficiency and require less time, but cannot be used for high-activity sources, which leads to poorer statistical characteristics. Rod-shaped sources rotate through the entirety of the acquisition, thus requiring more time to complete. However, rod-shaped sources have lower levels of random and scatter coincidences and can therefore be used for high-activity sources, making up for the longer acquisition time while also providing more accurate data. Acquisition errors caused by scatter are usually minimized using a technique known as "rod windowing," which identifies the LORs that pass through the source to effectively suppress scatter and random coincidence events. Current integrated PET/computed tomography (PET/CT) scanners use X-rays to perform penetrating acquisitions, which can improve the accuracy of attenuation correction.

2.1.5.4 Random Coincidence Correction

In the quantitative analysis of PET images, it is necessary to eliminate counts of scatter and random coincidences. A common method for this is to calculate and subtract the random coincidence counts on each LOR. The random coincidence rate for each LOR is given as follows:

$$R = 2\tau R_1 R_2 \tag{2.7}$$

where τ is the coincidence resolution time, and R_1 and R_2 are the single count rates of the detectors corresponding to the LOR. Since τ is known, R_1 and R_2 can be measured and used to calculate the random coincidence rate. As the single count rates are generally much higher than the coincidence count rates, the random coincidence rates measured using this method tend to have a small statistical error.

Another more commonly used method is the "delayed window" technique. Since true coincidence events only occur within the specified time window, whereas random coincidences are randomly distributed across any time period, we can extend the coincidence time of single detectors beyond the coincidence time window, and the coincidence counts obtained within this "delayed window" can be considered the random coincidence counts. The "delayed window" shares similar dead-time properties to the coincidence time window, thus avoiding the measurement errors caused by differences in dead-time. However, the coincidence count rate is lower in this "delayed window," which can also give rise to statistical error.

2.1.5.5 Scatter Correction

In 2D PET scans, the vast majority of scattered rays are shielded by the inter-ring septa, which means that the scattered coincidence rate is negligible. However, in 3D mode, the absence of inter-ring septa significantly increases the detectors' sensitivity to scattered coincidences, resulting in an extremely high count rate for scattered coincidences, and requiring scatter correction.

In scintillation detectors, the detection of γ photons is based on the conversion of high-energy photons which enter the scintillator into visible light. These photons undergo energy conversion through photoelectric absorption and Compton scattering, subsequently generating energetic electrons. These electrons excite surrounding electrons as they pass through the scintillator, and as the excited electrons release energy, they generate visible light. Photoelectric absorption and Compton scattering produce photoelectrons of various energy levels. During photoelectric absorption, all the photon energy is transferred to the photoelectrons, which causes their energy to be concentered within a high and narrow energy spectrum, producing a sharp energy peak.

The photoelectron energy produced by Compton scattering varies depending on the scattering angle, and therefore is distributed at a lower energy spectrum. Detectors with good energy resolution can separate scattered coincidences from true coincidences using the "dual- or multi-energy window" method, thereby removing the majority of the scattered coincidence counts. The "dual-energy window" method divides the energy window into the "main energy window" and the "Compton energy window," which is a simple and practical correction method, but is unable to discriminate sections where Compton coincidences intersect with true coincidences. The "multi-energy window" method is able to obtain the count rates for Compton and true coincidences at different energy spectra, and to discriminate between the distribution functions of the two types of coincidence counts, thereby effectively correcting for scattered coincidences. Other effective methods of scatter correction include the Monte-Carlo correction method, the convolution-subtraction method, and the model computation method, among others.

2.1.5.6 Dead-Time Correction

System dead-time refers to the time required by the system to process each event, and depends on a variety of factors, including the temporal characteristics of the detectors and electronics, the speed of the data processor, and the performance of the random buffer. Dead-time losses occur when the system is unable to finish processing one annihilation event before the next event occurs, which results in the loss of both events. System dead-time leads to the loss of coincidence counts, and these losses become more severe with increasing count rates, thereby affecting the accuracy of the quantitative analysis. Therefore, it is necessary to perform dead-time correction on the acquired data. One of the effective correction methods is to perform the model-based testing of dead-time count losses under different count rates, which involves obtaining the parameter of the corrected model through repeated testing and calculations. Dead-time correction can make up for the count losses caused by dead-time, while also effectively reducing the positioning error due to pulse pile-up at high count rates, especially in 3D mode.

2.1.6 Performance Evaluation of PET Systems

The parameters used for evaluating the performance of PET systems focus primarily on describing detector performance. The most important of these indicators include energy resolution, spatial resolution, temporal resolution, noise equivalent count rate, sensitivity, and maximum count rate.

2.1.6.1 Energy Resolution

For any PET detector, energy resolution is a critical indicator that has a direct impact on all other aspects of its performance. The physical definition of energy resolution is the ability of a detector to resolve the energies of incoming radiation. It is expressed using the full width at half maximum (FWHM) of the energy distribution curve for a given radiation as a percentage of the peak value of the curve, as follows:

$$E_{\mathrm{Res}} = \left(E_{\mathrm{FWHM}} / E_P\right) \times 100\% \quad (2.8)$$

where E_{Res} is the energy resolution, E_{FWHM} is the FWHM, and E_P is the peak value of the energy distribution curve.

The quality of energy resolution affects the performance of spatial resolution, noise equivalent count rate, and other indicators, while also reducing the ability of the detector to discriminate scattered coincidences, thereby affecting image quality and decreasing the accuracy of the quantitative analysis of PET images.

2.1.6.2 Spatial Resolution

Spatial resolution is one of the most important indicators in clinical practice, as the quality of spatial resolution directly impacts the ability to use the image for lesion detection. The physical definition of spatial resolution is the smallest object that the detector is able to resolve in the X, Y, and Z directions. It is expressed as the FWHM of the spatial distribution function curve for a point source image, and its unit is given in millimeters (mm). On the X-Y (cross-sectional) plane, the spatial resolution is highest at the center of the FOV and gradually deteriorates toward the edges. This is because when the photons originate from the edge of the FOV, one of the photons travels a longer distance through the adjacent tissue, whereas the other travels a smaller distance, and this asymmetry reduces the spatial resolution. Furthermore, due to the limitations of the maximum distance travelled by positrons and the angle of deviation between photon pairs travelling in opposite directions, there is a physical limit of about 2 mm in the spatial resolution of PET images. Above this physical limit, the inherent resolution of the detectors depends on the conversion efficiency of the crystals when converting high-energy (511 keV) photons into low-energy photons, the dimensions of individual detector modules, and the quality of coupling between the PMTs and the crystals.

2.1.6.3 Temporal Resolution

The temporal resolution of PET detectors is determined by the length of the detector's response time to γ photons, which generally follows a Gaussian distribution. The temporal resolution is expressed as the FWHM of the time-response curve, and its unit is given in nanoseconds (ns). In physical terms, it is the shortest time interval between a pair of γ photons that can be counted by the positron detector. During PET imaging, the coincidence window is set according to the temporal resolution. A coincidence window that is too wide will increase the random counts in the system, whereas one that is too narrow will cause the system to miss true coincidence counts. In general, the coincidence window is set at twice the FWHM of the time-response curve.

2.1.6.4 Noise Equivalent Count Rate

The coincidence counts of the PET system always consist of true coincidence, scatter, and random counts. If all counts other than true coincidence counts are classified as noise, then the noise equivalent count rate (NECR) can be used as a standard for measuring the signal-to-noise ratio. Its physical definition is as follows: for each set of coincidence data, the NECR equals the true coincidence count rate when it has the same signal-to-noise ratio in the absence of scattered and random coincidences. A higher NECR value implies a higher signal-to-noise ratio in the acquired data, resulting in better contrast in the PET images, and a higher imaging quality. Measurements indicate that NECR tends toward saturation as the radiation intensity increases. As the radiation intensity gradually increases, the true coincidence count rate will initially be higher than the scatter and random count rates. However, since the increase in the scatter and random count rates is directly proportional to the square of the total count rate, the increase in the scatter and random count rates will eventually overtake that of the true coincidence count rate as radiation intensity continues to increase. This leads to a decline in the signal-to-noise ratio of the acquired data, and a deterioration of image quality. Therefore, in coincidence detection, it is not necessarily better to use an imaging agent with higher levels of radioactivity; rather, the optimal radioactivity has the highest NECR.

2.1.6.5 System Sensitivity

System sensitivity measures how many counts the detector is able to acquire under the same conditions. Its physical definition is the coincidence count acquired per unit of radiation dose within a given unit of time. PET detectors with higher sensitivity require a shorter length of time or a smaller radiation dose to obtain one frame of coincidence image with the same quality.

2.1.6.6 Maximum Count Rate

The maximum count rate refers to the maximum count value measured by the detector in a given unit of time. The count rate measured by the detector increases with an increasing dose of radiation. However, due to the effects of dead-time, when the detector reaches higher count rates, its response time limits the increase in count rate, leading to missed counts. This is the point at which the count rate has reached saturation and no longer increases with further increases in radiation intensity, while NECR begins to decline, which generally occurs at 3000–5000 kcps.

2.2 Post-processing of PET Data

Once PET image acquisition is complete, the data need to be processed and analyzed in order to extract quantitative values, which can then be used for the diagnosis of diseases.

2.2.1 Image Pre-Processing

Raw PET image data are usually stored as Digital Imaging and Communications in Medicine (DICOM) files, as this format is able to meet the requirements of clinical data exchange and is one of the most widely used image formats used in medicine. In neuroimaging research, DICOM files are often converted to the Neuroimaging Informatics Technology Initiative (NIfTI) format for data processing. NIfTI is a format generated for digital medical imaging data, which aims to enhance the functions of various neuroimaging data processing software and the sharing of these processed data. The file extension of standard NIfTI images is .nii, which includes both the header file and image data. However, separate image (.img) and header (.hdr) files can also be used. Due to the differences between individual PET images, it is typically necessary to pre-process the images prior to analysis. Common steps for pre-processing include head motion correction, registration, correction for partial volume effect, spatial normalization, and smoothing. Common pre-processing tools include Statistical Parametric Mapping (SPM) and FMRIB Software Library (FSL).

2.2.1.1 Head Motion Correction

Since any movement of the head during the acquisition process may cause motion artifact that affects subsequent image analysis, the first step in image pre-processing is to perform head motion correction. The most common approach currently used is interframe correction, and in particular, the interframe difference method.

2.2.1.2 Registration

The registration of PET images to magnetic resonance (MR) images is a crucial pre-processing step. The majority of registration studies perform co-registration using the normalized mutual information (NMI) algorithm, which is based on a cost function that minimizes the registration error between the two types of images (e.g., least squares or mutual information). The cost function usually aligns the images based on information shared between the data (e.g., the cortical boundary), which ensures that it relies, to some extent, on the intensity distribution and resolution of the acquired data. A minority of studies employ the boundary-based registration (BBR) algorithm, which performs co-registration of T1-weighted MR images and PET images. However, since the registration is dependent on the spatiotemporal distribution of the PET images, and is extremely sensitive to the cost function selected, the BBR algorithm is not the best algorithm with which to capture the cortical folding pattern, especially when limited by the resolution of the PET scanner.

2.2.1.3 Partial Volume Correction

The partial volume effect (PVE) occurs when there are two or more substances with different densities in the same scan slice, causing the measured value to be average of the signals from these substances and therefore not truly reflecting the signal value of either substance. PVE can affect the accuracy of PET images; hence, it is necessary to perform partial volume correction (PVC). Here, we introduce two of the more mature PVC algorithms: (1) the voxel-based method (MG method) proposed by Müller-Gärtner et al. in 1992, and (2) the geometric transfer matrix method, based on regions of interest (ROIs), and proposed by Rousset et al. in 1998.

MG Method

The MG method is a three-compartment PVC method that extends the two-compartment method, as the latter only differentiates between the brain parenchyma and surrounding cerebrospinal fluid (CSF) signals. The MG method is currently the most widely implemented PVC method. This approach assumes that the PET signals observed in any given gray matter (GM) voxel are the spatially weighted average of the true radiotracer uptake signals in GM voxels and the signals originating from the white matter (WM) and CSF, while the spatial weighting is determined by the point spread function (PSF) of the PET scanner. Therefore, the proposed PVC algorithm corrects for the signal spillover from surrounding tissues into GM, and the spillover from GM into surrounding tissues:

$$C_{\text{PVC-GM}} = \frac{C_{\text{obs}} - C_{\text{WM}}\left(\text{WM} \oplus \text{PSF}\right) - C_{\text{CSF}}\left(\text{CSF} \oplus \text{PSF}\right)}{\text{GM} \oplus \text{PSF}} \tag{2.9}$$

where C_{obs} equals the GM signals observed in the PET scan; *GM*, *WM*, and *CSF* are the respective tissue compartments obtained using the scanner PSF; and C_{WM} and C_{CSF} are the radiotracer activity in the WM and CSF (these tissue types are assumed to be uniform).

ROI-Based PVC

The ROI-based PVC method attempts to determine the average radiotracer signal in a set of non-overlapping ROIs, which represents different brain structures and tissue types, and are generally segmented as prior information in MRI (or CT). The actual radiotracer uptake is assumed to be uniformly distributed within each ROI, while the spillover effect between different ROIs is estimated using the convolution between the binary mask of the ROI and the PSF of the PET scanner. We can estimate the relative effects of the signal of a given ROI, "A," on the signals measured in the adjacent ROI, "B," by convolving the ROI binary mask of "A" with the PSF to obtain the regional spread function (RSF), and calculating the probability weighted sum of the voxels in ROI "B." Then, each voxel is divided by the sum of the voxels in ROI "B." ω_{ij} describes the estimated spillover effect between each pair of ROIs, constituting the geometric transfer matrix (GTM), as follows:

$$\omega_{ij} = \frac{1}{v_j} \int_{\mathrm{ROI}_j} PSF_i(r)\,dr \tag{2.10}$$

where ω_{ij} is the overlapping part of the ROI with volume v_j, and r is the spatial coordinates in the image space. The observed regional intensity (t_j) reflects the change in true regional radiotracer concentration (T_j) due to spillover effects between regions with different intensity distributions. The true radiotracer concentration (T_j) of each region can be given below:

$$T_j = \mathrm{GTM}^{-1} * t_j \tag{2.11}$$

The GTM method is considered the reference numerical method of PVC for PET images. However, the most significant drawback of this method is that it only provides the average value of radioactivity in the correction region, and not the PVE-corrected images.

2.2.1.4 Spatial Normalization

Due to variations in the anatomy of the brain between different subjects, it is necessary to perform a spatial normalization of different brain images, converting them into normalized images with the same size and orientation. In other words, this process places brains of varying volumes and shapes into the same standard space and uses a common coordinate system to describe specific positions. The quality of spatial normalization depends directly on the extent to which the scan images matches the template. Common coordinate systems include the Talairach–Tournoux (TT) atlas used in Analysis of Functional NeuroImages (AFNI), and the Montreal Neurological Institute (MNI) atlas used in SPM. The TT system is based on a classic, standardized anatomical system, and its data is derived from a post-mortem brain dissection. The MNI system is a coordinate system established by the MNI using a series of MR images of normal human brains. Therefore, it is the new standard brain based on the magnetic resonance imaging (MRI) scans from a large number of healthy subjects.

2.2.1.5 Smoothing

The spatial smoothing of PET data can increase the signal-to-noise ratio to a certain extent, in order to ensure a greater conformity of the data to distributional assumptions, thereby enhancing the effectiveness of statistical analysis and satisfying the analytical requirements of the Gaussian random field theory. However, a major shortcoming of this technique is the reduction of image resolution and associated loss of detailed information. When performing the spatial filtering of PET images, a Gaussian kernel is often used to convolve the image. The size (smoothing range) of this smoothing kernel is determined by the FWHM and is usually 2–3 times the voxel resolution.

2.2.2 Quantitative Analysis

PET images display the distribution of the concentration of the radiotracer throughout various body tissues. In order to obtain physiologically significant parameters, it is still necessary to conduct further quantitative or semi-quantitative analyses on the images.

2.2.2.1 Absolute Quantitative Analysis

Kinetic compartmental modeling can be used to accurately measure the distribution of radiotracers throughout the body. It is a kinetic mathematical model based on the metabolic processes of the radiotracer in humans or animals and includes three factors: the input function, output function, and kinetic parameters. The input function is the time activity curve (TAC) of concentration of the radiotracer in arterial blood, and the values of its discrete time-series are usually obtained via frequent sampling of arterial plasma. The output function is the TAC of radiotracer concentration in an ROI, and its discrete values can be obtained via PET dynamic scanning. The kinetic parameters reflect the various rate constants of radiotracer metabolism and represent the physiological process of radiotracer metabolism. Based on the compartmental model of the radiotracer metabolism, we can adopt the appropriate mathematical algorithms, insert the measured values of the input and output functions, and use the relevant computational software to calculate the individual kinetic parameters of the mathematical model. These parameters can then be used to obtain physiologically significant quantitative indicators.

Here, we will use 18F-fluorodeoxyglucose (^{18}F-FDG) as an example to carry out the quantitative analysis of tissue glucose metabolic rate based on a three-compartment kinetic model. Glucose is an important energy source in the human body, while the level of glucose metabolism in tissues and organs can reflect their functional status to a certain extent. FDG is a glucose analog that can freely enter the interstitial fluid through the capillary walls and continue into the cell via glucose transporters, where it is phosphorylated via enzymatic action. According to the three-compartment kinetic model of FDG metabolism (Fig. 2.3), the metabolic transport of FDG in brain tissues can be expressed as follows:

$$\frac{dC_E(t)}{dt} = K_1 C_P(t) - (K_2 + K_3) C_E(t) + K_4 C_M(t) \tag{2.12}$$

$$\frac{dC_E(t)}{dt} = K_3 C_P(t) - K_4 C_M(t) \tag{2.13}$$

where C_p is the concentration of FDG in arterial plasma, C_E is the concentration of unphosphorylated FDG in tissues, C_M is the concentration of phosphorylated FDG in tissues, K_1 is the rate at which blood crosses the blood-brain barrier into brain tissue, K_2 is the rate at which FDG returns from brain tissue to the blood, K_3 is the rate at which FDG is phosphorylated under the catalysis of hexokinase in brain tissue, and K_4 is the rate at which phosphorylated FDG is converted back into FDG under the catalysis of phosphatase. The parameters K_1, K_2, K_3, and K_4 are the individual rate constants or microparameters and are given as the reciprocal of the time dimension.

K_1 and K_2 denote the rate constants for the forward and reverse transport of FDG between plasma and tissues, respectively; K_3 and K_4 denote the rate constants for the phosphorylation and dephosphorylation of FDG in cells, respec-

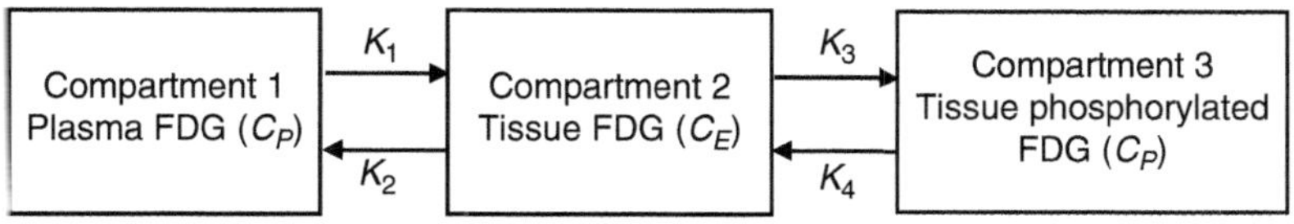

Fig. 2.3 ^{18}F-fluorodeoxyglucose (^{18}F-FDG)-based three-compartment kinetic model

tively; C_p is the concentration of FDG in arterial plasma; C_E is the concentration of unphosphorylated FDG in tissues; and C_M is the concentration of phosphorylated FDG in tissues.

In this model, the input function is the time-varying function $C_p(t)$ of FDG concentration in arterial plasma (C_p). Since the decay properties of radionuclides are unrelated to their chemical environment, there is no difference in the radioactivity between FDG and phosphorylated FDG at the time of measurement. Therefore, it is not possible to make separate measurements of FDG concentrations for $C_E(t)$ and $C_M(t)$. Instead, we can only measure the total radioactivity of tissues $C_i(t)$, as given below:

$$C_i(t) = C_E(t) + C_M(t) \tag{2.14}$$

Therefore, the output function is the total concentration of radioactivity in the tissues $C_i(t)$. When performing actual image quantitative analysis, the quantitative analysis can be carried out on either the TAC of a single voxel, or on the TAC of a specific ROI (i.e., the arithmetic of the TAC for all voxels included).

Images acquired through dynamic PET sequences can be used to obtain data on FDG concentration changes in local tissues $C_i(t)$, while arterial blood can be sampled at multiple time points and centrifuged to obtain data on changes in plasma FDG $C_p(t)$. The TACs obtained for changes in tissue and plasma FDG can then be substituted into Eq. (2.15):

$$C_i(t) = \frac{K_1}{a_2 - a_1}\left(\left(K_3 + K_4 - a_1\right)e^{-a_1 t} + \left(a_2 - K_3 - K_4\right)e^{-a_2 t}\right) \otimes C_P(t) \tag{2.15}$$

where $\otimes$ represents the convolution operation, while α_1 and α_2 can be calculated using the equations below:

$$a_1 = \sqrt{K_2 + K_3 + K_4 - \left(\left(K_2 + K_3 + K_4\right)^2 - 4 \times K_2 \times K_4\right)^{\frac{1}{2}}} \tag{2.16}$$

$$a_2 = \sqrt{K_2 + K_3 + K_4 + \left(\left(K_2 + K_3 + K_4\right)^2 - 4 \times K_2 \times K_4\right)^{\frac{1}{2}}} \tag{2.17}$$

The various rate constants can be fitted using the non-linear generalized least squares method. When glucose metabolism reaches an equilibrium, it is assumed that there is no synthesis or decomposition of glycogen. Since hexokinase is the only rate-limiting step in glycolysis, the rate of glucose phosphorylation is equal to the rate of glucose metabolism. Thus, the fitted rate constants above can be substituted into Eq. (2.18) to calculate the glucose metabolism rate of the target tissue:

$$R = \frac{C_P}{\mathrm{LC}} \times \frac{K_1 K_3}{K_2 + K_3} \tag{2.18}$$

where R denotes the glucose metabolism rate of the target tissue, C_p is the plasma glucose concentration, and LC is the lumped constant used to correct for the difference in transport and phosphorylation rates between FDG and glucose, which is given by the equation below:

$$\mathrm{LC} = \frac{\dfrac{K_1^*}{K_2^* + K_3^*} \times V_m^* K_m}{\dfrac{K_1}{K_2 + K_3} \times V_m K_m^*} \tag{2.19}$$

where V_m^* and V_m are the maximum phosphorylation rates of FDG and glucose, respectively, and K_m^* and K_m are the Michaelis constants for the phosphorylation of FDG and glucose, respectively.

Absolute quantitative analysis based on kinetic compartmental modeling is the gold standard for PET quantification, as it can give accurate measurements of radiotracer uptake values in various tissues. The computation of quantitative information in this complex kinetic model can be carried out using the PKIN tool in the PMOD image quantitative analysis software. However, despite the ability to produce accurate results using this approach, each subject must undergo dynamic acquisition, which is a complicated and time-consuming process, while the frequent blood sampling after radiotracer injection is especially inconvenient in routine clinical practice. Therefore, the discovery of new methods to reduce the number of blood samples and to acquire the input and output functions are currently key topics of focus in research on PET quantitative analysis.

2.2.2.2 Semi-Quantitative Analysis

Owing to the limitations of the clinical application of absolute quantitative analysis, semi-quantitative analysis is often utilized in clinical practice. This approach involves using the ratio of the radiation count between a given local ROI in the brain and a specific region in the body. This method can facilitate the discovery of abnormal regions that are difficult to identify visually, improve the sensitivity of the diagnosis, enhance the effectiveness of information for the clinical diagnosis, treatment, and efficacy evaluation, and provide a basis for comparison among different patients. Common semi-quantitative methods include the standardized uptake value (SUV) and standardized uptake value ratio (SUVR).

The SUV is the ratio of the concentration of radioactivity exhibited in the image itself to the whole-body concentration of the injected radiotracer. However, the absolute amount of the tracer taken up by local tissues depends not only on the radioactivity in the tissues themselves, but also on the radioactivity of the tracer injected into the body and the individual's body weight. Therefore, the tracer radioactivity and body weight are used to standardize the absolute amount of radiotracer processed by the tissues, in order to obtain the SUV of the target tissues:

$$SUV = \text{radioactivity of target tissue}\left(\text{kBq / mL}\right) / \text{injection dose}\left(\text{MBq}\right) / \text{body weight}\left(\text{kg}\right) \tag{2.20}$$

SUV is relatively simple to calculate and does not require multiple arterial blood sampling; therefore, the SUV of target tissues has been extensively utilized in clinical practice to describe the uptake of the radiotracer. However, the accuracy of this method is affected by factors such as body weight, blood glucose levels, scan time, and blood clearance rates of different tracers, all of which need to be taken into consideration during implementation.

Another common method of semi-quantitative analysis is the use of ROI-based techniques to calculate the ratio of radioactivity between target and non-target tissues. This approach uses the radiotracer uptake of normal tissues to standardize the uptake of target tissues, thereby reflecting the tracer uptake of the latter to a certain extent. The most commonly used quantitative indicator for this method is the SUVR:

$$SUVR = \text{uptake in target tissue / uptake in non-target tissue} \tag{2.21}$$

The SUVR is easy to implement and can directly obtain the uptake parameters of the corresponding tissues from the image itself, thereby attracting widespread attention. However, the selection of non-target tissues or reference brain regions has a substantial impact on the calculation of SUVR results, as the selection of different locations can give rise to significant variations in SUVR, thereby affecting its accuracy. Therefore, selecting a stable reference region that is not targeted by the radiotracer is the most critical step in this method.

In the quantitative analysis of PET images of the brain, absolute quantitative analysis, which involves directly measuring the uptake values of target tissues, is a more accurate approach, but requires frequent arterial blood sampling to obtain the arterial input function. Despite the availability of various simplified blood sampling techniques, there are still significant challenges in the clinical application. As for the methods of semi-quantitative analysis, although this approach allows us to measure the relative uptake values of target tissues, its results can be influenced by a variety of factors, and it is therefore necessary to weigh its pros and cons during clinical applications.

2.2.3 SPM

SPM, which involves the statistical analysis of images at the voxel level, is an internationally recognized method utilized in functional imaging research of the brain. As a method of image information analysis, the main advantages of SPM compared to the more traditional ROI-based analysis include its good repeatability, strong objectivity, clear differences in voxel comparison, clear regional localization, and lack of influence from analyst's subjectivity. ROI-based methods are not able to accurately discriminate focal changes within a group of images, whereas these changes can be easily distinguished using SPM. Furthermore, SPM can account for different confounding factors, while also performing statistical analysis on images acquired from different states of disease and time points within the same patient, or on images from different patients, and still providing statistical inferences.

When comparing the PET images of subjects who have received different numbers of scans or those in different groups, linear or non-linear transformation can be utilized in SPM to register the PET images to the same space, thereby ensuring that statistical testing can be performed within the same reference space. Therefore, the effects of individual differences can be minimized through spatial normalization and standardization, in order to ensure that the results have greater comparability. As for subjects with nonuniformities caused by motion artifact of the head across multiple acquisitions, SPM can employ the Realign correction module, based on volume fusion, to perform motion and position correction for multiple PET images, ensuring the same head position for multiple PET scans of the same subject. SPM can also analyze all voxels in the entire 3D image to obtain the amount of activity within each voxel, followed by the statistical testing of the numerical values in each voxel, and mapping based on the extraction of statistically significant voxels. Statistically significant brain regions can be fused with the standard MRI space, in order to present these significant regions as topographic maps and obtain their statistical parameters. Additionally, SPM can be used to accurately register the corresponding anatomical position of each voxel, and to determine the statistically significant coordinates and functional brain areas according to the TT atlas.

2.2.4 Other Methods of Image Analysis

2.2.4.1 Spatial Covariance Analysis

In PET image processing, quantitative analysis and SPM can easily be used to analyze PET images from different groups, providing corresponding statistical differences. These methods can produce good statistical results for two groups of PET images with pronounced differences, but are not as reliable when processing more minute differences. To address this issue, methods of multivariate analysis can be utilized for the analysis of PET images. Data-driven methods of multivariate analysis, such as principal component analysis (PCA), independent component analysis (ICA), and supervised learning, can be utilized to reveal metabolic patterns and various abnormalities. For example, a PCA-based spatial covariance method has been applied to the computation of metabolic PET images of the brain in the resting state, thereby uncovering the abnormal covariance relationships between brain region functions.

The scaled subprofile model (SSM) is a PCA-based spatial covariance method that can be used to identify metabolic abnormalities between the PET images of the brain in patients and healthy subjects, and can be used to derive topographic maps of specific brain areas for early disease diagnosis. Using spatial covariance analysis based on PET images, expression scores can be obtained for each subject, which are used as imaging markers to discriminate between healthy and disease groups, and to provide metrics related to disease severity. In this section, we will use spatial covariance analysis as a representative method to introduce the application of multivariate analysis in PET images.

Pre-processed PET images should first undergo the removal of low-intensity voxels, noise-related artifacts, and regions unrelated to brain activity (e.g., WM and ventricles) through the appropriate methods. Masking is performed to define the area within the mask as the ROI, and only voxels within the ROI are included in subsequent analyses. Masking involves setting a percentage threshold $T_{\text{percentage}}$, based on which the voxel threshold, *T*voxel, of each sample is determined. The *T*voxel is equal to the product of the sample's maximum voxel value Maxvoxel and $T_{\text{percentage}}$, and the area within the sample with a voxel value greater than T_{voxel} is considered the sample's mask region.

$$\text{mask} = \begin{cases} 1, \left(\text{voxel} \geq T_{\text{voxel}}\right) \\ 0, \left(\text{voxel} < T_{\text{voxel}}\right) \end{cases} \quad (2.22)$$

The masks from all of the subjects are multiplied to obtain a common mask, in which the non-zero region is defined as the final PET ROI. Finally, the common mask is multiplied with the PET images of each subject to obtain the voxels located within the mask region for subsequent analyses. The masked voxel values in the PET images of each subject are arranged into a row vector according to their continuous spatial positions, after which the row vectors of healthy controls and patients are combined into a data matrix, *D*. The first half of this matrix consists of the row vectors for the control group, while the second half consists of the row vectors for the patients, or vice versa. Each row in data matrix *D* represents all the masked voxel values for one subject, and each column represents the voxel values for a corresponding spatial position.

Diseases may only appear as slight deviations between normal and abnormal values, and it may not be possible to distinguish between minute deviations based on scaling alone. Furthermore, the patient's average voxel value may obscure small potential deviations. Therefore, by performing a log transformation and centering of the data, we can effectively eliminate the effects of the sample average value (which is a global scaling factor) and highlight potential differences. The steps used for data processing include applying the log transformation to data matrix *D* (log*D*), followed by the row- and column-centering of log*D*. This global normalization can effectively remove the effects of the global scale factor, which facilitates the extraction of true structure contained within the data. Row-centering is carried out by subtracting the mean row value (or the sample's average voxel value) from each row element. After row-centering, the matrix is averaged across all columns to obtain the group mean profile (GMP), which is also the row vector. Column-centering is achieved by subtracting the GMP from each row of the row-centered matrix. The size of the subject residual profile (SRP) after row- and column-centering is the same size as the original data matrix, and the SRP represents the difference image of the group, with each element denoting the deviation from the respective mean sample value and the mean value of the group. The GMP is also used for the column-centering of data from newly added subjects to ensure that they are placed within the same reference space after pre-processing, as shown in Eq. (2.23):

$$\text{SRP}_{SV} = \log D_{SV} - \text{mean}_s - \text{GMP}_v \quad (2.23)$$

where *s* and *v* represent the columns and rows of the data matrix, respectively.

The residual matrix, SRP, obtained after global normalization can be used to construct the covariance matrix between samples, S_{sub}. In S_{sub}, the value of the *i*th and *j*th column is equal to the value obtained by multiplying all the voxels of the *i*th sample with the *j*th sample in the SRP, and vice versa. This covariance matrix is a symmetric matrix, and its size is equal to the number of subjects:

$$S_{ij} = \sum_{\text{voxel}} \text{SRP}_{ij} \times \text{SRP}_{ji} \quad (2.24)$$

The above can also be expressed as:

$$S_{\text{sub}} = \text{SPR}\,"\text{SPR}^T \quad (2.25)$$

This covariance matrix can be decomposed using singular value decomposition (SVD) to obtain the eigenvalues λ_k, $k = 1, 2, \ldots, M$ and eigenvectors e_k, $k = 1, 2, \ldots, M$ (where M is the number of subjects). Each element in e_k corresponds to the scaling factor of each sample.

$$S_{\text{sub}} e_k = \lambda_k e_k \quad (2.26)$$

Both the left and right sides of the equation above can be multiplied by SRP^T to give:

$$\text{SRP}^T S_{\text{sub}} e_k = \text{SRP}^T \lambda_k e_k = \lambda_k \text{SRP}^T e_k \quad (2.27)$$

Substituting Eq. (2.25) into the above gives:

$$\left(\text{SRP}^T \cdot \text{SRP}\right)\text{SRP}^T e_k = \lambda_k \text{SRP}^T e_k \quad (2.28)$$

where $\text{SRP}^T{\cdot}\text{SRP}$ is the covariance matrix between the voxels. We can see from Eq. (2.28) that $\text{SRP}^T e_k$ is the eigenvector and λ_k is the eigenvalue of $\text{SRP}^T{\cdot}\text{SRP}$. This equation can be simplified to give:

$$S_{\text{voxel}} \text{GIS}_k = \lambda_k \text{GIS}_k \quad (2.29)$$

where $S_{\text{voxel}} = \text{SRP}^T \cdot \text{SPR}$, $\text{GIS}_k = \text{SRP}^T e_k$. The eigenvalues are sorted in descending order according to variance size, and the contribution corresponding to each eigenvalue vaf_k is calculated, with larger contributions indicating a greater importance of the eigenvector corresponding to the eigenvalue.

$$\text{vaf}_k = \lambda_k / \left(\lambda_1 + \lambda_2 + \ldots + \lambda_M\right) \quad (2.30)$$

Each element in e_k corresponds to the scaling factor of each sample. The e_k vector is weighted based on the square root of its corresponding λ_k value to obtain the score vector, score_k, of each sample. Each element in score_k represents the expression score of each sample relative to the pattern vector, GIS_k, and is given by the equation below:

$$\text{score}_k = \sqrt{\lambda_k} \cdot e_k \quad (2.31)$$

Due to the orthogonality of the GIS_k vectors, we can evaluate the sample score derived from any linear combination of GIS_k vectors. The sample score is obtained from the inner dot product of the sample's corresponding row vector in the difference matrix SRP and the GIS_k vector:

$$\text{score}_{ks} = \text{SRP}_S^T \text{GIS}_k \quad (2.32)$$

This equation can also be applied to prospective experimental validation by calculating the sample score of newly added subjects using Eq. (2.32). When calculating the sample score, the difference matrix SRP is calculated based on Eq. (2.25). When performing column-centering on the newly added data, the GMP image calculated based on the previous group can be used for subtraction (as this GMP is considered to be an invariant population characteristic), or the value of the GMP image can be recalibrated based on another batch of reference patient and control groups. Following PCA analysis, we can derive the GIS vectors of disease-related spatial covariance patterns. The GIS vectors are normalized, which involves subtracting their mean value and then dividing by their standard deviation. The normalized GIS vectors represent the voxel maps of standard deviations above and below the mean voxel weight, reflecting the deviations in regional brain function from corresponding component mean values derived from the combined control and patient dataset.

SSM/PCA is a simple and practical technique of spatial covariance analysis that can be applied to PET data analysis. Its main advantage lies in its ability to identify the sources of differences in the disease group relative to the control group, and decompose these differences into spatial orthogonal components. Only a handful of key principle components are needed to reflect abnormalities in disease, which substantially reduces the volume of data, demonstrating that PCA can be used for data compression. In certain neurodegenerative diseases, the disease-induced differences in PET images are often miniscule when compared to normal PET images and can easily be obscured by larger global factors. The application of spatial covariance analysis, specifically SSM/PCA, allows us to effectively identify the minute differences in the images between the patient group and the control group, while also deriving a series of different topographic maps that can reflect disease-related spatial covariance patterns. These patterns can serve as imaging biomarkers of diseases, to assist in early clinical diagnosis and efficacy evaluation.

2.2.4.2 Metabolic Brain Network Analysis

PET imaging based on the specific binding of radiotracers has evolved into a mature method of medical imaging in clinical practice. We can now conduct measurements of neurodegenerative diseases by measuring the level of brain metabolism or the specific binding of neuroreceptors and transmitters. The clinical methods of PET image analysis are predominantly based on visual/quantitative analysis, which involves evaluating the level of metabolism or specific binding (relative decrease/increase) within a specific region. These methods of local, quantitative univariate analysis have been extensively utilized in clinical settings, owing to the interpretability of their results and direct inference framework. However, these methods can lead to the loss of information on interactions between various regions of the brain, and overlook a large number of meaningful metabolic changes. Metabolic brain network analysis can be used to extract the metabolic interconnections within the images and reflect the changes in metabolic function during neurodegenerative processes. This approach is now widely used in the early diagnosis, risk prediction, pathogenesis research, and other areas of neurodegenerative diseases. In this section, we will briefly introduce metabolic brain network analysis.

The theoretical advantage of metabolic brain network analysis is that it can address the issue of brain connectivity by analyzing the network characteristics between brain regions and eliminate the impact of individual differences on statistical analysis through correlation and permutation testing. Due to the limited temporal resolution of PET imaging, methods of metabolic brain network analysis utilizing PET images are generally based on cohort construction. Seed-based analysis, which involves estimations based on metabolic connectivity at the voxel level, was the earliest proposed method of metabolic brain network analysis. First, PET images are acquired from the cohort targeted for metabolic network construction. After performing spatial normalization and other pre-processing operations on the images, quantitative or semi-quantitative analysis is performed to standardize the uptake values and obtain quantitative parameters such as the SUVR, in order to eliminate the effects of the individual differences in metabolic levels. Second, ROI-based techniques are utilized to create a seed region, and the uptake values of this ROI are extracted from the PET images of subjects within the group to form the seed metabolic time-series $x_1, x_2, \ldots, x_m$, where m is the number of subjects within the group. Third, the metabolic time-series of other voxels are extracted, $y_1^k, y_2^k, \ldots, y_m^k$, where k is the voxel at the kth position, and a generalized liner model or correlation model is used to calculate the metabolic correlation between the seed region and other voxels. Finally, the steps above are performed sequentially on all voxels to obtain the voxel-based metabolic brain network model. By employing seed-based analysis, we can measure the metabolic relationships of key brain regions with other brain regions using PET images, which can be used to analyze the abnormalities of metabolic relationships in patient populations, and potentially uncover the pathogenesis of diseases.

In recent years, ROI-based brain network analysis has also been widely used for PET image analysis. This method is also based on cohort construction, and its calculation process is divided into the construction of nodes in the brain network and the estimation of metabolic connectivity between the nodes. First, brain network nodes are designated for each subject to be included in the metabolic network, which can be accomplished, for example, by using standard brain atlases, such as Automated Anatomical Labelling (AAL), to delineate the

ROIs and to predefine the ROIs as nodes in the metabolic brain network V, $V \subset v_1, v_2, \ldots, v_m$. Second, the metabolic time-series is extracted from the pre-processed PET images, y_1^k, y_2^k, …, y_m^k, where m is the fold number of the cohort, and k is the selected node number. Third, Pearson's correlation or generalized linear model is used to estimate the metabolic correlations between the nodes. Finally, the adjacency matrix of the metabolic brain network is obtained. In order to minimize random errors caused by the enrolled subjects, the bootstrap method can be utilized to resample the subjects multiple times, with the adjacency matrix being calculated in turn for each resampling, according to the steps listed above. Then, the median connectivity value for each pair of brain regions is taken as the stable metabolic connectivity for a given node, which is used to create a stable adjacency matrix of the metabolic brain network, thereby producing the metabolic brain network for a given cohort.

The two methods above are both cohort-based construction methods of metabolic brain networks. In contrast, individual-based construction methods of metabolic brain networks can further elucidate individual differences, which is of crucial clinical value to precision medicine. Individual-based metabolic connectomics, based on Kullback–Leibler divergence estimation (KLS), can be applied to the construction and analysis of individual metabolic brain networks using PET images. As in cohort-based analyses, ROIs are first predetermined using a prior anatomical template in the pre-processed PET images as nodes in the brain network, V, $V \subset v_1, v_2, \ldots, v_m$. Following the pre-determination, the uptake values within the ROIs are extracted, and the probability density function (PDF) of a given ROI is estimated using non-parametric kernel density estimation (KDE). The kernel width of the KDE is estimated by solving the equation bandwidth estimation, in which the characteristic function is given by:

$$\varphi(t) = \frac{1}{n}\sum_{j=1}^{n} e^{itx_j} \tag{2.33}$$

where x_j is the series of voxel values in each ROI. The Gaussian function is applied as a damping function to avoid the problem of integral divergence:

$$\psi(t) = e^{-\pi t^2} \tag{2.34}$$

Next, the Fourier transform is used to derive the PDF within the given ROI:

$$\begin{aligned} f(x) &= \frac{1}{2\pi}\int_{-\infty}^{+\infty}\varphi(t)\psi(t)e^{-itx}dt = \frac{1}{2\pi}\int_{-\infty}^{+\infty}\frac{1}{n}\sum_{j=1}^{n}e^{it(x_j-x)}\psi(ht)dt = \frac{1}{nh}\sum_{j=1}^{n}\frac{1}{2\pi}\int_{-\infty}^{+\infty}e^{i(ht)\frac{x_j-x}{h}}\psi(ht)dht \\ &= \frac{1}{nh}\sum_{j=1}^{n}K\left(\frac{x-x_j}{h}\right) \end{aligned} \tag{2.35}$$

where K is the Fourier transform of the damping function. Then, symmetric KLS is utilized to evaluate the similarity between each pair of brain regions:

$$D_{KL}(P|Q) = \int_X P(x)\log\frac{P(x)}{Q(x)} + Q(x)\log\frac{Q(x)}{P(x)}dx \tag{2.36}$$

where $P(x)$ and $Q(x)$ denote the PDFs of any two ROIs, respectively. Following this, the equation below is used to calculate the metabolic correlation between different brain regions:

$$KLS(P|Q) = e^{-D_{KL}(P|Q)} \tag{2.37}$$

Finally, KLS performed on the metabolic series for all regions of the brain to obtain the individual's metabolic adjacency matrix, and hence construct the metabolic brain network.

Once the cohort- or individual-level metabolic brain network has been constructed, network parameters based on graph theory can be used to evaluate abnormal topological network connections and disturbances. Network parameters, such as clustering coefficients, characteristic path length, small-world parameters, local efficiency, and global efficiency, are commonly used to describe the performance of metabolic brain networks. Statistical methods such as permutation tests and post hoc tests can be used to verify the statistical significance of the metabolic brain networks, while the stability of the brain network can be determined using variance parameters, similarity parameters, and other parameters. Additionally, neurological diseases can be detected by comparing the topological network parameters of the diseased and healthy brain.

2.3 Research Applications of PET Imaging in Neuroscience

PET imaging techniques are currently widely used for the early diagnosis and treatment evaluation of neurodegenerative diseases. In this section, we will focus on three common neurodegenerative diseases, namely dementia, movement disorders, and epilepsy, and introduce the clinical applications of PET imaging for these diseases.

2.3.1 Dementia

Dementia is a syndrome that mainly refers to the decline of cognitive function (i.e., thinking abilities) beyond the expected range of normal aging. This condition can affect memory, thought, sense of direction, comprehension, calculation abilities, learning abilities, language, and judgement. Cognitive impairment is often accompanied by the deterioration of emotional control, social behavior, and/or motivation. Dementia involves a wide range of clinical presentations. The most common form of dementia is Alzheimer's disease (AD), and other major forms include vascular dementia, dementia with Lewy bodies (DLB), and frontotemporal dementia.

AD, commonly known as senile dementia, is estimated to account for 60–80% of dementia cases, and is characterized by three main pathological features: abnormal beta (β)-amyloid (Aβ) deposition, tau protein aggregation, and neurodegeneration. Aβ deposition can lead to the extracellular formation of neural plaques, while the hyperphosphorylation of tau protein can give rise to the intracellular formation of neurofibrillary tangles (NFTs). Neurodegeneration can be mapped to NFT distribution and is characterized by brain atrophy at the macroscopic level, as well as the loss of neurons and neuronal processes at the microscopic level.

Due to the involvement of multiple pathological processes and reactive changes of the brain in AD, a variety of CNS targets are available for PET imaging. Table 2.3 summarizes the most common PET targets, their respective radiotracers, and typical imaging findings in AD.

2.3.1.1 ^{18}F-FDG PET

^{18}F-FDG PET can be used to evaluate local brain metabolic abnormalities in AD patients and is an effective imaging method for detecting functional changes in the brains of AD patients, identifying early-stage AD, and differentiating AD from other causes of dementia.

Patients with early-stage AD often present with reduced glucose metabolism in the temporoparietal association cortex, posterior cingulate cortex, and precuneus (Fig. 2.4). As the disease progresses, these regions of hypometabolism will spread to the frontal cortex, whereas the metabolism of the thalamus, primary sensorimotor cortex, visual cortex, and cerebellum will remain relatively unchanged.

Bilateral temporoparietal hypometabolism is a classic regional metabolic abnormality associated with AD. In fact, if the ^{18}F-FDG PET findings of dementia patients exhibit metabolic patterns that do not include bilateral temporoparietal hypometabolism, then the causes of dementia other than AD should be suspected in these

Table 2.3 PET targets, radiotracers, and imaging findings

Target	PET tracer	PET imaging findings in AD
Neuronal/synaptic activity	^{18}F-FDG	Hypometabolism in the anterior and/or posterior cingulate cortex during the mild cognitive impairment (MCI) stage; further reduction in the bilateral temporoparietal cortex during the dementia stage
β-amyloid plaques	^{11}C-PiB, ^{18}F-florbetapir, ^{18}F-florbetaben, ^{18}F-flutemetamol	Increased neocortical amyloid plaques already present in the pre-symptomatic stage
Tau aggregates	^{11}C-PBB3, ^{18}F-THK5117, ^{18}F-]AV-1451	Increased tau protein in medial temporal region during MCI/ early dementia, and increase in the neocortical region in later stages
Translocator protein 18 kDa (TSPO)	^{11}C-R-PK11195	Microglial activation in brain areas affected by neurodegeneration during the MCI stage
Cholinergic system	^{11}C-PMP, 2–^{18}F-A85380	Decrease in α4β2 nicotinic acetylcholine receptor (nAChR) in brain areas affected by neurodegeneration in the MCI stage
Dopaminergic system	^{18}F-FDOPA, ^{11}C-raclopride	No related changes in dopamine synthesis
Serotonergic system	^{11}C-DASB, ^{18}F-MPPF	Decrease in serotonin transporter (SERT)

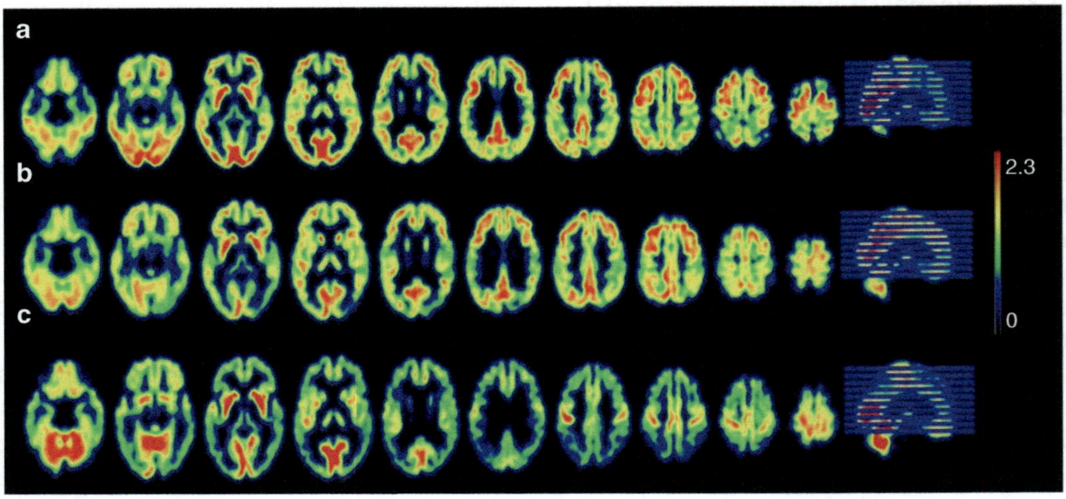

Fig. 2.4 ^{18}F-FDG PET images in normal aging and AD patients. In ^{18}F-FDG PET scans, the standardized uptake value ratio (SUVR) is calculated using the whole brain as the reference region (range: 0–2.3). Compared to a healthy 77-year-old control (**a**) and a 77-year-old AD patient with mild dementia (**b**), a 60-year-old patient with severe AD (**c**) showed significant regional hypometabolism in the temporoparietal cortex, with more pronounced reductions found in the patient with severe AD (**c**) compared to mild AD (**b**)

cases. Silverman et al. analyzed 146 patients undergoing evaluation for dementia, of whom 97 were histopathologically diagnosed with AD, while PET findings for these cases showed focal parietal, temporal, or frontal hypometabolism, or global hypometabolism. In patients with mild cognitive impairment (MCI), ^{18}F-FDG PET was superior to other imaging modalities in diagnosing and predicting the conversion of MCI to dementia. Del Sole et al. evaluated the ^{18}F-FDG PET images of 16 MCI patients and 14 other patients. Their findings indicated that the regions of glucose hypometabolism in AD patients included the posterior cingulate cortex, precuneus, inferior parietal lobule, and middle temporal gyrus, whereas MCI patients only had glucose hypometabolism in the posterior cingulate cortex. Compared to MCI patients, those with AD showed a wider area of glucose hypometabolism in the posterior cingulate cortex, which extended to the precuneus. Furthermore, hypometabolism of the lateral parietal cortex was found only in AD patients. Another important application of ^{18}F-FDG PET in the evaluation of MCI patients is its ability to predict the progression to dementia. Compared to normal controls and stable MCI patients, MCI patients who developed AD within one year exhibited cerebral glucose hypometabolism in the temporoparietal, inferior parietal, medial temporal, and posterior cingulate cortices. They found that as the disease progressed, the glucose uptake in those regions continued to decline, and new hypometabolic regions began to appear, including the lateral prefrontal cortex. In their assessment of 67 MCI patients, Anchisi et al. found that patients who converted to AD showed bilateral hypometabolism in the inferior parietal, posterior cingulate, and medial temporal cortex, whereas patients with stable MCI presented with hypometabolism in the dorsolateral frontal cortex. In addition, a number of studies based on ^{18}F-FDG PET imaging have been used to assist clinicians in differentiating between the different types of dementia. Gilman et al. examined ^{18}F-FDG PET images of 25 AD patients, 20 DLB patients, and 19 normal controls (NCs). Their results indicated that compared to AD patients, DLB patients showed significantly lower cerebral metabolic rates for glucose in the visual cortex (Brodmann areas 17, 18, and 19), but indicated no significant differences between the two groups in the posterior cingulate cortex, superior parietal lobe, lateral temporal lobe, and prefrontal region.

SPM analysis, which can be used to explore the specific topographic patterns related to a decline in cognitive function, has also been utilized to evaluate cerebral metabolic changes in neurodegenerative diseases. In a study of 67 patients diagnosed with amnestic MCI (aMCI), 48 patients attended regular follow-ups for at least a year to evaluate the extent of their progression to dementia. Their findings, which were based on the voxel-by-voxel SPM of PET images, revealed that 14 subjects with aMCI who developed AD within one year showed bilateral hypometabolism in the inferior parietal and posterior cingulate cortices.

Spatial covariance analysis has also been successfully utilized in ^{18}F-FDG PET image analysis for the detection of dementia. Habeck et al. performed SSM/PCA on ^{18}F-FDG PET images to identify AD, and proposed the concept of AD metabolic patterns. SSM was utilized in their study to identify the network-correlates of early dementia and age, capture the major sources of intra- and inter-group variation, produce a series of principal components using PCA, and apply Akaike's information criterion for goodness-of-fit estimation to determine the optimal number of principal components (these principal components should be included as predictors in a linear regression). Their results indicated that relative to the NC group, the AD group showed increased metabolism in the frontal lobe and decreased metabolism in the parietal, temporal, and prefrontal lobes. Using the sparse inverse covariance estimation method, Li et al. identified functional brain connectivity networks based on PET images. Their experimental results indicated that compared to the NC group, the AD group showed a decrease in interregional functional connectivity within the temporal lobe, especially in the parahippocampal area, as well as increased connectivity within the frontal lobe and between the parietal and occipital lobes. Additionally, compared to the NC group, AD patients showed weaker inter- than intra-lobe connectivity, and weaker inter-hemispheric connectivity.

^{18}F-FDG PET can also be used to measure the functional connectivity of changes in neuronal glucose metabolism, in order to evaluate local cerebral activity. Studies comparing fluctuations in ^{18}F-FDG uptake and blood-oxygen-level-dependent (BOLD) signals reported a close association between local metabolic activities and functional connectivity, thus indicating that ^{18}F-FDG PET is a feasible and reliable method for analyzing brain functional connectivity. Therefore, brain network analyses based on graph theory have been applied to study the connectivity patterns in AD and their potential topographic characteristics. Studies involving large-scale brain networks have shown that AD patients exhibit abnormal connectivity patterns with isolated brain regions, and disruptions in system integrity. Sanabria-Diaz et al. (2013) characterized complex brain networks based on glucose metabolism rates, and found, using global and local network attributes (global and local efficiency, clustering index, etc.), that patients with AD and MIC showed abnormal patterns compared to NCs. Furthermore, the attributes of the MCI network were located at an intermediate position between NC and AD, validating MCI as a transitional stage from normal aging to AD. Additionally, Wang et al. proposed an individual metabolic connectome method, which uses KLS to characterize and predict an individual's risk of transitioning from MCI to AD. This method involves comparing the intra- and inter-group similarities and differences between the KLS and group-level matrices, followed by the evaluation of KLS network stability and inter-individual variation. Their findings indicated that the KLS method captured more pathological connectivity in the parietal and temporal lobes compared to typical group-level methods, while also showing greater network stability.

2.3.1.2 Aβ PET

Although the etiology of AD remains to be confirmed, there is evidence to support the crucial role of Aβ in the pathogenesis of AD. The aggregation of Aβ fibers to form amyloid plaques is a neuropathological hallmark of AD-induced dementia. More importantly, Aβ deposition is believed to precede clinical cognitive symptoms in AD and is therefore considered a potential preclinical biomarker of AD.

Over the past decade, Aβ PET imaging probes have undergone extensive development, and the most common Aβ PET radiotracers include ^{11}C-Pittsburgh compound B (PiB), ^{18}F-florbetapir (^{18}F-AV45; amyloid), ^{18}F-florbetaben (AV1), and ^{18}F-flutemetamol.

Studies based on Aβ PET imaging have shown that the typical regional distribution of Aβ in AD patients is consistent with the regions of Aβ deposition in post-mortem examinations. Aβ deposition first occurs in the precuneus, orbitofrontal cortex, inferior temporal gyrus, and posterior cingulate gyrus, and then slowly extends into the prefrontal, lateral temporal, and parietal cortices with time. In contrast, Aβ deposition is relatively sparse in the sensorimotor areas, occipital lobe, and medial temporal lobe (Fig. 2.5). Negative findings in Aβ PET scans indicate a lower likelihood of AD-induced cognitive impairment, but positive scan results cannot be used to confirm AD. Therefore, Aβ PET imaging can only be performed in cases of suspected AD, as its specificity is relatively low.

Grundman et al. evaluated the impact of Aβ PET imaging on the diagnostic results of 229 AD

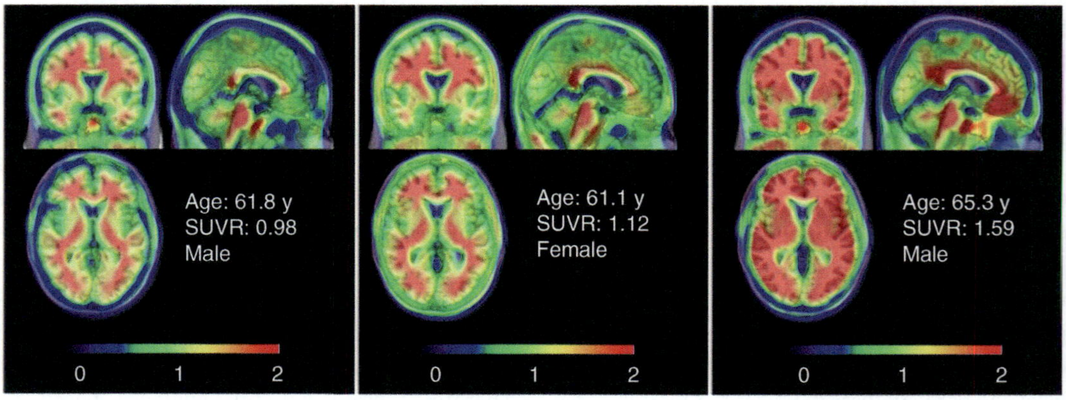

Fig. 2.5 Florbetapir-PET imaging of AD patients. The horizontal bar represents the range of the ratio of cortical to cerebellar signal scores (i.e., SUVR) in semi-automatic quantitative analysis; the maximum value (red) corresponds to an SUVR of approximately 2.3

patients and found that Aβ PET findings changed the diagnosis in 54.6% (95% confidence interval [CI], 48.1–60.9%) of patients and increased the diagnostic confidence by an average of 21.6% (95% CI, 13.3–24.8%). In an evaluation of 218 patients, Jack et al. found that positive Aβ PET scans were significantly correlated with a higher likelihood of progression to AD, with a risk ratio of 3.2 ($P = 0.004$). In contrast, less than 10% of MCI patients with negative Aβ PET scans developed AD, although about 20% developed other types of dementia, such as DLB or frontotemporal dementia.

Kemppainen et al. examined 17 AD patients and 11 NCs using the radiotracer ^{11}C-PiB, followed by SPM and ROI-based analysis to evaluate the group differences in ^{11}C-PiB uptake. Their findings showed increased uptake in the frontal, parietal, and lateral temporal cortices, as well as the posterior cingulate and striatum ($P < 0.001$). In addition, voxel-based analysis revealed widespread distribution of elevated ^{11}C-PiB uptake in AD patients. These findings are consistent with the distribution of amyloid pathology previously reported in post-mortem examinations.

Current studies have also applied SSM/PCA to ^{18}F-florbetapir PET imaging. Blazhenets et al. performed PCA based on ^{18}F-florbetapir PET and ^{18}F-FDG PET images to establish pattern expression scores associated with the transition of MCI to AD. Their results suggest that on the basis of the independent validation dataset, the ^{18}F-FDG PET model yielded significantly higher predictive value than the Aβ PET model, but both were inferior to the non-imaging model. Therefore, ^{18}F-FDG PET, Aβ PET, and non-imaging variables can serve as mutually complementary predictors of MCI progression to AD.

Although Aβ deposition is one of the key pathological features of AD, the level of Aβ plaques also gradually increases with age among elderly individuals with normal cognition, which is one of its limitations as a biomarker. Another limitation is that positive Aβ PET findings are not unique to AD and can be observed in other diseases as well, such as DLB or cerebral amyloid angiopathy. Therefore, it must be stressed that positive Aβ PET findings cannot be used to confirm a differential diagnosis between AD and other Aβ diseases. Furthermore, Aβ PET imaging is unable to provide useful information for identifying diseases unrelated to Aβ (e.g., frontotemporal dementia) or detecting rare forms of AD (in which ligand binding is substantially reduced to due to abnormal forms of Aβ).

2.3.1.3 Tau PET

Tau PET imaging is in the early phases of human trials for the optimization of tracer properties. These radiotracers have different affinities to the paired helical filaments of hyperphosphorylated tau aggregates. As tau PET findings are closely associated with cognitive status, tau PET is considered a potential surrogate marker of disease progression. For many years, the gold standard for quantifying tauopathies has been the histopathological analysis of post-mortem tissues, or the invasive collection of t-tau and p-tau from CSF via lumbar puncture. Compared to Aβ ligands, which have greater specificity, fewer studies have been conducted using in vivo PET radioligands to detect the progression of tauopathies in the human body. Unlike Aβ, tau exists intracellularly, which implies that potential ligands must be able to cross the blood-brain barrier and neuronal membrane. Moreover, compared to amyloidopathies, the total concentration of tau aggregates in the entire brain is lower, which imposes even greater requirements for specificity in tau ligands. Additionally, tau has a wide range of protein conformations and isomers, which may adversely affect the ligand binding site. Current commonly used tau PET radiotracers include ^{11}C-PBB3, ^{18}F-AV-1451, and the THK series (e.g., ^{18}F-THK5351 and ^{18}F-THK5317).

^{11}C-PBB3 is from the same family of radiotracers as ^{11}C-PiB and has shown significant potential in the evaluation of AD and MCI. Maruyama et al. validated the use of ^{11}C-PBB3 in AD patients and animals. They examined 3 AD patients and 3 NCs and found that AD patients showed higher radiotracer retention in the medial temporal region, especially the hippocampus, than NCs. Other studies have found that radiotracers from the THK series had different binding sites than ^{11}C-PBB3. The tau distribution seen on imaging with the former was closely associated with brain atrophy, CSF tau, and neuropsychological functions, whereas the latter was more selective for tau aggregates that were spatially related to Aβ deposition. In the THK series, ^{18}F-THK5351 and ^{18}F-THK5317 showed greater specificity in clinical practice compared to other radiotracers. ^{18}F-THK5351 had a relatively high retention rate in the temporal region. ^{18}F-THK5317 performed well at discriminating AD and MCI patients from NCs, and its regional uptake patterns included the temporal, frontal, occipital, and parietal lobes and the precuneus.

^{18}F-AV-1451, also known as ^{18}F-T807, has a clearer cortical uptake pattern in AD patients than ^{18}F-THK5317 and a lower level of non-target binding, but greater cerebellar uptake effects than ^{18}F-THK5351. A study on ^{18}F-AV-1451 found that its classification accuracy when discriminating between AD and MCI was 85.7%, while also showing high levels of sensitivity and specificity when discriminating AD patients from NCs. In addition, there is evidence to suggest that measurements of tauopathy manifestations based on ^{18}F-AV-1451 were associated with dementia-related cognitive impairment. Pontecorvo et al. showed that in a mixed group of Aβ-positive subjects, the increase in tau ligand binding was related to overall cognitive decline.

2.3.2 Movement Disorders

Movement disorders refer to a group of nervous system (neurological) degenerative diseases in which neuronal abnormalities lead to a decline in motor function. Common movement disorders include Parkinson's disease (PD), Huntington's disease, functional movement disorder, progressive supranuclear palsy (PSP), and tardive dyskinesia, of which, PD is the most common. The main pathological feature of PD is dopamine deficiency caused by the loss of neurons in the substantia nigra, thereby hindering the nigrostriatal dopaminergic pathway or inducing the formation of Lewy bodies. Clinical presentations of PD can be divided into motor and non-motor symptoms. The former includes resting tremors, muscle rigidity, postural abnormalities, and dyskinesia, whereas the latter includes anxiety, depression, sleep disorders, autonomic dysfunction, and olfactory disorders. PET imaging can be used to identify cerebral changes in patients with early-stage movement disorders, providing valuable assistance with the early diagnosis of these conditions.

2.3.2.1 Dopaminergic Imaging

The presynaptic, synaptic vesicle, and postsynaptic dopaminergic imaging of the substantia nigra can provide a wealth of information for the diagnosis of PD. 6-^{18}F-fluoro-L-DOPA (^{18}F-DOPA) is a presynaptic PET radiotracer used to quantify the density of presynaptic dopamine. ^{18}F-DOPA can be enzymatically converted to ^{18}F-dopamine and can indirectly reflect the status of dopamine storage. A large number of studies have found that the uptake of ^{18}F-DOPA in the posterior putamen, anterior putamen, and caudate nucleus in PD patients decreased successively. Furthermore, ^{18}F-DOPA uptake decreased further as PD progressed and was related to the extent of deterioration of the patient's motor functions. The recently developed PET radiotracer ^{18}F-FE-PE2I can also be used to evaluate the reduction of nigrostriatal dopamine in PD patients, with a shorter capture time and superior kinetic characteristics.

The function of the vesicular monoamine transporter 2 (VMAT2) is to encapsulate and store dopamine in presynaptic vesicles, after which it is released from the presynaptic membrane to the synaptic cleft, and visualized using radiotracers. VMAT2 is a membrane protein located on the synaptic vesicles of monoaminergic neurons, and its activity can be measured using ^{11}C-dihydrotetrabenazine (^{11}C-DTBZ). Imaging which utilizes this radiotracer has revealed a reduction in VMAT2 due to striatal degeneration in PD patients.

^{11}C-raclopride (RAC) is a PET radiotracer that binds to the postsynaptic dopamine receptor D2 (the D2-like receptor family includes D2, D3, and D4) in the striatum. In the early stages of PD, patients exhibit an increase in the number of RAC complexes in the striatum. This is due to the lower level of endogenous dopamine, which occupies fewer D2 receptors, causing an upregulation in the number of D2 receptors. As the disease progresses, or with the use of dopaminergic medications, the number of RAC complexes gradually decreases.

2.3.2.2 ^{18}F-FDG PET

Differences in glucose metabolism can be seen between PD and other atypical parkinsonian disorders, implying that ^{18}F-FDG PET imaging can be utilized for the differential diagnosis. The results of SPM analysis based on ^{18}F-FDG PET images suggest that PD patients show relatively intact glucose metabolism in the lentiform nucleus and thalamus, but exhibit hypometabolism in the bilateral frontal premotor and supplementary motor cortices. Furthermore, the glucose metabolism of the basal ganglia is relatively well-preserved in PD patients, but is reduced in PSP patients. Therefore, this feature can be used to differentiate between PD and PSP.

Additionally, there has been growing awareness among researchers about the presence of abnormal connections in the neural circuits of PD patients; therefore, studying metabolic brain networks can facilitate the investigation of pathological mechanisms in PD. SSM/PCA has been utilized when exploring the disease patterns of PD. The Parkinson's disease-related pattern (PDRP) proposed by Eidelberg et al. has now been verified by a number of independent samples. The PDRP is characterized by a relative increase in the metabolism of the globus pallidus, putamen, thalamus, cerebellum, pons, and sensorimotor cortex, as well as a relative decrease in the metabolism of the posterior frontal lobe and parieto-occipital junction. These changes exhibit a linear relationship with the motor function assessment of PD patients and can therefore be used to differentiate between PD and atypical parkinsonism. Wu et al. studied the cerebral glucose metabolic network of Chinese PD patients based on ^{18}F-FDG PET images. Their findings indicated that the increased metabolism of PD patients in the globus pallidus, pons, and cerebellum relative to NCs was related to the decrease in the premotor and posterior parieto-occipital cortex. Moreover, the split-sample analysis revealed that the pattern expression scores of PD patients were significantly higher than NCs. Other studies have also shown that PDRP is significantly correlated with the clinical symptoms and pathophysiological characteristics of patients. Pattern expression scores are positively correlated with the patient's disease severity and the severity of hypokinesia and rigidity, but negatively correlated with presynaptic dopaminergic markers in the posterior striatum.

2.3.2.3 Molecular Pathology Imaging

The main pathological changes in PD involve not only a decrease in dopaminergic neurons in the substantia nigra as described above, but also the deposition of synuclein, Aβ, and tau protein, and radionuclide markers used to label these proteins have gradually been applied in clinical practice. However, synuclein is deposited within nerve cells, which implies that although some markers, such as ^{11}C- and ^{18}F-labelled benzoxazole, can bind with synuclein, they lack specificity.

PD patients generally experience cognitive impairment, which often needs to be differentiated from other atypical parkinsonian disorders with cognitive impairment. A number of studies have shown that Aβ deposition is associated with the extent of cognitive impairment in PD. A previous study revealed that there was no significant difference in the ^{11}C-PiB uptake between patients with PD and PD dementia, but comparisons between Aβ-positive and Aβ-negative patients indicated that Aβ had an impact on the cognitive function of PD patients. Since Aβ deposition may precede cognitive impairment by many years, it can be used as a tool to predict cognitive impairment in PD patients.

The application of tau PET imaging is challenging in PD, due to the intracellular aggregation of tau proteins and different conformations of tau isomers in the brain. Moreover, the tracers for tau imaging must have high selectivity, high affinity, and superior pharmacokinetics. Only a handful of studies have employed tau imaging to investigate PD over the past few years. For example, ^{18}F-AV1451 tau imaging was performed to observe neuromelanin-pigmented neurons, which revealed significant reductions in ^{18}F-AV1451-positive neurons in the midbrain of PD patients.

2.3.3 Epilepsy

Epilepsy is a CNS (neurological) disorder characterized by abnormal brain activity that can induce seizures, abnormal behaviors, and sensations for a period of time, or even the loss of consciousness. The International League Against Epilepsy classifies epileptic seizures into generalized seizures and partial seizures (PS), with the former affecting the entire brain and the latter affecting only part of the brain. PS is the most common form of epilepsy (accounting for about 50% of epilepsy diagnoses), and mainly involves the temporal, frontal, parietal, and occipital lobes, of which, temporal lobe epilepsy (TLE) is the most common form. There are numerous causes of epilepsy, including traumatic brain injury, stroke (the main cause of epilepsy in the population aged over 35 years), dementia, or other vascular and genetic or neurological diseases. In recent years, PET imaging techniques have been widely used in the diagnosis of epilepsy. The various PET imaging methods can also be applied in epilepsy research, including the measurement of glucose, serotonin, and oxygen metabolism, cerebral blood flow, and receptor binding.

2.3.3.1 ^{18}F-FDG PET

^{18}F-FDG PET is the most well-established method of functional imaging for patients with epilepsy. However, owing to the long duration of steady-state glucose uptake, the scan usually encompasses multiple states, including the interictal, ictal, and postictal periods.

Preoperative ^{18}F-FDG PET scans for epilepsy are generally performed during the interictal period in order to detect local regions with reductions and relative reductions in metabolism, as these regions are thought to reflect the focal dysfunction in brain activity related to epileptic tissues. Considerable research has shown that even in patients with normal MRI scans, interictal PET imaging can be used to delineate the seizure onset zone. Although interictal PET imaging is an extremely sensitive technique for the unilateral location of seizure foci, the hypometabolic zone is often more extensive than the epileptogenic zone and therefore cannot be used to accurately determine the surgical margin. ^{18}F-FDG PET is superior to other methods for the evaluation of medically refractory patients with clinically suspected TLE. The classic disease pattern detected by ^{18}F-FDG PET imaging in LTE (no other lesions except for mesial temporal sclerosis) shows relative hypometabolism in the medial temporal, temporal pole, and lateral temporal neocortical regions. The sensitivity of ^{18}F-FDG PET in detecting relative temporal lobe hypometabolism in TLE is 80–90%. Even in cases without hippocampal sclerosis, ^{18}F-FDG PET can still reliably lateralize the epileptogenic temporal lobe. However, ^{18}F-FDG PET cannot accurately differentiate between medial and lateral TLE because the reduction in glucose metabolism may extend laterally to the abnormal temporal lobe. In addition to visual assessment, several studies have utilized SPM for image analysis. Kim et al. performed a comparative study on the use of visual assessment and SPM analysis to evaluate the sensitivity of ^{18}F-FDG PET imaging in localizing the epileptogenic zones in TLE. They found that the difference pattern was sensitive in localizing epileptogenic zones, and that SPM analysis was more sensitive than visual assessment, with no statistically significant differences between the two. This implies that SPM may be more sensitive than visual assessment and can be used to diagnose the epileptogenic zones in TLE. Shim et al. analyzed changes in the metabolic brain network of TLE patients based on ^{18}F-FDG PET images. Their results showed that the metabolic changes in TLE patients with hippocampal sclerosis were more severe than those without hippocampal sclerosis and NCs.

Research on ictal ^{18}F-FDG PET in epilepsy is scarce. A study involving ictal ^{18}F-FDG PET scanning of patients with status epilepticus (SE) or induced/triggered epilepsy found that when there are inconsistencies between clinical features and MR images with respect to the origin of SE, ^{18}F-FDG PET imaging can help to confirm the patient's diagnosis. Another study found in a case of suspected non-convulsive frontal SE that ictal ^{18}F-FDG PET imaging showed hypermetabolism in the left orbitofrontal cortex, and that the hypermetabolic foci disappeared after treatment with oxcarbazepine for 5 days.

Postoperative ^{18}F-FDG PET studies performed at different time points after epileptic seizures indicate that whether hyper- or hypometabolism is detected are determined by the injection time after seizures. A study found that the most severe regional hypometabolism occurred more than 48 h following seizures, and the least severe occurred 24–48 h after seizures. Within the first 24 h after seizures, metabolism was at an intermediate state, which implies that the brain may require more than 24 h after PS to return to its baseline state.

2.3.3.2 Neuroreceptor Imaging

Epilepsy involves a wide range of neurotransmitters (GABA, glutamate, opioids, serotonin, dopamine, acetylcholine, and adenosine) and receptor subtypes. Patients with epilepsy have either abnormally high levels of excitatory neurotransmitters or abnormally low levels of inhibitory neurotransmitters. PET neuroreceptor imaging has helped us to understand the role of neurotransmitters in epilepsy, identify epileptic foci, and discover new treatment methods. Research on PET neuroreceptor imaging has demonstrated reduced binding with ^{11}C-flumazenil ($GABA_A$-cBDZ) and ^{18}F-MPPF (5-HT1A serotonin), and increased binding with ^{11}C-carfentanil (μ opioid) and ^{11}C-MeNTI (δ opioid). It has been reported that ^{11}C-flumazenil is more sensitive than ^{18}F-FDG PET in identifying epileptic foci. Furthermore, $GABA_A$-cBDZ and opioid receptor images tend to have smaller areas of abnormalities compared to the areas of hypometabolism on ^{18}F-FDG PET images. In addition, studies have shown that ^{11}C-α-methyl-L-tryptophan PET (used to study the synthesis of serotonin) can detect epileptic foci within malformations of cortical development, facilitating the differentiation of epileptogenic and non-epileptogenic tubers in patients with tuberous sclerosis. ^{15}O-H_2O PET imaging has also been reported to have comparable sensitivity to ^{18}F-FDG PET imaging in the detection of epileptic foci. The application PET radiotracers in the neuroreceptor imaging of epilepsy patients is shown in Table 2.4.

Table 2.4 PET imaging findings of seizure foci in epileptic patients

PET studies	Imaging findings
Interictal ^{18}F-FDG	Metabolism generally declines
Ictal ^{18}F-FDG	Increased and decreased metabolism (complex pattern)
Postictal ^{18}F-FDG	Complex pattern, metabolism may increase or decrease
$GABA_A$-cBZR receptor	Decreased binding
Opioid receptors	Increased binding with μ and δ receptors
Serotonin receptors	Decreased binding
Dopamine receptors	Decreased binding
^{11}C-α-methyl-L-tryptophan PET	Increased binding
Interictal ^{15}O-H_2O	Perfusion generally declines
Ictal ^{15}O-H_2O	Increased perfusion

Studies using ^{11}C-flumazenil (FMZ) PET imaging to target the $GABA_A$-central benzodiazepine receptor ($GABA_A$-cBZR) complex have demonstrated reduced radiotracer binding in the epileptic foci of patients with PS. Furthermore, FMZ-PET imaging was more sensitive and accurate than ^{18}F-FDG PET in detecting the cortical region of seizure onset among patients with TLE and extra-TLE seizures. Patients with PLE showed reduced FMZ binding in the medial temporal structures, which was limited to the area of hippocampal sclerosis, whereas no abnormalities were detected in the temporal neocortex or other regions in the neocortex.

PET studies on opioid receptors support the relationship between the availability of opioid peptide receptors and epileptic seizures. Interictal PET studies with ^{11}C-cerfentanil (CFN) and ^{11}C-N1'-methylnaltrindole (MeNTI) found increased binding with μ and δ receptors in the temporal lobe ipsilateral to the epileptic foci. The regions of increased opioid receptor binding were smaller than the regions of reduced ^{18}F-FDG uptake. Increased μ receptor uptake was limited to the middle aspect of the inferior temporal cortex, while increased δ receptor binding was limited to the mid-inferior temporal cortex and anterior aspect of the middle and superior temporal cortices.

PET studies using 5-HT1A receptor antagonists (^{18}F-FCWAY, ^{11}C-WAY100635, and ^{18}F-MPPF) showed reduced 5-HT1A receptor binding in the epileptogenic temporal lobe. Apart from reduced binding in the medial temporal lobe, the remaining temporal regions and other cortical and limbic regions were also involved. PET studies based on a dopamine receptor antagonist, ^{18}F-fallypride, showed reduced D2 and D3 receptor binding in the pole and lateral aspects of the epileptogenic temporal lobe in TLE patients. Furthermore, patients with juvenile myoclonic epilepsy showed a decrease in D2 and D3 receptor binding that was limited to the bilateral posterior putamen, indicating that the dopaminergic system may have undergone specific changes.

2.3.3.3 Other PET Imaging Methods

^{11}C-α-methyl-L-tryptophan (AMT) is a radiolabelled tryptophan analog used to study the synthesis of serotonin in the brain. Research on interictal PET imaging in epilepsy has shown increased AMT uptake in the epileptogenic zones of patients with TLE, cortical dysplasia, cryptogenic partial epilepsy, tuberous sclerosis complex, and cortical development malformations. Most patients with tuberous sclerosis complex experience seizures, and AMT PET can facilitate the differentiation between epileptogenic and non-epileptogenic tubers in these patients. Furthermore, AMT PET imaging can also be used to detect epileptic foci within cortical development malformations. The focal increase in AMT uptake among children was less sensitive than the corresponding ^{18}F-FDG PET hypometabolism, but was more specific to the lobe of seizure onset and was generally associated with epileptogenic malformations of cortical development. In pediatric patients with intractable neocortical epilepsy with or without cortical development malformations, the specificity of AMT PET was equally high in detecting the lobe of seizure onset for the lesion (97%) and non-lesion (100%) groups, but the sensitivity was higher in the lesion than the non-lesion group (47% vs. 29%).

$^{15}O\text{-}H_2O$ is an inert, diffusible flow tracer. $^{15}O\text{-}H_2O$ PET can be utilized for the preoperative identification of the language dominant hemisphere and lateralization of epileptic foci in patients with complex partial seizures. Additionally, interictal $^{15}O\text{-}H_2O$ PET imaging of patients with bilateral TLE showed hypoperfusion of the temporal lobe relative to the whole brain.

Suggested Readings

Anchisi D, Borroni B, Franceschi M, et al. Heterogeneity of brain glucose metabolism in mild cognitive impairment and clinical progression to Alzheimer disease. Arch Neurol. 2005;62(11):1728–33.

Blazhenets G, Ma Y, Sörensen A, et al. Predictive value of ^{18}F-Florbetapir and ^{18}F-FDG PET for conversion from mild cognitive impairment to Alzheimer dementia. J Nucl Med. 2020;61(4):597–603.

Del Sole A, Clerici F, Chiti A, et al. Individual cerebral metabolic deficits in Alzheimer's disease and amnestic mild cognitive impairment: an FDG PET study. Eur J Nucl Med Mol Imaging. 2008;35(7):1357–66.

Eidelberg D, Moeller JR, Dhawan V, et al. The metabolic topography of parkinsonism. J Cereb Blood Flow Metab. 1994;14(5):783–801.

Gilman S, Koeppe RA, Little R, et al. Differentiation of Alzheimer's disease from dementia with Lewy bodies utilizing positron emission tomography with [^{18}F]fluorodeoxyglucose and neuropsychological testing. Exp Neurol. 2005;191(Suppl 1):S95–S103.

Grundman M, Pontecorvo MJ, Salloway SP, et al. Potential impact of amyloid imaging on diagnosis and intended management in patients with progressive cognitive decline. Alzheimer Dis Assoc Disord. 2013;27(1):4–15.

Habeck C, Foster NL, Perneczky R, et al. Multivariate and univariate neuroimaging biomarkers of Alzheimer's disease. NeuroImage. 2008;40(4):1503–15.

Hansen AK, Knudsen K, Lillethorup TP, et al. In vivo imaging of neuromelanin in Parkinson's disease using ^{18}F-AV-1451 PET. Brain. 2016;139(7):2039–49.

Holtbernd F, Ma Y, Peng S, et al. Dopaminergic correlates of metabolic network activity in Parkinson's disease. Hum Brain Mapp. 2015;36(9):3575–85.

Jack CR, Lowe VJ, Senjem ML, et al. ^{11}C PiB and structural MRI provide complementary information in imaging of Alzheimer's disease and amnestic mild cognitive impairment. Brain. 2008;131(3):665–80.

Kemppainen NM, Aalto S, Wilson IA, et al. Voxel-based analysis of PET amyloid ligand [^{11}C]PIB uptake in Alzheimer disease. Neurology. 2006;67(9):1575–80.

Kim YK, Lee DS, Lee SK, et al. (18)F-FDG PET in localization of frontal lobe epilepsy: comparison of visual and SPM analysis. J Nucl Med. 2002;43(9):1167–74.

Lee DS, Kang H, Kim H, et al. Metabolic connectivity by interregional correlation analysis using statistical parametric mapping (SPM) and FDG brain PET; methodological development and patterns of metabolic connectivity in adults. Eur J Nucl Med Mol Imaging. 2008;35(9):1681–91.

Leiderman DB, Albert P, Balish M, et al. The dynamics of metabolic change following seizures as measured by positron emission tomography with fludeoxyglucose F-18. Arch Neurol. 1994;51(9):932–6.

Li Y, Liu J, Huang J, et al. Learning brain connectivity sub-networks by group- constrained sparse inverse covariance estimation for Alzheimer's disease classification. Front Neuroinform. 2018;12:58.

Maruyama M, Shimada H, Suhara T, et al. Imaging of tau pathology in a tauopathy mouse model and in Alzheimer patients compared to normal controls. Neuron. 2013;79(6):1094–108.

Passamonti L, Vázquez Rodrgíuez P, Hong YT, et al. ^{18}F-AV-1451 positron emission tomography in Alzheimer's disease and progressive supranuclear palsy. Brain. 2017;140(3):781–91.

Petersen RC. Mild cognitive impairment: transition between aging and Alzheimer's disease. Neurologia. 2000;15(3):93–101.

Pontecorvo MJ, Devous MD, Navitsky M, et al. Relationships between flortaucipir PET tau binding and amyloid burden, clinical diagnosis, age, and cognition. Brain. 2017;140(3):748–63.

Sanabria-Diaz G, Martníez-Montes E, Melie-Garcia L. Glucose metabolism during resting state reveals abnormal brain networks organization in the Alzheimer's disease and mild cognitive impairment. PLoS One. 2013;8(7):e68860.

Shim HK, Lee HJ, Kim SE, et al. Alterations in the metabolic networks of temporal lobe epilepsy patients: a graph theoretical analysis using FDG-PET. Neuroimage Clin. 2020;27:102349.

Silverman DH, Small GW, Chang CY, et al. Positron emission tomography in evaluation of dementia: regional brain metabolism and long-term outcome. JAMA. 2001;286(17):2120–7.

Stayman A, Abou-Khalil B. FDG-PET in the diagnosis of complex partial status epilepticus originating from the frontal lobe. Epilepsy Behav. 2011;20(4):721–4.

Titov D, Diehl-Schmid J, Shi K, et al. Metabolic connectivity for differential diagnosis of dementing disorders. J Cereb Blood Flow Metab. 2017;37(1):252–62.

Wakamoto H, Chugani DC, Juhász C, et al. Alpha-methyl-l-tryptophan positron emission tomography in epilepsy with cortical developmental malformations. Pediatr Neurol. 2008;39(3):181–8.

Wang M, Jiang J, Yan Z, et al. Individual brain metabolic connectome indicator based on Kullback-Leibler divergence similarity estimation predicts progression from mild cognitive impairment to Alzheimer's dementia. Eur J Nucl Med Mol Imaging. 2020; https://doi.org/10.1007/s00259-020-04814-x.

Wu P, Wang J, Peng S, et al. Metabolic brain network in the Chinese patients with Parkinson's disease based on ^{18}F-FDG PET imaging. Parkinsonism Relat Disord. 2013;19(6):622–7.

3 Research Applications of Functional Magnetic Resonance Imaging (fMRI) in Neuroscience

Feng Xiong, Yizhen Pan, and Lijun Bai

3.1 Principles of Blood Oxygen Level-Dependent (BOLD) Imaging

3.1.1 Overview of Functional Magnetic Resonance Imaging (fMRI)

The human brain, which contains approximately 100 billion neurons and more than 100 trillion synapses, is the most complex system in the human body. With the rapid advancement of related disciplines and technologies, a number of new concepts, techniques, and methods have emerged, significantly contributing to the substantial growth in the neurosciences. Contemporary research in neuroscience is mainly characterized by two basic features. The first is that neuroscience research has shifted from the macroscopic to the microscopic level, integrating functional and structural research at the cellular and molecular levels, while also investigating the activity of neurons, synapses, and neural networks. The second is that neuroscience research no longer focuses solely on the control of general physiological (sensory and motor) functions, but has now incorporated complex and advanced mental functions and consciousness under its purview, to explore the relationships between the brain, behavior, and thinking. In neuroscience research, therefore, issues regarding the overall function of the brain must be assessed using in-depth localized knowledge. Numerous methods are available for researching brain function, and functional neuroimaging techniques can be divided into three major categories: (1) Techniques for measuring compounds within the brain, including single-photon emission computed tomography (SPECT), positron emission tomography (PET), and magnetic resonance spectroscopy (MRS); (2) Techniques for measuring local metabolic and blood oxygen changes—an increase in the neuronal activity leads to corresponding changes in local blood flow, oxygen metabolism, and glucose metabolism, thus enabling the study of the neuronal activity of a given brain region by measuring the associated secondary reactions, such as blood flow and metabolism. The primary methods for measuring secondary reactions include PET, fMRI, and optical imaging, techniques which have been utilized most extensively in cognitive science, and are primarily used in research regarding functional localization and the characterization of local brain responses; and (3) Techniques for measuring neuronal activity within the brain—

F. Xiong · Y. Pan · L. Bai (✉)
The Key Laboratory of Biomedical Information Engineering, Ministry of Education,
Department of Biomedical Engineering,
School of Life Science and Technology,
Xi'an Jiaotong University,
Xian, Shaanxi, China
e-mail: bailijun@xjtu.edu.cn

J. Lu, G. Zhao (eds.), *PET/MR: Functional and Molecular Imaging of Neurological Diseases and Neurosciences*, https://doi.org/10.1007/978-981-19-9902-4_3

these techniques directly measure the neuronal activity of human brains—including electroencephalography (EEG), magnetoencephalography (MEG), and event-related potential (ERP), which was developed based on EEG and MEG.

Specific sequences utilized in conventional MRI include T1- and T2-weighted imaging. T1-weighted imaging (T1WI) uses the longitudinal relaxation times of various brain tissues to visualize the fine anatomical structure of the brain, whereas T2-weighted imaging (T2WI) uses differences in transverse relaxation times to reveal minute differences between normal tissue and lesions, and can therefore be used to detect abnormalities such as edema and leukoaraiosis. In recent years, fMRI of the brain has been shown to reliably reflect functional activities in the cerebral cortex that have been elicited by external stimuli. BOLD fMRI, in particular, can demonstrate the morphology and location of numerous functional structures of the brain, from the sensory and motor to the cerebral cortical centers of mental and cognitive activities, and as such, has now become a crucial technique for studying the higher level functional cognitive activities of the human brain in vivo. Moreover, it is non-invasive and non-ionizing, has a high image resolution, can easily be combined with conventional MR images, and is readily accepted by patients and volunteers. These advantages have made BOLD-fMRI the most used technique for cognitive neuroscience and psychology research. Additionally, advanced multimodal MRI sequences, such as susceptibility-weighted imaging (SWI), diffusion tensor imaging (DTI), and fMRI, have also attracted growing attention from researchers. SWI is highly sensitive to microbleeds; DTI can be used to map the direction of white matter tracts and delineate their microstructures; fMRI can be used to calculate the voxel-based intrinsic connectivity network of the brain. In theory, all MRI sequences that aim to reflect the functional state of organs should be encompassed under the term fMRI. At present, fMRI techniques commonly employed in the clinical setting include perfusion-weighted imaging (PWI), diffusion-weighted imaging (DWI), MRS, and BOLD imaging. Broadly, fMRI methods are broken down into three categories: (1) measurement techniques for cerebral blood flow, such as contrast-enhanced imaging, PWI, and BOLD imaging; (2) measurement techniques for cerebral metabolism, such as ^{1}H and ^{31}P chemical shift imaging; and (3) nerve fiber tracking techniques, such as DTI and magnetization transfer imaging. Given its spatial and temporal resolution, non-invasiveness, and practicality, BOLD-based fMRI is currently the most widely used technique and is generally what people refer to when they mention fMRI.

3.1.2 Principles of BOLD-fMRI

BOLD-fMRI is currently the most frequently used technique for fMRI. Its core concept was proposed in 1990 by Seiji Ogawa et al., who experimentally demonstrated that in vivo changes in blood oxygen could be detected using MRI. fMRI signals are usually referred to as BOLD signals, because the images produced are dependent on the changes in cerebral oxygen levels induced by changes in blood flow. Ogawa et al. verified that hemoglobin exhibits different magnetic field properties in its oxidized and reduced forms, both of which can be displayed using MRI. Therefore, BOLD-fMRI is a functional brain imaging technique that indirectly measures neuronal activity based on blood oxygen levels. When T2*WI is utilized in BOLD imaging, MRI has the ability to detect both paramagnetic deoxyhemoglobin and diamagnetic hemoglobin. Traditional imaging techniques such as computed tomography (CT) are only able to display variations in patient's brain structure and morphology, i.e., from traumatic brain injury (TBI), but cannot characterize the patient's functional brain damage. BOLD-fMRI, on the other hand, is a dynamic imaging technique that can indirectly measure the metabolic levels of the brain and reflect the correlations of time-dependent cortical signals over the course of various neurophysiological processes, thus providing a reliable technique for evaluating changes in the functional networks of the brain. Early fMRI was based on the increased blood flow during neuronal activity and relied on the injection of paramagnetic contrast agents. As imaging techniques continued to evolve, BOLD-fMRI preserved the high temporal-spatial resolution of traditional MRI, while also conferring the ability to acquire physiological signals based on blood oxygen levels; therefore, this technique has significant value and potential in clinical applications, and has been widely used in neuropsychological research for investigating the underlying mechanisms of human language, thought, and sensory perceptions. In addition, BOLD-fMRI has been applied to the fields of psychology, rehabilitation medicine, cognitive science, and clinical neurology, where it serves as a potential biomarker in neuroimaging.

The external stimulation of neurons leads to the generation of electrical signals and increased oxygen consumption, which causes the concentrations of oxyhemoglobin and deoxyhemoglobin in the capillaries to decrease and increase, respectively, thereby increasing the ratio of deoxyhemoglobin to oxyhemoglobin. To return the neurons to their original polarized state, glucose is utilized as a source of energy to maintain the active transport of ion pumps, while blood flow is rapidly increased via perfusion, subsequently decreasing the ratio of deoxyhemoglobin to oxyhemoglobin in and around the nervous system tissues. Studies on oxyhemoglobin and deoxyhemoglobin have found that when oxyhemoglobin in arterial blood carries oxygen to local brain tissues, the magnetic susceptibility of the latter decreases and manifests as hyperintense signals on MRI. Once oxygen is consumed by the brain tissues, oxyhemoglobin is converted to deoxyhemoglobin, which increases the magnetic susceptibility of local brain tissues, and manifests as hypointense signals on MRI. It has been previously demonstrated that oxyhemoglobin is diamagnetic, whereas deoxyhemoglobin is paramagnetic (Fig. 3.1).

Deoxyhemoglobin is a powerful paramagnetic substance that can generate a small gradient field around the blood vessels through which it flows, leading to local magnetic field inhomogeneity and rapid proton dephasing, thus resulting in the shortening of T2 relaxation time. Conversely, oxyhemoglobin is a diamagnetic substance simi-

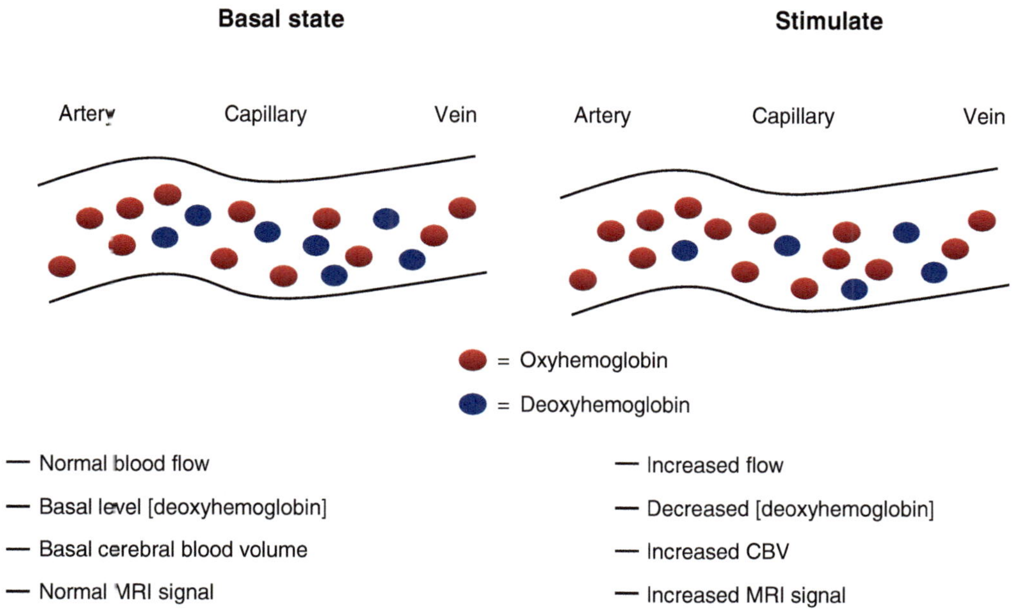

Fig. 3.1 Schematic diagram of BOLD: In the presence of neuronal activity, adjacent blood flow increases to replenish the consumed oxygen, which causes changes in the hemodynamics. When blood oxygen is overcompensated, the level of oxyhemoglobin increases, and the level of paramagnetic deoxyhemoglobin decreases, forming a local gradient magnetic field and strengthening the BOLD signals

lar to brain tissues. In physiology, it is believed that when the human body receives external stimuli, functional brain activity is triggered, leading to increases in local cerebral blood flow velocity, blood flow volume, and oxygen consumption. Based on this belief, Fox discovered that the oxygen consumption during functional brain activity is lower than the increase in oxygen that results from the increase in cerebral blood flow velocity and blood flow volume. This explains why the oxyhemoglobin concentration in the capillaries and venules of stimulated brain tissues is significantly higher than that of surrounding tissues. When the human body performs a specific behavior, the local blood flow in the associated functional areas of the cerebral cortex increases, and the extent of the increase in microcirculatory blood flow exceeds that of oxygen consumption, causing a decrease in the relative ratio of deoxyhemoglobin to oxyhemoglobin. The change in this ratio alters the magnetic properties of the blood, causing a transient increase in the local magnetic susceptibility, which is followed by a decrease, accompanied by a similar trend in the phase dispersion induced by magnetic susceptibility, which in turn causes an initial increase and subsequent decrease in the acquired signal. The decrease in the concentration of deoxyhemoglobin reduces the extent of magnetic field inhomogeneity, resulting in a relatively prolonged T2 or T2* compared to the resting state, and a relative increase in T2WI or T2*WI signals, which appears as local signal increases in BOLD imaging, known as activation.

The change in T2* relaxation times caused by variations in blood oxygen concentration is the foundation of BOLD-fMRI. By comparing the task- and non-task-related states, we can infer the corresponding areas of brain activity. BOLD-fMRI shows the difference between these two states by continuously acquiring brain images, which are then subjected to statistical analysis. T2WI, when implemented in the BOLD-fMRI system, can detect paramagnetic deoxyhemoglobin and diamagnetic oxyhemoglobin. In other words, BOLD can be used to detect the different magnetic susceptibilities of oxyhemoglobin and deoxyhemoglobin. Deoxyhemoglobin molecules are magnetically susceptible, which causes the rapid dephasing of protons; therefore, deoxyhemoglobin appears as hypointense signals on T2WI compared to oxyhemoglobin, which appears as hyperintense signals. Thus, an area with more oxyhemoglobin will display a higher signal intensity in T2*WI than that of surrounding areas with lower oxyhemoglobin levels. In MRI, this phenomenon is interpreted as follows: brain areas with a higher inflow of arterial blood exhibit hyperintense signals, which are considered to be related to functional brain activity.

In short, BOLD-fMRI is a relative measure that requires a comparison of two different states to create a meaningful image. As the process of image acquisition is very rapid (e.g., a 15-frame sequence of brain slices can be acquired in 3 s), an adequate number of images can be obtained for each study, and individual data can then be subjected to statistical analysis and measurement, to determine the differences between the two states. Under ideal conditions, the two states should differ in only one aspect; apart from the factor under investigation, any other factors that may lead to differences between the two states should be controlled.

A key concept in the field of fMRI techniques is the BOLD-fMRI paradigm, which involves presenting a given number of alternating baseline and task-related states and then comparing all images produced during the task-related state with those of the baseline state (images produced within 3–6 s after starting the scan are generally discarded due to delays in hemodynamic response). In recent years, BOLD-fMRI has been extensively utilized for the research of higher level cognitive functions, such as language, vision, hearing, pain, and movement, where it has produced numerous successful results. For example, when language and music stimuli were presented to the auditory channel, the functional brain activity of different areas was activated on both sides of the brain. More specifically, language stimuli activated both the superior and inferior temporal gyri, while music stimuli activated only the superior temporal gyrus. This implies that the superior temporal gyrus is related to music signal processing, while the inferior temporal gyrus is associated with semantic comprehension. A number of different studies have discussed the shortcomings of BOLD-fMRI. For instance, BOLD-fMRI is extremely sensitive to movement, meaning that subjects are restricted to tasks that do not cause motion of the head. BOLD-fMRI is also susceptible to artifacts in certain parts of the brain (e.g., the sinuses) due to the air-tissue interface, which can cause problems when observing certain areas of the brain at the cranial base, such as the orbitofrontal and medial temporal cortices. Despite the advantage of having a high spatial resolution (1–3 mm^3), the temporal resolution of BOLD-fMRI is somewhat limited, mainly due to the delay in hemodynamic response, which only reaches its peak value 4–5 s after the onset of neural activity.

In summary, once the brain is stimulated, excitation occurs in the local brain tissues, which causes arterial blood (oxyhemoglobin) to flow into the excited region, increasing the local oxygen level, resulting in a local increase of diamagnetic substances. At the same time, no changes are observed in the oxygen level of the surrounding brain tissues, due to the lack of neural activity, and hence the local area is dominated by paramagnetic substances. By comparing these two types of signals and performing associated image post-processing, we can determine the location and range of brain activity, which is the basic working principle of BOLD-fMRI.

3.1.3 Applications of BOLD-fMRI

The brain is the most structurally and functionally complex organ in the body. It is the hub for the acquisition, storage, organization, processing, and integration of information from the internal and external environments. Cognition and behavior are determined by the integration of information on multiple spatial and temporal scales; hence, research on cognitive brain functions must be performed on the basis of connections and networks. Currently, there are two different fMRI paradigms for research on cognitive impairment: resting-state fMRI and task-based fMRI, which can be further divided into active and passive task-based fMRI. Active task-based fMRI requires the subject to complete specific tasks (e.g., cognitive function-related tasks or limb movements) while MRI data are acquired, whereas passive task-based fMRI involves presenting the subject with specific external stimuli, such as visual, auditory, or sensory stimuli, in order to observe the enhancement of regional brain activity stimulated by neuronal responses under different task-related states. The acquisition of resting-state fMRI is relatively simple: the subject is scanned for several minutes while lying still and remaining awake with their eyes closed (or opened), without being asked to perform specific cognitive tasks or mental activities. For task-based fMRI, subjects are required to complete more complex cognitive tasks, which in patients with cognitive impairment, can more accurately elucidate the structural and/or functional changes that have caused the impairment.

In 1992, Kenneth and colleagues utilized a gradient-echo planar imaging (EPI) sequence at a magnetic field strength of 1.5 Tesla (T) to study the activation of the visual cortex. In 1995, Biswal et al. found correlations among the spontaneous neural activity of the bilateral motor cortices, and proposed that the correlations of low-frequency signal fluctuations between different brain regions (i.e., temporal correlations on a more distant spatial scale) indicate that there are quantifiable internal and external connections in neural networks with extensive and dispersed distributions, which can reflect the interactions among neurons in the absence of external stimuli. In 1998, McKeown et al. first introduced independent component analysis into BOLD data analysis, which subsequently enabled the separation of several common functional brain networks, such as the default mode (the task-negative network, responsible for the processing of internal information including introspection); central executive (the task-positive network, responsible for the processing of external information, including task execution, stimulus response, etc.); frontoparietal control, visual, auditory, and sensorimotor networks. Moreover, these networks exhibited excellent stability among different individuals. BOLD images have also provided substantial support in elucidating the potential pathology of post-injury sequelae and neuropsychiatric abnormalities in patients with mild traumatic brain injury (mTBI). Studies have shown that mTBI patients have significantly reduced functional connectivity in their default mode network, which has a significant negative correlation with the patient's recovery of consciousness. Patients who recovered consciousness showed significantly higher functional connectivity between the posterior cingulate cortex and the medial prefrontal lobe than patients who did not. These findings have a profound significance for predicting a patient's recovery of consciousness based on the functional connectivity of their default mode network. Other researchers have designed a working memory paradigm to study the complex relationship between cognitive load and brain activation. Their results revealed that under a moderate task load, mTBI patients showed increased functional connectivity between the right dorsolateral prefrontal and parietal cortices, but exhibited decreased activation under a low or high task load, implying that the brain network has the potential to perform compensatory activation.

BOLD-fMRI has laid a solid foundation for research on functional brain networks, although it has several limitations. Resting-state fMRI is highly susceptible to the effects of head motion and baseline scan, as well as the interference of physiological noise, such as breathing, heartbeat, and eye movement. Therefore, most studies of functional brain networks require the application of bandpass filters, which enable the selection of low-frequency signals (0.01–0.1 Hz) for analysis to minimize the impact of physiological signals on the result. Based on a comparison of intracranial EEG signals with the corresponding fMRI signals from the visual cortex of monkeys, Logothetis et al. found that BOLD signals were synchronous and similar with the local field potentials, indicating that BOLD-fMRI signals are a direct reflection of intracranial neuronal responses elicited by external stimuli. Additionally, BOLD-fMRI plays a critical role in clinical diagnosis, monitoring, and treatment, and can be applied to basic research on the underlying mechanisms of mTBI as well as in-depth investigations on the neurophysiological characteristics of other diseases, including depression, post-traumatic stress disorder, dementia, and addiction. Moreover, it can serve as an auxiliary tool for patient rehabilitation and drug intervention, as well as a potential imaging biomarker for the prognostic prediction of a patient's cognitive level.

3.2 Post-Processing of BOLD Data

fMRI of the brain primarily involves the detection of specific physiological signals (e.g., cerebral blood oxygen levels, cerebral blood flow, cerebral glucose metabolic rate) and task-related data sequences. The smallest unit in the resultant images is the voxel. To ensure sufficient spatial and temporal resolution, fMRI collects a massive amount of data, which in turn, requires relatively complicated data processing methods. fMRI data analysis methods can be categorized into region of interest (ROI) analysis or voxel-based analysis. ROI analysis involves the identification of specific regions of the brain through manual localization, and the subsequent statistical analysis of the data from these regions, aiming to ascertain the functional information from each region. This method is direct, straightforward, and very effective for experiments that are only evaluating the brain functions of specific regions. However, given the arbitrary nature of placing the ROI(s) and the difficulties of computer-based localization, this approach is not suitable for experiments aiming to identify task-related brain activation areas, and voxel-based analysis should be performed instead in these cases. Voxel-based analysis uses voxels as the basic unit for statistical analysis of fMR images, in order to obtain the brain activation map at a given significance level, which can then be used to create the time-dependent changes or task-related curves of physiological signals in certain (or all) activation areas. Since the analysis is based on the voxels themselves, this approach does not involve human factors, and can therefore be processed

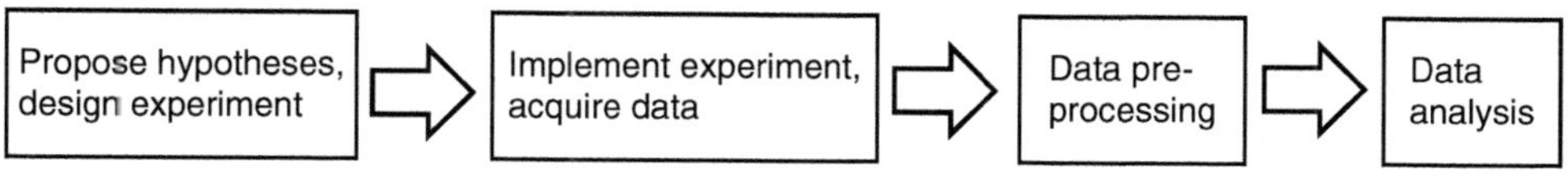

Fig. 3.2 General workflow of functional neuroscience research

automatically by a computer; hence, it has been widely adopted.

A typical brain fMRI study includes the following five steps: (1) formulate the hypotheses and design an experiment; (2) implement the experiment and acquire raw data; (3) perform pre-processing on the acquired data; (4) analyze the data; (5) make inferences based on the results (Fig. 3.2).

3.2.1 Pre-Processing of BOLD-fMRI Data

Since fMRI only provides an indirect measurement of functional brain activity, the resulting signals are relatively weak and susceptible to a variety of noise during the scanning process. Therefore, it is crucial that data undergo pre-processing prior to analysis. The primary sources of noise during data acquisition throughout the scan include (1) movement (motion) of the head; (2) differences in slice number/scan time; and (3) inhomogeneity of the external magnetic field. The most important thing to note is that there are various sources of noise, and the amount of signal variation is only 0.5–2%, which taken together give fMRI images a relatively low signal-to-noise ratio. It is therefore necessary to perform pre-processing on these images prior to statistical analysis, which includes the following steps:

3.2.1.1 Removal of Images from the First Few Time Points

To ensure the stability of fMRI data from longer scans, images from the first 5–10 time points should be discarded for each subject.

3.2.1.2 Slice Timing Correction (STC)

During the acquisition of fMRI data, a complete picture of the entire brain is usually acquired through interleaved or layer-by-layer scanning within one repetition time (TR). Due to the differences between scanning modes, each slice is acquired at a different time within the TR, resulting in time phase differences. STC involves the use of interpolation and other methods to process slice timing in order to ensure that the acquisition time for each slice is consistent.

3.2.1.3 Motion Correction (MC)

The acquisition of fMRI data takes a relatively long time (generally more than 30 min), and although subjects are instructed to remain as still as possible during acquisition and scanners are equipped with head stabilization devices, subjects inevitably exhibit slight head movements, which manifest as motion artifacts on fMRI images, diminishing image quality and affecting the accuracy of any subsequent analysis. Therefore, the first step in the processing of fMRI data is to mitigate the effects of motion artifacts. In MC, the displacement of the brain is regarded as a rigid-body motion, i.e., the combination of translation and rotation transformations. Hence, based on rigid-body transformations, we can calculate the translation parameters along the x, y, and z directions, and the rotation parameters around the x, y, and z axes, to realign the images.

3.2.1.4 Registration

Due to typical differences between individuals, there are variations in the size and shape of brains in different subjects. Therefore, to ensure that the anatomical structure represented by each voxel is consistent across the images of every subject, and that the signals measured accurately express their physiological significance, we can register the fMRI images of all subjects to the MNI152 template formulated by the Montreal Neurological Institute (MNI), on which both linear and non-linear registration can be implemented. To accomplish this, the fMRI data is first registered to the individual space, i.e., to three-dimensional (3D) T1 data, and then the individual T1 data is registered to the MNI152 standard space. Based on this two-step registration process, we can map functional data to a standard space, allowing us to register the fMRI data to that standard space.

3.2.1.5 Segmentation

3D T1 data are stripped of non-brain tissues, such as the skull and fascia, and subjected to probabilistic segmentation to obtain three tissue probability components: gray matter (GM), white matter (WM), and cerebrospinal fluid (CSF). Then, a threshold is selected to extract GM, WM, and CSM with a tissue probability greater than 80% to generate the corresponding mask.

3.2.1.6 Filtering

In order to eliminate the effects of physiological factors such as breathing and the heartbeat, studies generally adopt a 0.01–0.1 Hz bandpass filter in the frequency domain to process fMRI data.

3.2.1.7 Covariate Regression

In order to minimize the impact of other factors (e.g., head motion, WM, whole-brain signals etc.) on fMRI signals, linear regression can be applied to eliminate the effects of 18 covariates, including three translational displacement signals, three rotational displacement signals, WM signals, CSF signals, whole-brain signals, and the first-order derivatives of the nine parameters listed above. The residual data generated is then re-registered to the individual space and standard space after cortical reconstruction.

3.2.1.8 Spatial Smoothing

Spatial smoothing is performed using a Gaussian kernel function with the appropriate full width at half maximum (FWHM) in order to reduce the impact of random noise on image quality and improve the image signal-to-noise ratio. The results of intermediate steps in fMRI data pre-processing are shown in Fig. 3.3.

In addition to following the standard pre-processing procedures to ensure that the fMRI data accurately and genuinely reflect the levels of metabolic activity in the brain, strict quality control is required to eliminate subjects who have been significantly affected by motion or random noise artifacts. Using the mean temporal signal-to-noise ratio (*t*SNR) as the quality control indicator, subjects with a head motion parameter >1 mm (or rotational head motion >1°) and *t*SNR <80 should be excluded.

The mean head motion parameter is used to measure the amount of the subject's motion displacement. It is defined by averaging the absolute

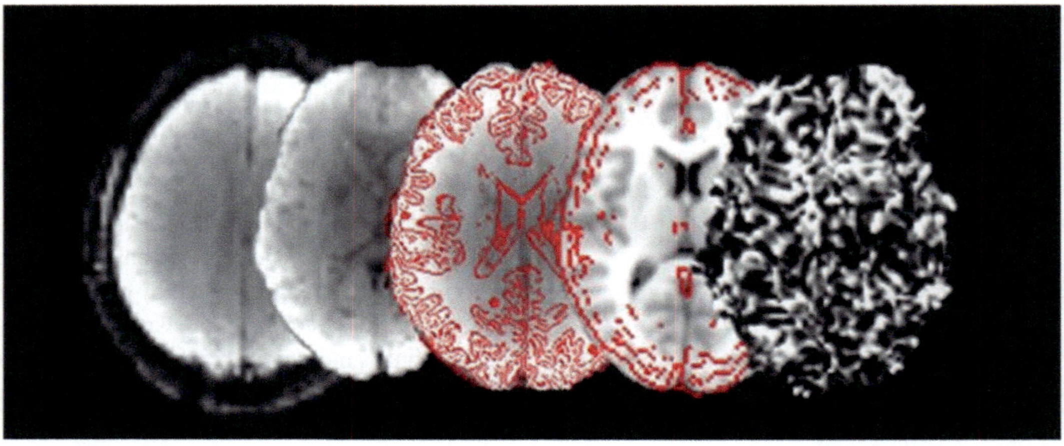

Fig. 3.3 fMRI pre-processing: The images, from left to right, are the raw BOLD image, skull-stripped BOLD image, BOLD image registered to the individual structural image, BOLD image registered to the MIN152 standard space, and smoothed BOLD image

values for the relative displacement of one image compared to the previous image and is given by Eq. (3.1) below:

$$m = \frac{1}{N-1}\sum_{i=1}^{N}\sqrt{\left(x_i - x_{i-1}\right)^2 + \left(y_i - y_{i-1}\right)^2 + \left(z_i - z_{i-1}\right)^2} \tag{3.1}$$

where m is the mean head motion parameter, N is a given time point in the fMRI scan, x_i, y_i, and z_i are the locations of the image at the ith time point, and x_{i-1}, y_{i-1}, and z_{i-1} are the locations of the image at the $(i-1)^{th}$ time point.

The tSNR refers to the ratio between the mean value and standard deviation of the image over time. It can be used to measure the stability of images and is calculated based on Eq. (3.2):

$$t\text{SNR} = \frac{\mu}{\sigma} = \frac{\mu}{\sqrt{\frac{1}{N}\sum_{i-1}^{N}\left(\mu_i - \mu\right)^2}} \tag{3.2}$$

where N is a given time point in the fMRI scan, μ_i is the mean value of the signal intensity for a single image (only the mean signal of the brain is calculated, and excludes the signal values of the background, skull, meninges, and other areas), μ is the mean value of the image across all time points, and σ is the standard deviation of μ_i.

3.2.2 Statistical Analysis of BOLD-fMRI Data

fMRI of the brain mainly involves detecting the spatial distribution of certain physiological signals in the brain or task-related data sequences. Therefore, data analysis is meant to analyze the correlations or other properties between the brain activity, as recorded on the fMRI, and the tasks performed by or stimuli presented to the subjects during the scan. However, the information about the subject's brain activity is encoded as the grayscale values of numerous images recorded in a given time-series, which implies that the researchers are unable to directly, or conveniently, acquire the required information about brain activity. This, therefore, necessitates the processing and analysis of the acquired data to extract relevant information and obtain images of brain activity.

Functional statistical processing refers to the use of appropriate algorithms after data preprocessing to extract voxels that truly represent functional brain activity. In early fMRI studies, data analysis used the simple approach of image subtraction to present task-dependent brain regions. This method is based on the principle of cognitive subtraction, which arises from the assumption of pure insertion in psychology, whereby the baseline image is subtracted from the task-related image, and high grayscale values in the resulting (difference) image represent the areas effectively activated by the task. This method cannot sufficiently set a threshold to distinguish between active and non-active voxels, and is especially sensitive to motion-related and other unknown artifacts. The currently preferred methods include parametric and non-parametric estimation.

Over the past decade or so, substantial progress has been made in the application of fMRI technology in the fields of cognitive and clinical neuroscience. fMRI data analysis has mainly focused on two aspects: the localization of functional areas of the brain and the analysis of brain connectivity. The localization of functional areas of the brain is also known as activation detection, and its purpose is to identify brain areas activated in relation to external tasks based on certain algorithms. This sometimes involves further quantitative analysis of changes in the time-series curve within the activated areas, in order to examine the signal changes during the activity of each activated brain area. Algorithms for activation detection in the brain can be divided into two basic categories: model-driven and data-driven algorithms. In model-driven algorithms, the brain areas are generally regarded as a linear, invariant system, in which prior knowledge about the stimulus sequence is used to detect activated brain areas. Examples of this approach include correlation analysis, the general linear model, and the deconvolution model. Data-driven algorithms, on the other hand, are completely based on information from the data itself, and do not account for prior knowledge about the stimulus sequence.

Common data-driven methods include principal component analysis (PCA) and independent component analysis (ICA), among others. Data-driven algorithms use a larger proportion of information that is contained within the data itself, whereas model-driven algorithms appear to have a more complete theoretical framework. The latter, however, may not show a perfect correspondence between brain activation and stimulus sequence for certain complex stimulus sequences or neuronal activity of certain regions of the brain (especially regions engaged in higher-order brain activity).

Studies involving brain connectivity analysis can be divided multiple ways, based on their different research objectives. When categorized based on brain regions, studies on brain connectivity analysis can be divided into interregional and intraregional brain connectivity. Interregional connectivity is mainly focused on examining the relationships between different regions of the brain, whereas intraregional connectivity mainly involves measuring the level of brain activity within a specific region under a variety of conditions. When categorized based on how the relationships between different regions of the brain are measured, studies on brain connectivity analysis can be divided into functional and effectivity connectivity. When categorized based on whether external stimuli or tasks are presented, studies on brain connectivity can be divided into task-related and resting-state functional connectivity.

The human brain is an incredibly complex information processing system composed of approximately 101.2 billion neurons. According to cytoarchitecture research, the brain can be divided into roughly more than 50 areas with distinct functions. By coordinating the different activities of these areas, the human brain is able to process and integrate information to accomplish high-level functions, while these different functional cortical areas are connected via a network of nerve fibers. Interregional brain connectivity exhibits different characteristics according to changes in external conditions. Typical examples include the impact of learning on interregional brain connectivity, and the strengthening or weakening of certain brain connections due to diseases. Abnormal interhemispheric connectivity, such as the dysgenesis of the corpus callosum, can lead to "disconnection syndrome," as well as impairments in motor, visual, auditory, and higher-order cognitive functions (e.g., semantic function). Furthermore, studies involving resting-state brain activity in patients with schizophrenia have shown abnormal connectivity between the prefrontal cortex (PFC) and the cingulate gyrus. Therefore, measuring the interregional connectivity of the human cerebral cortex plays a valuable role in our understanding of brain function under normal and diseased states.

3.2.2.1 General Linear Model (GLM)

The application of the GLM to the field of fMRI dates back to Friston's work from 1994 to 1995. Friston not only introduced the GLM framework but also continuously made improvements, which encouraged the gradual maturation of the GLM technique, which eventually gave rise to the Statistical Parametric Mapping (SPM) software, with GLM serving as the core of the entire software algorithm. GLM is a voxel-based model that expresses the observed data found within a voxel as a linear combination of several explanatory variables, based on which the statistical parameters can be mapped. This mapping is able to reflect statistical significance and special regional responses, while the factors of ROIs and non-ROIs can be included in the design matrix. If sufficient consideration can be given to the temporal and spatial autocorrelation between time-series, then this technique can be utilized for the analysis of fMRI data. The GLM addresses two major issues: (1) the estimation of unknown parameters and (2) testing the hypotheses of unknown parameters. Based on the research focus, GLMs can be divided into linear regression, analysis of variance (ANOVA), and analysis of covariance (ANCOVA) models. Linear regression focuses on the estimation of unknown parameters, ANOVA emphasizes the hypothesis testing of unknown parameters, while ANCOVA is a combination of the two.

When applying the GLM, let X (the $N*T$ matrix) be the fMRI data matrix, where N is the number of voxels, T is the duration of the time-series, and $X_n(t)$ is the signal of voxel n at time t. Thus, the following assumptions can be made about this model: (1) the system response elicited by the stimulus is linear and time-invariant; (2) the hemodynamic response function of each voxel is consistent; (3) noise, ε_n, is an independent and identically distributed variable that follows a normal distribution with a variance of σ^2 and expectation of 0, denoted as $\varepsilon_n \sim N(0, \sigma^2)$. The basic signal model is as follows:

$$X_n(t) = b_0 + \sum_{m=1}^{M} b_m(n) h^* P_m(t) + \varepsilon_n(t) \quad (3.3)$$

where $P_m(t)$ is the time-series of the stimulus function, h is the hemodynamic response function, $b_m(n)$ is the amplitude of the stimulus response, and $\varepsilon_n(t)$ is noise. In the remainder of this section, we will assume that the signal has been centered, i.e., $b_0 = 0$.

Let $g_m(t) = h^*P_m(t)$, $m = 1,2,\ldots.M$, which will give the following expression:

$$X = G\beta + \varepsilon \quad (3.4)$$

where $G = \{g_m(t)\}$ is the design matrix, and includes the explanatory variables related to the experimental conditions. If and only if the design matrix has full rank, the minimum variance estimate of β can be uniquely given by the equation below:

$$\hat{\beta} = \left(G^T G\right)^{-1} G^T X \quad (3.5)$$

According to the Gauss-Markov theorem, when the error is normally distributed, the minimum variance estimate is also the maximum likelihood estimate, as well as the optimal unbiased estimate. In other words, for all unbiased estimates, the minimum variance estimate has the smallest variance. The residual variance can be estimated using the following equation:

$$\hat{\varepsilon}^2 = \frac{\varepsilon^T \varepsilon}{T-p} \sim \hat{\sigma}^2 = \frac{\chi^2_{T-p}}{T-p} \quad (3.6)$$

where $p = \text{rank}(G)$. The minimum variance estimate is normally distributed, $\beta^\wedge \sim N(\beta, \sigma^2(G^TG)^{-1})$, thus the following relationship holds for a column vector c containing L weights:

$$c^T \hat{\beta} \sim N(c^T \beta, \sigma^2 c^T \left(G^T G\right)^{-1} c \quad (3.7)$$

$C^T\hat{\beta}$ can then be estimated using the equation below:

$$\frac{c^T \beta - \hat{c}^T \beta}{\sqrt{\hat{\sigma}^2 c^T \left(G^T G\right)^{-1} c}} \sim t_{T-p} \quad (3.8)$$

where t_{T-p} is a T distribution with T-p degrees of freedom. In SPM, all hypotheses to be tested are expressed as $C^T\beta = 0$, and all tests based on the T distribution are one-tailed.

Assuming that the parameter vector of the model is denoted as β and takes the form $\beta^T = [\beta^T{}_1 | \beta^T{}_2]^T$, then the hypothesis to be tested will be H:$\beta = 0$. If the corresponding design matrix is $G = [G_1, G_2]$, then the entire model can be given below:

$$X = \left[G_1 \vdots G_2\right] \begin{bmatrix} \beta_1 \\ \cdots \\ \beta_2 \end{bmatrix} + \varepsilon \quad (3.9)$$

If hypothesis H is true, then the model can be simplified as: $X = G_2\beta_2 + \varepsilon$. Assuming that the residual errors of the original model and the simplified model are $g(\beta)$ and $g(\beta_2)$, respectively, then when β_2 is known, the error caused by β_1 can be expressed as $s(\beta_1|\beta_2) = s(\beta_2) - s(\beta)$. If we assume that H is true, then $s(\beta)$ and $s(\beta_1|\beta_2)$ are independent, and $s(\beta_1|\beta_2) \sim \sigma^2\chi^2_p$, where the degree of freedom p is rank(G) − rank(G_2). Thus, the hypothesis can be tested using the equation below:

$$F = \frac{\left(s(\beta_2) - s(\beta)\right) / \left(p - p_2\right)}{s(\beta) / T - p} \sim F_{P-P_2, T-P} \quad (3.10)$$

where $p = \text{rank}(G)$, $p_2 = \text{rank}(G_2)$, and T is the total number of sequences scanned.

SPM-based fMRI statistical analysis utilized a larger number of univariate approximation methods (based on GLM), and involves the following steps: (1) modeling, which specifies the GLM design matrix, fMRI data files, and filtering; (2) estimation of the GLM parameters using canonical or Bayesian approximation; (3) inference, which uses the contrast vector to review the results and plot the results as statistical graphs.

The GLM and Gaussian random field theory utilize statistical parametric images for the statistical analysis and inference of spatially extended data. The GLM is utilized for parametric estimation, and the resulting parameters are used to describe the properties of spatially continuous data. Gaussian random field theory is used to solve the multiplicity problem in statistical inference, while the statistical processes regarded as spatially extended in SPM primarily refer to the randomness of the Gaussian field. The earliest established classes of SPM, such as ANOVA, correlation coefficients, and *t*-tests, are all based on linear models. In this sense, they can also be considered as special cases of the GLM, differing only with respect to the design matrix in the experimental design.

When building a model, we must consider whether the experimental design is event- or time-related. The only difference between the two is the duration of the input and stimulus functions, which express a series of events or a series of time points by convolving an $\delta_{(t)}$ or square wave function. First-order convolution or generalized convolution (second-order derivative) is generally applied to convolve the input parameters with hemodynamics. Hemodynamic or dynamic causal modeling can be used for the same input.

Time-dependent designs may be either random or deterministic. In a random design, one of the trial types may occur within a continuous period of time at a given probability, and this probability can either be fixed or time-dependent. The most effective design is achieved when the probability of each trial type is the same. The judgment criterion in random designs does not consider whether zero events are included. In order to evaluate the response elicited by a certain period of time, a zero event must be included.

Once the fMRI data has been processed and analyzed, it should be presented in an intuitive form to facilitate the interpretation and utilization of the results. After statistical inference, the *t*-values and the corresponding threshold can be used to set the *t*-values of voxels lower than the threshold as 0, and retain the *t*-values of voxels greater than the threshold, thereby obtaining the brain activation map at the confidence level corresponding to the threshold. As this map is obtained based on the statistical analysis of the model parameters, and presents the images related to the thresholded *t*-values, it is known as the statistical parametric map, and can be denoted according to the selected *t*-value as SPM$\{t\}$. Additionally, since the corresponding degree of freedom is still needed to give the confidence level after the *t*-value is obtained, SPM also provides the parametric value z of the $\{0, 1\}$ normal distribution corresponding to the confidence level of the *t*-values and their corresponding degrees of freedom. Thus, the images related to the z-values are obtained and denoted as SPM$\{z\}$. The functional activation maps of the brain can be overlaid onto structural maps of the brain (T1WI or CT maps) to generate fused images that can clearly display which brain areas are involved in the function being studied. Furthermore, based on these activation maps, SPM can also produce the response curves for physiological signals such as cerebral blood flow, as well as the response characteristics of different states.

In addition to overlaying anatomical images with SPM maps, we can also perform cortical reconstruction to obtain information about the anatomic structure and geometric features of the cortical surface, which can, in turn, be used for the cortical localization of activated functional areas. Standard T1 anatomical images can be segmented into GM, WM, and CSF for cortical anatomical reconstruction. fMRI retinotopic mapping allows the sulci and gyri of the occipital lobe to be unfolded and evaluated as a two-dimensional (2D) image. Although there are a number of reconstruction methods, such as voxel-based methods and 2D contour reconstruction, the key point of these is to maintain the anatomic topological structure of the cortex throughout the reconstruction.

Brodmann's classification is currently widely utilized for the localization of the functional areas of the brain. As the structure of the cerebral cortex is specific to each individual, apart from the primary motor and sensory cortices, which remain relatively constant, variations are commonly found in the relationships between other functional areas and anatomical structures. Therefore, unless one is familiar with both neuroanatomy and the Talairach-Tournoux system, it is generally difficult to perform functional localization of the brain regions involved through a simple visual identification. After normalizing the brain map of the individual to the standard brain structure in pre-processing, we can easily confirm the coordinates of the regions involved according to Brodmann's classification or implement automatic processing using professional software.

In addition to SPM, other programs, such as MRIcro, can also be used to display and process fMRI data. This step further addresses two key issues: (1) the presentation of regions with significant activation and (2) finding the coordinates of activated regions in order to accurately identify the anatomical location of these regions. Different methods can be utilized to control the activation of a certain voxel or cluster of voxels. The activation is dependent on the threshold chosen for the significance level, so that different thresholds will give different activations. The activated regions can also be controlled by adjusting the confidence level. In fMRI data, the appearance of multiple excitation points in marginal regions of the brain implies that some of these points may actually be motion artifacts. Once the precise coordinates of the activated regions have been obtained, a non-linear transformation can be applied to convert MNI coordinates to Talairach coordinates, based on the relationship between the MNI and Talairach atlases, which then allows us to identify the anatomical location of each activated region.

For the majority of the data acquired using imaging modalities (e.g., fMRI, PET, EEG, etc.), there is always one major issue—that of which statistical model should be used for data processing and analysis. This is because we do not know distribution type of the acquired data, and the spatial resolution of these techniques are insufficiently high, meaning each voxel also contains information from surrounding tissues. Moreover, performing registration during data preprocessing can also give rise to greater correlations between each voxel and its surrounding voxels. Due to these factors, ordinary statistical distribution models (e.g., Poisson distribution, Gaussian distribution, etc.) should not be used to process these data, necessitating the introduction of the GLM.

Analysis using the GLM utilized a large number of univariate, rather than multivariate, statistical methods, primarily because: (1) multivariate methods cannot be used to infer region-specific effects, and (2) multivariate methods require the number of observations (i.e., the number of scans) to be greater than the number of response variables (i.e., the number of voxels), which is difficult to achieve. Parametric methods require us to make prior assumptions about data distribution, whereas certain non-parametric methods avoid this problem. Non-parametric methods, however, are less convincing than parametric methods, although they can be used to evaluate the assumptions of parametric methods. There is also another class of methods known as Bayesian methods. Traditional methods first need to assume that the effect to be tested is not present (i.e., effect equals 0), whereas the Bayesian method employs posterior probability maps (PPMs) to infer the effects, thereby avoiding the problems of statistical inference encountered when using traditional statistical methods. Hence, this class of methods has significant potential for utilization in the analysis of fMRI data.

3.2.2.2 Deconvolution Model

In the deconvolution model, the whole system is assumed to be a linear, time-invariant system. Therefore, for an arbitrary input of a linear time-invariant system, the corresponding output can be determined using the impulse response function. The impulse (Dirac) function $\delta(t)$ is given as follows:

$$\delta(t)=\begin{cases}+\infty, t=0\\ 0, \ t\neq 0\end{cases} \tag{3.11}$$

where the area under the curve is given by:

$$\int_{-\varepsilon}^{+\varepsilon}\delta(\tau)d\tau = 1, \forall\varepsilon > 0 \quad (3.12)$$

Let $f(t)$ be:

$$f(t) = \int_{-\varepsilon}^{+\varepsilon} f(\tau)\delta(t-\tau)d\tau \quad (3.13)$$

Its discrete form is given by:

$$f(t) = \lim_{\Delta t \to 0}\sum_{-\infty}^{+\infty} f(n\Delta t)\delta(t-n\Delta t)\Delta t \quad (3.14)$$

Let $h(t)$ be the impulse function:

$$h(t) = T(\delta(t)) \quad (3.15)$$

Thus, for any input $f(t)$, let $y(t)$ be its corresponding output:

$$y(t) = T(f(t)) \quad (3.16)$$

Given the linearity of the system, the equation above can be transformed into:

$$y(t) = \lim_{\Delta t \to 0}\sum_{-\infty}^{+\infty} f(n\Delta t)T(\delta(t-n\Delta t))\Delta t \quad (3.17)$$

Furthermore, given the time-invariance of the system, we can obtain the following equation:

$$y(t) = \lim_{\Delta t \to 0}\sum_{-\infty}^{+\infty} f(n\Delta t)h(t-n\Delta t)\Delta t \quad (3.18)$$

Its corresponding integral form is as follows:

$$y(t) = \int_{-\infty}^{+\infty} f(\tau)h(t-\tau)d\tau \quad (3.19)$$

Based on the concept of the convolution integral, we arrive at the following equation:

$$\int_{-\infty}^{+\infty} f(\tau)h(t-\tau)d\tau \equiv f(t)\otimes h(t) \quad (3.20)$$

In reality, all actual physical systems are causal, that is, the system output at time t_0 is only related to the system input at time $t \le t_0$, while all inputs at time $t < 0$ are 0, which gives the following equation:

$$y(t) = \int_{0}^{t} f(\tau)h(t-\tau)d\tau \quad (3.21)$$

Its discrete form is given as follows:

$$y(n\Delta t) = \sum_{m=0}^{n} f(m\Delta t)h(n\Delta t - m\Delta t)\Delta t \quad (3.22)$$

Its numerical solution is given by:

$$y_n = \sum_{m=0}^{p} f_{n-m}h_m, n \ge p \quad (3.23)$$

Naturally, for all actual systems, the observed values will contain a certain amount of noise. If we let Z_n be the real observed signals, then:

$$Z_n = \sum_{m=0}^{p} f_{n-m}h_m + \varepsilon_n, n \ge p \quad (3.24)$$

For fMRI data, we have the following equation:

$$Z = X\beta + \varepsilon \quad (3.25)$$

Where:

$$Z = \begin{bmatrix} Z_p \\ Z_{p+1} \\ \vdots \\ Z_{N-1} \end{bmatrix}, X = \begin{bmatrix} 1 & p & f_p & \cdots & f_0 \\ 1 & p+1 & f_{p+1} & \cdots & f_1 \\ \vdots & \vdots & \vdots & \vdots & \vdots \\ 1 & N-1 & f_{N-1} & \cdots & f_{N-p-1} \end{bmatrix}, \beta = \begin{bmatrix} \beta_0 \\ \beta_1 \\ h_0 \\ \vdots \\ h_p \end{bmatrix}, \varepsilon = \begin{bmatrix} \varepsilon_p \\ \varepsilon_{p+1} \\ \vdots \\ h_p \end{bmatrix}$$

The minimum mean square error estimation of β is given by:

$$\hat{\beta} = \left(X^T X\right)^{-1} X^T Z \quad (3.26)$$

At this point, various statistical tests (e.g., t-test, F-test, etc.) can be implemented for hypothesis testing, and brain activation areas can be determined according to a given threshold.

3.2.2.3 Functional Connectivity

Basic Definition of Functional Connectivity

In traditional task-based fMRI studies, the resting state is usually taken as the baseline, and attention is rarely paid to the corresponding functional activities of the brain in the resting state. However, in the resting state, there are significant correlations in the low-frequency components ($f < 0.1$ Hz, known as "low-frequency oscillations") of BOLD signals from the primary motor areas of the left and right hemispheres.

The human brain processes information through the coordination of multiple cortical areas, which are paired to accomplish high-level functions. The concept of functional brain connectivity first emerged in electrophysiological research. In the early 1990s, Friston et al., at the Welcome Department of Cognitive Neurology (now the Welcome Center for Human Neuroimaging), expanded this concept to the field of functional imaging and divided it into functional and effective connectivity. Functional connectivity evaluates whether there are connective relationships between various regions of the brain, and commonly used algorithms include correlation analysis and PCA. Effective connectivity evaluates how transmission occurs within the relationships between the various regions of the brain, and commonly used algorithms include structural equation modeling and dynamic causal modeling. Generally speaking, the former measures whether functional connections exist between different regions of the brain without considering the directionality of these interactions, while the latter considers the directionality of the interactions between the regions of the brain, i.e., it examines the issue of how information is transmitted between these regions. In 2004, Sporns et al. proposed a more precise definition of functional connectivity: "Within the neuroanatomical substrate (structural connectivity), the non-linear dynamics of neurons and neuronal populations result in patterns of statistical dependencies (functional connectivity)." Based on Sporns' definition, we can identify the four characteristics of functional connectivity: (1) anatomical connectivity serves as its material basis; (2) it is dynamic relative to anatomical connectivity; (3) it is a pattern of dependencies, which embodies a form of interrelationship; (4) it exists in a statistical sense.

As such, the presence and strengths of interregional connections evaluated using functional connectivity are model-free. Researchers, therefore, determine the ROIs in each model as required, and then establish the model by comprehensively considering the constraints of neuroanatomy, neurophysiology, and functional imaging data.

The vast majority of studies on functional connectivity analysis (task-related/resting-state) utilize methods of correlation analysis to measure the functional connectivity among brain regions. The procedures usually involve selecting a specific ROI as the seed, and obtaining the BOLD response time-series of this region, $r(i), i = 1,2,\ldots,n$, where n is the length of the time-series, following which the correlational methods are implemented to calculate the correlation between the time-series for the region with that of other voxels in the brain. There are currently two widely used methods for functional connectivity analysis. The first involves selecting a nucleus that is closely related to the research question, and using the average time-series of this nucleus as a reference sequence, after which the correlation analysis is performed using the reference sequence with the corresponding time-series of other nuclei in the whole brain, and a threshold is defined. Nuclei greater than this threshold are considered to be functionally correlated with the reference nucleus, and therefore, these nuclei together constitute a brain network that can perform the corresponding function. This approach is known as seed-based correlation analysis. The second method does not involve the prior selection of a reference nucleus, and largely utilizes multivariate methods such as PCA and ICA.

Functional connectivity analysis is of crucial significance to neuroscience. Current fMRI-based functional connectivity analyses have been extensively applied to the study of perceptual, cognitive, and affective mechanisms, and the organizational structure of functional networks in the human brain. Functional connectivity analysis is also valuable to the pathological research of neurological and psychiatric diseases. At present, functional connectivity analysis has been widely utilized in the pathological research of various diseases, such as schizophrenia, depression, autism, and post-traumatic stress disorder, in the hope of uncovering their etiology and pathogenesis.

Interest in fMRI-based functional connectivity analysis has been growing among neuroscientists; however, due to the complexity of the human brain, as well as the inherent limitations of the temporal and spatial resolutions of MRI equipment, there is still room for growth in research involving the network of functional brain connectivity.

3.2.2.4 Common Steps in Functional Connectivity Analysis

Seed-based correlation analysis in the temporal region is currently the most widely used indicator to evaluate whether interdependencies are present between regions of the brain. Functional connectivity analysis generally involves the following steps: first, a specific ROI is selected as the seed, and the BOLD response time-series for this region, $x(i)$, $I = 1, 2, \ldots n$, is obtained, where n is the length of the time-series; then, correlational methods are used to calculate the correlation between the average time-series of voxels in the seed region with those of other voxels in the whole brain, $y(i)$, $i = 1, 2, \ldots n$. Further details on the procedure are presented below.

Data Pre-Processing

Common pre-processing steps include slice timing alignment, image sequence alignment, joint registration, standardization (or normalization), spatial smoothing and filtering, and temporal smoothing and filtering.

ROI Selection

Seed selection is a critical topic in functional connectivity analysis. The seed is generally selected based on anatomical knowledge of an area anticipated to become activated, but ROIs can also be extracted as seeds in experiments with a strong prior hypothesis once the activated areas of the brain have been obtained. First, standard GLM analysis is performed on the fMRI data of each subject to obtain their individual activation maps. Second, within-group random effects analysis is performed on the activation maps to determine the significant activation areas within each group. Third, the voxel with the largest t-value is selected, along with several surrounding voxels, to form the ROI. Finally, the group ROI is used as a mask, and the voxel with the maximum t-value within the mask on the t-statistic map of each subject is selected as their peak voxel. The peak voxel and a predetermined number of surrounding voxels (determined based on the size requirements of the ROI) are then selected as the subject's ROI.

Correlation Analysis

For each subject, a correlation analysis is performed between the reference time-series within the ROI and the other voxels of the entire brain. The correlation coefficient can be given by the equation below:

$$r = \frac{\sum_{i=1}^{n}(x_i - \bar{x})(y_i - \bar{y})}{\sqrt{\sum_{i=1}^{n}(x_i - \bar{x})^2}\sqrt{\sum_{i=1}^{n}(y_i - \bar{y})^2}} \tag{3.27}$$

Where x_i is the reference time-series, and y_i is the given time-series, and $\bar{x}$ and $\bar{y}$ are the mean values of the reference and given time-series, respectively. If the calculated r-value exceeds a predetermined threshold, then the two nuclei are considered to by functionally connected; if the

r-value falls below this threshold, then they are considered to not be functionally connected.

$$F = \frac{1}{2}\ln\frac{1+r}{1-r} \tag{3.28}$$

We know that an fMRI time-series contains both temporal and spatial information; Therefore, since the method of image acquisition is the underlying cause for endogenous and spatial correlation, we expect the distribution of the correlation coefficients to exhibit certain characteristics. In correlation analysis, this distribution may vary, depending on the ROIs selected, the spatial sampling frequencies, or physiological factors such as myocardial coupling and respiration. In order to normalize the distribution, the r-correlation coefficient map calculated using the equation above needs to be standardized using the Fisher transformation to approximate a normal distribution, which is then converted to a standard normal distribution using the method proposed by Lowe. Since the data from each time point are not mutually independent, the degree of freedom needs to be corrected based on Bartlett's theorem, following which random effects analysis is performed on each subject's correlation map (single-point t-test) to discern which voxels that are significantly correlated with the seed region at the group level.

3.2.2.5 Independent Component Analysis (ICA)

ICA emerged as a novel method from the field of signal processing in the late 1990s. As the name suggests, this method involves decomposing a given signal into a number of mutually independent components. If the signal itself is originally a mix of several independent sources, then the ideal situation would be to decompose the signal into each individual source. In principle, it would be impossible to achieve such a decomposition based on a single channel of observation, and simultaneous observations via a set of multiple channels that combine these sources according to their constituent ratios would be necessary. In other words, ICA is a method of multi-channel signal processing. However, the results obtained from decomposing a group of observation signals into their various independent components will almost certainly not be unique. Therefore, certain constraints must be specified for the decomposition to ensure that the solution is close to the expected results.

The development of ICA was closely connected blind source separation (BSS), a concept illustrated in Fig. 3.4. In BSS, only the output data (X) of a multi-channel system is available to determine its input function (S) and system transfer function (H). BSS is "blind" because, in principle, it does not require prior knowledge about S and H, and the solution is clearly not unique. Therefore, it is generally necessary to assume that the components of the multi-channel input (S) are mutually independent, have a zero-mean, and have a variance of one. Thus, it is apparent that the formulation of the BSS is very similar to that of ICA, although the former has a broader research scope, with more methods available to resolve the issue.

Since ICA can effectively detect certain activated regions that cannot be detected by other methods without any prior model assumptions about the time-series, it is a novel approach to fMRI data processing with promising prospects.

Traditional methods using model-based assumptions (e.g., correlation analysis) are only able to detect activated regions that are consistent with the stimulus-based models being utilized, while disregarding the remaining regions. Therefore, the most obvious problem with model-driven methods is that they are unable to extract certain signals that are somewhat unrelated to the model, such as transient task-related components, quasi-periodic patterns, or sudden head movements, and since these signals are all considered noise in the model-based assumptions, they are completely excluded from the final results.

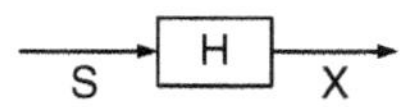

Fig. 3.4 Brief explanation of blind source separation (BSS): BSS uses only the output data (X) of a multi-channel system to determine its input function (S) and system transfer function (H)

By comparing ICA with a typical model-driven method (i.e., correlation analysis), we can see that ICA not only allows the discovery of consistently task-related areas of the brain, by identifying slightly larger regions that include the results of correlation analysis (i.e., left parieto-occipital junction and Brodmann areas 18 and 19), it also enables the detection of other task-related activated regions (i.e., PFC and temporal cortex).

3.2.2.6 Graph Theory Analysis

Many systems in nature are composed of highly interactive, dynamic subsystems. One approach to determine the global characteristics of these systems is to analyze them using network models, in which the dynamic subsystems are regarded as nodes, and the interactions between the subsystems are regarded as edges. Graph theory models are approximate descriptions of these systems. Unlike more traditional methods, network models ignore the structure and dynamic processes of the subsystems themselves, focusing instead on the interactions among the subsystems, and whether such interactions are present, while simultaneously ignoring the spatiotemporal changes of these interactions over time as well as other details.

Over the past decade, the most remarkable discovery in modern network theory has been the universality of network topology. More specifically, a surprising number of actual network systems, from cells to the Internet, have been shown to converge into similar structures that are unrelated to their age, mode, and size. It is precisely this universality that allows researchers from different disciplines to study network theory using a common paradigm. The topological similarities of network systems, a topic of high scientific import, have been corroborated beyond doubt in a wide range of scenarios, from molecular protein interactions to social networks and from the interconnected network of file links on the World Wide Web to the back-end hardware of the Internet. This solid foundation is derived not only from good structure charts and databases but also from the consistency between empirical data and model analyses that can predict network structure.

There is a consensus among numerous studies that the cerebral cortex is composed of neural clusters with local functional specificity, which interact dynamically and form different neural circuits depending on the cognitive activity being performed. A good equilibrium in brain function is achieved between widely-distributed regional functional specializations and interregional interactions, i.e., between functional segregation and integration. Furthermore, studies on neuroanatomy and electrophysiology have gathered a considerable amount of data on large-scale inter-cortical channels in the brain. However, the quantification and measurement of the overall characteristics of brain networks are still in their nascent stages, which necessitates the adoption of novel computational methods to analyze and examine the massive volume of information obtained on brain connectivity. Complex networks are a useful approach to address this issue, through which the brain activity recorded during cognitive tasks can be regarded as the result of interactions among different areas of the brain, which are regarded as nodes in a complex network, while the interactions and functional correlations between the different areas of the brain can be regarded as edges within the network. Based on this, the brain can be described using a model of the complex network, from which functional brain networks for different cognitive tasks can be established.

Neural networks are characterized by small-world network properties. Complex networks have been utilized to quantify the neural network of *Caenorhabditis elegans*, in which a directed network was established, with each neuron serving as a node and each synaptic connection an edge. These studies have found that the topological structure of this network is neither a random nor a regular network, but a small-world network. The whole brain can be segmented into 90 ROIs (45 in each hemisphere, covering the entire cerebral cortex), based on the brain structure, and the functional brain network can be constructed based on the degree of correlation between the

BOLD signals of any two brain regions in the resting state. Based on this network, we can analyze the network clustering coefficient and average shortest-path length, which will lead us to the following conclusion: the resting-state functional brain network is characterized by small-world network properties. Furthermore, cluster analysis has revealed that there are sub-networks within the functional brain network, with remote functional connectivity among the sub-networks.

3.2.2.7 Algorithms for State-Related fMRI Time-Series Analysis Based on Change-Point Theory

Current fMRI studies mostly utilize voxel-based GLM methods for analysis. This model is suitable for detecting whether the time-series changes of a given voxel can be explained by a set of regressors corresponding to different physiological stimuli. The application of this method is based on the premise of full compliance of the signal changes in the fMRI time-series with the prior conditions of the experimental design. However, for research areas such as the mechanisms of acupuncture, we do not know the precise prior conditions for the temporal changes in neural activations. This, therefore, necessitates new statistical models for the in-depth analysis of state-related changes in fMRI time-series, especially physiological states with unknown onset times, temporal intensity profiles, and end times. Such statistical models should be more data-driven, and enable us to estimate the timing and duration of state changes.

A method involving a previously published algorithm for state-related time-series analysis based on change-point theory that has previously been published in the literature has been derived from classic quality control theory (algorithm framework seen in Fig. 3.5), and is suitable for examining the neural response mechanisms of physiological and psychological processes with unknown dynamic functions. It has broad application prospects in the field of functional brain imaging, with the ability to analyze fMRI time-series, detect state changes, and estimate the timing and duration of these changes. As with other data-drive methods, this algorithm involves the construction of statistical models based on existing data. It is also semi-model-driven, incorporating the advantages of both model- and data-driven algorithms. Prior to analysis though, we must first specify the time period which corresponds to the baseline stage in which no activation is found in the fMRI time-series, following which a noise model is constructed based on the data from this baseline stage. The noise model is then used to determine whether the fMRI time-series in the

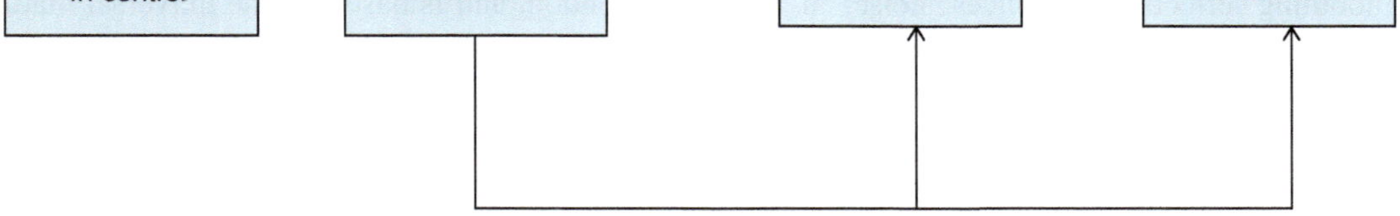

Fig. 3.5 Functional block diagram of algorithms for time-series analysis based on change-point theory: Algorithms for time-series analysis based on change-point theory divide the data from the time-series into baseline and change states, and based on the data characteristics of the baseline state, the corresponding time periods of the change states are obtained. Estimations of the onset times and durations of the change states are performed, which are then used to complete the feature extraction of the temporal patterns for the fMRI time-series

subsequent time periods deviates from the baseline state, i.e., the occurrence of state changes. As shown in Fig. 3.5, the algorithm divides the data from the time-series into baseline and change states. Based on the data characteristics of the baseline states, the corresponding time periods of the change states in the time-series are obtained. The onset times and durations of the change states are then estimated, which are used to complete the feature extraction of the temporal patterns for the fMRI time-series.

3.2.2.8 Algorithms for Multi-Voxel Pattern Analysis

One of the most challenging aspects of cognitive neuroscience is understanding how cognitive activity is reflected in the patterns of neural activation. Researchers have recently begun turning toward utilizing complex pattern recognition algorithms to analyze the multi-voxel distribution patterns of fMRI data, with the aim of decoding the information contained within the subject's brain at a given time point. Algorithms for multi-voxel pattern analysis provide a new means by which to gather this information.

Algorithms for multi-voxel pattern analysis are a type of data-driven method for fMRI data analysis, which can further validate fMRI research at the level of activation pattern analysis, rather than limiting it to the voxel level. This method is more focused on how to integrate information from multiple voxels, in order to enhance its ability to extract activated areas. It is worth noting, however, that in order to avoid signal loss, these algorithms generally do not include the spatial smoothing of voxel signals in the preprocessing stage of fMRI data. Although spatial smoothing effectively reduces noise, it also weakens two types of meaningful activation signals: the first includes signals that themselves contain information about the presence of stimuli, but have relatively weak activation intensity, while the second includes certain subtle textural features in the spatial patterns that have been blurred by spatial smoothing, which may diminish the amount of meaningful information that can be used to distinguish the activation patterns under different stimuli.

The choice of classifier is an integral step in the application of algorithms for multi-voxel pattern analysis, as the fundamental theories of machine learning have provided an extensive variety of classifier algorithms for multi-voxel pattern analysis. Linear classifiers are utilized in most cases, such as neural networks, linear discriminant analysis, and linear support-vector machines. These classifier algorithms all involve computing the weighted average of the grayscale values of the voxels, then inputting these weighted averages into a discriminant function, which determines the specific category to which a given voxel belongs based on an effective threshold. Some studies have also utilized non-linear classifiers. Although these classifiers are more powerful than linear classifiers with respect to the decision model for classification, studies on multi-voxel pattern analysis have not conclusively demonstrated that non-linear classifiers are more suitable than linear ones. Moreover, other studies have also shown that the precise results obtained by non-linear classifiers are more difficult to interpret than those obtained by linear vectors.

3.2.3 Software Related to BOLD Data Processing

3.2.3.1 SPM

SPM is currently the most widely used software for voxel-wise analysis. This software system was developed by Friston et al. at the University of London, and is based on the universal mathematical software package Matlab. It is equipped with powerful statistical functions, and the original purpose of this software package was to process fMRI, PET, and SPECT data using statistical methods. SPM is a free, open-source software package that runs on the Matlab platform, and was specifically designed to analyze

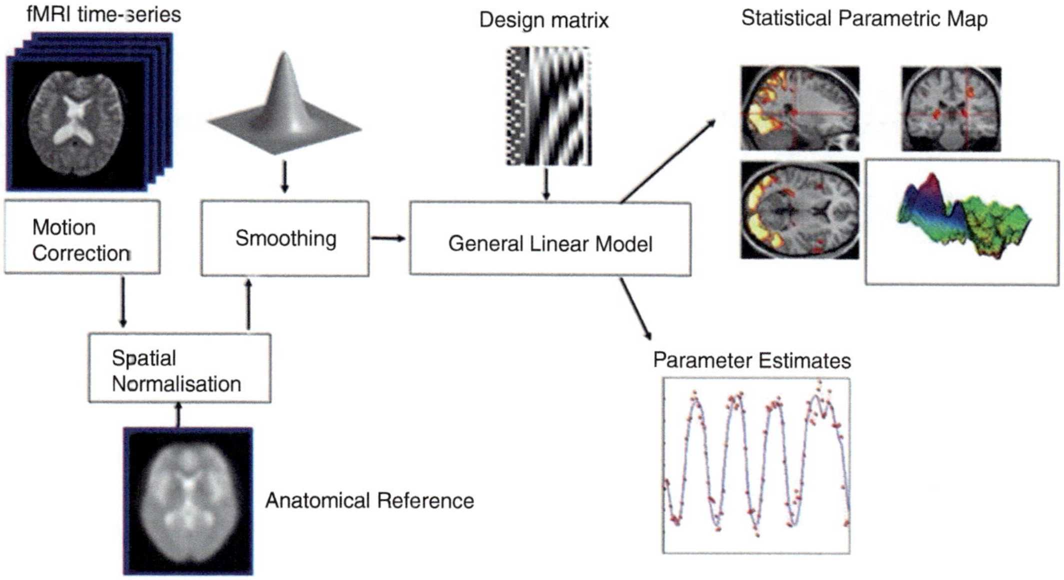

Fig. 3.6 General workflow for processing fMRI data in SPM: Motion correction, fusing the images from different imaging modalities, normalization of the images across different subjects, and spatial smoothing to enhance signal-to-noise ratio and eliminate subtle differences in brain structure

brain imaging data sequences. The data sequences can be a series of images from different groups or a time-series from the same subject. The current version was designed specifically for the analysis of fMRI, PET, SPECT, EEG, and MEG data.

Data processing and analysis in SPM are divided into two parts: pre-processing and statistical analysis. SPM is equipped with pre-processing functions for correction, smoothing, registration, and segmentation, as well as other functions for the statistical analysis and visualization of brain images. As functional brain imaging experiments require multiple subjects and measurements, one key issue to address is the fusion of experimental data for processing and analysis. First, we must perform the unification of the brain space, that is, the same voxels in the images obtained from multiple subjects and measurements should correspond to the same location in the brain space. Additionally, to enhance the data's signal-to-noise ratio and eliminate subtle differences in brain structure among different subjects, pre-processing should also be performed on the data prior to statistical analysis. Data pre-processing includes motion correction, fusing the images of different imaging modalities, normalization of the images across different subjects, and spatial smoothing to enhance signal-to-noise ratio and eliminate subtle differences in brain structure (Fig. 3.6).

3.2.3.2 Motion Correction

The diligent cooperation of subjects is needed when conducting fMRI studies, particularly with regards to keeping their body, and especially their heads, as still as possible, since experimental data with severe head motion must be discarded. Due to the long duration of functional imaging of the brain, head movements resulting from physiological factors such as breathing and blood flow pulsations are unavoidable. Therefore, to prevent deviations in the results, such motions can be effectively corrected through rotation, translation, and other methods.

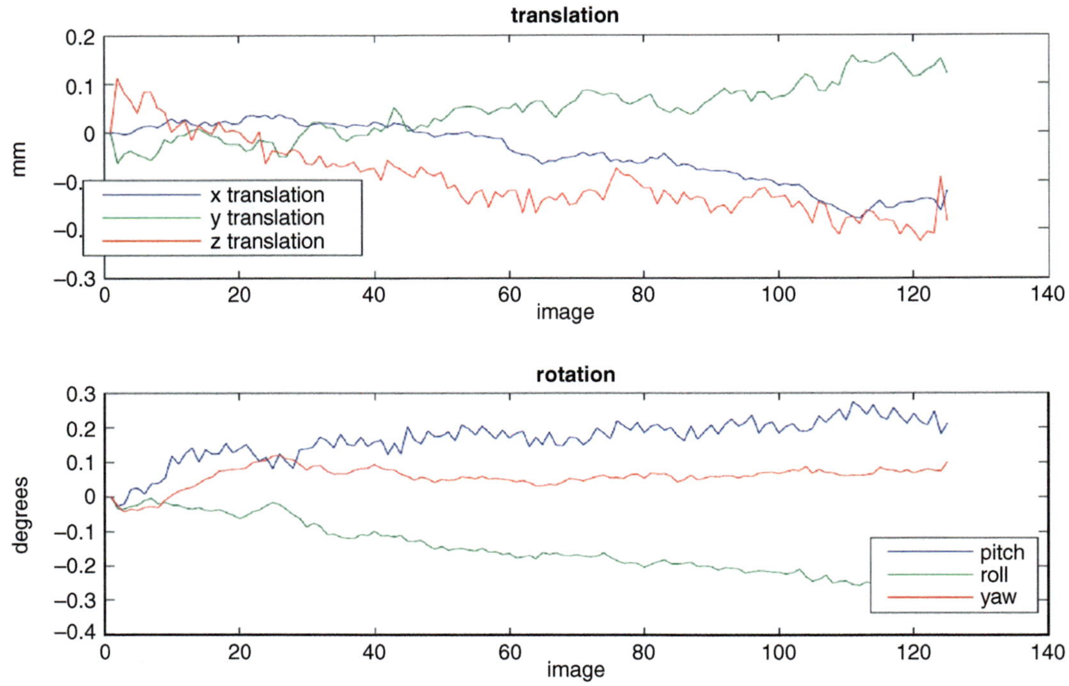

Fig. 3.7 Parameter diagram of rigid body motion: Translation refers to the translational motion of the subject's head in the *X*, *Y*, and *Z* directions, which are represented using red, green, and blue lines, respectively. Rotation refers to the rotational motion of the subject's head around the X, Y, and Z axes. The horizontal axis represents all images acquired in this series, while the vertical axis represents the offset and deflection angle in millimeters and degrees, respectively

When considered within the same subject, motion correction can be performed using rigid transformation (Fig. 3.7). For a given voxel with original coordinates (x, y, z), corrected coordinates (x', y', z'), rotational angle (ψ, φ, θ), and translation along the x-, y-, and z-axes of Δx, Δy, and Δz, the relationship between the original and corrected coordinates can be given by Eq. (3.29).

$$\begin{bmatrix} x' \\ y' \\ z' \\ 1 \end{bmatrix} = \begin{bmatrix} r_{11} & r_{12} & r_{13} & S_1 \\ r_{21} & r_{22} & r_{23} & S_2 \\ r_{31} & r_{32} & r_{33} & S_3 \\ 0 & 0 & 0 & 1 \end{bmatrix} \begin{bmatrix} x \\ y \\ z \\ 1 \end{bmatrix} = \begin{bmatrix} 1 & 0 & 0 & t_{x1} \\ 0 & \cos\Psi & -\sin\Psi & t_{x2} \\ 0 & \sin\Psi & \cos\Psi & t_{x3} \\ 0 & 0 & 0 & 1 \end{bmatrix} \begin{bmatrix} \cos\Phi & 0 & \sin\Phi & t_{y1} \\ 0 & 1 & 0 & t_{y2} \\ -\sin\Phi & 0 & \cos\Phi & t_{y3} \\ 0 & 0 & 0 & 1 \end{bmatrix} \begin{bmatrix} \cos\Theta & -\sin\Theta & 0 & t_{z1} \\ \sin\Theta & \cos\Theta & 0 & t_{z2} \\ 0 & 0 & 1 & t_{z3} \\ 0 & 0 & 0 & 1 \end{bmatrix} \begin{bmatrix} x \\ y \\ z \\ 1 \end{bmatrix}$$

$$= \begin{bmatrix} \cos\Phi\cos\Theta & -\cos\Phi\sin\Theta & \sin\Phi & S_1 \\ \sin\Psi\sin\Phi\cos\Psi + \cos\Psi\sin\Theta & -\sin\Psi\sin\Phi\sin\Theta + \cos\Psi\cos\Theta & -\sin\Psi\cos\Phi & S_2 \\ -\cos\Psi\sin\Phi\cos\Theta + \sin\Psi\sin\Theta & \cos\Psi\sin\Phi\sin\Theta + \sin\Psi\cos\Theta & \cos\Psi\cos\Phi & S_3 \\ 0 & 0 & 0 & 1 \end{bmatrix} \begin{bmatrix} x \\ y \\ z \\ 1 \end{bmatrix} \tag{3.29}$$

Calculating the parameters above allows us to correct the spatial location of functional data from the brain. There are a number of methods by which these parameters can be obtained, although the current methods of choice include the absolute value method of minimizing the grayscale values of the difference image and automatic image registration. The latter is typically utilized when using the SPM software.

Automatic image registration is based on the assumption that if the second image acquired using the same imaging technique is completely coincident with the first image, then the ratio of the corresponding grayscale values should equal to r for any given voxel. In other words, if the grayscale value of voxel i in the first image is a_i, and that of the second image is b_i, then when the two images are completely coincident, the ratio of the grayscale values $r_i = a_i/b_i$ should be consistent for all voxels. To this end, automatic image registration first involves calculating the ratio of the grayscale values for all corresponding voxels between the two images, and the optimal parameters can be determined when the variance of this ratio is minimized.

3.2.3.3 Image Registration

Owing to the individual differences in brain structure, rigid transformation is no longer applicable when performing the spatial unification of images acquired from different subjects using the same imaging method. Therefore, it is necessary to carry out an affine transformation with global swapping and local non-linear transformation to normalize the images onto a standard brain template. The SPM software uses the spatial transformation based on the brain atlas defined by Talairach and Tournoux.

The first step in image standardization is to perform an affine transformation with global swapping. The SPM software uses this method, followed by non-linear transformation, to remove minor local differences. The limitation of non-linear transformation is that is requires the warping function to be smooth. In SPM, a linear combination of predefined smooth spatial basis functions, such as a low-frequency 3D discrete cosine transform (DCT), is selected to satisfy this limitation. The specific procedure is as follows: after registering the original image to the shape of the template image using a 12-parameter affine transform, the local non-linearity is used to determine the parameters of the image and template; then, a linear combination of low-frequency basis functions is used to express non-linearity. The spatial transformation of coordinates x_i to coordinates y_i is given by:

$$y_{1i} = x_{1i} + u_{1i} = x_{1i} + \sum_j q_{j1} d_j\left(x_i\right)$$

$$y_{2i} = x_{2i} + u_{2i} = x_{2i} + \sum_j q_{j2} d_j\left(x_i\right)$$

$$y_{3i} = x_{3i} + u_3 = x_{3i} + \sum_j q_{j3} d_j\left(x_i\right) \quad (3.30)$$

where q^{jk} is the jth coefficient of the kth dimension, $d_j(x)$ is the jth bias function at location x.

3.2.3.4 Spatial Smoothing

Spatial smoothing involves deconvolving the data using a smooth function (usually a Gaussian function) in space, known as a convolution kernel function. Spatial smoothing performs a few functions. (1) It improves the signal-to-noise ratio: the neurophysiological signals detected by functional imaging of the brain originate from changes in cerebral blood flow at a scale of a few millimeters; therefore, image reconstruction corresponds to the component with the lowest spatial frequencies, whereas noise corresponds to the higher-frequency component. Thus, spatial smoothing ensures significant noise suppression. (2) It meets the requirements of a Gaussian random field, which is critical for statistical inferences based on Gaussian random field theory. This is because the theory requires: (a) the autocorrelation function to be twice differentiable, and (b) the spatial correlation to be stable. After spatial smoothing, i.e., after convolution with the Gaussian function, the data will roughly satisfy the two conditions of a Gaussian random field. (3) It eliminates minor variations in the brain structure of different subjects. As mentioned above, subtle variations will remain after performing image standardization to unify the brain maps of different subjects onto the standard brain map. However, for studies that require the average results across different subjects, these minor differences may have a serious impact on their findings. Hence, these differences are blurred after spatial smoothing.

A low-pass Gaussian filter is often applied to smooth functional images of the brain, the 2D Gaussian distribution function for which is given by the equation:

$$G(r) = \frac{1}{2\pi\sigma^2} e^{-\frac{r^2}{2\sigma^2}} \quad (3.31)$$

where i is the radius from the origin and σ is the standard deviation. Smoothing an image using a Gaussian filter eliminates all image structures small than σ.

3.2.3.5 FMRIB Software Library (FSL)

The FSL platform can be used for the pre-processing of fMRI data. FSL is a software library developed at the University of Oxford which contains tools for the comprehensive analysis of fMRI, T1 structural, and DTI data, mainly providing functions for data pre-processing, ICA-based analysis, and model-based task-related fMRI data analysis, among others. It runs on both Apple and PC (via virtual machines for Linux and Windows) computers, and is very easy to install. Most tools can be run from the command line or as graphical user interfaces (GUIs) as "point and click" functions.

The following tools are available in FSL:

1. fMRI: FEAT, MELODIC, FABBER, BASIL, and VERBENA
2. Structural MRI: BET, FAST, FIRST, FLIRT&FNIRT, FSLVBM, SIENA&SIENAX, and fsl_anat
3. Diffusion MRI: FDT, TBSS, EDDY, and TOPUP
4. GLM/Stats: GLM general advice, Randomize, Cluster, FDR, Dual Regression, Mm, and FLOBS
5. Others: FSLView, Fslutils, Atlases, Atlasquery, SUSAN, FUGUE, MCFLIRT, Miscvis, POSSUM, and BayCEST

Commonly used tools include FSL-BET (for skull stripping and brain surface extraction) and FSL-FAST (for brain tissue segmentation).

3.2.3.6 DPABI/Data Processing Assistant for Resting-State fMRI (DPARSF)

The DPABI computing platform is a key component of the Resting State-fMRI (R-fMRI) Maps Project (led by Yan Chao-Gan and his research team), part of the Human Brain Data Sharing Initiative launched by the Institute of Psychology at the Chinese Academy of Sciences. The goal of the R-fMRI Maps Project is to collate big data on intrinsic brain activity maps that encompass populations with a wide range of individual differences (including healthy individuals and individuals with various neurological and psychiatric diseases), so as to improve our understanding on the working mechanisms of the healthy human brain as well as the abnormal mechanisms of brain functions on the spectrum of different neurological and psychiatric diseases. Using the DPABI computing platform, this project undertakes the processing of public- and user-uploaded R-fMRI data in accordance with standard procedures, and the resulting brain activity indices are shared with researchers in the global scientific community, allowing the continuous accumulation of big data from intrinsic brain activity maps.

The DPABI computing platform incorporates DPARSF, an integrated data processing tool that encompasses the latest research advances in head motion control, noise suppression, data standardization, and other relevant aspects. This tool emphasizes test-retest reliability and quality control in the data processing of brain images and provides the corresponding computation modules. It can also serve as a user-friendly data processing pipeline tool for animal R-fMRI data (e.g., rats and non-human primates). In addition, this platform also includes modules for task-related data processing, structural morphometric analysis, statistical analysis, and result presentation. Therefore, it can reduce manual data processing, shorten processing time, decrease technical difficulties, minimize the probability of error, and ensure a greater comparability among the results of different studies.

3.2.3.7 Analysis of Functional NeuroImages (AFNI)

AFNI was originally developed at the Biophysics Research Institute of the Medical College of Wisconsin, primarily by Professor Cox, and is an interactive software for the analysis of functional brain imaging data. It allows researchers to overlay the experimental results of low-resolution functional imaging data onto high-resolution structural images for 3D visualization. By selecting specific data points, the software can convert experimental data into 3D localization coordinates. Furthermore, AFNI can simultaneously display the 2D images from the three orthogonal planes, allowing the user to switch views between the various functional and anatomical data. Its add-on program package also enables users to operate and fuse 3D image datasets.

AFNI version 1.0 was released in 1995, and later evolved to AFNI version 2.01 in February 1997, and a new version will be released in the near future. There are currently more than 100 organizations globally that are registered to use AFNI. Although AFNI is free for non-commercial research purposes, permission must be obtained from the Medical College of Wisconsin for clinical and commercial use.

AFNI runs in the UNIX workstation environment, and the operating system must have more than 32 MB of RAM, the X11R5 Window System, Motif1.2 toolbox, ANSIC compiler, and sufficient hard disk space for data storage. At present, AFNI cannot run on the Microsoft Windows or Apple Macintosh platforms.

3.2.3.8 FreeSurfer

FreeSurfer is a software package for the analysis and visualization of structural and functional neuroimaging data from cross-sectional or longitudinal studies. It provides a complete processing stream for structural MRI data, including the following functions: skull stripping, B1 bias field correction, GM-WM segmentation, reconstruction of cortical surface models (GM-WM boundary surface and pial surface), labeling of regions on the cortical surface and subcortical structures, non-linear registration of an individual's cortical surface onto a stereotaxic atlas, and statistical analysis of group morphometric differences.

3.3 Research Applications of BOLD Imaging in Neuroscience

Owing to the ongoing advancement of imaging modalities, it is now possible to provide extensive descriptions for the complex paradigms of the human brain. fMRI is a newer imaging technique that is based on BOLD signals. This non-invasive, exploratory method has enabled us to measure each individual response of the brain in a relatively direct manner, so as to obtain an overview of a complete brain network, and examine its cognitive mechanisms. Compared with other functional imaging techniques, BOLD-fMRI has a relatively high spatial and temporal resolution, which allows us to track time courses and describe functional brain processes in detail.

3.3.1 Research Applications of BOLD-fMRI in Perceptual Mechanisms

An individual's neurophysiological response to stimuli in the environment is known as perception. Perception occurs through sensory organs, and is commonly referred to as the "senses," which include hearing, sight, taste, smell, and touch. The process of perception involves the detection and recognition of stimuli. It begins when an object in the real world stimulates a sensory organ, for example, when light is reflected off the surface of an object and stimulates the eyes, or when a hot beverage stimulates the sense of touch. These stimuli are then converted into neurogenic energy and transmitted to the cerebral cortex.

BOLD-fMRI is a valuable method for studying perception, as it can acquire functional (dynamic, time-variant) information that occurs simultaneously with the (intracerebral) signal sources. The images generated when the subject is in a given cognitive state can be directly compared with the images generated when they are in a different cognitive state. Based on this, the changes in image intensity and differences in cognitive states can provide information about the potential changes in the physiological state and neuronal activity of the relevant brain tissues.

3.3.1.1 Audition

Of all the human senses, auditory stimulation is the most continuous and persistent. In the last thirty years, fMRI has been extensively utilized in the field of auditory neuroscience. The key contribution of early fMRI studies was the emphasis of the distributed and parallel processing of language in the human brain. These early studies showed that the classic model, which favors a serial processing stream, cannot fully capture the complex processing structure of the brain. Aside from the number of streams involved in the processing of complex sounds, fMRI studies have also further explored the strict lateralization model of language processing, and stressed the bilateral activation of language stimuli in different populations. In addition to helping us understand the fundamentals of how the healthy brain processes language-related information, fMRI also provides information on changes in language perception within the context of nervous system disorders. In the clinical setting, auditory studies conducted using fMRI can illustrate the possible consequences of resecting or damaging the auditory cortex and surrounding regions of the brain during neurosurgery. Furthermore, fMRI studies on individuals who are deaf or who use hearing aids have demonstrated the remarkable plasticity of the cerebral cortex among congenitally deaf patients who use cochlear implants, thus providing crucial neurological evidence for clinical treatment. In summary, fMRI has substantial scientific and clinical potential in the field of auditory perception.

3.3.1.2 Vision

Human visual perception is derived from the sensory system that includes retinal photoreceptor cells and the thalamus, among others. The cortical regions primarily involved in visual processing are the occipital lobe and its adjacent temporal and parietal lobes, with cortical and subcortical pathways interconnecting the visual cortex. Clinically, fMRI can be used to plan surgical procedures involving the central visual pathway, thus facilitating pre-operative surgical planning and surgical guidance. With the aid of fMRI-acquired activation maps related to the visual cortex, neurosurgeons can plan the optimal resection method and scope, thereby maximizing the success of treatment while preventing damage to the visual cortex. In the clinical setting, therefore, fMRI can provide key information for the planning of neurosurgery in patients with lesions in the occipital, temporal, and parietal visual cortices.

3.3.1.3 Pain

As individuals interact with the environment, their brains receive incoming information from the activation of cutaneous receptors. In a pain study that recruited a group of veterans with chronic pain, task-related fMRI with quantitative sensory testing was performed to assess brain activation in response to noxious and non-noxious heat stimuli. The results of the study revealed strong activation in the thalamus and cerebellum in response to noxious heat stimuli, which indicated specific changes in brain function when subjects experienced pain. Another study on physical and emotional pain stimuli discovered the synchronous activation of the subgenual cingulate cortex when subjects were presented with the both stimuli. These results implied that experiencing an event that poses a major threat to social relations will activate the pain-related networks in the brain. In a clinical study on autism, alterations in cutaneous perception under synchronized stimulation were measured in autistic patients. The results of that study revealed local functional disconnections when compared to healthy controls, thus providing crucial information for clinical interventions in autistic patients. Whether in social psychology research or clinical research, fMRI has provided valuable insights into the neural and underlying genetic basis of perception.

The application of BOLD-fMRI in neuropsychology and clinical medicine has deepened our understanding of perception, enabling us to grasp the interactions of perception with cognition and diseases, thereby providing new ideas for further exploration of physiological function and clinical research.

3.3.2 Research Applications of BOLD-fMRI in the Mechanisms of Working Memory

The ability to retain and manipulate information even in the absence of external stimuli is a prerequisite for goal-oriented interactions between humans and the external environment. This ability, known as working memory, is a core concept in cognitive psychology and neuroscience that is closely related to clinical, intelligence, and neuroscience research.

The results of BOLD-fMRI studies have indicated that working memory has a specific activation pattern in the brain, which primarily includes the frontal and parietal cortices. The coordination between these regions forms the neural basis of working memory. Furthermore, studies in cognitive psychology and neuroscience have shown that working memory training and ability can affect BOLD activity in the related brain areas. These results imply that the increase and decrease of BOLD signals can reflect information about stimuli related to working memory, indicating its excitatory and inhibitory responses to working memory stimuli. In summary, improvements in working memory are related to changes in fMRI activation patterns.

Functional connectivity is a relatively new computational method for studying brain networks. Apart from seed-based functional connectivity analysis and multivariate statistics of connectivity data, this field also includes the extraction of functional connectivity features at the whole-brain level based on graph theory. Task-related functional connectivity analysis has demonstrated that brain areas activated by working memory-related tasks form a functionally connected network. Thus, the involvement of this working memory-related network in working memory tasks can be used to identify individual differences, as well as facilitate clinical diagnoses and treatment. Resting-state fMRI has been widely adopted in the study of functional connectivity. Typically, the acquisition of resting-state fMRI data does not require subjects to perform specific tasks. Nevertheless, even in the absence of task constraints, there is still a high degree of stability in functional brain connectivity. The importance of the PFC in working memory has been verified by resting-state fMRI studies on monkeys, in which researchers found that lesions in the dorsolateral PFC severely impaired the monkeys' working memory. Furthermore, by performing and evaluating resting-state fMRI scans, Owen et al. further confirmed the role of the lateral PFC in maintaining working memory.

The applications of fMRI in working memory have gradually expanded into the field of neurophysiology. A previous fMRI study demonstrated that stress-induced short-term deficits in working memory are related to the decreased PFC activation. The study also found, using fMRI, that medical students exposed to exam stress exhibited weaker functional connectivity in the PFC. In addition, another study found that alcoholism can cause brain damage and working memory deficits. The imaging findings of that study showed that when executing working memory tasks, alcoholic subjects exhibited alterations in the BOLD activation patterns of the relevant brain regions. Moreover, the study also found significant deficits in the working memory of alcohol-dependent young women, with negative brain activations in the parietal and frontal cortices. When compared with male subjects, female subjects performed better at verbal working memory tasks after consuming alcohol but worse at spatial working memory tasks.

Working memory research based on BOLD-fMRI has also been extended into neurological and psychiatric diseases, such as Alzheimer's disease (AD), where it has provided robust evidence for early diagnosis. Working memory is a key aspect that affects patients with early-stage AD, and previous fMRI studies have reported alterations in brain activation elicited by working memory tasks. These alterations can be used to distinguish between the brain activation patterns of patients with AD and those with mild cognitive impairment (MCI), thus enabling us to differentiate between the two conditions and improve our understanding of neural connections in memory impairments.

By combining the applications of BOLD-fMRI in neuroscience and clinical practice, we will gain a more profound understanding of the relationships between working memory and disease, thereby providing new ideas for future investigations on cognitive function and clinical research.

3.3.3 Research Applications of BOLD-fMRI in the Mechanism of Executive Function

In the past decade, there has been keen interest on executive function in the clinical and scientific fields. Executive function is an important cognitive process that is generally considered to encompass a broad cognitive domain, as it is a type of "high-level" cognitive function with a "supervisory" role. Executive function can control and coordinate other more basic cognitive functions, such as language, memory, and visuospatial processing. Miyake et al. conceptualized executive function as "general-purpose control mechanisms that modulate the operation of various cognitive subprocesses and thereby regulate the dynamics of human cognition." Therefore, executive function is not a single brain function, but rather it encompasses the ability to plan, initialize, organize, and supervise complex goal-oriented behaviors.

Neuroimaging is an effective means by which to comprehend the neural structure and function of cognitive processes; therefore, a wealth of groundbreaking studies have been conducted on executive functions using neuroimaging techniques. BOLD-fMRI can display the physiological and metabolic activation of brain regions during executive function tasks, and has been widely used in this field. Nowrangi et al. stated in a review on neuroimaging and executive function that the frontal, parietal, and cerebellar regions of the brain were consistently associated with executive functions across a variety of neurological and psychiatric disorders. A meta-analysis by Rottschy et al. confirmed this finding, as their results demonstrated the correlation mentioned above occurring among the activated regions on fMRI during working memory tasks. These results suggest that there is a distribution network in the brain that involves executive function. Additionally, relevant fMRI studies have also found that impairment in executive function tasks is caused by damage to the ventromedial and/or dorsolateral PFCs. Therefore, the cognitive processes of executive function spans multiple cortical regions, which are connected to the frontal lobe via afferent and efferent projections, and interact with each other, implying that the implementation of executive function tasks requires the participation of multiple regions of the brain.

In recent years, a number of studies have confirmed the occurrence of executive function impairment in various neurological and psychiatric diseases. Aging involves fundamental changes in multiple domains of brain function, and although the decline of memory and sensory abilities is inevitable, fMRI studies have shown that the reduced functional connectivity of the frontal cortex among the elderly is significantly associated with the decrease in executive function. Furthermore, fMRI studies on other neurological disease, including neurodegenerative diseases, TBI and vascular diseases, have also found strong evidence supporting the correlation of frontal and parietal lobe damage with executive function deficit. As for psychiatric diseases, such as schizophrenia and depression, fMRI studies have demonstrated a significant correlation between brain activation and executive function during the course of these diseases.

In summary, changes in executive function have significant implications for the clinical diagnosis and treatment of neurodegenerative diseases. As a non-invasive technique, fMRI can help us to identify more specific functional areas within large-scale brain networks, which will facilitate the formulation of better diagnostic, treatment, and management strategies.

3.3.4 Research Applications of BOLD-fMRI in the Mechanisms of Language

Language processing requires the coordination of multiple regions of the brain and involves multiple steps such as the input, integration, comprehension, and expression of information. Task-based BOLD-fMRI is currently widely used in the study of pre-operative functional language localization and lateralization. During task-based BOLD-fMRI, subjects are instructed to perform certain tasks related to language processing, which stimulate their neuronal activity and cause hemodynamic changes in the brain. The resulting changes in deoxyhemoglobin levels indirectly reflect the activated areas related to language processing. Language paradigms adopted in task-based BOLD-fMRI can be divided according to the steps of language processing into three categories: language reception, semantics, and production.

Language reception paradigms aim to activate the cortical regions associated with language comprehension, including reading and listening comprehension tasks. In fMRI-based language reception tasks, the primary activated region is Wernicke's area (which includes the superior temporal, middle temporal, supramarginal, and angular gyri), but activation can also be detected in the fusiform gyrus and parietal areas. In fMRI-based semantic tasks, the primary activated regions include the inferior frontal gyrus, inferior temporal gyrus, and inferior parietal lobule. As for fMRI-based language production tasks, the supplementary motor and frontal areas are activated, including Broca's area (pars opercularis, pars triangularis, and pars orbitalis of the left inferior frontal gyrus) and the precentral, superior frontal, and middle frontal gyri.

Task-based BOLD-fMRI primarily involves the localization and lateralization of language areas, whereas resting-state fMRI reveals the functional architecture of language networks. For example, Hampson et al. found that during the resting conditions, subjects exhibited significant functional connectivity between Broca's area with the left angular gyrus and left occipito-temporal junction, while the strength of this functional connectivity was positively correlated with the subject's reading ability. Thus, these findings have demonstrated the functional significance of specific language networks of the brain in language processing. Other researchers have also performed resting-state fMRI with Broca's and Wernicke's areas as seed regions to explore language networks. Their findings revealed the presence of significant functional connectivity among the left fusiform gyrus, left temporo-parietal junction, left precentral gyrus, and left inferior occipital gyrus, as well as a significant correlation between reading ability and the functional connectivity of language networks. Furthermore, when compared with children, adults exhibited a more significant positive correlation between their reading ability and strength of functional connectivity among the left fusiform gyrus, inferior parietal lobule and Broca's area, as well as a more significant negative correlation between their reading ability and strength of functional connectivity between the left fusiform gyrus and the default state network. Therefore, this study has further elucidated the relationship between the resting-state language network and reading ability.

3.3.5 Research Applications of BOLD-fMRI in the Mechanisms of Attention

Attention is a high-level cognitive function in humans that refers to the process of orienting and concentrating one's consciousness toward specific external information. From a functional and anatomical perspective, Posner and Petersen divided the attention network into three relatively independent sub-networks, which can be used to describe the operational modes of the human attention system. The sub-networks proposed in this theoretical model include the alerting, orienting, and executive control networks.

The alerting network serves to elicit and sustain persistent attention toward emerging stimuli, and is characterized by high arousal and alertness. For example, it is involved in switching from the drowsiness of sleep to a state of readiness for dealing with unexpected events. The alerting network is mainly measured using vigilance tasks, in which a cue is presented before the target stimulus in order to signal the appearance of the target, and subjects are required to respond as quickly and accurately as possible when the target is presented. Studies have shown that the brain regions activated during vigilance tasks primarily include the frontal lobe, thalamus, and parts of the parietal lobe. These regions are relatively distributed, and the thalamus is also closely associated with the maintenance of vigilance. Additionally, some researchers have proposed that the posterior parietal cortex (PPC) is also involved in alertness.

The orienting network is involved in selecting specific information from a large stream of input stimuli. Attention orientation consists of three basic processes: disengagement, shift, and re-engagement. More specifically, it involves disengaging attention from the current point of focus, shifting the attention to a new target or channel, and then engaging the attention on the new target or channel. Studies on attention orientation often employ tasks where the subject's attention is guided toward a spatial cue before the target stimulus is presented, and then requires the subject to respond to the location of the target. Visual attention orientation is primarily related to the parietal lobe (superior and inferior parietal lobules), pars orbitalis of the inferior frontal gyrus, and certain subcortical areas (superior colliculus, thalamic reticular nucleus, etc.). Some studies have also demonstrated the involvement of the cerebellum in spatial attention orientation.

The executive control network is primarily responsible for supervising and resolving conflicts among expectations, stimuli, and responses; therefore, it is generally measured using tasks involving conflicts among different stimuli or responses. A classic example is the Stroop task, in which subjects are required to respond to the color dimension of the stimulus, while ignoring interference arising from conflict with its semantic dimension. BOLD-fMRI results indicate that the Stroop task can activate the dorsolateral PFC and posterior cingulate gyrus. Another task that is frequently used is the lateral inhibition task, in which the target is presented with two flanking distractors, and the subject is required to ignore the effects of the distractors while responding only to the target. Studies have shown that executive control is primarily associated with the anterior cingulate cortex and lateral PFC. Other studies have also found that it may be related to the cerebellum.

Attention is the regulatory mechanism for all cognitive activity in humans, and patients with cognitive impairments have been found to exhibit varying extents of attention deficits, as seen, for example, in the most common neurodevelopmental disorder in childhood—attention deficit hyperactivity disorder (ADHD). In China, the incidence of ADHD among school-age children is about 3–10%, and its main symptoms include hyperactivity, impulsivity, and deficits in attention. A task-based BOLD-fMRI study on ADHD found that the severity of behavioral symptoms during cognitive shifting tasks was negatively correlated with the activation intensity of the striatum, parietal lobe, cerebellum, and other regions of the brain. Using resting-state fMRI, children with ADHD were found to have reduced amplitude of low-frequency fluctuations (ALFFs) in the right inferior frontal gyrus, left sensorimotor cortex, and bilateral cerebellum, as well as increased ALFFs in the right anterior cingulate gyrus, when compared with healthy children. The results of functional connectivity among different regions of the brain have also confirmed that patients with ADHD have stronger connectivity among the anterior cingulate gyrus, pons, insula, cerebellum, and thalamus, as well as weaker connectivity among the putamen, posterior parietal lobe, and superior parietal lobe. Furthermore, they exhibit functional abnormalities in the cortical-striatal-thalamic circuit and the default mode network, as well as altered node efficiency in the prefrontal, temporal, and occipital lobes. Additionally, when performing neuropsychological tasks, ADHD patients often exhibit higher rates of response error, longer response time, and greater response variability. The dysfunction in these areas of the brain and the impairments in their associated high-level cognitive neural circuits may form the neural basis for behavioral abnormalities in ADHD. This also highlights the critical role of attention networks in the cognitive activities of ADHD.

3.3.6 Research Applications of BOLD-fMRI in the Mechanisms of Numerical Cognition

Numerical cognition is a high-level cognitive activity of the human brain. It is a form of abstract thinking and occupies an important position in the cognitive function of the brain. The abilities and processes involved in numerical cognition have always been a topic of concern in the fields of psychology, cognitive science, neuroscience, and pedagogy, among others. With ongoing advances in imaging technology, brain fMRI can be used to effectively evaluate cortical activity, determine the brain areas involved in specific cognitive functions, and uncover the connections between functional areas. Thus, it is an important research method that has been rapidly utilized in all domains of cognitive neuroscience.

In 1999, Dehaene et al. proposed the Triple Code Model, which posits that numerical cognition is composed of three functional modules, which are based on different representational codes for numbers with corresponding channels among them modules to facilitate switching between cognitive functions. In 2004, Ryuta et al. compared the activated brain areas between adults and children when performing simple arithmetic of single digits. Their results indicated that the activation of the right frontal cortex was detected during addition and multiplication tasks in the adult group but not in the children group, and activation was observed in the intraparietal cortex of the adult group during each task. Moreover, despite the slight differences in activation patterns during the different tasks and between the different groups, only a small number of areas showed statistically significant differences. Therefore, the activation patterns for simple arithmetic operations are similar between the two groups, and do not differ significantly. Wang et al. studied the effects of abacus-based mental calculation training on visuospatial working memory and its neural correlates in 67 boys. They found that the training group showed greater activation than the control group in the frontal, parietal, and occipital regions, which implied that the frontal region may be the neural basis for the transfer effects of abacus-based mental calculation training to visuospatial working memory. In a study by Wood et al., the number bisection task activated the bilateral frontoparietal network, including the intraparietal cortex, supplementary motor area, and dorsolateral and ventrolateral PFCs. In another task-based fMRI study, 28 healthy volunteers were asked to perform training tasks for number and physical line bisection (the respective baselines were also measured), and whole-brain analysis revealed that both types of bisection tasks shared neural connections in the bilateral parietal and frontal regions. Furthermore, compared to the physical line bisection task, the number bisection task elicited stronger activation in the bilateral parietal region, right cerebellum, left insula, and left supplementary motor area.

The application of fMRI has provided a new approach for studying numerical cognition, which has not only corroborated previous findings in neuropsychological and behavioral research, but also provided new discoveries. Although cognitive science is an extremely complex field with numerous aspects that remain poorly understood, ongoing advances in imaging technology, including fMRI, will continue to deepen our understanding of the mechanisms underlying numerical cognition, and provide key technological support for clinical research.

Suggested Readings

Benjamin CF, Walshaw PD, Hale K, et al. Presurgical language fMRI: mapping of six critical regions. Hum Brain Mapp. 2017;38:4239–55.

Benjamin CFA, Li AX, Blumenfeld H, et al. Presurgical language fMRI: clinical practices and patient outcomes in epilepsy surgical planning. Hum Brain Mapp. 2018;39(7):2777–85.

Cao X, Cao Q, Long X, et al. Abnormal resting-state functional connectivity patterns of the putamen in medication-naive children with attention deficit hyperactivity disorder. Brain Res. 2009;1303:195–206.

Cordes D, Haughton VM, Arfanakis K, et al. Mapping functionally related regions of brain with functional connectivity MR imaging. AJNR Am J Neuroradiol. 2000;21(9):1636–44.

Dardo T, Volkow ND. Abnormal Functional connectivity in children with attention-deficit/hyperactivity disorder. Biol Psychiatry. 2012;71(5):443–50.

Dehaene S, Spelke E, Pinal P, et al. Sources of mathematical thinking: behavioral and brain-imaging evidence. Science. 1999;284(5416):970–4.

Dronkers NF, Plaisant O, Iba-Zizen MT, et al. Paul Broca's historic cases: high resolution MR imaging of the brains of Leborgne and Lelong. Brain. 2007;130(5):1432–41.

Fan J, Flombaum JI, Mccandliss BD, et al. Cognitive and brain consequences of conflict. Neuroimage. 2003;18(1):42–57.

Fox MD, Snyder AZ, Vincent JL, et al. The human brain is intrinsically organized into dynamic, anticorrelated functional networks. Proc Natl Acad Sci U S A. 2005;102:9673–8.

Friston KJ. Functional and effective connectivity: a review. Brain Connect. 2011;1(1):13–36.

Hampson M, Tokoglu F, Sun Z, et al. Connectivity-behavior analysis reveals that functional connectivity between left BA39 and Broca's area varies with reading ability. Neuroimage. 2006;31(2):513–9.

Lindquist MA, Waugh C, Wager TD. Modeling state-related fMRI activity using change-point theory. Neuroimage. 2007;35(3):1125–41.

Logothetis NK, Pauls J, Augath M, et al. Neurophysiological investigation of the basis of the fMRI signal. Nature. 2001;412(6843):150–7.

Lowe MJ, Mock BJ, Sorenson JA. Functional connectivity in single and multislice echoplanar imaging using resting-state fluctuations. Neuroimage. 1998;7(2):119–32.

MacDonald AW, Cohen JD, Stenger VA, et al. Dissociating the role of the dorsolateral prefrontal and anterior cingulate cortex in cognitive control. Science. 2000;288(5472):1835–8.

Miyake A, Friedman NP, Emerson MJ, et al. The unity and diversity of executive functions and their contributions to complex "Frontal Lobe" tasks: a latent variable analysis. Cogn Psychol. 2000;41(1):49–100.

Nowrangi MA, Lyketsos C, Rao V, et al. Systematic review of neuroimaging correlates of executive functioning: Converging evidence from different clinical populations. J Neuropsychiatry Clin Neurosci. 2014;26(2):114–25.

Owen AM, McMillan KM, Laird AR, et al. N-back working memory paradigm: a meta-analysis of normative functional neuroimaging studies. Hum Brain Mapp. 2005;25(1):46–59.

Posner MI, Petersen SE. The attention system of the human brain. Annu Rev Neurosci. 1990;13:25–42.

Quigley M, Cordes D, Turski P, et al. Role of the corpus callosum in functional connectivity. AJNR Am J Neuroradiol. 2003;24(2):208–12.

Rottschy C, Langner R, Dogan I, et al. Modelling neural correlates of working memory: a coordinate-based meta-analysis. Neuroimage. 2012;60(1):830–46.

Ryuta K, Masato T, Katsuo O, et al. A functional MRI study of simple arithmetic-a comparison between children and adults. Brain Res Cogn Brain Res. 2004;18(3):225–31.

Smith K. Traumatic brain injury: CT scan does not predict outcome of mild traumatic brain injury. Nat Rev Neurol. 2012;8(9):474.

Smits M, Dippel DWJ, Houston GC, et al. Postconcussion syndrome after minor head injury: Brain activation of working memory and attention. Hum Brain Mapp. 2009;30(9):2789–803.

Sporns O, Chialvo DR, Kaiser M, et al. Organization, development and function of complex brain networks. Trends Cogn Sci. 2004;8(9):418–25.

Wang C, Xu T, Geng F, et al. Training on abacus-based mental calculation enhances visuospatial working memory in children. J Neurosci. 2019;39(33):6439–48.

Wood G, Nuerk H, Moeller K, et al. All for one but not one for all: how multiple number representations are recruited in one numerical task. Brain Res. 2008;1187:154–66.

Wu CY, Ho MR, Chen SH. A meta-analysis of fMRI studies on Chinese orthographic, phonological, and semantic processing. Neuroimage. 2012;63(1):381–91.

Xydakis MS, GSF L, Mulligan LP, et al. Epidemiologic aspects of traumatic brain injury in acute combat casualties at a major military medical center: a cohort study. Ann Neurol. 2012;72(5):673–81.

Zhang Q, Luo Y. Functional brain imaging of mathematical cognition. Chin J Med Imag Technol. 2004;20(10):1607–9.

Zhou Y, Liang M, Jiang TZ, et al. Functional dysconnectivity of the dorsolateral prefrontal cortex in first-episode schizophrenia using resting-state fMRI. Neurosci Lett. 2007;417(3):297–302.

4 Research Applications of Cerebral Perfusion Magnetic Resonance Imaging (MRI) in Neuroscience

Fan Yu, Chunxue Wu, Yayan Yin, Xia Wei, Xiyue Yang, Su Lui, and Jie Lu

4.1 Principles of Perfusion MRI

4.1.1 Overview of Perfusion MRI

Perfusion refers to the flow of blood through the capillary network, which enables the transport of oxygen, nutrients, and waste to or from the tissues surrounding each capillary bed. Cerebral perfusion is the process by which blood transports oxygen and nutrients to the brain tissues, where they are utilized for various functions. This process is generally considered equivalent to the blood flow process in the brain. Cerebral perfusion imaging can provide information on cerebral hemodynamics at the level of the microvasculature and is therefore a valuable approach for identifying and monitoring the pathophysiological processes of neurological diseases. Perfusion MRI has been widely used for the evaluation of tumors, cerebrovascular diseases, and neurodegenerative diseases. Compared to nuclear medicine and computed tomography (CT) perfusion imaging studies, the greatest advantage of perfusion MRI is the absence of ionizing radiation, which allows repeat examinations within a short period of time without exposing patients to multiple doses of radiation. Current perfusion MRI techniques can be divided into two categories, based on the type of contrast agent used: (1) techniques involving the intravenous (IV) injection of an exogenous, non-diffusible contrast agent—gadopentetate dimeglumine—to induce dynamic changes in MRI signal intensity that are recorded and analyzed to obtain cerebral perfusion parameters, such as dynamic susceptibility contrast (DSC) and dynamic contrast-enhanced (DCE) imaging; and (2) techniques involving the use of water in the human body as an endogenous, diffusible contrast agent to perform imaging and obtain cerebral perfusion parameters, such as arterial spin labelling (ASL).

4.1.2 Principles of DSC Imaging

DSC MRI can create an image of cerebral perfusion by recording the dynamic changes of signal intensities in T_2 or T_2* sequences; it is based on the first-pass effect of the contrast agent. This technique involves a short scan time and has broad clinical applications. Gadolinium-based contrast agents are paramagnetic; therefore, the IV injection of gadopentetate dimeglumine

F. Yu · C. Wu · Y. Yin · J. Lu (✉)
Department of Radiology and Nuclear Medicine, Xuanwu Hospital, Capital Medical University, Beijing, China

X. Wei · X. Yang · S. Lui (✉)
Department of Radiology, Huaxi MR Research Center (HMRRC), West China Hospital of Sichuan University, Cheng du, China

J. Lu, G. Zhao (eds.), *PET/MR: Functional and Molecular Imaging of Neurological Diseases and Neurosciences*, https://doi.org/10.1007/978-981-19-9902-4_4

induces local changes in magnetic susceptibility differences, which in turn leads to transient changes in the magnetic field and shortening the T_2 or T_2* relaxation time of the surrounding tissues, consequently causing transient attenuation or loss of signal. These transient and minute changes can be measured based on the signal changes in MR images. The rapid imaging sequences used in DSC, such as single-shot echo planar imaging (EPI), in which data is acquired once every 1–2 s, have high temporal resolution, and can therefore accurately measure the changes in the T_2 or T_2* signal intensities. The sequences most frequently utilized in DSC MRI include spin-echo EPI (SE-EPI) and gradient-echo EPI (GRE-EPI), in which time-signal intensity curves are generated based on T_2- or T_2*-weighted images, respectively, and then converted into time-concentration curves for subsequent model computations. A key premise in DSC imaging is the basic assumption of an intact blood-brain barrier. This enables the gadolinium-based contrast agent, which has a relatively large molecular weight, to be retained within the blood vessels during the first pass, which is the basis for susceptibility-induced contrast.

4.1.3 Principles of DCE Imaging

DCE perfusion imaging requires the injection of an exogenous gadolinium-based contrast agent. The difference between DSC and DCE is that DCE exploits the ability of the paramagnetic contrast agent to shorten the T_1 relaxation time of the surrounding tissues, which induces a transient increase in signal intensity. Therefore, the dynamic acquisition of time-signal intensity curves can be combined with pharmacokinetic modeling to obtain the quantitative perfusion parameters. For this reason, DCE is also known as "T_1 perfusion" or "permeability MRI."

From a physiological perspective, injecting a bolus of a paramagnetic contrast agent leads to the rapid increase in its plasma concentration. At the same time, some of the contrast agent will penetrate the vascular wall as it flows through the vessel and permeates the surrounding interstitial space, causing an increase in the amount of contrast in the surrounding tissues and subsequent gradual decline in the plasma concentration (due to extravasation). The recirculation of the intravascular contrast agent is also involved in this process (Fig. 4.1). By converting the DCE time-signal intensity curves into time-contrast agent

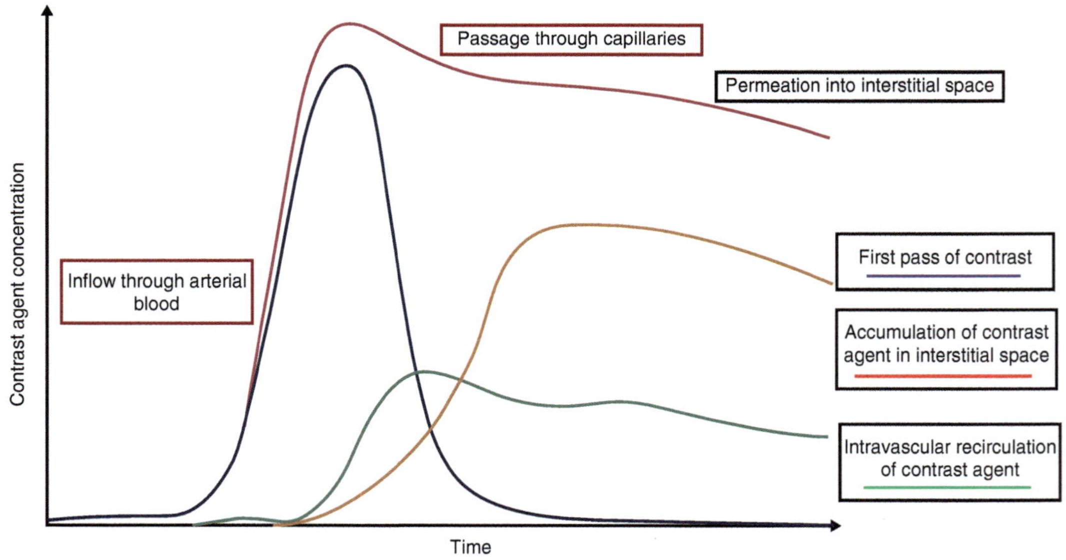

Fig. 4.1 Time-contrast agent concentration curves: The blue line represents the plasma concentration of the contrast agent; the orange line represents concentration of the contrast agent in the interstitial space; the green line represents the intravascular recirculation of the contrast agent; and the red line represents the final intracerebral concentration of the contrast agent

concentration curves, we can observe the comprehensive effects of the extravasation and recirculation of the intravascular contrast agent, as well as the accumulation and removal of contrast agent in tissues, thus reflecting the process of contrast agent extravasation from blood vessels to the interstitial space over time.

The pharmacokinetic models commonly used in DCE imaging can be divided into two major categories: compartmental models and spatial distribution models. The former include the Tofts, Brix, and Larsson models, while the latter include the tissue homogeneity (TH) and adiabatic approximation of TH (AATH) models. The Tofts model is currently the most widely used, simplest, and most classic model utilized in clinical applications. This model comprehensively considers the intravascular distribution and extravascular permeation of the contrast agent, offering a close approximation to the true pathophysiological state of the human body. Commonly used parameters for this model include the following: volume transfer constant (K^{trans}), rate constant (K_{ep}), fractional volume of the extravascular extracellular space (V_e), and fractional volume of the plasma space (V_p).

4.1.4 Principles of ASL Imaging

ASL imaging, first proposed in 1992, is a method of perfusion imaging that does not require the use of an exogenous contrast agent. Unlike the gadolinium-based contrast agent, which is confined to the extracellular space and used in DSC and DCE imaging, ASL perfusion imaging uses the water molecules in the arterial blood as an endogenous tracer. Since the water molecules in arterial blood are diffusible, they can move freely within the capillaries, brain parenchyma, and even brain cells, thereby providing a true reflection of the entire perfusion process. In ASL imaging, the carotid artery is selected as the "magnetically labelled plane," and the water molecules in the arterial blood are magnetically labelled using a radiofrequency pulse to serve as an endogenous tracer. Data acquisition is performed before and after labelling the arterial blood, after which the two sets of images are subtracted to obtain a picture of the cerebral perfusion. Based on the labelling method used, ASL can be classified as continuous ASL (CASL), pulsed ASL (PASL), and pseudo-continuous ASL (pCASL), from which the respective territorial ASL (tASL) techniques can then be derived.

4.1.4.1 CASL Perfusion MRI

CASL MRI uses the water molecules in the arterial blood of the magnetically labelled plane and continuous radiofrequency pulses as an endogenous contrast agent. The labelling plane is set at a point prior to where the arterial blood enters the cerebral tissues (usually the carotid artery plane), where the longitudinal relaxation of the water protons is inverted. The intracranial region of interest (ROI) is selected as the control plane, and dynamic acquisition is performed twice using EPI sequences. The first scan is performed before the inverted water protons arrive at the ROI, to generate the control images. The second scan is performed after the inverted water protons arrive at the ROI, to generate the labelled images. Subtraction is then performed between the labelled and control images to obtain the perfusion-weighted images. CASL has a high signal-to-noise ratio and high contrast, but its drawbacks include a lengthy labelling time and large amount of energy deposition in tissues.

4.1.4.2 PASL Perfusion MRI

Unlike the labelling for continuous and pseudo-continuous, PASL MRI uses labelling pulses with a very short duration, typically around 10–20 ms. Based on the different positional relationships between the labelling pulses and the imaging plane, PASL can be further divided into the following: EPI with signal targeting and alternating radiofrequency (EPISTAR) sequence, in which the labelling pulses are located below the imaging plane; and the flow-sensitive alternating inversion recovery (FAIR) sequence, in which the labelling pulses overlap the imaging plane. Despite the different descriptive terms used in PASL, the basic principles are similar.

EPISTAR-based PASL MRI involves labelling the blood using radiofrequency pulses, via numerous methods, within a thick slab proximal to the imaging plane and performing imaging

Fig. 4.2 Defining the labelled and control planes in the three types of ASL imaging: CASL, continuous arterial spin labelling cerebral perfusion MRI; pCASL, pseudo-continuous arterial spin labelling cerebral perfusion MRI; PASL, pulsed arterial spin labelling cerebral perfusion MRI

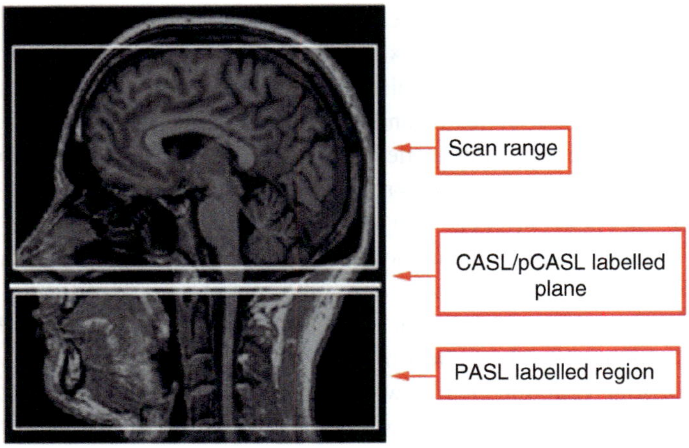

once the labelled blood is fully mixed with the tissues in the ROI (Fig. 4.2). Other common techniques include the FAIR and flow-sensitive alternating inversion recovery with an extra radiofrequency pulse (FAIRER) sequences, which invert the initial magnetization state of the tissues to obtain labelled blood. Compared to CASL, PASL is a simple technique that is less affected by the effects of tissue magnetization transfer (MT), and has less radiofrequency energy deposition, but its labelling efficiency is significantly lower than that of CASL.

4.1.4.3 pCASL Perfusion MRI

pCASL, which combines CASL and PASL while also taking into account the issues of signal-to-noise ratio and energy deposition, was first proposed in 2007. Unlike CASL (in which a single plane is labelled continuously for 1–3 s) or PASL (in which a thick slab is labelled in short pulses lasting 10–20 ms), pCASL employs a train of ≥1000 modulated radiofrequency pulses at a frequency of 1 pulse per millisecond, which prolongs the labelling duration while also significantly reducing the effects of MT, thereby improving the labelling efficiency and signal-to-noise ratio of images. The 2014 expert consensus on the clinical application of ASL recommends pCASL as the first choice for perfusion imaging.

4.1.4.4 tASL Perfusion MRI

tASL MRI comprises different techniques derived from CASL, PASL, and pCASL for the selective labelling of individual blood vessels to reflect the blood flow volume in the vascular networks of individual blood vessels. The two most common tASL methods currently used are vessel-encoded ASL (VE-ASL) and super selective AS (ss-ASL).

VE-ASL MRI involves the application of additional transverse gradient fields on the labelled plane to alter the labelling efficiency of different points within the same plane, thereby allowing for the selection of different brain-supplying arteries. This technique is characterized by the ability to simultaneously select multiple blood vessels, which allows the cerebral blood flow (CBF) distribution maps of multiple blood vessels to be acquired in a single scan within 3.5–5.0 min, significantly enhancing the labelling speed (Fig. 4.3). In addition to selecting the internal carotid artery as the labelled vessel, VE-ASL also enables the selective labelling of arteries superior to the circle of Willis.

In ss-ASL MRI, time-varying gradients are applied perpendicular to the labelled plane to produce a labelling focus that is located in the artery of interest, thereby achieving the selective labelling of individual arteries. Therefore, even when the labelled blood vessel is in close proximity to the surrounding vessels, ss-ASL is able to precisely select labelled blood vessel. Early studies utilized ss-ASL to label arterioles (diameter≈1.2 mm) distal to the circle of Willis, with a distance of 5.0 mm from the surrounding blood vessels. However, ss-ASL has several drawbacks, including the need for additional magnetic resonance angiography (MRA) for the pre-scan planning of each blood vessel, a long

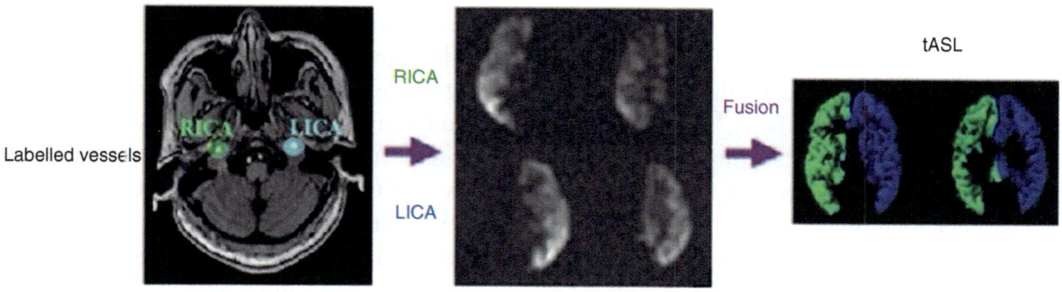

Fig. 4.3 Principles of VE-ASL imaging: The simultaneous labelling of the bilateral internal carotid arteries, which allows the cerebral blood flow distribution maps of the bilateral internal carotid arteries to be acquired in a single scan. RICA, right internal carotid artery; LICA, left internal carotid artery; tASL, territorial pulsed arterial spin labelling cerebral perfusion MRI

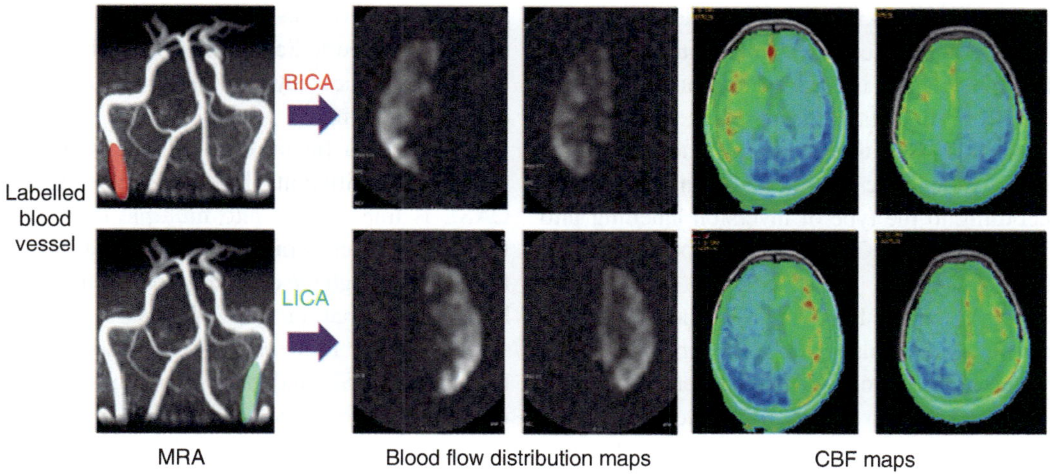

Fig. 4.4 Principles of ss-ASL imaging: The bilateral internal carotid arteries are labelled on the respective MRA images to obtain their cerebral blood flow distribution maps. RICA, right internal carotid artery; LICA, left internal carotid artery; CBF, cerebral blood flow

scan duration, and sensitivity to subject motion. Unlike VE-ASL, ss-ASL involves selecting and scanning each individual blood vessel and is therefore generally utilized in cases involving only a few arteries of interest (Fig. 4.4).

4.2 Post-Processing of Perfusion MRI Data

ASL MRI is a completely non-invasive perfusion imaging technique that does not require the injection of contrast agents. This technique was first used by Detre et al. in 1992 to acquire cerebral perfusion images of rats via the continuous labelling of carotid artery blood. In 1994, Roberts et al. acquired cerebral perfusion images of humans using a 1.5 Tesla (T) MRI scanner. As ASL continued to advance in regard to sequence design, acquisition time, image quality, and post-processing methods, it became widely used in clinical research. To further understand the basic principles of ASL perfusion imaging and to improve its clinical applications, this section will introduce the post-processing of ASL images.

4.2.1 Overview of ASL

ASL MRI exploits the fact that blood flows dynamically through the body, whereas tissues remain static. Therefore, labelling the inflowing blood via inversion pulses can be applied to a specific plane, followed by image acquisition after the labelled blood has entered the ROI, which provides the sum of signals from the tissues and blood. In order to obtain the perfusion signals, we must first acquire control images (without labelling inversion pulses), and then acquire labelled images after a delay. The second acquisition produces labelled images, which are the sum of the signals from the static tissues and the labelled blood, acquired after blood upstream of the ROI has been inverted and has entered the ROI. The control images are the sum of the signals from the static tissues and non-inverted blood in the ROI that can be used to remove the signals from static tissues. ASL can be classified according to the type of inversion labelling into CASL, PASL, pCASL, and velocity-selective ASL (VS-ASL).

CASL utilizes long and continuous inversion radiofrequency pulses to label a narrow plane on the carotid artery to invert the magnetization of the blood flowing into this narrow plane. If inversion labelling is performed only in the carotid artery, then the effects of MT will occur in the brain tissues of the scan region—that is, saturation transfer will occur during the interaction between water and other large molecules in the tissues. Therefore, the control images are generally acquired by selecting an area that is symmetric relative to the imaging region to perform the same labelling process. Although the labelling efficiency of CASL is higher than that of PASL, CASL has increased hardware requirements for the MRI equipment owing to the need to generate long and continuous radiofrequency pulses (duration≈1–2 s), which involves a relatively large specific absorption rate (SAR), and is susceptible to the effects of MT. Due to these shortcomings, CASL has limited applicability in clinical practice.

PASL uses single short radiofrequency pulses to invert and label the water protons within a thick slab through the carotid artery, and its typical pulse duration is 2–5 ms (usually 10–20 ms). This labelling method can be implemented using three different techniques: EPISTAR, FAIR, and proximal inversion with control of off-resonance effects (PICORE). Compared to CASL, PASL has fewer hardware requirements, higher inversion efficiency, lower energy deposition, and lower susceptibility to the effects of MT, but its signal-to-noise ratio is lower than that of CASL by 30–50%. Moreover, the thick-slab labelling method causes blurring at the distal edges, resulting in a systematic bias in the quantification of CBF. The implementation of techniques such as quantitative imaging of perfusion using a single subtraction (QUIPSS II) and QUIPSS II with thin-slice T_1 periodic saturation (Q2TIPS) can improve the accuracy of PASL for quantitative perfusion imaging.

pCASL is a fusion of PASL and CASL, in which the continuous labelling pulse used in CASL is transformed into multiple short high-frequency pulses, which are then used to label a thin slice through the carotid artery. Some studies have shown that in a 3T magnetic field, the signal-to-noise ratio of pCASL is 50% higher than that of PASL, and that its labelling efficiency is 18% higher than that of CASL. Owing to fewer hardware requirements, high labelling efficiency, high signal-to-noise ratio, and good repeatability, pCASL has been widely utilized in clinical settings. In 2008, a team of researchers developed a 3D whole-brain perfusion MRI technique based on pCASL, which has provided a solid foundation for the clinical application of ASL.

VS-ASL involves labelling based on flow velocity, which differs from the spatial labelling approach adopted in conventional ASL techniques. In VS-ASL, labelling is based on a predefined cutoff velocity (only blood flowing above this velocity is labelled), rather than just labelling areas proximal to the acquisition slice, thereby avoiding the errors caused by transit delay. In reality, however, VS-ASL has a low signal-to-noise ratio and the cutoff velocity is difficult to define, which can result in inaccurate information on local perfusion.

4.2.2 Computation of ASL Perfusion-Weighted Maps and Quantitative CBF Maps

Cerebral perfusion is an important physiological indicator that can reflect the status of brain function and is primarily measured on MRI after the administration of exogenous or endogenous contrast agents. In this section, we will discuss the quantitative post-processing of PASL and pCASL data, primarily focusing on perfusion-weighted and quantitative CBF images.

Perfusion-weighted images are obtained by performing subtraction between the control and labelled images, the signals for which are derived from the difference between the inversion recovery and non-inverted signals of blood flow. The majority of perfusion disorders result in easily visualized lesions. However, certain diseases will cause global changes, necessitating the utilization of quantitative CBF maps. CBF refers to the volume of blood flowing through the vasculature of 100 g of brain tissue per unit time and is expressed as mL/100 g/min. CBF is calculated differently for different ASL techniques. In pCASL-based CBF quantification, the voxel-based CBF map is given using the following equation:

$$\mathrm{CBF}=\frac{6000\times\lambda\times\left(S_{\text{control}}-S_{\text{label}}\right)\times\exp\left(\frac{\mathrm{PLD}}{T_{1,\text{blood}}}\right)}{2\times\alpha\times T_{1,\text{blood}}\times S_{\mathrm{PD}}\times\left(1-\exp\left(-\frac{\tau}{T_{1,\text{blood}}}\right)\right)}\left[\mathrm{mL}/100\,\mathrm{g}/\min\right] \tag{4.1}$$

PASL-based CBF quantification with QUIPSS II correction is calculated using the equation below:

$$\mathrm{CBF}=\frac{6000\times\lambda\times\left(S_{\text{control}}-S_{\text{label}}\right)\times\exp\left(\frac{\mathrm{TI}}{T_{1,\text{blood}}}\right)}{2\times\alpha\times T_{1,\text{blood}}\times S_{\mathrm{PD}}}\left[\mathrm{mL}/100\,\mathrm{g}/\min\right] \tag{4.2}$$

CBF quantification based on 3D ASL is given as follows:

$$\mathrm{CBF}=\frac{6000\times\lambda\times\left(S_{\text{control}}-S_{\text{label}}\right)\left(1-\exp\left(-\frac{\mathrm{TI}_{\mathrm{SAT}}}{\mathrm{TI}_{\mathrm{GM}}}\right)\right)\exp\left(\frac{\mathrm{PLD}}{T1_{1,\text{blood}}}\right)}{2\times\alpha\times T_{1,\text{blood}}\times S_{\mathrm{PD}}\times\left(45.25\text{nex}\right)\times\left(1-\exp\left(-\frac{\tau}{TI_{1,\text{blood}}}\right)\right)}\left[\mathrm{mL}/100\,\mathrm{g}/\min\right] \tag{4.3}$$

where λ is the brain/blood partition given in mL/g; S_{control} and S_{label} are the acquired control and labelled images, respectively; $T_{1,\text{blood}}$ is the longitudinal relaxation time of blood; TI_{SAT} and TI_{GM} are the saturation recovery time and correction parameter of the proton-density weighted image; nex is the number of weighted averages; a is the labelling efficiency; S_{PD} is the proton-density weighted image; τ is the labelling duration; PLD is the post-labelling delay; TI_1 is the time between the labelling and saturation pulses in QUIPSS II; and TI is the time between the inversion labelling pulse and start of image acquisition (Fig. 4.5). It should be noted that in 2D multi-slice acquisition, the TI duration should be adjusted for each slice. The specifications and levels of specific parameters can be found in the 2015 white paper on the clinical applications of ASL published in *Magnetic Resonance in Medicine*.

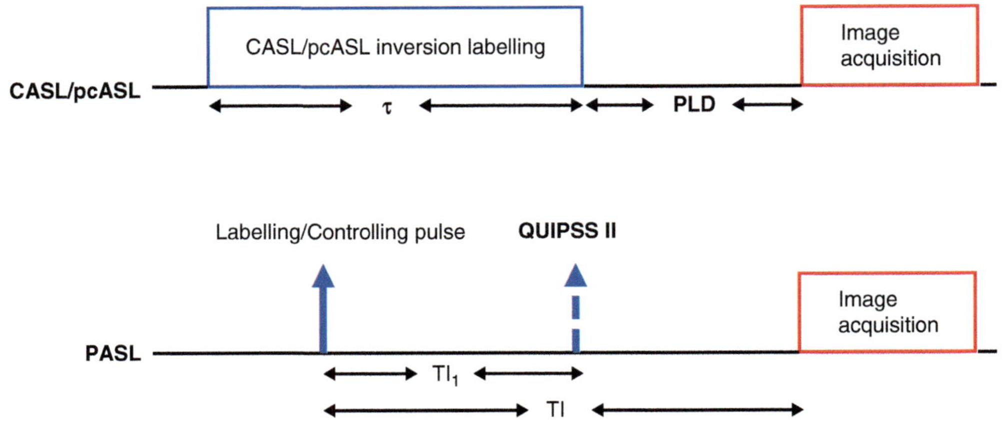

Fig. 4.5 Timing diagram for CASL, pCASL, and PASL: CASL/pCASL refers to continuous labelling where τ is the duration of continuous labelling; PLD is the delay between the end of labelling and the start of image acquisition; TI_1 in PASL is the time between inversion labelling and QUIPSS II saturation pulse, and TI is the time between the inversion labelling pulse and the start of image acquisition

4.2.3 Post-Processing of ASL Data

The post-processing of ASL data generally consists of two main steps: pre-processing and quantitative analysis, while quantitative analysis primarily involves the computation of perfusion-weighted maps and quantitative CBF maps. Pre-processing can be divided into two types, based on different research purposes: individual analysis and group analysis. The post-processing procedure of ASL data for individual analysis includes the following: head motion correction, pairwise subtraction between control and labelled images, averaging, segmentation of the 3D structural images, and computation of the CBF maps. The post-processing procedure of ASL data for group analysis includes the following: head motion correction, spatial normalization (registration of images to the MNI space, and normalizing voxel size to 3 mm), spatial smoothing, pairwise subtraction between control and labelled images, weighted averaging, and computation of the CBF maps.

The quantitative analysis of ASL data is primarily based on subtraction calculations, which implies that ASL computations are very sensitive to motion. Therefore, prior to calculating the average, the difference obtained by performing subtraction on the control and labelled images should be used to eliminate artifacts caused by motion to ensure the accuracy of the CBF computations. An important point to note here is that head motion correction cannot be performed on 3D ASL data; therefore, the subject's head should be secured in a fixed position during data acquisition. The software currently available for ASL data analysis includes the Bayesian Inference for Arterial Spin Labelling (BASIL) toolbox based on the FSL software (*https://fsl.fmrib.ox.ac.uk/fsl/fslwiki/BASIL*), the ASLtbx toolbox based on the Statistical Parametric Mapping (SPM) software (*https://www.cfn.upenn.edu/~zewang/ASLtbx.php*), and the ASL online data processing tool ASL-MRICloud.

4.3 Research Applications of Perfusion MRI in Neuroscience

Irrespective of whether scanning is done using DSC imaging, which requires the administration of an exogenous contrast agent, or ASL imaging, which uses labelled blood as an endogenous tracer, both these techniques can all be used to reflect the microvessel distribution and blood perfusion information from brain tissues. Cerebral perfusion MRI is a valuable reference for establishing the diagnosis and differential diagnosis of neurological diseases. With the advent of high-field MR scanners, ongoing improvements in perfusion models, and integration with other fMRI techniques, cerebral perfusion MRI has played an indispensable role in neuroscience research. In this section, we will discuss recent advances in the application of cerebral perfusion imaging in neuroscience research.

4.3.1 DSC Imaging

DSC perfusion imaging has a number of advantages, including fast scanning speed, high spatial resolution, large scan coverage, ability to assess a wide range of hemodynamic parameters, and the ability to be performed during routine MRI scans. Moreover, it has been extensively utilized in the differential diagnosis, prognostic assessment, and treatment efficacy evaluation of cerebrovascular diseases, brain tumors, epilepsy, and neurodegenerative diseases, and is currently the most widely used method for perfusion imaging in clinical settings. However, due to the non-linear relationship between MR signal intensity and contrast agent concentration, the effects of extravasation of the contrast agent into the extracellular space on tissue relaxation time remain poorly understood, which implies that the absolute CBF values cannot be obtained using DSC perfusion imaging. Furthermore, variations in DSC perfusion curves can occur due to factors such as the model of the MRI scanner and the strength of the gradient field. Additionally, DSC also requires the IV injection of an exogenous MRI contrast agent. Taken together, these factors have contributed to the limited utilization of DSC perfusion imaging in neuroscience research. Some researchers have used this technique to study the mechanism of post-stroke aphasia and found that reduced blood flow in the language areas of the brain can lead to aphasia. For example, hypoperfusion in the Broca's area can manifest as sensory aphasia; hypoperfusion in the anterior frontal lobe, inferior and posterior parietal lobes, and temporal gyrus can manifest as reading and writing abnormalities; while hypoperfusion in the parietal cortex, supramarginal gyrus, and angular gyrus can manifest as repetition deficits. Additionally, the degree of hypoperfusion in the language center is correlated with the severity of the aphasia. For example, Hillis et al. reported that when a cerebral infarction occurred in the dominant hemisphere, the volume of hypoperfused tissue had a significantly positive correlation with the severity of the aphasia. Fridriksson et al. also showed that more significant hypoperfusion in the language center was associated with more severe aphasia.

4.3.2 ASL Imaging

4.3.2.1 Advantages of ASL Imaging in Neuroscience

There are several advantages to utilizing ASL imaging, which uses arterial blood as an endogenous tracer, in neuroscience research. First, ASL can directly reflect changes in CBF; therefore, task-related activation areas can be localized based on CBF, which can be applied to sensory, motor, or cognitive tasks. In contrast, BOLD imaging is based on the complex interactions among multiple physiological variables induced by neuronal activity, including CBF, blood volume, oxygen extraction fraction, and metabolic changes. Furthermore, BOLD imaging must rely on changes in T_2* signals to indirectly reflect changes in CBF. Second, the endogenous tracer used in ASL is freely diffusible; thus, it can be used to accurately localize the activated cortical areas and implement real-time imaging, while measurements can also be performed using physiological units to monitor task-related CBF changes. In contrast, changes in task-related BOLD signal intensity cannot be directly quantified using physiological units. Third, ASL signals are comprised of information obtained by performing subtraction between pre- and post-labelling data. This paired subtraction can improve the noise characteristics of ASL by removing low-frequency noise, thereby enhancing its low-frequency sensitivity over longer scan times. A sensorimotor study demonstrated that ASL can still detect reliable CBF changes in the motor cortex 24 h after finger tapping, whereas

BOLD-induced activation only persisted for a few minutes after the task. Therefore, ASL-based functional brain imaging can replace BOLD imaging in studies involving brain activation over a longer duration and numerous neurophysiological states, such as motor learning, emotional or mental states, emotional changes, and natural vision. Despite the decreased sensitivity and temporal resolution of ASL compared with conventional BOLD, ASL is more sensitive to cohort effects, which may be caused by the reduced inter-subject variations in CBF compared with changes in BOLD signals.

4.3.2.2 Research Applications of ASL Imaging in Neurodevelopment

ASL can serve as a biomarker for evaluating brain development in both a healthy population and patients with developmental disorders. Children have higher CBF and brain water content compared to adults, which not only enhances their perfusion enhancement but also increases the concentration and half-life of the ASL endogenous tracer (i.e., water in arterial blood). A PASL-based cerebral perfusion study on children showed that the signal-to-noise ratio of ASL images acquired in children was 70% higher than that in healthy adults. Furthermore, studies using PASL or CASL to observe perfusion changes over the course of brain development found that among healthy children aged 4–5 years, whole-brain, gray matter, and white matter CBF decreased with increasing age, which is consistent with the results of single-photon emission computerized tomography (SPECT) studies. In addition, studies have also demonstrated that the regional CBF (rCBF) of the frontal cortex, cingulate gyrus, angular gyrus, and hippocampus increased with increasing age, which may reflect the delayed maturation of the cortical areas associated with executive function, cognitive control, and memory integration. Taki et al. calculated the gray matter density and cerebral perfusion of 22 brain regions in 202 healthy children, aged 5–18 years, to analyze the effects of the developmental process on brain structure and perfusion. Their study results revealed that the gray matter density of most areas of the brain gradually peaked with increasing age, and that its correlation with age increased gradually from the occipital to the frontal lobe via the temporal and parietal lobes, showing a U-shaped trajectory. In contrast, the correlation of cerebral perfusion with age showed an inverted-U shaped trajectory. ASL is able to provide quantitative CBF at baseline, without the need for external tasks, which can facilitate research in infants and young children. For example, a study found that the cerebral cortical perfusion levels in unsedated neonates were lower than those in adults, whereas perfusion in the basal ganglia was significantly higher than that in the cortical gray and white matter, which is consistent with positron emission tomography (PET) results. Another study compared the cerebral perfusion images of normally developing 7- and 13-month-old infants during unsedated sleep. The results demonstrated that the rCBF of infants increased with increasing age, with 13-month-old infants showing higher rCBF in the frontal lobe, hippocampus, anterior cingulate gyrus, amygdala, occipital lobe, and auditory cortex when compared with 7-month-old infants.

4.3.2.3 Research Applications of ASL Imaging in Pharmacology

ASL can also be used as a biomarker to investigate the pharmacological effects of numerous drugs. Pharmacological imaging enables the *in vivo* visualization of the effects of certain drugs and can be applied to preclinical drug trials and in human subjects. PET remains the most widely used method of pharmacological imaging, as it can image the radiotracer distribution of drugs or drug targets. However, PET requires the development of costly radiopharmaceuticals and involves the use of ionizing radiation. Non-specific PET tracers for neurophysiological activity, such as $^{15}O\text{-}H_2O$ and ^{18}F-FDG, have been used to perform pharmacological imaging. These non-specific methods are dependent on the regulatory effects of drugs on neuronal activity and the resulting changes in CBF and metabolism. ASL, on the other hand, can serve as a biomarker for studying pharmacological effects that have a high reproducibility and is suitable for investigating orally administered drugs and treatment of chronic diseases.

Black et al. used ASL to study the mechanism of action underlying the novel adenosine A_{2a} receptor antagonist, SYN115, in patients with Parkinson's disease (PD) receiving levodopa infusions. The patients received SYN115 treatment twice daily for one week, and then underwent ASL scanning. After the initial (control) scan, they underwent a one-week washout period, followed by one week of placebo administration, and then underwent another ASL scan. Furthermore, to obtain the dose–response curves, the patients were divided into two groups and were randomly administered either 20 or 60 mg of SYN115. The findings of this study indicated that in addition to a slight decrease in whole-brain CBF induced by SYN115 (4% and 7% for 20 mg and 60 mg, respectively), there was a significant decrease in thalamic CBF, which supports the hypothesis that A_{2a} antagonists inhibit the basal ganglia pathway. In another study by Chen et al., pCASL was used to detect the effects of a single dose of citalopram on CBF. Twelve healthy subjects randomly received either a placebo or 20 mg citalopram. Baseline pCASL was acquired prior to drug administration, and further post-medication pCASL scans were performed at 30 min, 1 h, and 3 h after drug administration. The results of their study showed significant drug-induced CBF reductions in the amygdala, fusiform gyrus, insula, and orbitofrontal cortex. Moreover, mixed-effects analysis on data extracted from ROIs in the aforementioned study indicated significant drug effects in serotonergic areas. Taken together with the findings that that the same regions show elevated CBF in patients with depression, as well as in subjects genetically prone to depression, we can uncover the potential mechanisms of citalopram in treating depression. Fernandez-Sear et al. used ASL to detect the effects of a single dose of metoclopramide. In their study, 18 healthy subjects randomly received 10 mg metoclopramide or a placebo and underwent pCASL ASL scanning before and 1 h after medication. The results of their study showed an increase in CBF in the bilateral putamen, globus pallidus, and thalamus, as well as reduced CBF in the bilateral insulae extending to the anterior temporal lobes. These findings are consistent with those from PET studies involving other antipsychotic medications and are similar to the pathologically hyperperfused areas observed in PD patients.

4.3.2.4 Research Applications of ASL Imaging in Neuropsychiatry

As ASL can quantify brain functional states and display brain functional areas related to pharmacological effects using CBF changes, it is a particularly valuable technique in the research and treatment of neuropsychiatric disorders. In fact, preliminary studies have demonstrated the effectiveness of utilizing ASL in several fields, including tobacco and alcohol addiction.

By exploiting the temporal stability of ASL, Franklin et al. compared the changes in brain function during smoking and non-smoking sessions, while also controlling for withdrawal effects by allowing subjects to smoke before each scan. The results of their study demonstrated greater CBF in the smoking sessions, compared to the non-smoking sessions, in the ventral striatum, amygdala, orbitofrontal cortex, hippocampus, medial thalamus, and left insula, while cue-induced craving was positively correlated with CBF changes in the dorsolateral prefrontal cortex and posterior cingulate gyrus. Wang et al. used ASL to examine smokers after smoking satiety or abstinence and found that abstinence was associated with increased CBF in the anterior cingulate, medial orbitofrontal, and left orbitofrontal cortices. Furthermore, abstinence-induced cravings to smoke could be predicted by CBF increases in the brain's visual circuitry, which includes the right orbitofrontal cortex, right dorsolateral prefrontal cortex, occipital cortex, anterior cingulate cortex, ventral striatum, thalamus, amygdala, bilateral hippocampus, left caudate, and right insula. These craving responses are associated with functional genetic variations related to nicotine dependence. Subjects with genotypic variants in the dopamine D2 receptor and catechol-*O*-methyltransferase exhibited a significant correlation between CBF and smoking addiction, suggesting that the neural mechanisms of these genetic variants may be linked to nicotine dependence.

Tolentino et al. utilized PASL to investigate the effects of alcohol intake on CBF. Their study involved 88 healthy young adults who were placed in either a high- or low-response group based on their sensitivity to alcohol. The subjects then randomly received 0.70–0.75 mL/kg of ethanol or placebo (in the form of a decaffeinated beverage), followed by PASL scanning 22 min after ingestion. The results of their study indicated elevated CBF in the frontal brain regions after ethanol intake, which is consistent with the CBF findings based on other modalities (e.g., PET, SPECT, and ^{133}Xe uptake). Furthermore, subjects with a lower response to alcohol showed smaller increases in CBF, which is consistent with the results of previous fMRI studies.

In addition to the above, ASL imaging has also been used to study other neuropsychiatric syndromes and neurodegenerative diseases. ASL studies on depression and schizophrenia have revealed reduced CBF in the prefrontal cortex. In patients with attention deficit hyperactivity disorder, ASL imaging demonstrated that cranial electrotherapy stimulation can achieve its therapeutic effects by normalizing hyperperfused cortical and subcortical regions. Lui et al. utilized ASL imaging to assess focal cerebral perfusion in 24 patients with refractory depressive disorder (RDD), 37 patients with non-refractory depressive disorder (NDD), and 42 healthy controls; the results of their study showed that compared with the control group, NDD patients showed decreased perfusion in the left prefrontal cortex and increased perfusion in the limbic-striatal areas, whereas RDD patients showed decreased perfusion in the bilateral frontal lobe and bilateral thalamic regions. Compared with RDD patients, those with NDD showed increased perfusion in the limbic-striatal areas (Fig. 4.6). These findings suggest that RDD and NDD patients exhibit different alterations in focal perfusion, which are consistent with the results of previous fMRI studies. Mild cognitive impairment (MCI) is a well-defined non-motor manifestation of PD that can seriously limit the patient's quality of life and social function. In a study by Suo et al. involving 22 PD patients with MCI (PD-MCI), 17 PD patients with normal cognition (PD-N), and 36 age- and sex-matched healthy controls, the included subjects underwent voxel-based brain analysis to examine the

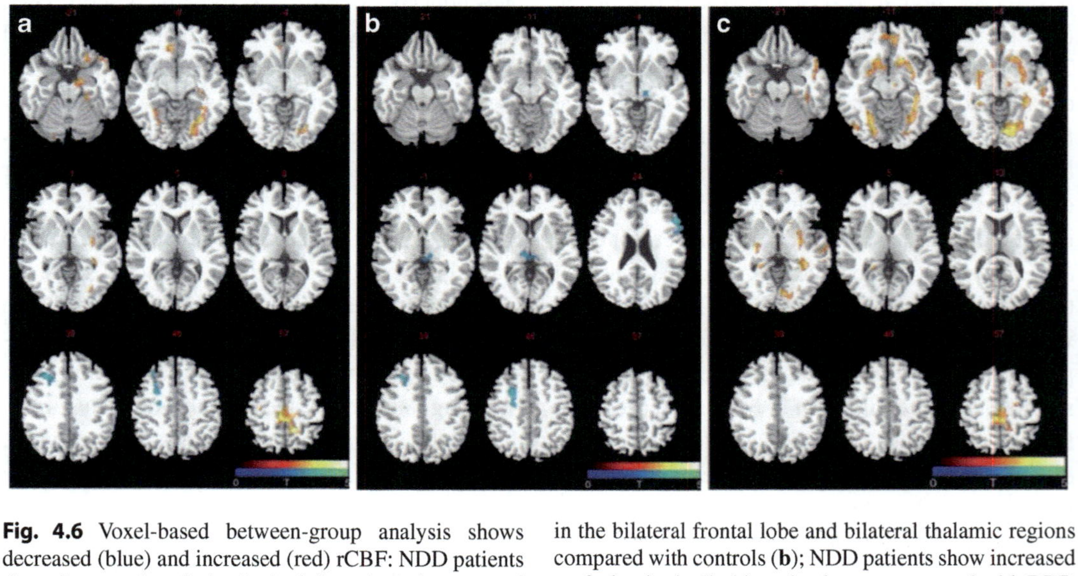

Fig. 4.6 Voxel-based between-group analysis shows decreased (blue) and increased (red) rCBF: NDD patients show decreased perfusion in the left prefrontal cortex and increased perfusion in the limbic-striatal areas compared with controls (**a**); RDD patients show decreased perfusion in the bilateral frontal lobe and bilateral thalamic regions compared with controls (**b**); NDD patients show increased perfusion in the limbic-striatal areas compared with RDD patients (**c**)

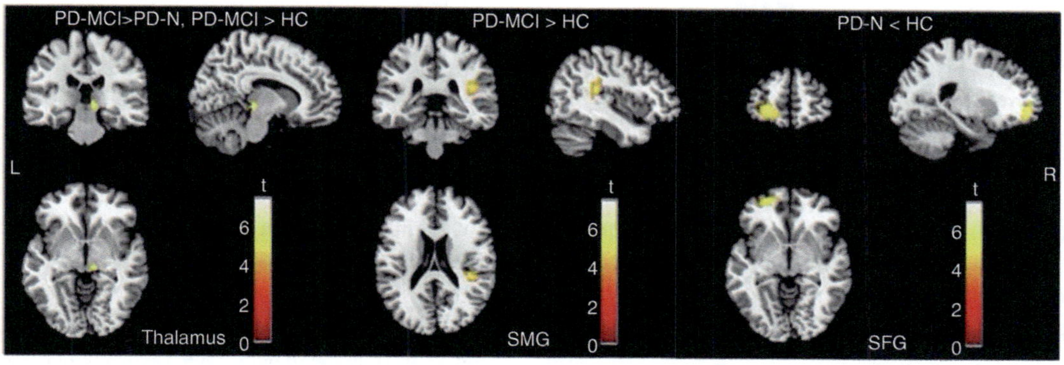

Fig. 4.7 Differences in arterial transit time (ATT) among PD-MCI, PD-N, and HC: PD-MCI shows prolonged ATT in the right thalamus compared with PD-N and HC, and prolonged ATT in the right SMG compared with HC; PD-N shows shorter ATT in the left superior frontal cortex compared with HC. PD, Parkinson's disease; PD-MCI, PD with mild cognitive impairment; PD-N, PD with normal cognition; HC, healthy control; L, left; R, right; SFG, superior frontal gyrus; SMG, supramarginal gyrus

between-group differences in two perfusion parameters, CBF and arterial transit time (ATT). The PD-MCI group showed prolonged ATT in the right thalamus, whereas the PD-N group showed a shorter ATT in the left superior frontal cortex (Fig. 4.7). This suggests that ATT is a more sensitive marker for MCI than CBF and highlights the potential role of the thalamus and inferior parietal region in early-stage PD.

As ASL can be utilized for the absolute quantification of the biological parameter of CBF, it has become a valuable technique in longitudinal and cross-sectional research, with increasing applications in basic research and clinical neuroscience. Thus, not only can ASL help explore the neural mechanisms of behavioral disorders, it also has immense value in the development and validation of novel treatments for neurological diseases.

Suggested Readings

Aguirre GK, Detre JA, Alsop DC. Experimental design and the relative sensitivity of BOLD and perfusion fMRI. Neuroimage. 2002;15(3):488–500.

Alsop DC, Detre JA, Golay X, et al. Recommended implementation of arterial spin-labeled perfusion MRI for clinical applications: a consensus of the ISMRM perfusion study group and the European consortium for ASL in dementia. Magn Reson Med. 2015;73(1):102–16.

Biagi L, Abbruzzese A, Bianchi MC, et al. Age dependence of cerebral perfusion assessed by magnetic resonance continuous arterial spin labeling. J Magn Reson Imaging. 2007;25(4):696–702.

Black KJ, Koller JM, Campbell MC, et al. Quantification of indirect pathway inhibition by the adenosine A2a antagonist SYN115 in Parkinson disease. J Neurosci. 2010;30(48):16284–92.

Chen Y, Parrish TB. Caffeine dose effect on activation-induced BOLD and CBF responses. Neuroimage. 2009;46(3):577–83.

Duong TQ, Silva AC, Lee SP, et al. Functional MRI of calcium-dependent synaptic activity: cross correlation with CBF and BOLD measurements. Magn Reson Med. 2000;43(3):383–92.

Fan AP, Guo J, Khalighi MM, et al. Long-delay arterial spin labeling provides more accurate cerebral blood flow measurements in moyamoya patients. Stroke. 2017;48(9):2441–9.

Feng L, Yunsuo D, Bradley SP, et al. Resting state cerebral blood flow with arterial spin labeling MRI in developing human brains. Eur J Paediatr Neurol. 2018;22(4):642–51.

Fernandez-Seara MA, Aznarez-Sanado M, Mengual E, et al. Effects on resting cerebral blood flow and functional connectivity induced by metoclopramide: a perfusion MRI study in healthy volunteers. Br J Pharmacol. 2011;163(8):1639–52.

Franklin T, Wang Z, Suh JJ, et al. Effects of varenicline on smoking cue-triggered neural and craving responses. Arch Gen Psychiatry. 2011;68(5):516–26.

Franklin TR, Lohoff FW, Wang Z, et al. DAT genotype modulates brain and behavioral responses elicited by cigarette cues. Neuropsychopharmacology. 2009;34(3):717–28.

Franklin TR, Wang Z, Wang J, et al. Limbic activation to cigarette smoking cues independent of

nicotine withdrawal: a perfusion fMRI study. Neuropsychopharmacology. 2007;32(11):2301–9.
Fridriksson J, Holland AL, Coull BM, et al. Aphasia severity: association with cerebral perfusion and diffusion. Aphasiology. 2002;16(9):859–71.
Gillihan SJ, Rao H, Wang J, et al. Serotonin transporter genotype modulates amygdala activity during mood regulation. Soc Cogn Affect Neurosci. 2010;5(1):1–10.
Gogtay N, Giedd JN, Lusk L, et al. Dynamic mapping of human cortical development during childhood through early adulthood. Proc Natl Acad Sci U S A. 2004;101(21):8174–9.
Hillis AE, Barker PB, Beauchamp NJ, et al. MR perfusion imaging reveals regions of hypoperfusion associated with aphasia and neglect. Neurology. 2000;55(6):782–8.
Hillis AE, Heidler J. Mechanisms of early aphasia recovery. Aphasiology. 2002;16(9):885–95.
Huppert TJ, Hoge RD, Diamond SG, et al. A temporal comparison of BOLD, ASL, and NIRS hemodynamic responses to motor stimuli in adult humans. Neuroimage. 2006;29(2):368–82.
Li Y, Liu P, Li Y, et al. ASL-MRICloud: an online tool for the processing of ASL MRI data. NMR Biomed. 2019;32(2):e4051.
Lim J, Wu WC, Wang J, et al. Imaging brain fatigue from sustained mental workload: an ASL perfusion study of the time-on-task effect. Neuroimage. 2010;49(4):3426–35.
Lui S, Parkes LM, Huang X, et al. Depressive disorders: focally altered cerebral perfusion measured with arterial spin-labeling MR imaging. Radiology. 2009;251(2):476–84.
Miranda MJ, Olofsson K, Sidaros K. Noninvasive measurements of regional cerebral perfusion in preterm and term neonates by magnetic resonance arterial spin labeling. Pediatr Res. 2006;60(3):359–63.
Olson IR, Rao H, Moore KS, et al. Using perfusion fMRI to measure continuous changes in neural activity with learning. Brain Cogn. 2006;60(3):262–71.
Rao H, Wang J, Tang K, et al. Imaging brain activity during natural vision using CASL perfusion fMRI. Hum Brain Mapp. 2007;28(7):593–601.
Silva AC, Lee SP, Iadecola C, et al. Early temporal characteristics of cerebral blood flow and deoxyhemoglobin changes during somatosensory stimulation. J Cereb Blood Flow Metab. 2000;20(1):201–6.
Suo X, Lei D, Cheng L, et al. Multidelay multiparametric arterial spin labeling perfusion MRI and mild cognitive impairment in early stage Parkinson's disease. Hum Brain Mapp. 2019;40(4):1317–27.
Taki Y, Hashizume H, Sassa Y, et al. Correlation between gray matter density-adjusted brain perfusion and age using brain MR images of 202 healthy children. Hum Brain Mapp. 2011;32(11):1973–85.
Tolentino NJ, Wierenga CE, Hall S, et al. Alcohol effects on cerebral blood flow in subjects with low and high responses to alcohol. Alcohol Clin Exp Res. 2011;35(6):1034–40.
Wang DJ, Rao H, Korczykowski M, et al. Cerebral blood flow associated with different meditation practices and perceived depth of meditation. Psychiatry Res. 2011;191(1):6011t.
Wang J, Aguirre GK, Kimberg DY, et al. Arterial spin labeling perfusion fMRI with very low task frequency. Magn Reson Med. 2003;49(5):796–802.
Wang J, Korczykowski M, Rao H, et al. Gender difference in neural response to psychological stress. Soc Cogn Affect Neurosci. 2007;2(3):227–39.
Wang J, Licht DJ, Jahng GH, et al. Pediatric perfusion imaging using pulsed arterial spin labeling. J Magn Reson Imaging. 2003;18(4):404–13.
Wang Z, Faith M, Patterson F, et al. Neural substrates of abstinence-induced cigarette cravings in chronic smokers. J Neurosci. 2007;27(51):14035–40.
Wang Z, Ray R, Faith M, et al. Nicotine abstinence-induced cerebral blood flow changes by genotype. Neurosci Lett. 2008;438(3):275–80.
Welker K, Boxerman J, Kalnin A, et al. ASFNR recommendations for clinical performance of MR dynamic susceptibility contrast perfusion imaging of the brain. AJNR Am J Neuroradiol. 2015;36(6):E41–51.

Radiotracers for PET Imaging of the Brain

5

Hongwei Qiao and Jie Lu

PET radiotracers are functional compounds that are labeled with positron-emitting radionuclides and identifying a tracer with specific properties is a necessity for PET imaging. Radiotracers for brain imaging must have several important features, such as having clear targets, non-invasiveness, and quantifiability; therefore, they have consistently remained a hot topic in radiopharmaceutical development. Most radiotracers for PET imaging of the brain use nuclides with short half-lives, which commonly include ^{11}C, ^{13}N, ^{15}O, and ^{18}F, which have half-lives of 20.5, 10, 2.1, and 110 min, respectively. These elements are the building blocks of human life, and therefore, the metabolic processes of their radioactively labeled compounds can reflect changes in the body's physiological and biochemical functions. In this chapter, we will introduce the radiotracers frequently used for PET imaging of the brain.

H. Qiao · J. Lu (✉)
Department of Radiology and Nuclear Medicine, Xuanwu Hospital, Capital Medical University, Beijing, China

5.1 PET Radiotracers for Brain Tumors

Targeted radiotracers can be used for PET imaging to visualize and assess the molecular and functional characteristics of tumor tissues, which facilitates tumor grading, guides the formulation of effective treatment plans, and enables the prediction of patient prognosis. Diagnostic imaging agents for brain tumors can be divided as follows: agents for glucose metabolism, amino acid metabolism, cell proliferation, hypoxia, and other receptors (Fig. 5.1).

5.1.1 PET Radiotracers for Glucose Metabolism

Currently, the glucose analog ^{18}F-fluorodeoxyglucose (^{18}F-FDG) is the most commonly used PET radiotracer for the imaging of brain tumors. ^{18}F-FDG can pass through the blood–brain barrier (BBB) and enter nerve cells via glucose transporters (GLUTs). High-grade gliomas—World Health Organization (WHO) grades III and IV—exhibit significantly higher ^{18}F-FDG uptake, which is positively correlated with tumor malignancy, than low-grade tumors—WHO grade II—which do not exhibit significant changes in uptake. Furthermore, the relatively high physiological glucose metabolism in normal brain (such as in the cerebral cortex, basal gan-

J. Lu, G. Zhao (eds.), *PET/MR: Functional and Molecular Imaging of Neurological Diseases and Neurosciences*, https://doi.org/10.1007/978-981-19-9902-4_5

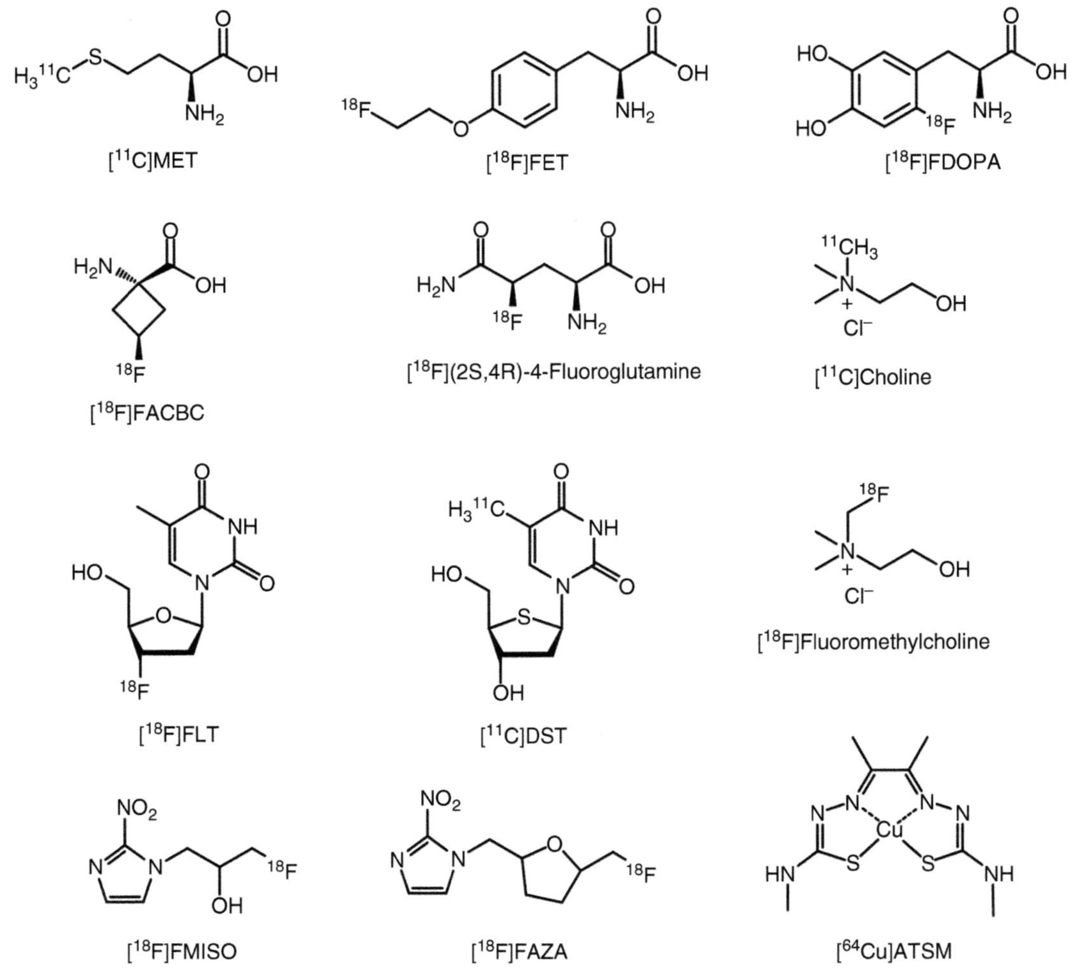

Fig. 5.1 Chemical structures of common PET radiotracers used for brain tumor imaging

glia, and thalamus) and inflammatory tissues can reduce the contrast between the tumor and surrounding tissue, making it difficult to accurately detect lesions within such tissues, and may even lead to a missed diagnosis or a misdiagnosis of smaller lesions. Therefore, optimized imaging strategies should be utilized to improve the detection of brain tumors with ^{18}F-FDG imaging. The first of these strategies is to fuse ^{18}F-FDG PET images with magnetic resonance (MR) images. Using this strategy, the MR images can be used to accurately delineate regions of interest (ROIs) and focus on regions of elevated ^{18}F-FDG uptake. The second strategy is to perform delayed imaging sequences. Due to the lower degradation rate constant of phosphorylated ^{18}F-FDG in tumor tissues, increasing the time between the ^{18}F-FDG injection and PET imaging enhances the sensitivity of tumor detection.

5.1.2 PET Radiotracers for Amino Acid Metabolism

Radionuclide-labeled amino acids can be transported through the BBB via amino acid transporters and have been used in PET imaging of brain tumors since 1983. L-[Methyl-^{11}C]methionine (^{11}C-MET) is currently the most commonly used agent for amino acid metabolic imaging, which reflects the protein synthesis and cell proliferation of gliomas. Clinical imaging studies have demonstrated a significantly increased ^{11}C-MET uptake in gliomas that appear negative on both magnetic resonance imaging (MRI) and ^{18}F-FDG imaging. ^{11}C-MET uptake is not only related to tumor microvessel density and blood volume, but is also associated with the expression levels of L-type amino acid transporter 1 (LAT1) in vascular endothelial and tumor cells. Furthermore, increased ^{11}C-MET uptake has been reported in oligodendrogliomas due to their high cellular density, as well as in fibrillary astrocytomas due to their elevated vascularization and high expression of amino acid transporters in vascular endothelial cells. It should be noted, however, that non-tumor lesions (including those from inflammation, infarction, and hemorrhage) may also exhibit elevated ^{11}C-MET uptake, which can result in false positive results.

^{18}F-fluoro-ethyl-tyrosine (^{18}F-FET) is an aromatic amino acid analog labeled using a radionuclide with a relatively long half-life, ^{18}F (half-life, 109.8 min), and its clinical applications have been rapidly expanding in recent years. It has been demonstrated in clinical practice that ^{18}F-FET has similar imaging effects to ^{11}C-MET, the difference being that the original compound of ^{18}F-FET has a slow blood clearance rate, which can lead to difficulties in distinguishing blood vessels and metabolically active tumor tissues. Therefore, in clinical applications, dynamic PET imaging is used to improve the accuracy of the differentiation between low- and high-grade gliomas. Another commonly used amino acid tracer is ^{18}F-fluorodopa (^{18}F-FDOPA), which can reveal the extent of the tumor and has a good tumor-to-background ratio. However, due to the high physiological uptake of ^{18}F-FDOPA in the striatum, it may not be possible to delineate the boundaries of tumor infiltration into the basal ganglia.

There has been continuous progress in the development of novel amino acid agents for the imaging of brain tumors, an example of which is the recently developed anti-1-amino-3-^{18}F-fluorocyclobutane-1-carboxylic acid (^{18}F-FACBC) tracer. Previous studies have demonstrated increased ^{18}F-FACBC uptake in gliomas compared to normal tissues and inflammatory areas. Another example is ^{18}F-(2*S*,4*R*)4-fluoroglutamine, which is an ^{18}F-labeled glutamine analog that can demonstrate the energy metabolism of tumor cells. Previous clinical studies have shown that ^{18}F-(2*S*,4*R*)4-fluoroglutamine exhibits a relatively high uptake in gliomas that were found to be negative using ^{18}F-FDG imaging. Given these examples, we should expect that the development of novel tracers and the optimization of the PET imaging process will further promote the utilization of PET imaging based on amino acid metabolism in the diagnosis and evaluation of brain tumors.

5.1.3 PET Radiotracers for Cell Proliferation

Radionuclide-labeled nucleoside analogs can show the status of cell proliferation. One example is 3′-deoxy-3′-^{18}F-fluorothymidine (^{18}F-FLT), a thymidine analog, the brain uptake of which is affected by multiple factors, including BBB permeability, intracellular phosphorylation rate, and cell proliferation markers. ^{18}F-FLT has a very high tumor-to-background ratio in tumors involving BBB damage but cannot be used to image tumors in patients with an intact BBB. Another thymidine analog is 4′-methyl-^{11}C-thiothymidine (^{11}C-DST), which can resist degradation due to thymidine phosphorylase and can be incorporated into deoxyribonucleic acid (DNA). Thus, ^{11}C-DST may produce a superior image compared to ^{18}F-FLT, but further investigation is needed to verify this claim. The elevated metabolism of choline in hyperplastic tumor cells implies that ^{11}C-choline and ^{18}F-fluorocholine can also be utilized in the imaging of gliomas. ^{11}C-choline has a decreased uptake in normal brain tissues and low-grade gliomas, but an increased uptake in high-grade gliomas, providing a good tumor-to-background ratio.

5.1.4 PET Radiotracers for Hypoxia

Hypoxic areas in malignant tumors are caused by insufficient blood supply due to the abnormal proliferation of tumor cells and associated blockages of intratumor blood vessels. Hypoxic tissues promote neovascularization through various molecular signals, which may drive the expansion of the tumor into surrounding tissues and may be associated with an insensitivity to radiotherapy and chemotherapy. Currently, 3-^{18}F-2-hydroxypropyl-2-nitroimidazole (^{18}F-FMISO), a nitroimidazole derivative, is the most widely used agent for the imaging of hypoxic areas. In normoxic tissues, the metabolism of ^{18}F-FMISO produces free radical anions that can be oxidized back to the parent compound and readily diffuse out of the cells. In hypoxic tissues, however, the free radical anions remain in the cells for a long time, allowing them to react with other substances and accumulate within hypoxic cells. Clinical studies have demonstrated the increased uptake of ^{18}F-FMISO in WHO grade IV gliomas, but not grade II or III. Further studies have also revealed that the level of hypoxia in pre-radiotherapy WHO grade II gliomas was closely associated with both disease duration and survival time. Based on the biological link between hypoxia and tumor-induced neovascularization, a significant correlation can also be found between ^{18}F-FMISO uptake and the intratumoral expression of vascular endothelial growth factors, making it possible for the latter to serve as markers for evaluating the efficacy of anti-angiogenic treatments in malignant gliomas. Furthermore, due to the insensitivity of hypoxic tissues to chemotherapy and radiotherapy, ^{18}F-FMISO PET imaging can also be used to evaluate the efficacy of these treatments in gliomas. Other PET tracers for hypoxia include ^{18}F-fluoroazomycin arabinoside (^{18}F-FAZA) and ^{64}Cu-diacetyl-bis(N^4-methylthiosemicarbazone) (^{64}Cu-ATSM), but further investigations are needed to verify their application value in the evaluation of gliomas.

5.1.5 Other PET Radiotracers for Brain Tumors

Somatostatin is a neuropeptide secreted by endocrine cells, neurons, and immune cells. Its functions include neuromodulation and cell growth inhibition, via paracrine and autocrine pathways. Somatostatin exerts its effects through a group of G-protein-coupled receptors known as somatostatin receptors (SSTRs), of which six subtypes have been discovered so far, including SSTR1, 2A, 2B, 3, 4, and 5. At present, a number of SSTR imaging agents have been utilized in clinical settings, such as ^{68}Ga-DOTA-TOC, ^{68}Ga-DOTA-NOC, and ^{68}Ga-DOTA-TATE. These imaging agents have a high affinity for SSTR2, but varying levels of affinity for the other subtypes, and different brain tumors express different SSTR subtypes. For gliomas, WHO grades I and II tumors exhibit higher levels of SSTR expression than grades III and IV, and for meningiomas, although SSTR can be detected in normal pia mater cells, its expression levels are even higher in meningioma cells. In medulloblastomas, SSTR2 and SSTR3 have the highest expression, which implies that ^{68}Ga-DOTA imaging may play a crucial role in the evaluation of medulloblastomas.

5.2 PET Radiotracers for Alzheimer's Disease (AD)

AD is the most common form of neurodegenerative dementia, and its pathological characteristics include extracellular plaques composed of β-amyloid (Aβ) peptides and intracellular neurofibrillary tangles (NFTs) composed of hyperphosphorylated tau proteins. Frontotemporal lobar degeneration (FTLD) is related to tau aggregation and encompasses several different pathologies of frontal and/or anterior temporal lobar degeneration and other related dementias, including frontotemporal dementia (FTD), semantic dementia, and progressive non-fluent aphasia.

5.2.1 PET Radiotracers for Aβ

Over the past 10 years, ^{11}C-labeled Pittsburgh compound-B (^{11}C-PiB) has been the most commonly used PET radiotracer for evaluating Aβ. However, due to its short half-life and the need for an on-site cyclotron and synthesis system, the clinical applications of ^{11}C are limited. The second-generation PET tracers for Aβ were therefore labeled with ^{18}F, which has a longer half-life. Examples of these include: ^{18}F-florbetapir (^{18}F-AV-45), ^{18}F-AZD4694, ^{18}F-florbetaben (^{18}F-AV-1), and ^{18}F-flutemetamol. These radiotracers have a greater potential for clinical application than ^{11}C-labeled tracers, and have been utilized for the diagnosis of AD and for the efficacy evaluation of new treatment measures. ^{11}C-PiB and second-generation ^{18}F-labeled tracers have a high affinity for the β-sheets of fibrillar Aβ (Fig. 5.2), which enables their specific localization within regions of Aβ deposition in the brain, without binding to other misfolded proteins (e.g., tau or α-synuclein).

^{11}C-PiB was the first Aβ-specific radiotracer to be used in PET imaging, and its structure is derived from the Aβ fluorescent dye, thioflavin T. ^{11}C-PiB exhibits significant radioactive uptake in the association cortices of AD patients, which have been previously shown to be areas with increased of Aβ deposition. Subsequent studies found that ^{11}C-PiB not only enabled the detection of Aβ deposition in AD patients, but also in certain non-dementia patients, suggesting that Aβ imaging can be used for the detection of preclinical AD. Furthermore, the results of a correlational study between ^{11}C-PiB uptake and Aβ deposition based on post-mortem examinations revealed a direct relationship between the two, thus supporting the effectiveness of ^{11}C-PiB PET in the detection of Aβ deposition.

^{18}F-florbetapir is a derivative of stilbene and its structure is based on the Aβ dye Congo red. It is the first Aβ radiotracer to be approved by the United States Food and Drug Administration (US FDA) and has fast in vivo kinetic properties. In AD patients, it begins to show a clear demarcation between cortical and cerebellar uptake around 30 min after the intravenous injection, meaning that PET scanning can start 30–50 min after the injection. Additionally, results from phase III clinical trials for this radiotracer showed a strong correlation between antemortem ^{18}F-florbetapir PET images and the distribution of Aβ deposits on post-mortem examinations.

^{18}F-florbetaben, approved by the FDA in 2014, shares a similar structure with ^{18}F-florbetapir, and has been shown to exhibit nanomolar binding affinity to synthetic Aβ fibrils and AD brain homogenates. Furthermore, sections of brains from AD patients have revealed that ^{18}F-florbetaben binds specifically to Aβ plaques, but not tau to protein or α-synuclein deposits, demonstrating the high specificity of this imaging agent for Aβ plaques. A study comparing ^{18}F-florbetaben with ^{11}C-PiB found that the two tracers were equally accurate at distinguishing between AD patients and healthy controls and showed a good correlation in the semi-quantitative analysis.

^{18}F-flutemetamol, approved by the FDA in 2013, is an ^{18}F-labeled PiB derivative with simi-

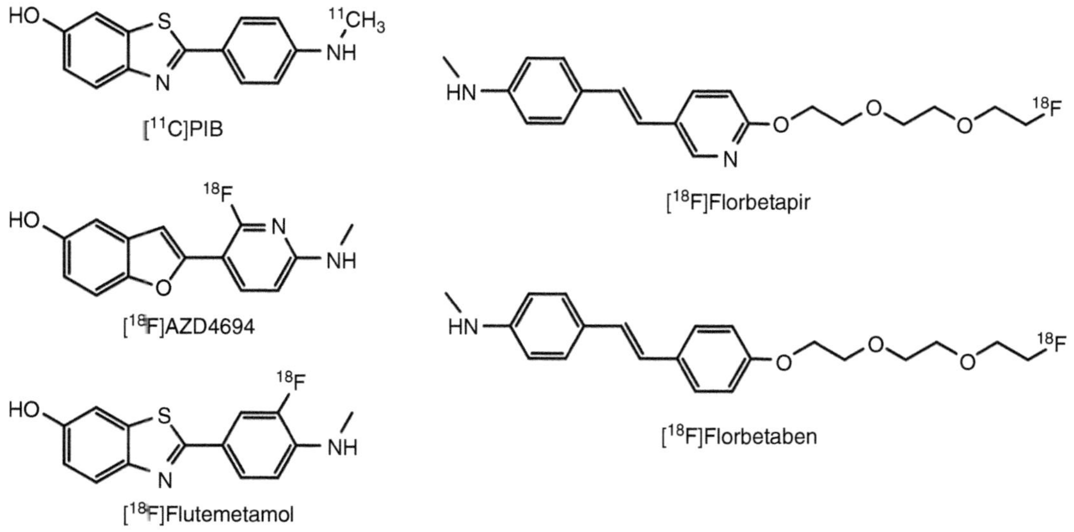

Fig. 5.2 Chemical structure of PET radiotracers for Aβ

lar kinetic properties to PiB. Studies involving the brain tissues of AD patients have revealed a strong correlation between the distribution of ^{18}F-flutemetamol and the localization of Aβ plaques in different regions of the brain. Furthermore, a dual-tracer clinical imaging study reported that the cortical uptake of ^{18}F-flutemetamol matched that of ^{11}C-PiB, while a phase III clinical trial demonstrated that ^{18}F-flutemetamol had a higher sensitivity and specificity for the detection of Aβ plaque densities in the brain.

In terms of Parkinson's disease dementia (PDD), ^{11}C-PiB PET imaging studies have detected Aβ deposition in early-stage dementia with Lewy bodies (DLB), more than the Aβ deposition of PDD but less than that observed in AD. This finding explains why DLB patients may exhibit symptoms of dementia at an earlier stage. Among patients with PDD, ^{11}C-PiB binding did not differ significantly from that in PD patients or healthy subjects. However, the detection of cortical ^{11}C-PiB uptake can predict a decline in cognitive function. Therefore, Aβ PET imaging may help us to explore the pathogenesis of PDD. As for FTLD, ^{11}C-PiB PET imaging studies revealed the absence of ^{11}C-PiB retention in the brains of FTD patients, which implies that Aβ PET imaging can be utilized to differentiate between FTD and AD.

5.2.2 PET Radiotracers for Tau Proteins

There are more challenges facing the development of tau protein tracers, including the following: (1) tau proteins have multiple subtypes and undergo different posttranslational modifications; (2) tau proteins are localized within neurons, which implies that tracers must be able to penetrate the cell membrane and the BBB; and (3) tau protein aggregates are often co-localized with Aβ plaques, but the concentration of tau protein is 5 to 20 times lower than that of Aβ plaques; therefore, not only do tau protein tracers need increased affinity but they must also have high selectivity for tau proteins over Aβ peptides. At present, a number of tau protein tracers have been utilized in clinical research, including ^{18}F-FDDNP, ^{11}C-PBB3, ^{18}F-THK5351, ^{18}F-T807, ^{18}F-MK-6240, ^{18}F-PI2620, ^{18}F-APN-1607, and ^{18}F-GTP1 (Fig. 5.3).

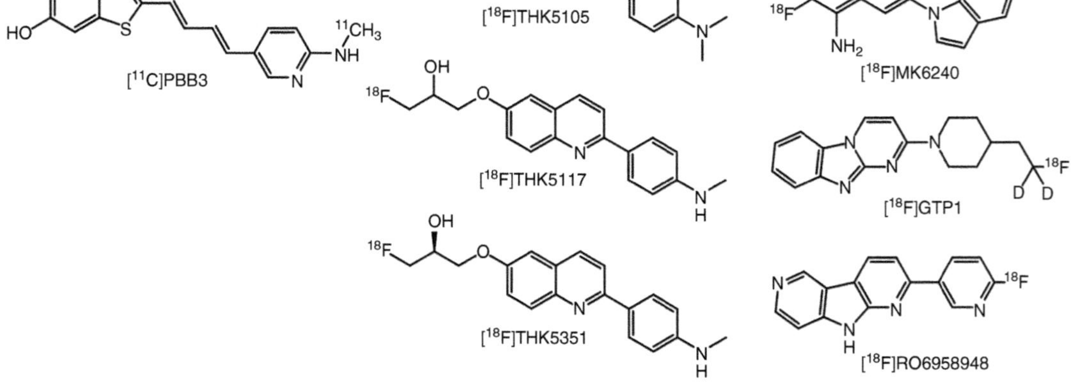

Fig. 5.3 Chemical structure of PET radiotracers for tau protein

^{18}F-FDDNP was the first tau protein PET radiotracer used for imaging the human body. However, this tracer does not bind specifically to tau protein; rather, it binds simultaneously to NFTs and Aβ plaques. PET imaging studies comparing ^{11}C-PiB and ^{18}F-FDDNP have shown that ^{18}F-FDDNP can discriminate AD patients and healthy controls, but the signal intensity of its specific binding is nine times lower than that of ^{11}C-PiB, which may have been due to the co-imaging of Aβ and tau protein.

^{11}C-PBB3 is another first-generation tau protein tracer. Based on the results of clinical studies, ^{11}C-PBB3 was found to discriminate AD patients and healthy controls, while its hippocampal uptake confirmed its ability to bind to NFTs. High ^{11}C-PBB3 binding was also detected in the medial temporal lobe, precuneus, and frontal lobe. Furthermore, ^{11}C-PBB3 uptake was found to correlate with cognitive decline and gray matter atrophy. Although PET imaging of Aβ plaques can be used to diagnose AD, this biomarker remains virtually unchanged after the appearance of clinical symptoms. ^{11}C-PBB3 PET imaging, on the other hand, successfully exhibited changes in uptake from normal aging to moderate AD, thus suggesting that tau protein PET imaging can serve as an objective indicator of disease progression. Apart from AD, ^{11}C-PBB3 imaging can also detect tau protein deposition in patients with non-AD dementia. Studies have reported that ^{11}C-PBB3 has a significant binding affinity with tau proteins in the basal ganglia of patients with corticobasal degeneration (CBD).

Quinoline derivatives (the THK series of compounds) are also considered first-generation tau protein tracers. In vitro studies involving ^{18}F-THK-523, ^{18}F-18F THK-5105, and ^{18}F-THK-5117 demonstrated high selectivity (relative to Aβ) and affinity of these compounds for tau proteins in brain sections from AD patients. In human PET imaging studies, ^{18}F-THK-523 did not clearly visualize tau protein deposition in the human brain, whereas increased ^{18}F-THK5105 and ^{18}F-THK5117 uptake was observed in common sites of tau pathologies among AD patients and was associated with the clinical severity of dementia. Furthermore, ^{18}F-THK-5117 exhibited a higher signal-to-noise ratio and superior pharmacokinetic properties. The problem with THK compounds is the high nonspecific retention in subcortical white matter, which may interfere with the visual analysis of PET images and reduce the sensitivity of tau protein deposition in early-stage AD. In order to reduce nonspecific uptake in white matter and to improve the signal-to-noise ratio of PET images, the structure of ^{18}F-THK5117 was further optimized to develop the tau protein tracer ^{18}F-THK5351. Human PET studies have found that ^{18}F-THK5351 has more rapid kinetic properties, higher contrast, and lower white matter retention. However, subsequent studies have also shown that monoamine oxidase (MAO) inhibitors can reduce ^{18}F-THK5351 uptake, thus suggesting the presence of off-target binding with MAO in the human brain, which is unfavorable for the quantitative analysis of PET images.

^{18}F-AV-1451 is currently the most widely used tau protein tracer in AD research and has been approved for marketing in the US. High ^{18}F-AV-1451 uptake can be detected in AD patients in brain regions with high tau protein aggregation and is correlated with disease severity. A phase III clinical trial found that the pattern of ^{18}F-AV-1451 uptake corresponded to NFT accumulation in patients with a Braak stage of V or VI and was consistent with the neuropathological changes of AD, as defined by the National Institute on Aging-Alzheimer's Association (NIA-AA) guidelines. However, it is worth noting that the reliability of ^{18}F-AV-1451 in lower Braak stages (e.g., stages III and IV) has yet to be confirmed. Furthermore, other studies have also demonstrated the considerable overlap in the results of tau protein imaging between healthy subjects with normal cognition and AD patients. Therefore, further research is needed to clarify the scope of application for this imaging agent.

One of the drawbacks of the first-generation PET tau protein radiotracers is that despite their predominant binding with tau protein in patients with AD, they exhibit varying levels of off-target binding. Thus, in order to improve their binding selectivity and pharmacokinetic properties, second-generation tau protein tracers were developed, which include ^{18}F-MK-6240, ^{18}F-RO6958948, ^{18}F-APN-1607, and ^{18}F-GTP1.

^{18}F-MK-6240 is a pyridine isoquinoline amine derivative that binds to paired helical filament-tau (PHF-tau) with high sensitivity and specificity, while also having excellent kinetic properties. In AD patients, ^{18}F-MK-6240 exhibits high uptake in regions with NFT accumulation (e.g., the hippocampus), but extremely low uptake in cerebellar gray matter, meaning that the latter can serve as a reference region in simplified quantitative image analysis. Preclinical studies confirmed that ^{18}F-MK-6240 does not exhibit off-target binding with MAO-A and -B, while further clinical studies have demonstrated that the distribution pattern of ^{18}F-MK-6240 in the brain is consistent with the neuropathological staging of NFTs. Furthermore, unlike ^{18}F-T807 and ^{18}F-THK5351, ^{18}F-MK-6240 does not engage in off-target binding in the basal ganglia and choroid plexus.

^{18}F-RO6958948 (RO-948) has a high affinity to the 3H-T808 binding site on tau aggregates in the brains of patient with advanced AD, while also demonstrating satisfactory pharmacokinetic and metabolic properties in mice and non-human primates. The results of preliminary clinical studies involving ^{18}F-RO6958948 PET imaging are consistent with preclinical data and show a good signal-to-noise ratio in AD patients. Another novel tracer, ^{18}F-PI-2620, has demonstrated low uptake in non-target regions, such as the choroid plexus, basal ganglia, striatum, amygdala, and meninges. Moreover, significant regional uptake was found in both patients with AD and those with progressive supranuclear palsy (PSP) compared to non-dementia controls. ^{18}F-APN-1607 (^{18}F-PM-PBB3) is an ^{18}F-labeled pyridinyl butadienyl benzothiazole (PBB) derivative with a higher signal-to-noise ratio and lower off-target binding signals than ^{11}C-PBB3. Another second-generation tau tracer, ^{18}F-GTP1, has demonstrated good in vivo stability, and its intracerebral uptake corresponds with AD pathology. In sum, the usefulness of second-generation tau tracers in clinical applications is gradually being verified through basic and clinical research.

5.2.3 PET Radiotracers for α-Synuclein

α-Synuclein is a key component of Lewy bodies, which are characteristic markers of PDD, DLB, and FTD. Thus, α-synuclein is an important pathophysiological target and a potential therapeutic target. Since α-synuclein is a type of amyloid, PET tracers that were originally developed to target Aβ (e.g., ^{11}C-PiB and ^{18}F-BF227) also had a certain level of affinity to α-synuclein. Although ^{11}C-PiB can bind to aggregated α-synuclein, it has a higher affinity to Aβ, while immunohistochemical studies have shown that ^{18}F-BF227 can bind to Lewy bodies in brain sections from PD patients. In post-mortem PD brain tissues, it was found that a novel α-synuclein tracer, ^{123}I-SIL23, could bind to α-synuclein fibrils, but this compound also exhibited high nonspecific binding in white matter, which has limited its application in imaging studies. To date, all α-synuclein tracers examined have shown off-target binding, with an especially high affinity to Aβ, and hence cannot be used for the quantitative in vivo detection of α-synuclein.

5.2.4 PET Radiotracers for the Cholinergic System

The cholinergic system is believed to play a critical role in cognition and the pathophysiology of dementia. The PET imaging targets of the cholinergic system include the presynaptic choline acetyltransferase (ChAT) and acetylcholinesterase (AChE), as well as postsynaptic muscarinic acetylcholine receptor (mAChR) and nicotinic acetylcholine receptor (nAChR).

The cholinergic hypothesis posits that the degeneration of cholinergic neurons and the subsequent reduction in cholinergic neural transmission contribute to cognitive and functional impairment in patients with AD. ^{11}C-PMP is a selective AChE tracer, and PET studies have revealed decreased AChE activity in the cortex, hippocampus, and amygdala of AD patients, which is consistent with the loss of ChAT and AChE found in AD patients upon post-mortem examinations. A PET imaging study using ^{11}C-MP4 found that carriers of the ε4 allele of apolipoprotein E (APOEε4) showed significantly higher cortical AChE activity than non-carriers, indicating that the APOEε4 allele may have protective effects against the widespread loss of AChE activity. ^{18}F-FEOBV is a novel presynaptic vesicular acetylcholine transporter (VAChT) tracer, which may serve as a potentially useful tool for studying the role of this transporter in AD patients.

^{18}F-2FA is a targeted α4β2 nAChR tracer that has been used to evaluate postsynaptic cholinergic dysfunction. In PET imaging studies, ^{18}F-2FA showed significantly reduced uptake in the frontal, parietal, and temporal lobes and the hippocampus of AD patients, which may be related to the decline in cognitive ability. However, other studies have also reported that patients with AD or mild cognitive impairment (MCI) did not exhibit a significant loss of nAChR activity compared with that in healthy controls. The novel tracer, ^{18}F-AZAN, has faster kinetic properties than ^{18}F-2FA, and can therefore better reflect cholinergic dysfunction. A PET imaging study using ^{11}C-nicotine revealed reduced nAChR binding in the frontal lobe, temporal lobe, and hippocampus of patients with moderate AD. However, ^{11}C-nicotine also has high levels of nonspecific binding and is strongly dependent on cerebral blood flow; therefore, further verification is needed for the findings of PET studies involving this tracer.

5.3 PET Radiotracers for Parkinson's Disease (PD)

PD is a chronic, progressive, neurological disease characterized by the degeneration of dopaminergic neurons and the formation of Lewy bodies in the substantia nigra. PD is considered a process of multi-system degeneration that not only targets the dopaminergic system, but also involves other central neurotransmitter systems, including the serotonergic, cholinergic, and opioid systems. In addition to patient with PD, patients with multiple system atrophy (MSA), PSP, and CBD also present with symptoms of motor dysfunction, including bradykinesia, muscle rigidity, and sometimes resting tremors. Collectively, these symptoms are known Parkinsonism. The differentiation of these diseases at the early stages is challenging, which can lead to higher rates of misdiagnosis. PET imaging has been utilized in the diagnosis and research of PD for several decades and has now become an important method of clinical examination.

5.3.1 PET Radiotracers for the Dopaminergic System

The dopaminergic neurons of the central nervous system are mostly located in the hypothalamus, substantia nigra, and ventral tegmental area, with projections into the pituitary gland (tuberoinfundibular pathway), striatum (nigrostriatal pathway), frontal cortex (mesocortical pathway), and limbic and olfactory regions (mesolimbic pathway). The nigrostriatal pathway is the main component of the dopaminergic system involved in motor control and is also the predominant pathological pathway involved in PD. Therefore, evaluating the integrity of the dopaminergic neurons in this pathway can facilitate the diagnosis and evaluation of PD. The molecular probes used to reflect the integrity of dopaminergic neurons can be divided into three categories based on their different targets: (1) probes that target aromatic L-amino acid decarboxylase (AADC) with tracers such as ^{18}F-fluoro-L-DOPA (^{18}F-FDOPA); (2) probes that target the dopamine transporter (DAT) and are primarily tropane compounds, including PET tracers such as ^{11}C-CFT, ^{18}F-FP-CIT, and ^{18}F-FE-PE2I, as well as single photon emission computed tomography (SPECT) imaging agents such as ^{123}I-FP-CIT and ^{99m}Tc-TRODAT-1; and (3) probes that target vesicular monoamine transporter 2 (VMAT2), with tracers including radiolabeled dihydrotetrabenazine derivatives, ^{11}C-DTBZ and ^{18}F-FP-DTBZ (^{18}F-AV133) (Fig. 5.4). These targets are all located on the presynaptic membranes of dopaminergic neurons, and therefore reflect the condition of neu-

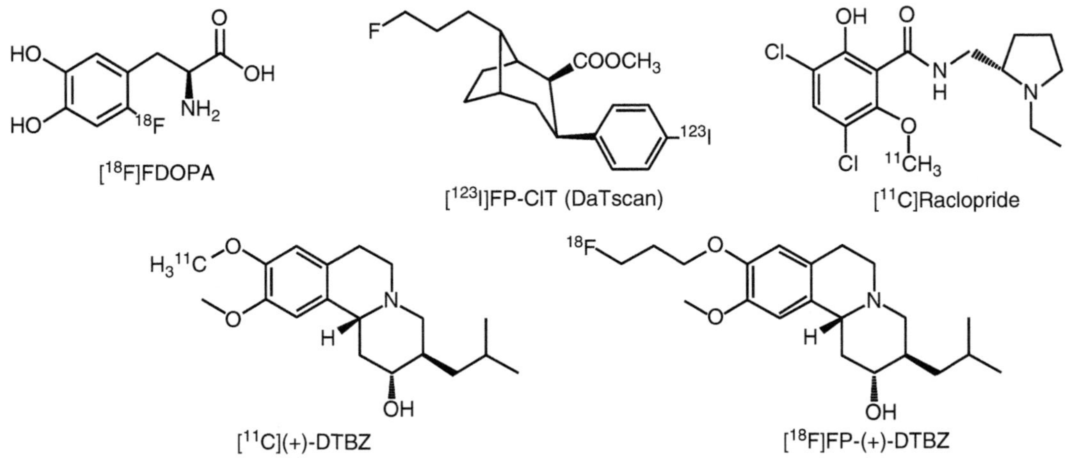

Fig. 5.4 Common PET radiotracers for the brain dopaminergic system

rons projecting from the substantia nigra to the striatum.

There are five processes involved in the striatal uptake of ^{18}F-FDOPA: (1) transport across the BBB; (2) uptake by dopaminergic neurons; (3) decarboxylation under the action of AADC to produce ^{18}F-dopamine; (4) storage of ^{18}F-dopamine in vesicles; and (5) degradation of ^{18}F-dopamine under the actions of MAO-B and catechol-*O*-methyltransferase (COMT). During these processes, AADC activity and axonal synaptic density are the major determinants of ^{18}F-FDOPA uptake. Post-mortem examinations have demonstrated that striatal ^{18}F-FDOPA uptake can reflect the number of residual dopaminergic neurons in the substantia nigra of PD patients and MPTP-induced monkey models. Nevertheless, it should be noted that due to the compensatory upregulation of residual terminal AADC, ^{18}F-FDOPA may underrepresent the extent of damage in early-stage PD.

By the time PD patients develop motor symptoms, their putamen ^{18}F-FDOPA uptake has been reduced by 50%. Several studies have revealed significant negative correlations of ^{18}F-FDOPA uptake with the Hoehn & Yahr stage and the severity of the movement disorder as measured by the Unified Parkinson's Disease Rating Scale (UPDRS). Further analyses revealed that putamen ^{18}F-FDOPA uptake is also inversely proportional to the extent of rigidity and bradykinesia, but not directly proportional to the severity of tremors. These results suggest that the pathogenic mechanism of tremors may not involve the nigrostriatal pathway. The process of neurodegeneration occurs non-uniformly across various regions of the brain in PD patients. The dopaminergic neurons projecting from the ventrolateral substantia nigra into the dorsal putamen are the first to be affected, followed by those projecting from the dorsomedial substantia nigra into the anterior part of the putamen and caudate nucleus. Therefore, in the striatum of PD patients, the greatest reduction in ^{18}F-FDOPA uptake is found in the posterior putamen, with smaller reductions in the caudate nucleus and the anterior putamen. It is worth noting that ^{18}F-FDOPA uptake does not strictly reflect residual synaptic density, as radiotracer uptake is a reflection of both neuronal loss and the effects of compensatory mechanisms, such as the upregulation of AADC activity. ^{18}F-FDOPA PET imaging can also serve as a biomarker for PD progression. When compared with age-matched controls, PD patients showed a faster rate of decrease in striatal ^{18}F-FDOPA uptake. Furthermore, among patients with early-stage PD, the amount of putamen uptake decreased by approximately 10% of the baseline level each year (compared to an average of 5% in healthy controls), whereas patients with advanced PD showed a slower rate of decline due to the floor effect.

Tracers targeting DAT are primarily tropane compounds based on the structure of cocaine. Currently, several imaging agents have been used in human imaging or for clinical application studies, of which the ^{123}I-labeled SPECT imaging agent, ^{123}I-FP-CIT, has been approved for marketing in Europe and the US (trade name: DaTScan™). Several studies have confirmed the value of utilizing DAT imaging to determine the correlation between PD and striatal dopamine deficiency, as DAT imaging has now become the most important method for detecting striatal dopamine deficiency. Despite the differences in the kinetic properties and target affinity among different DAT tracers, all of them provide similar information regarding presynaptic dopaminergic neurons. Nevertheless, it is worth noting that DAT imaging may underrepresent the density of nerve terminals, as DAT activity may be downregulated in the remaining neurons as a compensatory response to the reduced dopamine concentration in the synaptic cleft. Furthermore, DAT activity may also be affected by drugs, and therefore controversy remains over the use of DAT tracers to monitor disease progression and evaluate therapeutic efficacy.

^{11}C-DTBZ and ^{18}F-FP-DTBZ have been adopted as PET tracers for VMAT2 in clinical settings. PET studies of the brain in PD patients have revealed significant reductions in striatal ^{11}C-DTBZ uptake. In a PET study comparing the measurement of striatal dopaminergic nerve terminals using three imaging agents—^{11}C-DTBZ, ^{18}F-FDOPA, and ^{11}C-methylphenidate (^{11}C-MP, a DAT tracer)—the results indicated that when compared with ^{11}C-DTBZ, the measurements based on ^{18}F-FDOPA were slightly higher, whereas those based on ^{11}C-MP were slightly lower. These findings were interpreted as the relative upregulation of AADC and downregulation of DAT in the striatum of PD patients, which signifies that VMAT2-targeted PET imaging may be a more accurate method for measuring the density of dopaminergic nerve terminals.

PET imaging of dopamine receptors can be used to measure the dopaminergic status of the postsynaptic membrane, providing information related to dopamine transmission. The dopamine receptors on the postsynaptic membranes of dopaminergic neurons are classified into two main families: the D1-like family (including receptors D1 and D5) and the D2-like family (including receptors D2, D3, and D4). PET imaging studies of D1 receptors using the radiotracers ^{11}C-SCH23390 and ^{11}C-NNC112 found no significant differences in D1 receptor density between PD patients and healthy controls. However, this may have been due to the relatively low selectivity of the D1 receptor tracers; therefore, these findings will require further validation. More extensive research has been conducted on the PET imaging of D2 receptors. ^{11}C-raclopride has a moderate affinity to D2 receptors and can compete with endogenous dopamine; therefore, this tracer can be used to evaluate the concentration of dopamine in the synaptic cleft during disease and treatment. ^{18}F-fallypride and ^{11}C-FLB-457 have high target affinities and can be utilized for the quantitative analysis of postsynaptic dopamine receptor density in the striatum.

5.3.2 PET Radiotracers for the Serotonergic System

A wide range of radiolabeled molecular probes has been utilized in PET imaging studies of the serotonergic system. ^{11}C-DASB is a specific tracer for serotonin transporter (SERT) that can be used to evaluate the function of serotonergic nerve terminals. A ^{11}C-DASB PET study involving advanced PD patients found that ^{11}C-DASB uptake was lower than healthy controls in the orbitofrontal cortex, caudate nucleus, putamen, and midbrain regions, suggesting the involvement of serotonergic neurons in advanced PD, whereas the dorsolateral prefrontal regions associated with depression did not exhibit significant reductions. These findings are similar to the conclusions of ^{123}I-β-CIT SPECT imaging studies of PD patients with and without depressive symptoms.

^{11}C-WAY-100635 is a PET tracer for 5-HT1A receptors, which are primarily located at the presynaptic membranes in the raphe nuclei, where they serve to suppress the release of serotonin. On the contrary, 5-HT1A receptors in cortical pyramidal neurons and glial cells are mainly located at the postsynaptic membranes. The concentration of 5-HT1A receptors is highest in the hippocampus and limbic cortex, relatively low in the striatum, and absent in the cerebellum. A PET imaging study based on ^{11}C-WAY-100635 demonstrated that PD patients exhibited 25% lower ^{11}C-WAY100635 uptake in the raphe nuclei compared to healthy controls, while the extent of uptake reduction was similar between PD patients with and without depressive symptoms. These results suggest that serotonergic impairment may be unrelated to depression in PD. Another study found that the severity of overall tremors and resting tremors was associated with decreased 5-HT1A binding in the raphe nuclei. These results will help to further our understanding on the pathogenic mechanism of tremors in the midbrain tegmental area.

5.3.3 Other Targeted PET Radiotracers

^{11}C-diprenorphine is a molecular probe for the PET imaging of opioid receptors. This tracer is used to detect the striatal and extra-striatal binding of opioid receptors in patients with dyskinetic and non-dyskinetic PD, the results of which revealed significantly reduced striatal and thalamic uptake in dyskinetic patients, but no significant changes in non-dyskinetic patients. Furthermore, Statistical Parametric Mapping (SPM) analysis showed decreased radiotracer uptake in the cingulate gyrus and prefrontal cortex, which corresponds to the elevated endogenous opioid transmitters in the brains of dyskinetic PD patients.

^{11}C-SCH442416 is an imaging agent specific to the adenosine A2A receptor. PET imaging studies of dyskinetic and non-dyskinetic PD patients have revealed normal A2A binding in non-dyskinetic patients, but elevated striatal A2A uptake in the dyskinetic PD patients. These results suggest that the deficit in adenosine activity may play a role in causing levodopa-induced dyskinesia (LID) among PD patients.

Phosphodiesterases (PDEs), such as PDE10A, serve to mediate the metabolism of cyclic adenosine monophosphate (cAMP), in turn regulating striatal cAMP signaling. Animal models of PD have shown that dopaminergic lesions in the substantia nigra and striatum can lead to elevated cAMP levels, while treatment with levodopa can reduce the elevated cAMP levels in denervated striatum. Other animal model studies have also demonstrated that using PDE10A inhibitors for pharmacological regulation can mitigate the severity of LID. ^{11}C-IMA107 is a tracer targeting PDE10A. In clinical studies, PD patients showed reduced ^{11}C-IMA107 uptake in the caudate nucleus, putamen, and globus pallidus, which was associated with the severity of motor symptoms as measured by the UPDRS-Part III motor scores and Unified Dyskinesia Rating Scale scores. These findings indicate that the degeneration of nigrostriatal neurons can affect the expression of PDE10A.

Cannabinoid receptor type I (CB1) is a modulator of synaptic transmission and is considered a potential therapeutic target for LID, and ^{18}F-MK-9470 is a selective CB1 tracer. In a PET imaging study using ^{18}F-MK-9470, PD patients showed increased uptake in the nigrostriatal, mesolimbic, and mesocortical dopaminergic projection areas. However, CB1 availability did not differ significantly between patients with and without LID and did not correlate with LID severity.

Noradrenergic dysfunction may also play a crucial role in PD-related complications. A PET imaging study based on the noradrenaline transporter tracer, ^{11}C-MeNER, showed reduced uptake among PD patients, which may be associated with sleep behavior disorder, cognitive ability, and orthostatic hypotension. Therefore, noradrenergic impairment in PD patients may give rise to non-motor symptoms.

5.4 PET Radiotracers for Epilepsy

Epilepsy is a common neurological disease characterized by seizures. Its incidence, based on epidemiological surveys, is about 5–7%, while the total number of patients in China is approximately 6.5–9.1 million. The fundamental cause of epileptic seizures is the highly synchronized, abnormal electrical discharge of neurons in the brain induced by a variety of underlying causes. The utilization of ^{18}F-FDG PET imaging in epilepsy research began in the 1980s, and early studies revealed that focal gray matter hypometabolism was associated with the localization of epileptic foci. Thus, this technique was extensively implemented in the pre-operative assessment of epilepsy treatment. However, with the increasing utilization of high-resolution MRI, the use of PET imaging for the localization of epileptic foci began to decline. At the same time, however, the emergence and application of targeted tracers meant that PET imaging in epilepsy began shifting toward studying the neurochemical changes in the brain. In the following section, we will focus on targeted PET radiotracers that have been used for studying epilepsy in humans.

5.4.1 PET Radiotracers for γ-Aminobutyric Acid (GABA)

^{11}C-flumazenil (^{11}C-FMZ) has been widely used in PET imaging studies of epilepsy. This imaging agent binds to the benzodiazepine site on the $GABA_A$ receptor complex and has shown good results in the localization and lateralization of epileptic foci. ^{11}C-FMZ has shown decreased uptake in hippocampal sclerosis and vascular lesions and increased uptake in regions of dysgenesis. Among patients with non-lesional focal epilepsy, ^{11}C-FMZ PET imaging has revealed that the frequency of epileptic seizures is negatively correlated with uptake in the frontal piriform cortex. An alternative tracer, ^{18}F-FMZ, which has a longer half-life, has also shown promising imaging results, and has been used in a wide range of clinical applications.

5.4.2 PET Radiotracers for Glutamate

Glutamate is the main excitatory neurotransmitter of the central nervous system and is released during the preictal and ictal stages of epileptic seizures. The *N*-methyl-D-aspartate (NMDA) glutamate receptor is closely related to excitotoxic neuronal damage and epileptogenesis. PET imaging studies using ^{11}C-labeled ketamine have found reduced regional uptake in patients with temporal lobe epilepsy, which may have been due to the reduced NMDA receptor density, reduced perfusion, or focal atrophy. ^{18}F-GE-179 is a novel NMDA tracer. A prospective study based on this tracer found that epileptic patients not taking antidepressants showed significantly elevated uptake compared to the control group, and four of the eight patients had focally increased signals, whereas epileptic patients taking antidepressants exhibited significantly decreased global uptake. These results suggest that the NMDA receptor may play an important role in the pharmaceutical treatment of epilepsy.

5.4.3 PET Radiotracers for Synaptic Vesicle Glycoprotein 2A (SV2A)

SV2A-targeted PET tracers can reflect the integrity of synaptic connections in the brain, and their structures are based on the antiepileptic drugs brivaracetam and levetiracetam. The first SV2A tracers to be examined included ^{11}C-UCB-A, ^{11}C-UCB-J, and ^{18}F-UCB-H, of which ^{11}C-UCB-J has excellent pharmacokinetic properties with high brain uptake, rapid and reversible binding kinetics, and good metabolic properties; ^{11}C-UCB-A has relatively slow in vivo kinetic properties; and ^{18}F-UCB-H has poor target affinity. In human PET studies, ^{11}C-UCB-J showed ideal imaging characteristics and high specific binding signals; therefore, its application has been expanded to encompass research on epilepsy, AD, PD, and other diseases. A research team at Yale University subsequently developed ^{18}F-labeled SV2A imaging agents with longer half-lives, including ^{18}F-UCB-J, ^{18}F-SDM-2, and ^{18}F-SDM-8 (Fig. 5.5). A study involving ^{18}F-UCB-J in non-human primates found that it had similar pharmacokinetic properties, regional distribution, and target affinity to ^{11}C-UCB-J. ^{18}F-SDM-2 showed faster brain pharmacokinetics than ^{11}C-UCB-J and comparable regional dis-

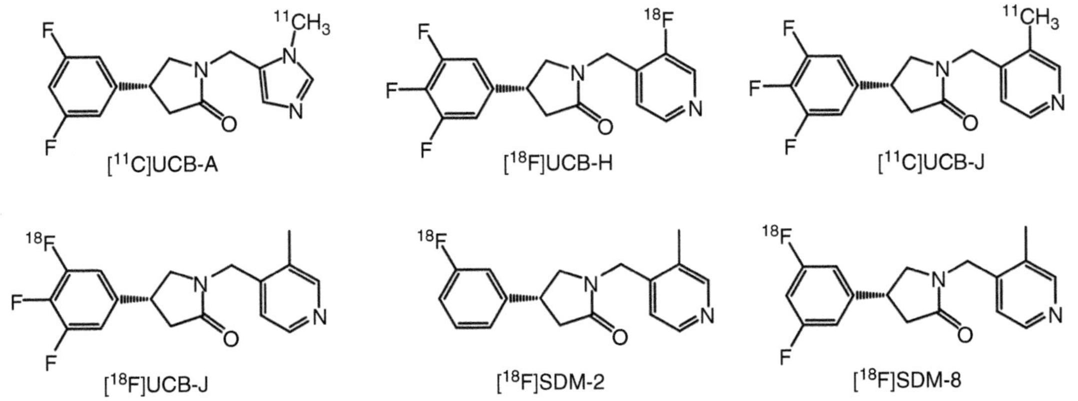

Fig. 5.5 Chemical structure of PET tracers for the SV2A receptor

tribution and regional target affinity. ^{18}F-SDM-8 exhibited similar pharmacokinetic properties to ^{11}C-UCB-J, with a higher regional target affinity.

5.5 PET Radiotracers for Depression

Depression, also known as major depressive disorder, is clinically characterized by marked and persistent low mood, loss of interest, and other emotional (mood) disorders. Approximately 20% of the Chinese population experiences depressive symptoms, of whom 7% have severe depression. PET imaging can be used to evaluate the brain functional metabolism and neurochemical changes based on glucose metabolism, receptor distribution, and receptor activity, enabling us to explore the pathogenic mechanisms of depression. Selective serotonin reuptake inhibitors (SSRIs) are an important class of antidepressants that can indirectly demonstrate the critical role of the serotonergic system in relation to the occurrence and development of depression. SERT is a target of SSRIs, and PET tracers targeting this receptor have been extensively utilized in research on depression.

5.5.1 PET Radiotracers for SERT

SERT is an Na^+/Cl^- dependent transporter that is distributed throughout the brain and spinal cord but is most densely localized in the raphe nuclei. SERT-specific inhibitors are an important class of antidepressant drugs and include fluoxetine, sertraline, and paroxetine, among others. SERT-targeting PET imaging agents can be divided, based on their chemical structures, into diaryl sulfide, tropane, quipazine, and isoquinoline compounds. Of these drugs, diaryl sulfide compounds have been most widely used in research and clinical use, examples of which include ^{11}C-DASB, ^{11}C-HOMADAM, ^{11}C-AFM, ^{11}C-ADAM, ^{11}C-MADAM, 4-^{18}F-ADAM, and ^{18}F-FPBM.

^{11}C-DASB is currently the most widely used SERT-targeted PET imaging agent. It was first reported in 2000, as exhibiting high uptake in the raphe nuclei and hypothalamus, where SERT is highly expressed, but with minimal uptake in the cerebellum, where SERT distribution is limited. Furthermore, PET imaging studies have shown that citalopram can competitively inhibit ^{11}C-DASB uptake in the raphe nuclei and hypothalamus; however, the widespread application of ^{11}C-DASB is restricted by its short physical half-life and low production yield. Another radiotracer, 4-^{18}F-ADAM, was introduced in 2003, and has a higher initial brain uptake and faster clearance in non-target regions. The first human imaging study using 4-^{18}F-ADAM was reported in 2013, the results of which showed that this compound could meet the requirements of clinical imaging, but clinical application was restricted due to its extremely low production yield. ^{18}F-FPBM was first reported in 2007, as exhibiting high affinity and selectivity to SERT, with a high production yield and successful application in the PET imaging of monkey brains.

5.5.2 PET Radiotracers for the Serotonin 1A (5-HT$_{1A}$) Receptor

Based on animal model studies, 5-HT$_{1A}$ receptor knockout mice exhibited anxiety- and depression-like behaviors under controlled conditions. Furthermore, the use of compounds targeting the 5-HT$_{1A}$ receptor as antidepressants is currently in the clinical trial phase. PET tracers targeting the 5-HT$_{1A}$ receptor have undergone more than 30 years of research and development, many of which have been applied in human imaging studies. PET tracers for 5-HT$_{1A}$ can be divided into antagonists and agonists. The antagonists include ^{11}C-WAY100635, ^{11}C-DWAY, ^{11}C-®-RWAY, ^{11}C-6FPWAY, ^{11}C-6BPWAY, ^{11}C-CPC-222, ^{18}F-MeFWAY, ^{18}F-MPPF, ^{18}F-FCWAY and ^{18}F-DMPPF; and the agonists include ^{11}C-MPT, ^{18}F-F15599, ^{18}F-F13714, and ^{18}F-FEMPT.

^{11}C-WAY100635 was the first antagonistic 5-HT$_{1A}$ PET tracer to be tested, but its radioactive metabolites could pass through the BBB and therefore affected quantitative image analysis. ^{18}F-MPPF is currently the most widely used 5-HT$_{1A}$ PET tracer, with human imaging studies demonstrating a target/non-target ratio > 3 in PET images and the absence of metabolite effects on image analysis. An ^{18}F-MPPF PET normative database of a variety of ages and genders has now been established, which has strongly promoted the application of this tracer in research studies. Agonistic 5-HT$_{1A}$ PET tracers only bind to G-protein coupled receptors in the high-affinity state, and hence can better reflect the 5-HT$_{1A}$ binding and activation of exogenous drugs compared to antagonistic tracers. ^{11}C-MPT was the first successful agonistic PET tracer reported, but it has a slow brain clearance rate, resulting in a low signal-to-noise ratio. Research is ongoing for other novel agonistic tracers, such as ^{18}F-F15599, ^{18}F-F13714, and ^{18}F-FEMPT.

5.6 PET Radiotracers for Neuroinflammation

Inflammation may play a key role in the process of neurodegeneration, as the activation of neuroimmune cells has consistently been observed in neurodegeneration involving different pathological mechanisms. This implies that neuroinflammation is not specifically related to any particular pathologies, but instead reflects a generalized neurodegenerative process. PET imaging agents targeting neuroinflammation have helped further our understanding on the role of neuroinflammation in the occurrence and development of diseases.

5.6.1 PET Radiotracers for the 18 kD Translocator Protein (TSPO)

TSPO is overexpressed on the mitochondrial membrane of activated microglia and is believed to be a PET tracer targeting neuroinflammation. The first-generation TSPO tracer, ^{11}C-PK11195, is the most widely used neuroinflammation imaging agent that reflects microglial activation. However, it has certain drawbacks, such as high levels of nonspecific binding and low brain uptake, which have resulted in its poor signal-to-noise ratio in imaging. Therefore, second-generation TSPO tracers were subsequently developed, including ^{11}C-PBR28, ^{11}C-DAA1106, ^{11}C-DPA-713, ^{18}F-DPA-714, ^{18}F-FEDAA1106, ^{18}F-FEPPA, ^{18}F-PBR06, and ^{18}F-PBR111. These tracers have higher specificity and affinity, but different sensitivities to a single nucleotide polymorphism (*rs6971*) in the TSPO gene, which affects their target affinity, leading to differences in PET imaging results. In recent years, third-generation TSPO radioligands that are insensitive to the *rs6971* polymorphism have been reported, including ^{11}C-ER176 and ^{18}F-GE180. ^{11}C-ER176 showed a high affinity to all *rs6971* genotypes in humans, allowing the quantification of TSPO levels in all subjects. Preliminary clinical studies on ^{18}F-GE180 showed lower brain uptake in healthy controls compared to ^{11}C-ER176, which may give rise to a higher signal-to-noise ratio, but further confirmation is needed in subjects with different *rs6971* genotypes.

5.6.2 Other Targeted PET Radiotracers

MAO-B has been found to be highly expressed among reactive astrocytes in certain neuroinflammatory diseases (e.g., AD). Thus, radiolabeled selective MAO-B antagonists have been utilized in the PET imaging of astrocytes, of which ^{11}C-deprenyl-D2 has been most commonly used. ^{11}C-deprenyl-D2 has excellent kinetic properties, but caution is advised when analyzing its PET findings, as MAO-B is also highly expressed in serotonergic and histaminergic neurons.

Cyclooxygenase-1 (COX-1) is upregulated in activated microglia, and targeted imaging using ^{11}C-KTP-ME has been performed in healthy volunteers. However, controversy remains as to whether COX-1 is only expressed microglia, so further research is needed to verify the selectivity and application of COX-1 tracers in diseases.

The adenosine A_{2A} receptor is involved in key neuroinflammatory processes, such as lipopolysaccharide-induced synaptic plasticity alteration and microglial retraction during activation. A ^{11}C-TMSX PET study of patients with secondary progressive multiple sclerosis found elevated uptake in normal-appearing white matter, and these regions were known to contain activated glial cells. Further analysis indicated that tracer uptake was negatively correlated with white matter integrity, as measured using MRI, thus suggesting that A_{2A} receptors are involved in the pathological alterations of white matter. It should be noted, however, that the A_{2A} receptor is expressed by all immune cells in the central nervous system. Hence, as with TSPO, it may be difficult to obtain specific information regarding glial cells through A_{2A} receptor imaging.

The nicotinic acetylcholine (nACh) system is responsible for regulating a number of important physiological functions and is closely related to neuroinflammation. In PET imaging studies on animal models, the α4β2-nAChR imaging agent, 2-^{18}F-A85380 showed similar distribution patterns to the TSPO imaging agent, ^{11}C-PK1119578. Furthermore, histological findings indicate that TSPO and α4β2-nAChR are upregulated simultaneously in activated microglia and astrocytes, suggesting that α4β2 may be an imaging agent for glial cell activation like TSPO. The targeted tracer ^{18}F-flubatine has been utilized in human imaging but is limited by its poor kinetic properties and long image acquisition time. Therefore, further investigations are needed to develop more superior PET tracers.

5.7 Summary

Radiotracers used for PET imaging of the brain have undergone decades of research and development, eventually yielding hundreds of different tracers targeting different receptors, enzymes, and proteins. These tracers can be used to fully exploit the non-invasiveness and high sensitivity of PET imaging in the research, diagnosis, assessment, and efficacy evaluation of various neurological diseases. Some PET techniques, such as Aβ imaging for AD diagnosis and DAT imaging for PD evaluation, have come to be widely accepted. They are now crucial methods in the clinical assessment of these patients and play an increasingly important role in the development of new treatment methods, including the screening of clinical research subjects and the evaluation of intervention outcomes. The development of novel PET radiotracers for brain imaging is inextricably linked with advances in pathophysiology. On the one hand, new pathophysiological discoveries can provide research directions for the development of novel tracers, while on the other hand, the clinical application of novel tracers can serve as a tool for pathophysiological research. Additionally, due to their complexity, it is generally not possible to use single tracers to achieve the comprehensive assessment of diseases. Therefore, the combination of multi-targeted molecular probes for disease evaluation will soon become an important research direction in PET imaging of the brain.

Suggested Readings

Albert NL, Weller M, Suchorska B, et al. Response assessment in neuro-oncology working group and European association for neuro-oncology recommendations for the clinical use of PET imaging in gliomas. Neuro Oncol. 2016;18(9):1199–208.

Albrecht DS, Granziera C, Hooker JM, et al. In vivo imaging of human neuroinflammation. ACS Chem Nerosci. 2016;7(4):470–83.

Cai Z, Li S, Matuskey D, et al. PET imaging of synaptic density: a new tool for investigation of neuropsychiatric diseases. Neurosci Lett. 2019;691:44–50.

Chauveau F, Van Camp N, Dolle F, et al. Comparative evaluation of the translocator protein radioligands ^{11}C-DPA-713, ^{18}F-DPA-714, and ^{11}C-PK11195 in a rat model of acute neuroinflammation. J Nucl Med. 2009;50(3):468–76.

Doraiswamy PM, Sperling RA, Johnson K, et al. Florbetapir F 18 amyloid PET and 36-month cognitive decline: a prospective multicenter study. Mol Psychiatry. 2014;19(9):1044–51.

Fan Z, Calsolaro V, Atkinson RA, et al. Flutriciclamide (^{18}F-GE180) PET: first-in-human PET study of novel third-generation in vivo marker of human translocator protein. J Nucl Med. 2016;57(11):1753–9.

Fedorova TD, Seidelin LB, Knudsen K, et al. Decreased intestinal acetylcholinesterase in early Parkinson disease: an ^{11}C-donepezil PET study. Neurology. 2017;88(8):775–81.

Galovic M, Koepp M. Advances of molecular imaging in epilepsy. Curr Neurol Neurosci Rep. 2016;16(6):58–69.

Hayashida Y, Hirai T, Morishita S, et al. Diffusion-weighted imaging of metastatic brain tumors: comparison with histologic type and tumor cellularity. AJNR Am J Neuroradiol. 2006;27(7):1419–25.

Kebir S, Khurshid Z, Gaertner FC, et al. Unsupervised consensus cluster analysis of -18F -fluoroethyl-L-tyrosine positron emission tomography identified textural features for the diagnosis of pseudoprogression in high-grade glioma. Oncotarget. 2017;8(5):8294–304.

Kobayashi K, Hirata K, Yamaguchi S, et al. Prognostic value of volume-based measurements on (11) C-methionine PET in glioma patients. Eur J Nucl Med Mol Imaging. 2015;42(7):1071–80.

Kratochwil C, Combs SE, Leotta K, et al. Intra-individual comparison of ^{18}F-FET and ^{18}F-DOPA in PET imaging of recurrent brain tumors. Neuro Oncol. 2014;16(3):434–40.

Krohn T, Verburg FA, Pufe T, et al. ^{68}Ga-PSMA-HBED uptake mimicking lymph node metastasis in coeliac ganglia: an important pitfall in clinical practice. Eur J Nucl Med Mol Imaging. 2015;42(2):210–4.

Louis DN, Perry A, Reifenberger G, et al. The 2016 World Health Organization classification of tumors of the central nervous system: a summary. Acta Neuropathol. 2016;131(6):803–20.

Malik D, Sood A, Mittal BR, et al. Nonspecific uptake of ^{68}Ga-prostate-specific membrane antigen in diseases other than prostate malignancy on positron emission tomography/computed tomography imaging: a pictorial assay and review of literature. Indian J Nucl Med. 2018;33(4):317–25.

Marquie M, Normandin MD, Vanderburg CR, et al. Validating novel tau positron emission tomography tracer F-18-AV-1451 (T807) on postmortem brain tissue. Ann Neurol. 2015;78(5):787–800.

Nahimi A, Sommerauer M, Kinnerup MB, et al. Noradrenergic deficits in Parkinson disease imaged with ^{11}C-MeNER. J Nucl Med. 2018;59(4):659–64.

Nandu H, Wen PY, Huang RY. Imaging in neuro-oncology. Ther Adv Neurol Disord. 2018;11:1756286418759865.

Niccolini F, Foltynie T, Reis Marques T, et al. Loss of phosphodiesterase 10A expression is associated with progression and severity in Parkinson's disease. Brain. 2015;138(Pt10):3003–15.

Okubo S, Zhen HN, Kawai N, et al. Correlation of L-methyl-^{11}C-methionine (MET) uptake with L-type amino acid transporter 1 in human gliomas. J Neurooncol. 2010;99(2):217–25.

Rocchi L, Niccolini F, Politis M. Recent imaging advances in neurology. J Neurol. 2015;262(9):2182–94.

Roussakis AA, Politis M, Towey D, et al. Serotonin-to-dopamine transporter ratios in Parkinson disease: relevance for dyskinesias. Neurology. 2016;86(12):1152–8.

Sharma P, Mukherjee A, Bal C, et al. Somatostatin receptor-based PET/CT of intracranial tumors: a potential area of application for ^{68}Ga-DOTA peptides. AJR Am J Roentgenol. 2013;201(6):1340–7.

Teipel S, Drzezga A, Grothe MJ, et al. Multimodal imaging in Alzheimer's disease: validity and usefulness for early detection. Lancet Neurol. 2015;14(10):1037–53.

Van Laere K, Casteels C, Lunskens S, et al. Regional changes in type 1 cannabinoid receptor availability in Parkinson's disease in vivo. Neurobiol Aging. 2012;33(3):620.e1–8.

Wilson WR, Hay MP. Targeting hypoxia in cancer therapy. Nat Rev Cancer. 2011;11(6):393–410.

Wu K, Politis M, O'Sullivan SS, et al. Single versus multiple impulse control disorders in Parkinson's disease: an ^{11}C-raclopride positron emission tomography study of reward cue-evoked striatal dopamine release. J Neurol. 2015;262(6):1504–14.

Ye L, Velasco A, Fraser G, et al. In vitro high affinity alpha-synuclein binding sites for the amyloid imaging agent PIB are not matched by binding to Lewy bodies in postmortem human brain. J Neurochem. 2008;105(4):1428–37.

6 Research Applications of Positron Emission Tomography/Magnetic Resonance (PET/MR) Imaging in Neurosurgery

Qiongge Li, Zhenming Wang, Penghu Wei, Guoguang Zhao, and Jie Lu

Over time, medical imaging has become an inextricable part of neurosurgery. In the past, the separation between the imaging space and operative space meant that surgeons could only observe the morphology and location of the lesion on the available images. They then had to combine this information with their anatomical knowledge and imagine the shape, texture, adhesions, blood supply, and adjacent areas of the lesion, as well as its relationship with surrounding structures. This limitation imposed exacting demands on neurosurgeons in terms of clinical practice.

With the rapid development of image-guided neurosurgery techniques, surgeons are now able to fuse the imaging and operative spaces using infrared, optical, and other methods, while also performing real-time interactions. This enables surgeons to determine the optimal surgical approach based on quantitative image information, thereby minimizing the risk of inflicting damage to functional areas and important structures. Although neuronavigation continues to drive the ongoing development of image-guided neurosurgery, there are still limitations that are yet to be overcome. In traditional surgical navigation, the intra-operative images are acquired pre-operatively, and the loss of cerebrospinal fluid following craniotomy may lead to shifting of the anatomical structures. Furthermore, in cases such as gliomas, surgical microscopes cannot be used to identify a clear boundary between diseased and healthy brain parenchyma. Subsequently, the adequacy of tumor resection cannot be determined quantitatively during neurosurgery guided by traditional navigation, and many patients cannot undergo repeat resection once the craniotomy is closed. These limitations have prompted further advances in intra-operative imaging technology; therefore, in this chapter, we will focus on PET molecular imaging and image-guided neurosurgical techniques.

Q. Li · Z. Wang · P. Wei · G. Zhao (✉) · J. Lu (✉)
Department of Radiology and Nuclear Medicine, Xuanwu Hospital, Capital Medical University, Beijing, China

6.1 Multimodal Image-Guided Neurosurgery

6.1.1 Combined MRI and Neuronavigation Techniques

Due to the lack of accurate and objective anatomical evaluation in the early days of neurosurgery, there was an urgent need to integrate the anatomical and functional data provided by imaging for post-processing. Stereotactic navigation laid the foundation for the development of modern neuronavigation systems, while the fusion of medical imaging with neuronavigation systems serves as an auxiliary tool for neurosurgeons.

J. Lu, G. Zhao (eds.), *PET/MR: Functional and Molecular Imaging of Neurological Diseases and Neurosciences*, https://doi.org/10.1007/978-981-19-9902-4_6

The introduction of computed tomography (CT) and MRI provided new options in the field of neurosurgery and provided the pre-operative imaging data for neuronavigation systems. The incorporation of pre-operative imaging data into neuronavigation systems enabled the visualization of stereotactic images of structures in diseased and normal brain tissues. In 1986, Robert et al. performed the fusion of CT images with a stereotactic navigation system to facilitate surgical procedures. In 1993, Barnett et al. incorporated ultrasound, CT, and MR images within their navigation system to reconstruct three-dimensional (3D) models. In 1998, Kelly and Watanabe proposed a new navigation technique for real-time intra-operative spatial monitoring. As imaging technology continued to improve, techniques such as functional MRI (fMRI), diffusion tensor imaging (DTI), and PET further promoted the rapid development and widespread application of neuronavigation techniques.

Neuronavigation consists of two systems: image processing and surgical localization. Medical imaging data can be imported into the neuronavigation system, in which image processing and analysis performed on the two-dimensional (2D) data are used to generate 3D stereotactic images. Skin surface markers are then placed on the patient, which are used to register the patient's head with the imported 3D data to implement surgical navigation for anatomical localization. Remarkable progress has been made in image-guided neurosurgery, as represented by microsurgery for the treatment of tumors, vascular malformations, and other intracranial diseases. Computer-aided neuronavigation utilizes high-resolution, multimodal pre-operative imaging for surgical guidance, identification of relevant anatomical structures, and production of 3D images of the patient's pathology. Based on the spatial relationship of the lesion within the anatomy obtained through the analysis of human–machine interactions, relevant data and basic grayscale values can be integrated into the navigation system through the processing of pre-operative data, facilitating the evaluation of tumor resection.

The identification of functional cortical areas around lesions can be challenging because of factors such as the displacement of anatomical structures caused by the space-occupying effect or the plasticity and reorganization of the cerebral cortex. Therefore, the integration of pre-operative blood oxygen level-dependent (BOLD)-fMRI data into the neuronavigation system allows the accurate localization of intracranial lesions and adjacent functional areas, facilitating both pre-operative assessment and intra-operative guidance. Task-based BOLD-fMRI involves the use of different tasks or sensory stimuli to stimulate the corresponding functional cortical areas, resulting in changes to the local concentration of oxyhemoglobin, which in turn cause changes in magnetic susceptibility seen on BOLD-fMRI. The functional areas of the cerebral cortex that are stimulated appear as local hyperintense areas of activation. Sommer et al. combined BOLD-fMRI with other imaging techniques to acquire the functional activation maps of 19 patients with tumors in functional areas of the brain. The maps were then used to perform pre-operative assessments and to guide surgical resection. Their results indicated that total resections were achieved in 14 patients, while 5 patients showed a significant decrease in tumor volume rather than a complete resection.

DTI depends on the anisotropic diffusion of water molecules in different brain regions, which causes water molecules to generate different magnetic fields as they diffuse outwards, to reflect the course of white matter tracts. In a study on ten patients with gliomas near the cortical language areas, pre-operative DTI was used to reconstruct six fiber bundles (including the arcuate, fronto-occipital, inferior longitudinal, and uncinate fasciculi, as well as two premotor tracts), which were validated through intra-operative electrical stimulation of the cortex. The results of their study showed that the patients' language functions remained intact. Cho et al. performed pre-operative DTI scans on 123 patients with brain tumors to reconstruct their corticospinal tract (107 cases), optic radiation (31 cases), and/or arcuate fasciculus (38 cases). The DTI scans were fused with the surgical navigation, to avoid damaging the corresponding fiber bundles. Postoperative examinations revealed that the patients' fiber bundles remained intact, and the incidence of postoperative neurologic symptoms decreased.

Although image-guided neuronavigation has a broad applicability and significant value in clinical applications, one major disadvantage of this technique is that it depends on MRI data acquired pre-operatively. A number of factors, however, may cause intra-operative brain shift, including changes in gravity, loss of cerebrospinal fluid, cerebral edema, and brain tissue or tumor resection, which may diminish the effectiveness of neuronavigation during the surgical process. Therefore, it is only through intra-operative imaging that neurosurgeons are able to obtain relevant real-time data, which enable them to perform true intra-operative image-guided neurosurgery. Intra-operative MRI (iMRI) has recently become the most accurate and reliable means of addressing intra-operative brain shift during neuronavigation. A meta-analysis found that patients who underwent iMRI combined with traditional surgical navigation had higher survival rates than those who underwent only traditionally navigated surgery. Thus, iMRI is an ideal method for intra-operative image guidance. PET-guided navigation techniques are also important tools for functional neurosurgery and the treatment of brain tumors, particularly gliomas, as they can provide the details of tumor infiltration beyond the hyperintensities. With the advances in PET techniques, integrated PET/MR-guided navigation has been utilized for needle biopsies in clinical settings. The gradual development of integrated PET/MR navigation in the setting of surgical craniotomy will contribute substantially to glioma surgery in the future.

6.1.2 Combined Application of Multimodal Imaging Data and Neuronavigation

The combined application of multimodal imaging data and neuronavigation techniques is gradually evolving, and is widely utilized in the field of neurosurgery, including brain tumor resection, cerebrovascular malformation surgery, epilepsy surgery, and brain biopsy. The implementation of iMRI systems has contributed to the widespread application of a surgical model involving the combination of pre-operative imaging data with neuronavigation for surgical planning. Furthermore, intra-operative real-time MRI is integrated with neuronavigation for the precise localization of tumor margins. Some studies have reported that multimodal imaging combined with intra-operative navigation offers significant clinical value with respect to the precise localization of lesions, selection of the optimal surgical path, improvement of total resection rates, and reduction of postoperative complications.

In terms of tumor characteristics, Xuanwu Hospital has formulated pre-, intra-, and postoperative multimodal MRI acquisition protocols on the basis of its existing 3.0 T iMRI technique, which include conventional T1- and T2-weighted imaging (T1WI, T2WI; Fig. 6.1), magnetic resonance spectroscopy (MRS, Fig. 6.2), DTI (Fig. 6.3), and fMRI (Fig. 6.4). This iMRI system is dependent on the ceiling-mounted intra-operative guide rail system, on which a 1.5-ton, 70 cm diameter magnet can be moved from the magnet room to the operating theater. This system allows the magnet to be shared between two operating theaters. The magnet room is separated from the operating room by a screen door, and when the magnet is not being used for intra-operative scanning, it can be used for routine diagnostic research.

Multimodal imaging allows the differentiation of anatomical and pathological changes in patients both before and during surgery, while also enabling the real-time observation of intra-operative brain shift and the status of the tumor resection. It contributes to the implementation of real-time intra-operative navigation, thus providing neurosurgeons with an intuitive and reliable imaging-based reference. MRS can be applied in clinical neurosurgery to differentiate recurrent and primary lesions, assist in tumor grading, confirm the tumor margins, and follow up on the prognostic outcomes of tumors. When combined with intra-operative DTI, shifts or damage to

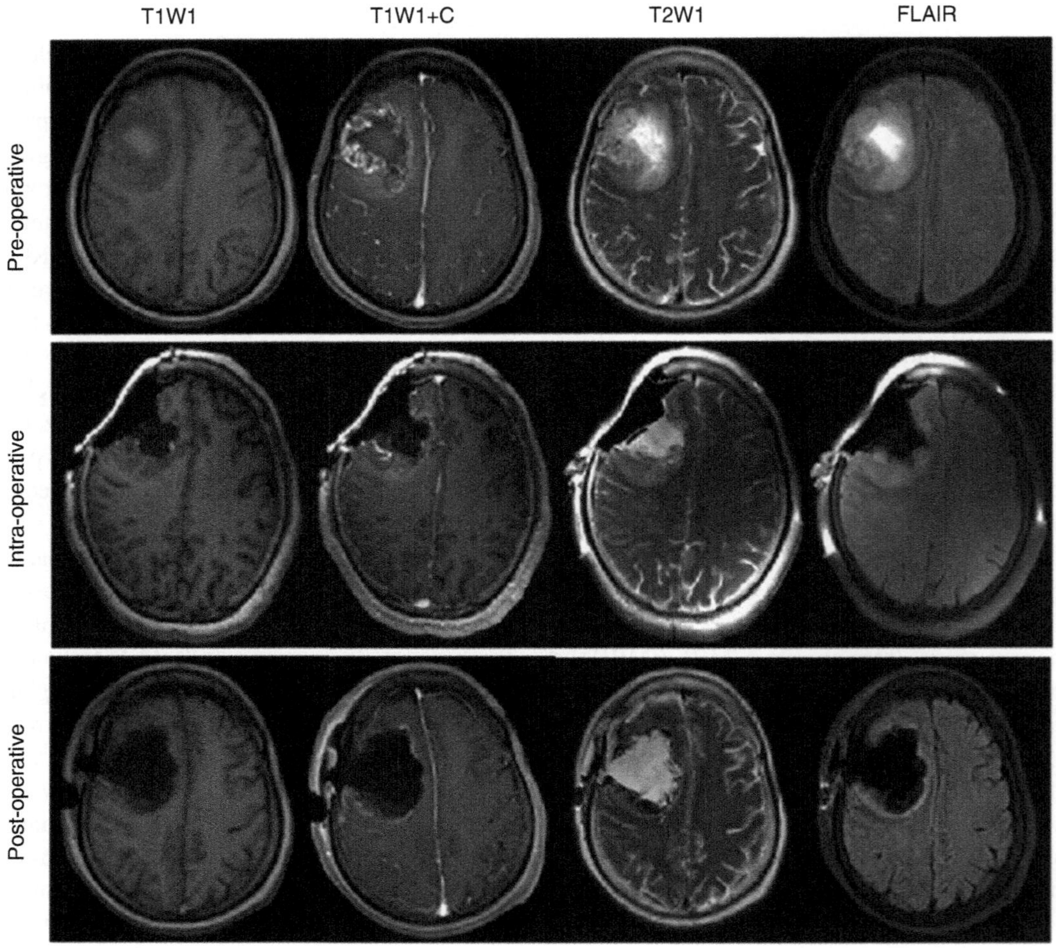

Fig. 6.1 A 70-year-old female patient admitted with memory loss for >7 months; postoperative pathological diagnosis: glioblastoma, WHO grade IV. The pre-operative MRI shows a right frontal lobe tumor. The patient's pre-operative imaging was used in pre-surgical planning to delineate the extent of the tumor. The intra-operative MRI shows a small amount of residual tumor, whereas the postoperative MRI after the repeat resection shows that the tumor has been completely resected

white matter tracts can be observed in a timely manner, and the intra-operative recovery of damaged white matter tracts can be monitored, thereby preventing postoperative neurological deficits. BOLD-fMRI is widely utilized in the pre-operative assessment of brain tumors, and can contribute significantly to both surgical planning and the minimization of intra-operative functional damage. When combined with neuronavigation systems, these multimodal imaging methods can provide targeted assistance to pre-operative planning in terms of brain structure and function. The combination of iMRI and neuronavigation allows real-time determination of the tumor resection status (Fig. 6.1) and potential damage to the white matter tracts. Postoperative MRI can then help to evaluate the postoperative recovery of the patient's brain tissues (Fig. 6.1) and fiber bundles (Fig. 6.3).

PET imaging has unique advantages in revealing the proliferation of gliomas, as well as delineating the tumor boundaries. Thus, its application in neuronavigation systems can facilitate precise biopsy localization and maximize tumor resec-

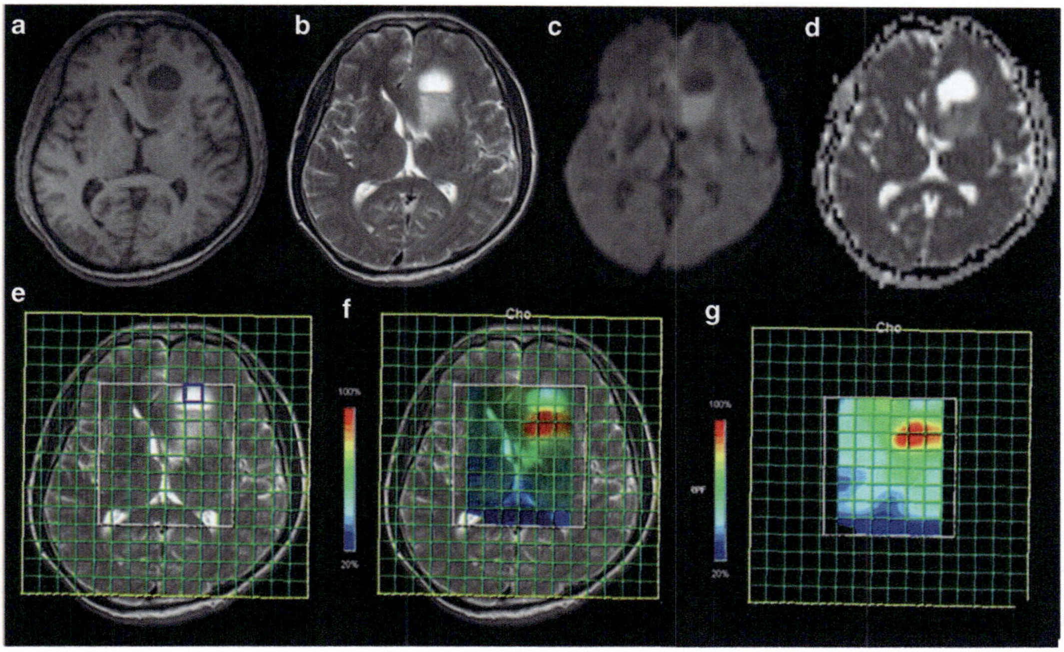

Fig. 6.2 A 67-year-old male patient admitted with recurrent seizures for >1 month; postoperative pathological diagnosis: glioblastoma in the left frontal lobe with IDH mutation, WHO grade IV. The pre-operative MRI (**a–d**) shows a left frontal lobe tumor. MRS (**e–g**) was performed with a threshold of Cho/NAA = 1 to confirm the boundaries of the solid part of the tumor

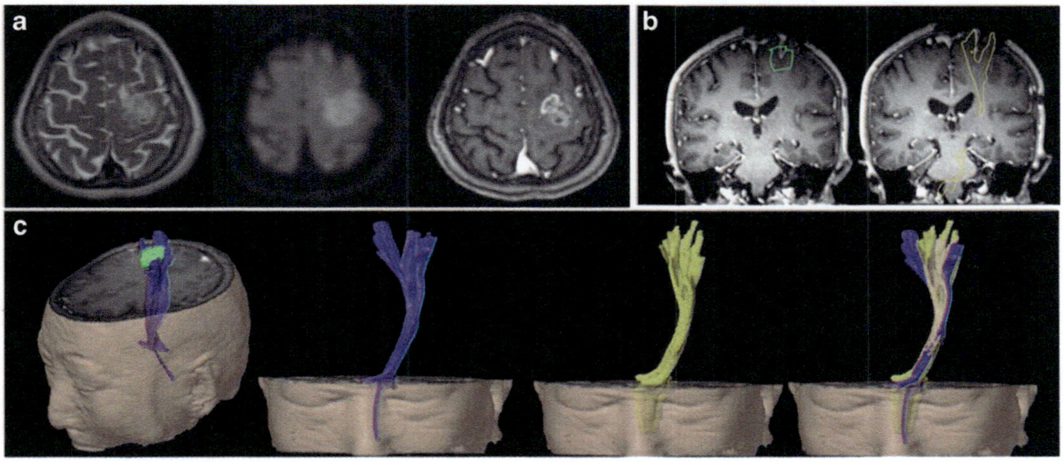

Fig. 6.3 A 65-year-old female patient admitted with intermittent epilepsy for 1 month; postoperative pathological diagnosis: left frontal lobe glioblastoma, WHO grade IV. The pre-operative MRI shows a left frontal lobe tumor (**a**). The green represents the tumor boundary drawn based on pre-operative images and the yellow represents the boundary of the left pyramidal tract drawn based on pre-operative DTI (**b**). The green represents the tumor location; purple, the pyramidal tract based on pre-operative DTI; and yellow, location of the pyramidal tract after tumor resection based on intra-operative DTI (**c**). Before surgery, the tumor is seen pushing against the adjacent pyramidal tract, whereas after surgery, the pyramidal tract has shifted. A significant difference can be observed when comparing the purple and yellow fiber bundles. After the surgery, the patient's motor functions were unimpaired, which suggested good intra-operative protection of the fiber bundles

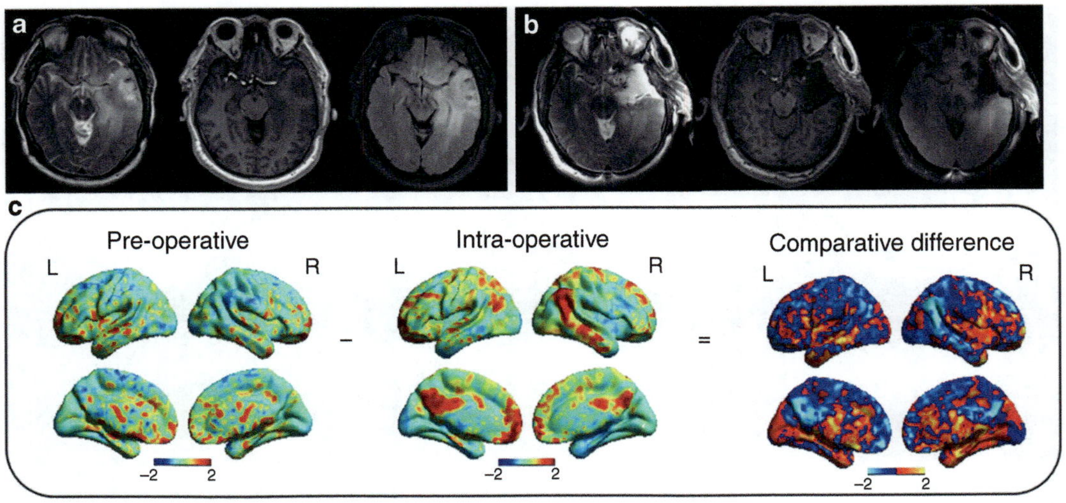

Fig. 6.4 A 40-year-old male patient with a right frontal lobe space-occupying lesion for 3 months; postoperative pathological diagnosis: left temporal lobe oligodendroastrocytoma, WHO grade III. Pre-operative MRI (**a**). Intra-operative imaging (**b**). The pre- and intra-operative levels of global functional connectivity, and their comparative differences (**c**)

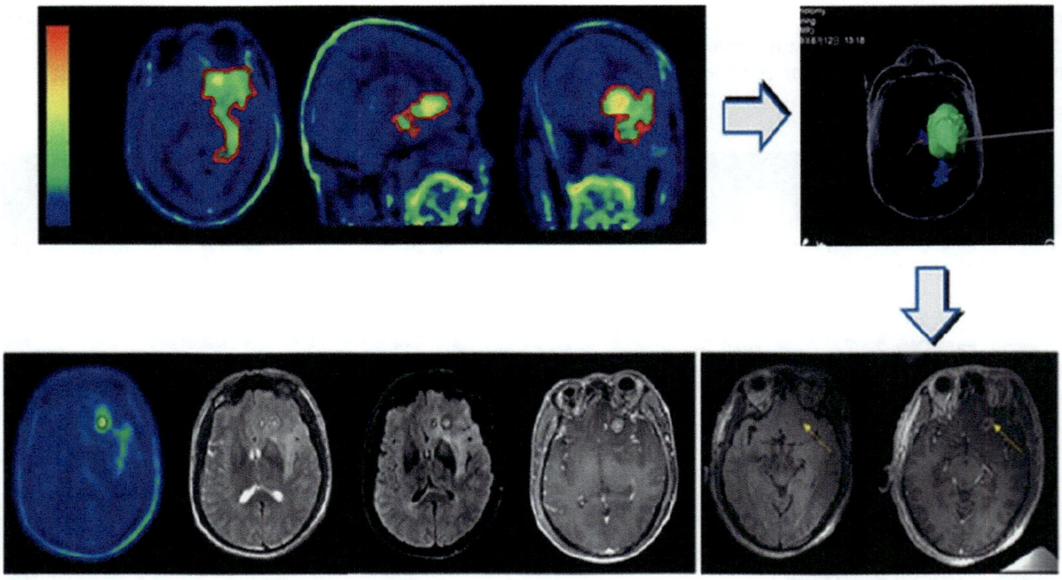

Fig. 6.5 A 46-year-old male patient with an anaplastic astrocytoma, WHO grade III. ^{18}F-fluoro-ethyl-tyrosine (FET) PET was utilized to display the extent and boundaries of the tumor, which were combined with intra-operative navigation for localizing the biopsy puncture site. iMRI was performed to detect the precise location of the biopsy puncture site

tion while protecting nerve function. In our hospital, PET imaging data are utilized in neuronavigation for tumor biopsy localization (Fig. 6.5), which enables the precise localization of tumors for biopsy guided by PET-integrated neuronavigation.

The combination of multimodal imaging with neuronavigation-based localization is currently one of the most advanced techniques in the field of neurosurgery, bringing together various imaging techniques for the pre- and intra-operative assessment of patients' anatomical and functional status, and therefore, is of great clinical and scientific value. The integrability of neuronavigation allows it to combine different forms of data, including anatomy, neuroimaging, molecular imaging, and neurophysiology, which can enhance the efficiency, effectiveness, and conclusiveness of clinical research. Although the combination of multimodal imaging and neuronavigation cannot replace the professional knowledge and clinical reasoning of neurosurgeons, it is a beneficial technological aid for the performance of neurosurgery.

6.2 Applications of PET Imaging in Deep Brain Stimulation (DBS) and Stereoelectroencephalography (SEEG)

Stereotactic electrode implantation can be performed through frame-based or frameless (stereotactic robot) methods. Based on the integration and unification of the imaging space with the physical space, recording or active stimulation electrodes can be embedded within target regions for structural/functional imaging, enabling therapeutic interventions involving the regulation, recording, and disruption of neural activity. At present, this approach is primarily used in DBS and SEEG. PET is another effective method of assessing neural activity that is inseparable from stereotactic diagnosis and treatment.

6.2.1 Applications of PET Molecular Imaging in DBS

The central nervous system is, at its core, a system of electrical activity. Within this system, information is encoded, processed, and transmitted in the form of electrical signals, while the pulsed transmission between neurons is essentially controlled by neuroelectrical activity. As the field of medicine advanced, researchers began noticing that many movement- or cognition-related diseases were associated with abnormalities in intracranial neuroelectrical activity. This observation, therefore, gave rise to the possibility of treating such diseases by intervening in these pathological electrical activities through neuroelectrophysiological means.

With this concept in mind, subsequent technological innovations led to the emergence of implantable interventional devices for neuroelectrical activity, such as DBS, in the field of neurosurgery. DBS is an invasive modulatory method that involves the stereotactic implantation of electrodes into anatomical targets (usually brain nuclei or fiber bundles) in an attempt to regulate the activity of the associated neural networks. PET molecular imaging is a crucial technique in functional brain research that facilitates the in vivo study of metabolism, perfusion, and neurotransmitter activity in neural circuits, thereby strongly supporting the development of invasive, modulatory neurosurgical interventions.

6.2.1.1 DBS and Molecular Imaging in Parkinson's Disease (PD)

PD is a chronic neurodegenerative disease, which presents with symptoms such as limb bradykinesia, postural instability, rigidity, resting tremor, and gait impairment. At present, the diagnosis of PD is largely based on parkinsonian symptoms. However, studies have shown that parkinsonian symptoms only appear when striatal dopamine levels have decreased by 80% and more than 50% of the substantia nigra cells are lost. Therefore, PD diagnosis and treatment are often initiated several years after the actual onset of the disease, when functional deficits have already emerged. Functional PET imaging of the brain is a valuable tool for the diagnosis of PD. PET tracers can bind to targets with relatively high specificity and resolution, which allows the measurement of dopaminergic, cholinergic, serotonergic, noradrenergic, phosphodiesterase, and other target areas.

Impact of DBS on Brain Metabolism

Metabolic research using ^{18}F-fluorodeoxyglucose PET (^{18}F-FDG-PET) in PD patients has revealed hypermetabolism in the globus pallidus, thalamus, and primary motor cortex, as well as hypometabolism in the premotor cortex and parieto-occipital region. DBS treatment of the subthalamic nucleus (STN) and medial globus pallidus enables the effective control of pathological network activities. Similar network improvements were also observed in PD patients who responded positively to treatment with levodopa. Thus, the common mechanism shared among treatment-responsive PD patients is as follows: STN stimulation reduces the neuroelectrical activity of the motor cortex and cerebellum, while increasing the metabolism of the limbic system, prefrontal association cortex, and parieto-occipital cortex. In the local DBS target area and other deeper subcortical regions, ^{18}F-FDG PET studies have found that DBS treatment of the STN decreased putamen metabolism, while significantly increasing STN and globus pallidus activity, indicating that the portion of the STN and the adjacent region (globus pallidus) covered by the DBS electric field are predominantly characterized by excitatory neuroelectrical activity.

Impact of DBS on the Dopaminergic System

STN-DBS therapy can block the glutaminergic excitatory effects (originating from the substantia nigra) on the STN but not the persistent damage that the disease inflicts on the dopaminergic system. A follow-up study of 30 PD patients found that within 1 year of undergoing DBS treatment, striatal uptake of ^{18}F-fluorodopa (FDOPA) still exhibited a progressive decline of approximately 9.5–12.9%. However, it is believed that STN stimulation can increase striatal dopaminergic projections.

Impact of DBS on the Motor Cortex

Oxygen 15-labelled water (^{15}O-H_2O) can be used to detect the perfusion of cerebral blood flow and the activation of functional areas of the brain. In a ^{15}O-H_2O PET study, patients who received STN-DBS therapy showed significantly enhanced perfusion from the thalamus to the dorsolateral prefrontal cortex (DLPFC), supplementary motor area (SMA), and anterior cingulate cortex (ACC) when performing motor tasks, while in the resting state, the pathological overexcitation of the primary motor cortex was reversed. Similar enhancements in perfusion were also observed in the SMA and ACC (but not the DLPFC) of patients who underwent DBS treatment of the globus pallidus internus (GPi). Gait impairment and postural instability are common problems experienced by PD patients, and low-frequency electrical stimulation of the pedunculopontine nucleus (PPN) significantly improves gait disturbances and freezing. A ^{15}O-H_2O study demonstrated that after PPN-DBS therapy, patients with significant improvements in lower limb symptoms also exhibited significantly higher SMA activation. The results of that study also revealed that PPN-DBS may potentially have a positive effect on complex voluntary movements, such as walking.

DBS and Language in PD

Language is a complex form of movement, and language impairments in PD patients are often accompanied by decreased activity in the motor cortex and cerebellum, as well as the overexcitation of the SMA and DLPFC. STN-DBS therapy can significantly improve the patient's language ability, while also reversing the aforementioned pathological activities.

DBS and Behavior and Cognition in PD

The STN consists of three components: the dorsolateral component connected to the sensorimotor areas, the ventral component connected to the association cortices, and the ventromedial component connected to the limbic system. Therefore, researchers now suspect that the non-motor loop of the basal ganglia, where the STN is located, may also be affected by STN-DBS. According to previous ^{18}F-FDG and ^{15}O-H_2O PET studies, STN-DBS significantly interferes with the activities of the frontal cortex. Although studies conducted on such patients generally have not reported global cognitive decline after DBS implantation, some patients still have cognitive deficits in specific domains.

In summary, molecular imaging can be used to evaluate neurotransmission, energy metabolism, and cerebral perfusion after DBS electrodes are implanted in PD patients, as physicians can utilize these electrodes for the in vivo evaluation of DBS efficacy. Therefore, molecular imaging has substantially expanded our understanding of PD and has contributed significantly to the lives of PD patients.

6.2.1.2 DBS and Molecular Imaging in Alzheimer's Disease (AD)

Although DBS was initially intended for the high-frequency stimulation therapy of tremor disorders, many researchers have recently begun to realize that neural circuit abnormalities may be involved in the underlying mechanisms of a number of neuropsychiatric disorders. Therefore, it may be possible to detect abnormal activities in specific nodes through metabolic, functional, and electrophysiological research, while the DBS treatment of these nodes may help to rectify pathological neural circuit activities.

From a histopathological perspective, the primary manifestations of AD are beta (β)-amyloidosis and tau (τ) protein deposition, which can damage the large-scale neural networks related to memory, executive function, and language. Therefore, in PET and fMRI studies, we can observe hypometabolism and network disruptions in the memory association cortices of the medial temporal and parietal lobes. From the perspective of neural circuits, AD patients often exhibit significant abnormalities in the activities of key memory- and cognition-related circuits (i.e., the cholinergic system). The primary targets of DBS treatment in AD patients include the columns of the fornix and the nucleus basalis of Meynert (NBM).

Fornix Column DBS

Anatomically, the columns of the fornix are the gateways leading in and out of the hippocampus. Approximately 1.2 million axons are projected via the fornix into the Papez circuit, which means that applying DBS to the fornix may stimulate the memory-related networks, thereby incidentally treating AD. Only a few studies have examined the treatment of AD via fornix DBS, with a total of 48 cases in phase I and II clinical trials. As an important technique for evaluating brain activity, PET can facilitate the observation of the therapeutic efficacy of DBS in AD patients.

Laxton et al. conducted a phase I clinical trial of fornix DBS in 6 patients with probable AD who exhibited mild cognitive impairment (MCI). PET imaging of these patients revealed increased metabolism in the temporal and parietal regions a month after the stimulators were activated, and these changes persisted for more than a year. Furthermore, based on the Mini-Mental State Examination (MMSE), five of the six patients showed a significant reduction in the rate of cognitive decline. Lozano et al. subsequently conducted a phase II clinical trial of fornix DBS in 42 patients with probable AD who exhibited MCI. Based on the patients' Alzheimer's Disease Assessment Scale – Cognitive Subscale (ADAS-Cog) scores at 1-year postoperatively, the experimental group did not show a significant improvement in cognitive ability compared to the control group. Based on PET imaging, however, the experimental group showed increased glucose metabolism 6 months after the stimulators were activated. It is noteworthy that despite the insignificant cognitive improvement in the experimental group, patients aged ≥65 years showed a significant reduction in cognitive decline and the most significant increase in PET metabolism.

NBM-DBS

The cholinergic neurons of the hippocampus, along with its connected network, play a critical role in memory encoding and consolidation, while the NBM plays a pivotal role in the neural projections from the neocortex into the medial temporal lobe structures. Furthermore, NBM-specific neuroapoptosis is often observed in AD patients. Therefore, similarly to the loss of dopaminergic neurons in PD, the cognitive decline in AD patients may be related to the dysfunction of the cholinergic circuit in the NBM. In the case of pharmacotherapy, some have suggested the use of cholinesterase inhibitors for the treatment of AD, while the NBM has been proposed as a therapeutic target for DBS. The application of NBM-DBS in AD was first reported in 1985 by Turnbull et al., involving one patient with early-stage AD. After 2 months of continuous stimulation to the left NBM, ^{18}F-FDG PET imaging indicated a significantly slower rate of metabolic decrease in the left temporal and parietal lobes compared to the contralateral side. However, the cognitive benefit of the treatment was inconclusive. In

2015, Kuhn et al. performed bilateral NBM-DBS therapy on six patients with mild-to-moderate AD. After 1 year of treatment, the patients' ADAS-Cog scores indicated that the cognitive function significantly improved in 1 patient, non-significantly worsened in 3, and continued to deteriorate in 2. Of the six patients, four underwent ^{18}F-FDG PET imaging before, and after treatment, three of whom exhibited significant increases in glucose metabolism.

In summary, DBS offers a new alternative treatment for AD but is still in the early stages of development, and more clinical studies are needed to evaluate its effectiveness. Additionally, as essential methods of observing brain function, PET, and molecular imaging will inevitably play an important role in evaluating the efficacy of DBS in patients with AD.

6.2.2 Applications of PET Imaging in SEEG

SEEG is utilized for the localization of intracranial epileptogenic foci, as well as the localization of functional areas. This technique is frequently utilized in patients with MRI-negative epilepsy, i.e., epileptic lesions that cannot be observed even with high-resolution 3D MRI without interslice gaps. Nevertheless, due to the high cost of single SEEG electrodes and the low number of sampling points, the ability to acquire SEEG signals of epileptic activity depends to a large extent on pre-operative localization.

PET has been utilized in recent years to optimize the implantation of intracranial electrodes, primarily by determining the epileptogenic and extension zones. Common PET radiotracers include ^{18}F- or ^{11}C-labelled flumazenil (FMZ), and ^{18}F-FDG, which can identify the epileptogenic origin by detecting regions of reduced radioactive uptake. Imaging agents for opioid receptors, such as ^{11}C-carfentanil, can identify areas affected by epilepsy by detecting regions of increased uptake. The most commonly used PET radiotracers are FDG and FMZ.

FDG is a glucose analog, and in an early study, FDG-PET imaging showed a relatively high sensitivity (up to 84%) for detecting epileptogenic foci in temporal lobe epilepsy (TLE), but its sensitivity decreased to only 33% for extra-TLE. In subsequent studies, the sensitivity of FDG PET imaging for TLE and extra-TLE was found to be 87–90% and 38–55%, respectively. In terms of lateralizing the seizure focus, FDG-PET imaging showed relatively high accuracies for both TLE and extra-TLE (95% and 84%, respectively). Furthermore, in 53% of cases involving MRI-negative epilepsy, FDG-PET imaging was useful for surgical decision-making. In children with refractory MRI-negative frontal lobe epilepsy, FDG-PET imaging showed a sensitivity of 92% and specificity of 62.5% in localizing the epileptogenic foci.

FMZ has a high affinity to benzodiazepine receptors, especially γ-amino butyric acid A (GABAA) receptors. FMZ PET imaging has also been utilized in the localization of epileptic foci. Studies have reported that patients with focal epilepsy exhibited decreased FMZ binding in regions of seizure onset. As this is a receptor-based radiotracer, FMZ has a higher specificity than that of FDG. In patients with medial TLE, FDG often shows hypometabolism in the entire anterior temporal lobe on the affected side, whereas FMZ more selectively reveals decreased binding in the hippocampus and amygdala, while showing normal binding in neocortical regions. When utilized for the localization of epileptic foci, FMZ PET imaging showed a detection rate of 94% in TLE and 50% in extra-TLE.

In summary, advances in PET and molecular imaging have substantially diversified the variety of stereotactic techniques for diagnosis and treatment. Further research in this area will continue to expand the role of PET molecular imaging in stereotactic diagnosis and treatment.

6.3 Applications of PET Imaging in Radiotherapy and Stereotactic Biopsy

Radiotherapy is now fully integrated into multidisciplinary cancer treatment, and it is estimated that 50% of cancer patients can benefit from radiotherapy. In fact, the efficacy of radiotherapy, both as a monotherapy and in combination with other treatment methods (e.g., surgery, chemotherapy, and other recently developed targeted biological therapy), has been confirmed by a large number of prospective or retrospective clinical studies.

6.3.1 PET-Guided Radiotherapy

Radiotherapy has most certainly transformed the treatment of brain metastases. In its preliminary stages, radiosurgery of the brain was limited to only a handful of medical institutions and required an invasive head frame. Nevertheless, the remarkable advances in technology and the ever-increasing demand for radiosurgery have enabled the widespread utilization of radiotherapy for cancer treatment. Technologies such as image-based navigation, intensity-modulated radiotherapy (IMRT), robotic technology, and micro-multileaf collimators frameless stereotaxis are rapidly becoming standard components of modern linear accelerators, allowing patients with brain metastases to receive standardized treatment.

PET imaging can accurately and sensitively display in vivo metabolic processes and radiotracer concentrations. Therefore, PET scans play an important role in improving the process of medical diagnosis and treatment. The combination of brain tumor therapy with PET imaging can provide metabolic and functional information for disease diagnosis and treatment. In recent years, the application of medical imaging, especially ^{18}F-FDG imaging, has been growing in the field of cancer therapy. With the continuous development of new radiotracers, PET-based molecular imaging facilitates the visualization of tumor metabolism, oxygen transport and consumption, and receptor or gene expression. PET can also serve as a tool for tumor staging, selecting or delineating radiotherapy target areas, evaluating the treatment response of tumors, detecting early recurrence, or evaluating post-treatment changes in organ function. Therefore, ^{18}F-FDG PET imaging is becoming increasingly important in radiotherapy planning, with a growing number of oncologists believing that target selection and delineation cannot be adequately completed without ^{18}F-FDG-PET.

A variety of methods are utilized in clinical settings to use the metabolic information provided by PET scans to guide neurosurgical interventions. From the visual information obtained from standard PET images to the PET-derived information and images used in stereotactic treatments, PET scans can provide data with relatively high levels of accuracy and convenience compared to other techniques. For example, CT-guided stereotactic biopsy may not provide sufficient information for a pathological diagnosis, whereas the hypermetabolic regions displayed by FDG-PET imaging have shown greater agreement with the affected tissues in the final diagnosis. In radiotherapy, the lesion extent delineated using FDG-PET is highly consistent with the subsequent diagnosis based on stereotactic biopsy specimens, with metastatic adenocarcinoma detected in hypermetabolic regions, and radiation necrosis detected in hypometabolic regions of the lesion. These findings indicate that PET, when combined with CT or MRI, can provide supplementary information for the selection of brain biopsy sites.

The visual localization techniques currently utilized are not very precise, and there is still much progress to be made in achieving precision-guidance neurosurgery, which may only be limited to guidance for biopsies in specific patients (e.g., patients with larger lesions). By utilizing image fusion techniques, frameless PET data can be registered with precise anatomical structures at a precision of 1 mm, elevating the accuracy and precision of radiotherapy to a new level. Certain commercial software designed for stereotactic planning can be used for registration, for example, between non-stereotactic MRI images and stereotactic CT images. If PET images can be easily imported into the relevant software, then the fusion of non-stereotactic PET images with stereotactic CT or MR images may help to provide greater convenience when utilizing metabolic information for brain tumors. Additionally, the simple registration of multimodal images, including PET images, will also improve the precision and accuracy of neurosurgery. In a case report by Thiel et al., ^{11}C-L-methionine (^{11}C-MET) PET and MRI registration was implemented in a patient with a brain tumor. The registration accurately discriminated between areas of radiation-induced necrosis and tumor recurrence, thereby guiding the formulation of the stereotactic plan.

It is not realistic to expect optimal outcomes from the current practice of using the same radiotracer for different types of brain tumors. From the perspective of neurosurgical navigation, an ideal tumor marker should detect with high sensitivity tumor cells exhibiting specific malignant characteristics, to ensure an accurate diagnosis and appropriate treatment. Regardless of the malignancy of the tumor cells, the delineation of the extent of the tumor will also improve with the increasing sensitivity of the PET radiotracers.

The stereotactic PET imaging utilized in neurosurgical navigation offers new prospects for the treatment of diseases other than cancer, and different types of functional neurosurgery can also benefit from this technique. For example, PET-guided neurosurgical techniques can be implemented in epilepsy surgery for the metabolism-based localization of epileptic foci. PET imaging can also be used to delineate functional areas in both resection surgery and gamma knife radiosurgery (GKR).

Advances in PET techniques will improve the resolution and sensitivity of PET-based neurosurgical navigation, as newer tomographic techniques utilize a higher number of detectors, which enhances the system's axial resolution, in particular, while also enabling the acquisition and storage of 3D data. This will not only improve the sensitivity of the system but also integrate PET information into a stereotactic 3D space, allowing the examination of frameless PET data acquisition techniques based on stereotactic MRI, as well as performing registration and integration within the surgical planning system, enabling the automatic integration of PET images into GKR planning systems.

6.3.2 PET-Guided GKR

GKR is the primary treatment method for brain metastases and an adjuvant treatment for recurrent malignant gliomas. Although MRI can provide good anatomical information and high spatial resolution for GKR treatment plans, other imaging methods are still needed to determine whether recurrence has occurred in the area targeted by radiotherapy. PET scans are generally used to localize abnormal metabolic regions in the brain, while MET PET can assess tumor recurrence and radiotherapy-induced alterations (e.g., radiation necrosis). MET PET can also be performed in GKR to identify malignant tumors that require treatment, despite the limited spatial resolution, which is due to partial volume effects. When implementing MET PET in GKR, these limitations in spatial resolution and precision should be considered. For example, by providing the same axial plane and window level as the MRI images, these MRI-based warped MET PET images can be used to identify tumors.

6.3.3 PET-Guided Stereotactic Biopsy

The first step in PET-guided neurosurgery is to perform a PET-guided stereotactic brain biopsy. Although CT and MRI are typically used to guide stereotactic surgery, even highly experienced physicians are unable to provide a pathological diagnosis for approximately 5% of patients. Hence, there is a need for PET-guided stereotactic biopsy techniques. Despite the high accuracy of CT- and MRI-guided biopsy, there is still a possibility of an inaccurate diagnosis or an underestimation of the histological grading of tumors. Therefore, given the histological heterogeneity of brain tumors, especially gliomas, an insufficient number of stereotactic biopsy specimens or an inaccurate localization may risk the acquisition of incorrect or inadequate tissues for an accurate diagnosis. PET imaging can provide independent metabolic information; therefore, some hospitals have begun routinely integrating PET data into stereotactic surgical planning to improve the success rate of diagnostic biopsies. By utilizing the techniques above, the target area selected based on stereotactic PET images can be accurately compared with CT or MR images, enabling neurosurgeons to obtain accurate biopsy specimens from abnormal metabolic regions in brain tumors.

The information provided by PET studies depends primarily on the radiotracers used, and FDG is one of the most commonly used radiotracers. Although FDG-PET-guided biopsy is relatively useful, it has certain drawbacks. For example, in cases with little or no FDG uptake, it is not feasible to perform biopsy target selection based on the PET images alone, and this situation is more commonly seen among low-grade tumor cases. Furthermore, when hypermetabolic lesions are closely related to cortical or subcortical gray matter, it becomes difficult to distinguish between the FDG uptake of the tumor and normal tissues. Radiolabeled amino acid tracers have been shown to be suitable for studying the delineation of brain tumors or the specific metabolism. The most commonly used amino acid tracer is ^{11}C-MET, which has relatively fast kinetics and a short half-life, offering the advantages of a shorter scan time and the ability to perform multi-tracer PET acquisition. MET PET shows a higher uptake than FDG-PET for visualizing tumors located in the gray matter and low-grade gliomas (e.g., astroglioma and oligodendroglioma). MET PET images indicate that lesions tend to exhibit higher uptake rates than normal gray matter in malignant tumors and other pathologies, as these diseases increase amino acid transport and protein synthesis. MET PET is a non-invasive examination that can display local metabolism, and can discriminate between non-tumor and tumor tissues with high sensitivity and specificity. Furthermore, the functional information provided by MET PET images can be utilized in the diagnosis of tumors and tumor recurrence, and to guide stereotactic biopsy and neurosurgical resection, monitor treatment status, and delineate the pre- and post-radiotherapy target areas. Stereotactic PET studies not only facilitate the selection of biopsy targets, but also link the tumor's metabolic information with its histopathological characteristics (Fig. 6.6).

New imaging techniques, such as PET molecular imaging and image-guided neurosurgery, have substantially improved neurosurgeons' abilities to visualize lesions, and enabled the intuitive depiction of crucial adjacent structures. Based on pre- and intra-operative imaging, neurosurgeons

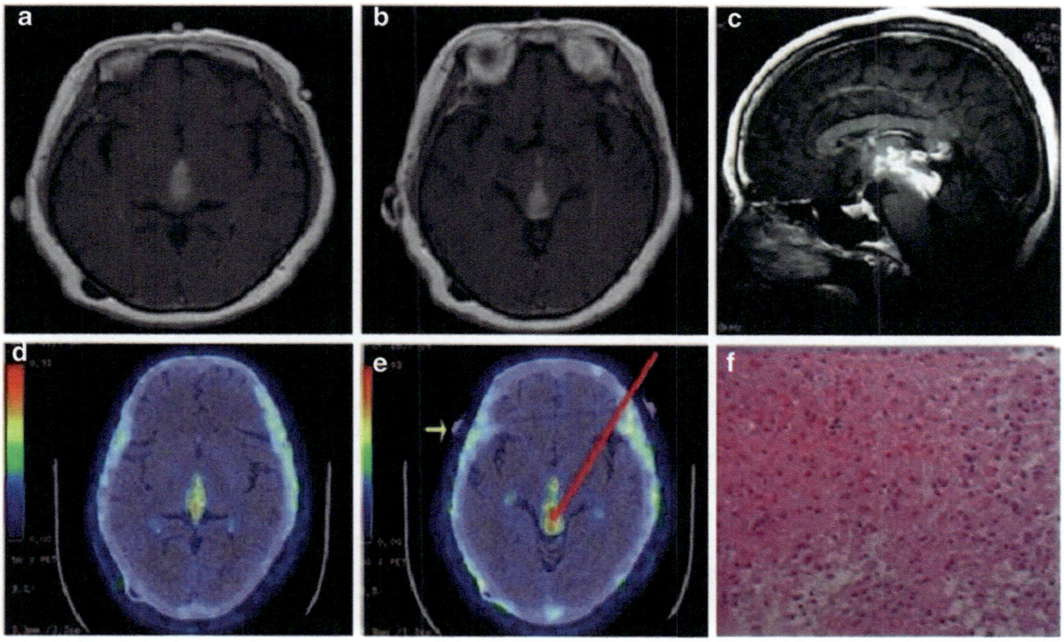

Fig. 6.6 Application of PET in the stereotactic biopsy of gliomas in the pineal gland: Contrast-enhanced T1WI MRI shows significant enhancement in the pineal gland, but uniform signal intensity, which cannot be used to determine the specific status of tumor activity (**a**–**c**). MET PET uses protein metabolism to fully display the tumor shape and differences in protein metabolism (**d**). MET PET-guided surgical path planning (**e**). Histological staining indicates successful acquisition of diseased brain tissue, which agrees with a diagnosis of glioma (**f**)

can determine the optimal surgical approach or stereotactic implantation path, thereby maximizing the resection or treatment of lesions while also minimizing the damage inflicted on functional brain tissues. This not only improves the accuracy and precision of targeted interventions, but also reduces surgical injury, and therefore represents the future direction of neurosurgery.

Suggested Readings

Adler CH, Beach TG, Hentz JG, et al. Low clinical diagnostic accuracy of early vs advanced Parkinson disease: clinicopathologic study. Neurology. 2014;83(5):406–12.

Barnett GH. The role of image-guided technology in the surgical planning and resection of gliomas. J Neurooncol. 1999;42(3):247–58.

Barnett GH, Kormos DW, Steiner CP, et al. Use of a frameless, armless stereotactic wand for brain tumor localization with two-dimensional and three-dimensional neuroimaging. Neurosurgery. 1993;33(4):674–8.

Bernier J, Hall EJ, Giaccia A. Radiation oncology: a century of achievements. Nat Rev Cancer. 2004;4(9):737–47.

Drzezga A, Arnold S, Minoshima S, et al. 18F-FDG PET studies in patients with extratemporal and temporal epilepsy: evaluation of an observer-independent analysis. J Nucl Med. 1999;40(5):737–46.

Fearnley JM, Lees AJ. Ageing and Parkinson's disease: substantia nigra regional selectivity. Brain. 1991;114(5):2283–301.

Fukuda M, Mentis M, Ma Y, et al. Networks mediating the clinical effects of pallidal brain stimulation for Parkinson's disease: a PET study of resting-state glucose metabolism. Brain. 2001;124(8):1601–9.

Galldiks N, Dunkl V, Kracht LW, et al. Volumetry of [11C]-methionine positron emission tomographic uptake as a prognostic marker before treatment of patients with malignant glioma. Mol Imaging. 2012;11(6):516–27.

Gelb DJ, Oliver E, Gilman S. Diagnostic criteria for Parkinson disease. Arch Neurol. 1999;56(1):33–9.

Glaudemans AW, Enting RH, Heesters MA, et al. Value of 11C-methionine PET in imaging brain tumours and metastases. Eur J Nucl Med Mol Imaging. 2013;40(4):615–35.

Gok B, Jallo G, Hayeri R, Wahl R, Aygun N. The evaluation of FDG-PET imaging for epileptogenic focus localization in patients with MRI positive and MRI negative temporal lobe epilepsy. Neuroradiology. 2013;55(5):541–50.

Grech-Sollars M, Vaqas B, Thompson G, et al. An MRS-and PET-guided biopsy tool for intraoperative neuronavigational systems. J Neurosurg. 2016;127(4):812–8.

Haslinger B, Kalteis K, Boecker H, et al. Frequency-correlated decreases of motor cortex activity associated with subthalamic nucleus stimulation in Parkinson's disease. Neuroimage. 2005;28(3):598–606.

Hasselmo ME. Neuromodulation: acetylcholine and memory consolidation. Trends Cogn Sci. 1999;3(9):351–9.

Hilker R, Voges J, Weber T, et al. STN-DBS activates the target area in Parkinson disease: an FDG-PET study. Neurology. 2008;71(10):708–13.

Hushek SG, Martin AJ, Steckner M, et al. MR systems for MRI-guided interventions. J Magn Reson Imaging. 2008;27(2):253–66.

Jacobs HI, Radua J, Lückmann HC, et al. Meta-analysis of functional network alterations in Alzheimer's disease: toward a network biomarker. Neurosci Biobehav Rev. 2013;37(5):753–65.

Jung TY, Min JJ, Bom HS, et al. Prognostic value of post-treatment metabolic tumor volume from 11C-methionine PET/CT in recurrent malignant glioma. Neurosurg Rev. 2017;40(2):223–9.

Kacher DF, Whalen B, Handa A, et al. The advanced multimodality image-guided operating (AMIGO) suite. Intraoperative Imaging and Image-Guided Therapy. New York: Springer; 2014. p. 339–68.

Kalbe E, Voges J, Weber T, et al. Frontal FDG-PET activity correlates with cognitive outcome after STN-DBS in Parkinson disease. Neurology. 2009;72(1):42–9.

Kato T, Shinoda J, Nakayama N, et al. Metabolic assessment of gliomas using 11C-methionine, [18F] fluorodeoxyglucose, and 11C-choline positron-emission tomography. AJNR Am J Neuroradiol. 2008;29(6):1176–682.

Kuhn J, Hardenacke K, Lenartz D, et al. Deep brain stimulation of the nucleus basalis of Meynert in Alzheimer's dementia. Mol Psychiatry. 2015;20(3):353–60.

Laxton AW, Tang-Wai DF, McAndrews MP, et al. A phase I trial of deep brain stimulation of memory circuits in Alzheimer's disease. Ann Neurol. 2010;68(4):521–34.

Levivier M, Wikler D Jr, Massager N, et al. The integration of metabolic imaging in stereotactic procedures including radiosurgery: a review. J Neurosurg. 2002;97(5):542–50.

Levivier M, Massager N, Wikler D, et al. Use of stereotactic PET images in dosimetry planning of radiosurgery for brain tumors: clinical experience and proposed classification. J Nucl Med. 2004;45(7):1146–654.

Lozano AM, Fosdick L, Chakravarty MM, et al. A phase II study of fornix deep brain stimulation in mild Alzheimer's disease. J Alzheimers Dis. 2016;54(2):777–87.

Meilinger T, Frankenstein J, Watanabe K, et al. Reference frames in learning from maps and navigation. Psychol Res. 2015;79(6):1000–8.

Momose T, Nariai T, Kawabe T, et al. Clinical benefit of ^{11}C methionine PET imaging as a planning modality for radiosurgery of previously irradiated recurrent brain metastases. Clin Nucl Med. 2014;39(11):939–43.

Navarro-Ramirez R, Lang G, Lian X, et al. Total navigation in spine surgery; a concise guide to eliminate fluoroscopy using a portable intraoperative computed

tomography 3-dimensional navigation system. World Neurosurg. 2017;100:325–35.
Rathore C, Dickson JC, Teotónio R, et al. The utility of 18F-fluorodeoxyglucose PET (FDG PET) in epilepsy surgery. Epilepsy Res. 2014;108(8):1306–14.
Ryvlin P, Bouvard S, Le Bars D, et al. Clinical utility of flumazenil-PET versus [18F] fluorodeoxyglucose-PET and MRI in refractory partial epilepsy: a prospective study in 100 patients. Brain. 1998;121(11):2067–81.
Seifert V, Zimmermann M, Trantakis C, et al. Open MRI-guided neurosurgery. Acta Neurochir. 1999;141(5):455–64.
Spencer SS. The relative contributions of MRI, SPECT, and PET imaging in epilepsy. Epilepsia. 1994;35(Suppl. 6):S72–89.
Spiegel EA, Wycis HT, Marks M, et al. Stereotaxic apparatus for operations on the human brain. Science. 1947;106(2754):349–50.
Tanaka Y, Nariai T, Momose T, et al. Glioma surgery using a multimodal navigation system with integrated metabolic images. J Neurosurg. 2009;110(1):163–72.
Turnbull IM, McGeer P, Beattie L, et al. Stimulation of the basal nucleus of Meynert in senile dementia of Alzheimer's type: a preliminary report. Appl Neurophysiol. 1985;48(1–6):216–21.
Vivash L, Gregoire M-C, Lau EW, et al. 18F-Flumazenil: a γ-aminobutyric acid A—specific PET radiotracer for the localization of drug-resistant temporal lobe epilepsy. J Nucl Med. 2013;54(8):1270–7.
Yordanova YN, Cochereau J, Duffau H, et al. Combining resting state functional MRI with intraoperative cortical stimulation to map the mentalizing network. Neuroimage. 2019;186:628–36.

7 Research Applications of Positron Emission Tomography/Magnetic Resonance (PET/MR) Imaging in the Brain Mechanisms of Acupuncture

Long Zhao, Yi Shan, Boci Shan, and Jiliang Fang

Acupuncture has been used as a form of therapy in China for more than 3000 years. It is a key component of Chinese medicine, arising from the combination of ancient Chinese philosophy and medicine. Acupuncture is an important discipline that involves the use of specialized techniques such as needling and moxibustion to act on certain sites in the human body (i.e., meridians and acupoints) to prevent and/or treat disease. Acupuncture has been adopted globally because of its rapid effects, simple and safe operation, low cost, virtual absence of side effects, and the wide range of clinical indications it can provide. The unique theory of meridians and acupoints, related to acupuncture, is intricately linked with modern medical anatomy, physiology, and pathology. However, the basic disciplines of modern medicine have yet to fully uncover the scientific characteristics of meridians and acupoints, due to the limitations of the various fields.

Medical imaging is a product of modern technology and medical theory. It combines morphological and functional imaging techniques with fundamental knowledge of anatomy, physiology, and pathology, to achieve the non-invasive in vivo visualization of the structure and function of human tissues and organs, as well as the progression of diseases. Medical imaging offers significant advantages in perfecting and elucidating the theory of acupuncture, while also playing an indispensable role in the clinical diagnosis and treatment of diseases and efficacy evaluation. Acupuncture imaging is an emerging multidisciplinary field that carries on the historical trend of medical imaging. On the one hand, modern diagnostic imaging has provided a wide range of objective medical evidence for the clinical practice of acupuncture. On the other hand, the rapid development of functional brain imaging over the last 20 years, especially functional MRI (fMRI) and PET imaging, has enabled numerous researchers to study the brain mechanisms of acupuncture using non-invasive functional imaging techniques. This research has produced fruitful results in a number of aspects, promoted the development of acupuncture, and increased its neuroscientific connotations. Therefore, medical imaging is now a crucial research method for studying the clinical diagnosis, treatment techniques, and scientific principles of modern acupuncture.

L. Zhao · J. Fang (✉)
Department of Radiology, Guang An Men Hospital, China Academy of Chinese Medical Science, Beijing, China

Y. Shan
Department of Radiology and Nuclear Medicine, Xuanwu Hospital, Capital Medical University, Beijing, China

B. Shan
Center for Nuclear Technology and Applications, Institute of High Energy Physics, Chinese Academy of Sciences, Beijing, China

J. Lu, G. Zhao (eds.), *PET/MR: Functional and Molecular Imaging of Neurological Diseases and Neurosciences*, https://doi.org/10.1007/978-981-19-9902-4_7

7.1 Acupuncture, Neurological Diseases, and Neurosciences

Acupuncture can be used to treat or assist in the treatment of multisystem diseases, and has been increasingly recognized and accepted internationally, owing to its beneficial therapeutic and minimal side effects. Modern studies have found that acupuncture can regulate systemic and local functional changes; however, given that acupuncture encompasses a wide variety of techniques and its therapeutic effects involve multisystem, multilevel regulation of human physical functions, its underlying mechanisms are complex and remain poorly understood. At present, acupuncture has been utilized in the treatment of 29 types of neurological diseases related to mental and behavioral disorders, primarily focusing on cerebral infarction, hemorrhage, ischemia, stroke rehabilitation, migraine, vertigo, insomnia, facial nerve palsy, depression, vascular dementia (VD), Alzheimer's disease (AD), epilepsy, Parkinson's disease (PD), anxiety, and neurosis. Research on the use of acupuncture to treat neurological diseases is advancing on multiple levels, from the microscopic level of molecular and cellular mechanisms, biomarkers, and molecular typing, to the mesoscopic level of network mechanisms, and further to the macroscopic level of imaging diagnosis and treatment strategies.

7.1.1 Research on the Mechanisms of Acupuncture Treatment for Cerebral Infarction

Cerebral infarction, also known as an ischemic stroke, is the result of localized cerebral ischemia and hypoxia, and associated brain cell damage induced by a number of factors. The results of the clinical practice of and basic research on acupuncture have demonstrated that treating patients in the early stages of cerebral infarction with acupuncture can improve cerebral blood flow (CBF) to the infarcted area, suppress cellular apoptosis, promote the recovery of neural function, enhance the energy metabolism of ischemic brain tissue, and improve patient health and safety.

A study on electroacupuncture found that this technique can increase the activity of superoxide dismutase (SOD), an enzyme which can inhibit the generation of free radicals and promote resistance against ischemia-reperfusion injury in rats. Other studies have also shown that acupuncture has regulatory effects on intraneuronal Ca^{2+}, enabling a reduction of intraneuronal Ca^{2+} in rats following cerebral ischemic injury. A middle cerebral artery occlusion (MCAO) stroke model was utilized in rats to investigate the effects of the Xingnao Kaiqiao, or "Consciousness-Restoring, Obstruction-Clearing," needling technique on free Ca^{2+} concentration in hippocampal neurons at different time points during cerebral ischemia. The results indicated that after a focal cerebral ischemic injury, the intracellular Ca^{2+} concentration in the hippocampal neurons of rats increased with time, suggesting that this needling technique can rapidly and effectively regulate the concentration of Ca^{2+} in the ischemic area, maintain Ca^{2+} homeostasis, and suppress a series of pathological responses caused by intracellular Ca^{2+} overload and its corresponding neuronal damage. By observing CBF, the number of brain microvessels, and the diameter of pial microvessels in rats, Chinese researchers discovered that treatment with acupuncture can expand the diameter of pial microvessels, increase CBF, and increase the number of brain microvessels. Studies have demonstrated that electrical stimulation of the cerebellar fastigial nucleus (FNS) in rats following focal cerebral ischemia can promote the proliferation of vascular endothelial cells and the expression of vascular endothelial growth factor (VEFGF), while also facilitating the formation of new capillaries in the area around the lesion. Furthermore, treatment with electroacupuncture after ischemia in rats can increase the gene and protein expression of erythropoietin (EPO), promote the phosphorylation of Janus kinase 2 (JAK2) and signal transducer and activator of transcription 5 (STAT5), and increase the protein levels of phosphorylated JAK2 (P-JAK2) and phosphorylated STAT5 (P-STAT5) in the brain, as well as promote regional CBF (rCBF) and micro-vascularization. Using single-photon emission computed tomography (SPECT) imaging, researchers have observed that performing scalp acupuncture at the motor areas in stroke patients led to improvements in cerebral perfusion and CBF within the area of the lesion. Moreover, the application of electroacupuncture to stimulate the Dazhui and Baihui acupoints in rat models of cerebral ischemia resulted in a decrease in the levels of endothelin (ET) and nitric oxide (NO) in the brain tissue, which prevented secondary nerve damage. Electroacupuncture stimulation of the Baihui and Shuigou acupoints in rats after focal cerebral ischemia can control the protein expression of c-Fos in the brain within a certain range, thereby reducing neuronal apoptosis during cerebral ischemia. Additionally, studies on the effects of acupuncture on patients' brain metabolism have found that acupuncture can increase deoxyglucose uptake in the primary auditory, prefrontal, tertiary association, and premotor cortices, thus suggesting that acupuncture can promote glucose metabolism in brain tissues.

In summary, acupuncture can induce the dilation of cerebral blood vessels, promote blood circulation, reduce blood viscosity, enhance neural conduction, regulate metabolism, and restore the immune system, thereby readjusting the physical functions of patients with cerebral infarction while promoting clinical rehabilitation.

7.1.2 Research on the Mechanisms of Acupuncture Treatment for Insomnia

Insomnia is a common sleep disorder, characterized by an insufficient duration and/or quality of sleep. Acupuncture can alleviate insomnia, as it can be used to achieve Yin-Yang regulation and meridian dredging. According to current research, the physiological pathogenesis of insomnia is thought to include the following aspects: (1) central nervous system (CNS) dysfunction, as the pathogenesis of insomnia stems from either the weakening of inhibitory effects or enhancement of facilitatory effects on neurophysiological function; (2) endocrine dysfunction, as the hypothalamic-pituitary-adrenal (HPA) axis is closely involved in the sleep-wake cycle, and (3) circadian rhythm disorders. Current studies on the mechanisms of acupuncture treatment for insomnia are primarily based on animal models, which have found that acupuncture acts by affecting CNS neurotransmission, immune cytokines, antioxidative defense systems, hormones, and neuroelectrophysiology.

Scalp acupuncture performed in animal models of insomnia inhibited the release of excitatory monoamine neurotransmitters, such as norepinephrine (NE) and dopamine (DA), effectively improving central inhibition during sleep. Studies also found that needling the Baihui and Shenmen acupoints significantly decreased, whereas needling at sham points significantly increased, serotonin (5-HT) levels in the brainstem, which induced cerebral excitation and led to wakefulness. These results imply that needling the Baihui and Shenmen acupoints can induce sleep regulation by modulating 5-HT levels in the brain stem. Furthermore, heat-sensitive moxibustion has been shown to alleviate symptoms of insomnia in rats, which may be related to the increase in SOD activity and decrease in malondialdehyde (MDA) levels. Researchers have also found that rats in the insomnia model group exhibited an absence of circadian rhythm, prolonged escape latency, reduced SOD activity, and elevated MDA levels, whereas those in the heat-sensitive moxibustion group showed an almost normal circadian rhythm, shorter escape latency, elevated SOD activity, and reduced MDA levels. Additionally, compared to the insomnia model group, rats that received heat-sensitive moxibustion had low serum corticosterone (CORT), thyroxine (T4), growth hormone (GH), and melatonin (MT) levels, and higher serum adrenocorticotropic hormone (ACTH) levels. Thus, it is speculated that the relief of insomnia provided by heat-sensitive moxibustion may be associated with hormonal regulation in the body.

The amplitude of low-frequency fluctuations from resting-state fMRI has been utilized to evaluate the effects of needling the Sanyinjiao acupoint in sleep-deprived but otherwise healthy individuals. Needle retention reportedly activated the emotion-related brain areas during the resting state. Furthermore, administration of the Tongdu Tiaoshen, or "Governor Vessel-Dredging, Spirit-Regulating," needling technique activated the thalamus, lentiform nucleus, and caudate nucleus in patients with insomnia, suggesting that these acupoints are related to the CNS regulation of sleep; therefore, the therapeutic effect of this technique is achieved by regulating the incoming and outgoing transmissions of the brain.

7.1.3 Research on the Mechanisms of Acupuncture Treatment for Depression

Depression is a common affective disorder that is related to a number of factors, including neurobiochemistry, neuroendocrine function, cellular signal transduction mechanisms, neurotrophic factors, and inflammatory cytokines. Compared to the antidepressants used in Western medicine, acupuncture has fewer side effects and a higher efficacy, which has led to its increasingly widespread utilization in clinical practice. In a chronic restraint stress (CRS) rat model of depression, electroacupuncture was found to regulate the expression of interleukin (IL)-1 and IL-6 in the cornu ammonis (CA) 3 region of the hippocampus and restore the level of brain-derived neurotrophic factor (BDNF). Furthermore, electroacupuncture reduced the level of Capase-3 and increased the B-cell lymphoma 2 (Bcl-2)/Bcl-2-associated X (BAX) ratio by affecting the Ras-MKK-JNK signaling pathway, thereby mitigating cellular apoptosis. By utilizing the Tongdu Tiaoshen needling technique, Sun et al. demonstrated that acupuncture treatment can produce behavioral improvements in a rat model of post-stroke depression, while also increasing plasma NE and 5-HT levels, indicating that acupuncture exerts its antidepressant effects by increasing plasma neurotransmitter levels. Needling of the Baihui, Yintang, and Sishencong acupoints in rats led to significantly elevated levels of cortical 5-HT, NE, and DA, as well as marked behavioral improvements in rat models of post-stroke depression, suggesting that acupuncture can induce antidepressant effects by increasing cerebral levels of monoamine neurotransmitters. In rat models of HPA axis hyperactivity, needling performed at the Baihui, Shenmen, and Taichonghou acupoints decreased the levels of ACTH and CORT, while also alleviating depressive behaviors. These results imply that acupuncture can induce the beneficial downregulation of ACTH and CORT expression, thereby inhibiting HPA axis hyperactivity while restoring the functions of the HPA and hypothalamic-pituitary-thyroid (HPT) axes. Furthermore, Rong et al. found that electroacupuncture at the auricular concha region led to the stimulation of the vagus nerve and the downregulation of the HPA axis, which significantly improved the depressive state induced by unpredictable chronic mild stress in rats combined with isolation, thereby normalizing their functional activity. This study also found that the Raf/ERK/RSK/CREB signaling pathway in the hippocampus may be involved in the antidepressant effect of electroacupuncture at the auricular concha, which may be inhibited, to a certain extent, by ERK blockers.

The hippocampus in the brain is involved in learning, memory, behavior, and emotion. It is also a key target in stress injury. Observations of the hippocampal neurons in rat models of depression before and after electroacupuncture treatment revealed the apoptosis of hippocampal neurons in models of chronic stress, but long-term electroacupuncture treatment was able to inhibit neuronal apoptosis. The underlying mechanism for this may involve the neuroprotective effects electroacupuncture, which inhibits neuronal apoptosis, therefore mitigating depression in rats. Another study found that the rats in a chronic stress model of depression exhibited significant increases in hippocampal BDNF and tropomyosin receptor kinase B (TrkB) expression during the early stages (seventh day) of electroacupuncture treatment, whereas such increases were not significant in the early stages of fluoxetine therapy. This rapid mechanism of antidepressant therapy may be the result of the upregulation of the cAMP-CREB pathway induced by electroacupuncture, which in turn promptly produced antidepressant effects. Furthermore, depressive rats being treated with acupuncture showed significantly lower hippocampal 5-HT, 5-hydroxyindoleacetic acid (5-HIAA), and glutamate (Glu) levels, as well as higher DA levels, than those treated with antidepressant medication alone. These results imply that the rapid alleviation by acupuncture treatment may be achieved through the upregulation of DA and γ-aminobutyric acid (GABA), and the downregulation of Glu, which suppresses neuronal damage induced by the excessive accumulation of Glu and alleviates its toxicological reactions in the body, thereby exerting an antidepressant effect. Additionally, behavioral studies of animal models have demonstrated that rats treated with acupuncture had better outcomes than the model group in terms of behavioral performance, body mass changes, and syrup consumption rate.

7.1.4 Research on the Mechanisms of Acupuncture Treatment for AD

AD is a common form of dementia, and studies have found that acupuncture treatment in AD patients primarily exerts its effects via the following: the reduction of β-amyloid (Aβ) deposition, inhibition of tau protein hyperphosphorylation, suppression of neuronal apoptosis, promotion of CNS transmission, improvement of energy metabolism, regulation of oxidative stress and inflammatory responses, and other pathways.

In one study, grain moxibustion was applied once daily at the Xinshu and Shenshu acupoints in amyloid precursor protein (APP)/presenilin 1 (PS1) double-transgenic mice. After 90 days of treatment, the Morris water maze test was performed, and the results showed that the treatment group had a shorter escape latency, higher number of platform crossings, higher percentage of time spent in the target quadrant, and lesser Aβ deposition in the frontal cortex and hippocampus than the model group. These findings indicate that the improvements in learning and memory that result from moxibustion may be related to the decreased Aβ deposition in the frontal cortex and hippocampus. Furthermore, APP/PS1 mice that received electroacupuncture at the Baihui and Yongquan acupoints once every other day for 6 weeks exhibited superior behavioral performance and lower cortical Aβ-42 levels than those of the model group, suggesting that the effects of electroacupuncture are associated with the reduction in cortical Aβ-42 levels. In a rat model of AD, electroacupuncture performed at the Baihui and Shenshu acupoints enhanced learning and memory. Moreover, the AD model group showed significantly higher levels of hyperphosphorylated tau protein in the hippocampus than that of the normal control group, whereas electroacupuncture led to a significant decrease in both groups. Thus, the enhancement in memory and learning may be associated with the downregulation of tau protein hyperphosphorylation to a certain extent.

Additionally, electroacupuncture, when performed at the Xiusanzhen acupoint, increased the density of muscarinic acetylcholine receptor (mAChR) in the hippocampi of rat models of AD, while also enhancing the affinity of the radioligands to mAChR, suggesting that the mechanism of action underlying the Xiusanzhen treatment in patients with AD may be related to the cholinergic neurons in the olfactory pathway. By utilizing PET imaging with ^{18}F-fluorodeoxyglucose (^{18}F-FDG), a glucose metabolism tracer, Lai et al. observed the effects of acupuncture at the Shenmen acupoint on the glucose metabolism of the hippocampus, thalamus, hypothalamus, and frontotemporal lobe in rat models of AD. They found that before treatment, the AD model group showed significantly lower glucose metabolism in these regions than the control group, whereas after treatment, the AD model group showed an increase in glucose metabolism and a significantly shorter total reaction time in the Y-maze test. These results indicate that acupuncture can improve cognition by increasing local levels of cerebral glucose metabolism. Furthermore, Jiang et al. proposed, based on an AD model in mice, that performing musical electroacupuncture produces a greater effect on glucose metabolism in the frontal lobe than electroacupuncture alone.

7.1.5 Research on the Mechanisms of Acupuncture Treatment for VD

VD refers to the loss of cognitive function due to ischemia, hypoxic damage in the ischemic tissue, and hemorrhagic brain damage. Acupuncture can lead to significant improvements in the short-term symptoms of VD through numerous mechanisms, including the mitigation of cerebral ischemia, regulation of neurotransmitter release, functional adjustment of vasoactive substances, alleviation of free radical damage, and inhibition of neuronal apoptosis.

Studies have shown that eye acupuncture can significantly improve the cognitive abilities of VD patients, as well as their whole blood viscosity, plasma viscosity, hematocrit, and fibrinogen concentration, thereby alleviating microcirculation disorders and their associated brain damage following ischemia-reperfusion injuries. rCBF measurements based on hydrogen peroxide scavenging in the parietal lobes and hippocampi of rats with VD revealed that the therapeutic effects of electroacupuncture could significantly improve rCBF in the parietal lobe and hippocampus, block the cerebral ischemic cascade, and restore the Papez circuit (neural basis of emotional expression in the limbic system). Furthermore, electroacupuncture at the Baihui and Dazhui acupoints revealed significant improvements in the ultrastructural alterations of the neurons in the electroacupuncture group, compared to the model group, suggesting that electroacupuncture has neuroprotective effects in ischemic rats.

Electropuncture can also reduce the protein expression of heme oxygenase-1 (HO-1) in cortical and hippocampal neurons, thereby mitigating the loss and/or protection of hippocampal neurons, alleviating the learning and/or memory impairments in rats with VD, and promoting the functional recovery of damaged neurons following an ischemic injury. In pre- and post-treatment comparisons of 30 VD patients who received acupuncture and Chinese herbal medicine, and in comparison with age-matched healthy controls, researchers found that treatment with acupuncture led to a significant decrease in the concentration of plasma thromboxane B2 (TXB2) and a significant increase in the concentration of 6-keto-prostaglandin $F_{1\alpha}$ (6-keto-$PGF_{1\alpha}$) in patients with VD. These changes re-established a dynamic balance between the two compounds, which subsequently led to cerebral arterial dilation, inhibited platelet aggregation, reduced blood flow resistance, and enhanced brain metabolic rate, thereby facilitating the recovery of brain function. Additionally, electroacupuncture treatment can significantly reduce ET levels, while also strengthening learning and memory abilities in rats, producing comparable effects to those of nimodipine. Some studies have also found that needling can upregulate the expression of copper-zinc-superoxide dismutase (CuZnSOD) at both the transcriptional and translation levels, thereby enhancing the effect of antioxidant enzymes on the effective clearance of free radicals and improving the cognitive status of rats with VD. Researchers performed acupuncture at the Baihui and Dazhui acupoints in rats with VD and found significant increases in the cerebral activity of glutathione peroxidase (GSH-Px) and catalase (CAT), improving the learning and memory abilities of rats with VD.

7.1.6 Research on the Mechanisms of Acupuncture Treatment for PD

PD is a neurodegenerative disease, in which acupuncture has shown promising results in improving symptoms, relieving adverse reactions to medications, slowing disease progression, and enhancing the patient's quality of life.

By performing Xiusanzhen acupuncture in mouse models of PD, researchers found that this technique could inhibit the expression of tumor necrosis factor α (TNF-α) and IL-6 in the olfactory bulb and substantia nigra, which subsequently inhibited the inflammatory process, mitigated or effectively blocked the degeneration of dopaminergic neurons, and produced therapeutic effects on PD symptoms. In a study including 96 patients with PD, the control group received levodopa and benserazide tablets, while the experimental group received the aforementioned drug therapy and additional treatments, including the Huangqi Bushen decoction and acupuncture. The results indicated that compared to the control group, the experimental group showed superior therapeutic efficacy, fewer adverse reactions, and lower levels of high-sensitivity C-reactive protein (hs-CRP), TNF-α, and IL-6.

7.1.7 Future Prospects

The pathogenesis and treatment of neurological diseases have always been both a focus and a challenge in medical research. Owing to the ongoing advances in molecular biology, genomics, proteomics, and neurophysiology, some progress has been made in studying the mechanisms underlying the use of acupuncture as a treatment for neurological diseases, which can serve as a solid foundation for future in-depth investigations. However, the limitations of existing studies imply that a large proportion of current findings cannot comprehensively reflect the complex mechanisms involved in this treatment. Furthermore, studies on the mechanisms of acupuncture should now shift from animal models to clinical trials in patient populations, which will provide more scientific, reliable, and objective evidence.

7.2 Research Applications of MRI in the Brain Mechanisms of Acupuncture

7.2.1 Acupoint Specificity of Brain Responses

The theory and practice of acupuncture posit that acupuncture, when performed at specific sites on the skin (i.e., acupoints), can treat diseases, and that performing acupuncture at a variety of acupoints allows the treatment of different diseases. In other words, performing acupuncture at different acupoints produces different effects, which is known as acupoint specificity. At present, the nature of meridians remains poorly understood. One popular view on the mechanism of acupuncture is that its effects may be related to the neuro-humoral-endocrine system, meaning that the effects of acupuncture on acupoints are primarily mediated through the nervous system. Acupoint specificity refers to the specific brain responses elicited when acupoints are stimulated through needling and other techniques. The most direct approach to address the question of whether acupuncture is mediated by the nervous system, or whether acupuncture has an impact on the nervous system, is to observe whether acupuncture is associated with changes in neuronal excitation. Functional brain imaging techniques, such as PET, fMRI, and SPECT, can be utilized for the non-invasive detection and evaluation of blood flow, metabolism, blood oxygen levels, and receptors in various brain regions. Thus, these techniques can be effectively used to observe the functional state of the brain and to demonstrate the acupoint specificity of brain responses. fMRI, in particular, is a popular technique due to its excellent spatial and temporal resolution.

As fMRI and data processing techniques continue to improve, a growing number of experimental paradigms and data analysis methods have been adopted in research on acupuncture, and researchers have proposed a wide range of hypotheses and viewpoints. The most influential theory, at present, is the theory of limbic system deactivation, proposed by Hui of Massachusetts General Hospital at Harvard University. This theory has been extensively confirmed by serial studies and meta-analyses conducted by numerous research teams.

7.2.1.1 Research on the Characteristics of Brain Responses to Single-Acupoint Stimulation

Performing acupuncture at a single acupoint is similar to presenting a single somatosensory stimulus, and block designs are generally selected for fMRI experimental studies. Due to the unique nature of performing fMRI studies of the brain during acupuncture, needle retention without rotation is considered the baseline state, whereas needle rotation is considered the activation state. During the activation state, acupoint stimulation is performed using the same needling depth and rotation technique across different trials.

In 2000, Hui et al. conducted the first experiment to detect, and hence propose, the deactivation effects of the limbic system elicited by needling the Hegu acupoint on the hand. They utilized fMRI to evaluate the effects of needling the Zusanli acupoint, and revealed that the experience of *deqi* (i.e., a composite of sensations elicited by acupuncture) in healthy subjects was accompanied by a significant deactivation of the amygdala, hippocampus, parahippocampal gyrus, hypothalamus, anterior cingulate cortex (ACC), caudate nucleus, putamen, temporal pole, and insula. Moreover, when the subjects experienced pain without *deqi*, increased activation was detected in the ACC, caudate nucleus, putamen, anterior thalamus, and posterior insula. These findings suggest that acupuncture, which elicits the *deqi* sensation, can produce analgesic effects, primarily by regulating the subcortical limbic regions. Subsequently, Fang et al. examined the brain responses of needling the Taichong and its adjacent acupoints, and concluded that the key feature of manual acupuncture is the modulation of the limbic-paralimbic-neocortical network (LPNN), thereby laying the foundation for research in this field (Fig. 7.1).

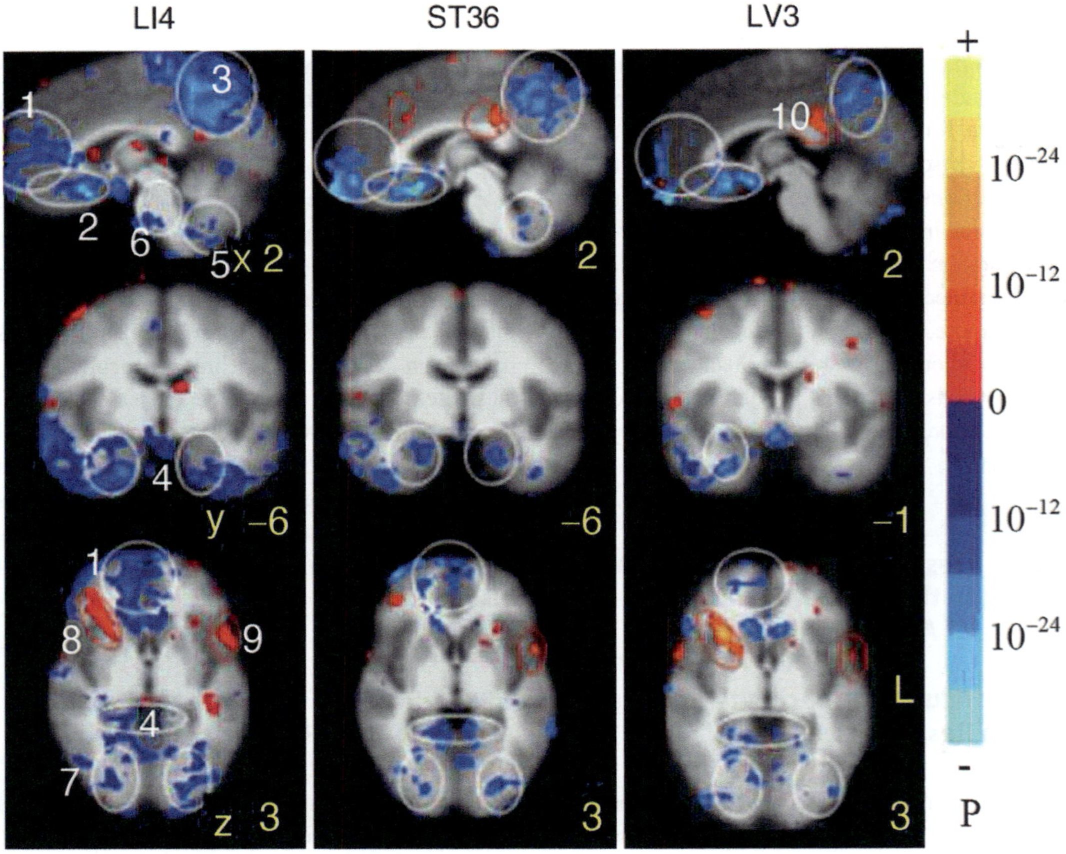

Fig. 7.1 The key feature of manual acupuncture is the modulation of the limbic-paralimbic-neocortical network: BOLD-fMRI functional maps of randomized manual acupuncture at the three major acupoints (Hegu acupoint, LI4: 64 experimental/37 healthy subjects; Zusanli acupoint, ST36: 74/43; Taichong acupoint, LV33: 63/37; $P < 0.0001$). Regions of deactivation are concentrated in the ventromedial prefrontal cortex (1, 2), medial parietal cortex (3), and medial temporal lobe (4), although deactivation is observed in the cerebellar tonsils and vermis (5), pontine nuclei (6), and lateral striatum (7). The overall pattern is similar for all three acupoints, but there are regional differences in the signal intensity and distribution. Overall, the strongest signal is from the Hegu acupoint at the frontal pole, and the weakest is from the ACC and cerebellum. Additionally, a few paralimbic regions are activated: the Hegu and Taichong acupoints activated the right anterior insula (8) and posterior cingulate gyrus-BA23d (9), while the superior temporal gyrus-BA22 (10) is activated for all three acupoints

A study evaluating hand acupuncture at the Neiguan acupoint (PC6) found that compared with the stimulation of adjacent sham acupoints and superficial acupoint stimulation, true acupoint needling elicited the specific activation of certain cerebellar areas. Thus, it was speculated that acupoint needling can also lead to specific cerebellar responses. Fang et al. performed needle rotation at the Taichong (LV3) and Qiuxu (G40) acupoints, and found significant overlap in cortical activation, whereas needle rotation at a sham acupoint adjacent to Taichong elicited only sporadic responses. The stronger response elicited by true acupoints compared to sham acupoints therefore illustrates the difference in the brain responses between the two, and demonstrates the relative specificity of acupoint effects. Additionally, the transcutaneous electrical stimulation of different acupoints can elicit brain activation in different regions. For instance, electrical stimulation of the Zusanli (ST36) and Sanyinjiao (SP6) acupoints increased the activation of the prefrontal cortex (PFC) and decreased the activation of the hippocampus, whereas electrical stimulation of the Yanglingquan (GB34) and Chengshan (B57) acupoints increased the activation of the dorsal thalamus and decreased the activation of the motor areas. Of note, the nerves for these four acupoints are located in similar spinal segments but elicit different brain responses. In another study, fMRI was used to observe the specific brain responses evoked by needling the Taichong and Hegu acupoints. Random effects analysis revealed that needling the Taichong acupoint led to more regions with increased than decreased activation, whereas the Hegu acupoint led to the opposite.

In summary, a number of studies have shown that compared to sham acupoints, the stimulation of true acupoints produces a range of regions with increased and decreased activation. The similarity among the different acupoints is that all of them elicit increased activation in the somatosensory areas, whereas decreased activation is mostly distributed in the limbic system or in the overlapping default mode network (DMN). However, there are differences in the extent and intensity of increased and decreased activation, which demonstrates the relative acupoint specificity of brain responses elicited by acupuncture.

7.2.1.2 fMRI Research on the Brain Responses to Multi-Acupoint Stimulation

The majority of fMRI-based studies on acupoints, conducted in both China and abroad, have focused on single acupoints, acupoint specificity, and acupoint correlations. However, single acupoints are rarely utilized in clinical settings for the treatment of diseases, as most needling is performed on groups of compatible acupoints. Acupoint combination refers to the combined application of two or more compatible acupoints, with the aim of increasing the physical stimulation of acupuncture and exploiting the synergistic effects among the acupoints, thereby improving the clinical efficacy. Many studies evaluating multiple acupoints have observed that the outcome is not a simple additive effect but does have relative specificity.

fMRI studies of the brain involving multiple acupoints are based on single acupoints as well as the comparison of true and sham acupoints. These studies generally utilize acupoint combinations commonly adopted in clinical practice, most of which involve the selection of two acupoints for combined acupuncture, and the experimental models are largely based on block designs.

Brain fMRI Research on the Siguan Acupoints

The Hegu and Taichong acupoints are both key for preserving health, with effects such as awakening the mind, opening the orifices, calming the heart, soothing the spirit, promoting *qi*, activating the blood, resolving stagnation, and relieving pain. The combination of the Hegu and Taichong acupoints is known as the "Siguan acupoints," which refers to the important gateways of human life, primarily serving to regulate Yin-Yang, expunge blocked heat, clear the heart, awaken the mind, and calm the spirit. These acupoints are commonly used in clinical practice and have achieved good outcomes in the treatment of psychiatric disorders. Xu et al. utilized fMRI techniques to study the brain responses to acupuncture at multiple acupoints. They found that needling the Hegu acupoint led to increased CBF and blood volume at the frontal and occipital lobes; the Taichong acupoint led to increased CBF and blood volume at the temporal lobe; and the combination of the Hegu and Taichong acupoints led to increased CBF and blood volume at the frontal and temporal lobes. Thus, the acupoint combination did not simply result in the summation of brain activation areas between the two single acupoints, but elicited a new distribution of brain hemodynamics. Additionally, by selecting sham acupoints that are at a certain distance from the true acupoints but not located on meridians, adopting the same needling technique as that for true acupoints, and comparing the differential brain activation between the two, it is possible to further validate the specificity of brain responses elicited by the Siguan acupoints. By performing fMRI while stimulating the true and sham Siguan acupoints, Shan et al. were able to observe differences in brain activity between the two conditions. Their findings revealed that the true Siguan acupoints could activate the somatosensory cortex, limbic system, vision-related areas, pain-related areas, and cerebellum, some of which may be related to the therapeutic efficacy of the Siguan acupoints in analgesia and regulating visceral movement. In contrast, the sham acupoints primarily activated the bilateral cingulate cortex, basal ganglia, insula, and cerebellum, the majority of which have been shown to be pain-related areas commonly activated during needling (Fig. 7.2). These results suggest that true acupoints elicit more widespread activation than sham acupoints, with significant differences in distribution characteristics, which can reflect the specificity of brain responses to needling the Siguan acupoints.

Brain fMRI Research on the Dazhong-Taixi Acupoint Combination

The Dazhong and Taixi acupoints are the connecting and source points, respectively, of the Kidney Meridian of Foot Shaoyin. These meridian acupoints are primarily used to treat diseases

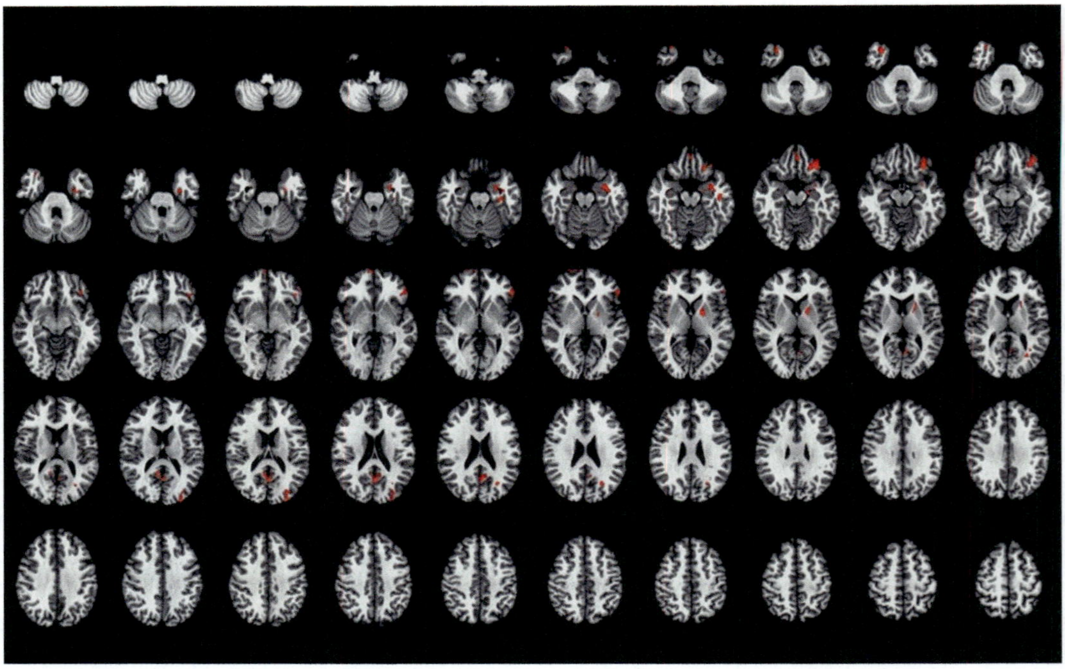

Fig. 7.2 Comparison of brain activation maps between the true Siguan acupoints and sham acupoints: Brain areas with greater activation for true rather than sham acupoints are located in the bilateral frontal lobes, right temporal pole, left parahippocampal gyrus, precuneus, basal ganglia, and occipital lobe

of the urogenital and nervous systems, and their clinical applications mainly involve the treatment of menopausal syndrome. The brain activations elicited by needling the Dazhong-Taixi acupoint combination did not simply result in the summation of the two individual acupoints but also led to relatively specific activations. The analgesic mechanism of this acupoint combination may be associated with the regulation of the pain matrix (PM) and midbrain activity, while its therapeutic mechanism for menopause may be related to the regulation of thalamic, especially hypothalamic, function.

7.2.2 *Deqi* Sensation in Acupuncture

7.2.2.1 Functional Brain Imaging of *Deqi*

The *deqi* needling sensation in acupuncture is a vital component of its therapeutic effects, and is also considered a key focus in brain fMRI research on the mechanisms of acupuncture. In a study on manual acupuncture at multiple acupoints, Hui et al. found that when subjects experienced *deqi* during acupuncture, they exhibited widespread decreased activation in the cerebrum, cerebellum, and brain stem, whereas the experience of pain mainly elicited patterns of increased activation. The results of their study showed that maximizing the degree of *deqi* experienced during acupuncture stimulation led to greater activation in the postcentral gyrus and limbic system. Additionally electroacupuncture studies have found that needling sensation was associated with the increased activation of cognitive processing and sensorimotor areas, as well as decreased activation of the DMN. Correlational studies between fMRI brain activity during acupuncture and the intensity of needling sensations revealed that during manual acupuncture at the Taichong acupoint on the right foot, the sensations of pressure, heaviness, fullness, numbness, and tingling were each correlated with specific brain areas. There were significant overlaps in these brain areas, which included the ACC, medial temporal cortex (MTC), and posterior parietal cortex (PPC). Pressure and fullness were positively correlated with the ACC, and negatively with the PPC. Heaviness was negatively correlated with the ACC and positively with the PPC. Numbness was positively correlated with the PPC and negatively with the hippocampus and parahippocampal gyrus. Tingling was the opposite, showing a negative correlation with the PPC and positive correlations with the hippocampus and parahippocampal gyrus. Tingling was also positively correlated with the bilateral posterior corpus callosum. Pressure contributed most extensively to the deactivation of the LPNN induced by acupuncture.

7.2.2.2 Differences in Functional Brain Imaging between *Deqi* and Sharp Pain

Fang et al. performed a comparative study of brain responses induced by *deqi* and *deqi* mixed with sharp pain during manual acupuncture at the Taichong acupoint on the right foot. Their results showed that *deqi* and sharp pain both activated the cortical somatosensory network, including the primary somatosensory cortex (SI), secondary somatosensory cortex (SII), motor cortex, supplementary motor area (SMA), thalamus, and insula, which is similar to the findings of previous fMRI studies on tactile and needling stimulations. More specifically, subjects who experienced *deqi* during acupuncture exhibited decreased activation in numerous regions of the LPNN, whereas sharp pain during acupuncture attenuated this deactivation or resulted in increased activation. Therefore, the findings suggest that *deqi* and *deqi* mixed with pain produced mutually antagonistic effects in the functional brain networks. The widespread deactivation of the LPNN and PM elicited by *deqi* may contribute to the central analgesic mechanisms of acupuncture.

Asghar et al. utilized two needling techniques, deep and superficial needling, to the right Hegu acupoint in order to compare the brain responses elicited by predominantly *deqi* with predominantly sharp pain sensations. Significant differences were found in the brain activation patterns between *deqi* and sharp pain for both deep and superficial needling. The *deqi* group exhibited deactivations in multiple brain areas, whereas the sharp pain group exhibited both deactivations and activations in multiple brain areas. For subjects who experienced *deqi* during deep needling, deactivations occurred primarily in the fusiform and lingual gyri; for those who experienced *deqi* during superficial needling, deactivations occurred primarily in the middle temporal and fusiform gyri. For subjects who experienced sharp pain during deep needling, deactivations occurred primarily in the posterior temporal lobe; while for those who experienced sharp pain during superficial needling, deactivations occurred primarily in the posterior temporal lobe and fusiform gyrus. When the *deqi* score was greater than the pain score, significant deactivations were detected in the bilateral insula, hippocampus, amygdala, thalamus, and cerebellum.

Despite the differences in the fMRI findings on the *deqi* sensation during acupuncture, the scans all showed that the *deqi* sensation is different from sharp pain, which also signifies the importance of recording needling sensations during fMRI studies on acupuncture. Few studies have been conducted regarding the correlation between complex *deqi* sensations and induced brain activity. Thus, this topic can serve as a future research direction, which may also provide objective, visualizable evidence for studying the utility of specific *deqi* sensations in clinical efficacy (Fig. 7.3).

7.2.3 Acupuncture-Induced Analgesia

7.2.3.1 Brain Areas and Networks Related to Acupuncture-Induced Analgesia

Imaging studies using fMRI, PET, SPECT, and other techniques have found that acupoints can elicit signals or metabolic changes in pain- or analgesia-related brain areas, such as the periaqueductal gray (PAG), thalamus, somatosensory cortex, insula, cingulate gyrus, and areas near the frontal lobe, suggesting that multiple brain regions or networks are involved in acupuncture-induced analgesia.

According to the results of preliminary research, peripheral nociceptive information can stimulate neuronal activity in the somatosensory cortex, and this neuronal activity can be attenuated by analgesics or acupuncture. The application of electroacupuncture at the Zusanli acupoint led to the significant attenuation of neuronal discharge elicited by noxious electrical stimulation, a phenomenon comparable to that evoked by intravenous analgesics, which implies that acupuncture can produce analgesic effects by regulating the activity of the somatosensory cortex. In a study by Fang et al., acupuncture at the right Taichong acupoint activated the somatosensory cortex (SI, SII), thalamus, and insula in both the *deqi* and pain groups. Therefore, acupuncture can regulate the CBF of SI and SII.

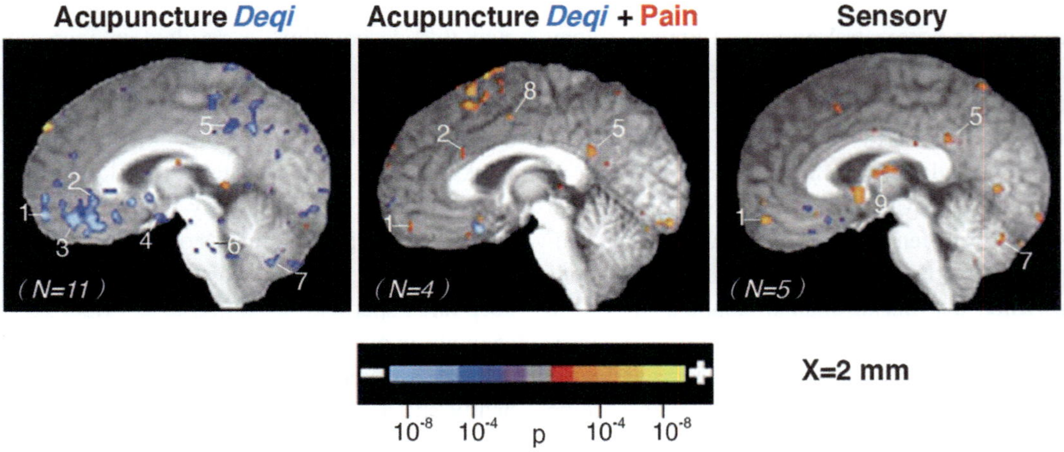

Fig. 7.3 Comparison of brain functional maps between *deqi* and *deqi* + pain with true acupuncture at acupoint ST36 and sham acupuncture (tactile stimulation with a Von Frey monofilament): The *deqi* group induced significant deactivation patterns in the prefrontal lobe and cingulate gyrus while the *deqi* + pain and sham acupuncture groups induced scattered activations in the prefrontal lobe, superior frontal lobe, and cingulate gyrus

Further studies by Kong et al. revealed that patients with migraine showed reduced functional connectivity of the PAG with the ACC and the medial prefrontal cortex (mPFC), while the magnitude of the reduction was closely related to migraine intensity. Acupuncture treatment was able to enhance the functional connectivity between the PAG and the ACC. Research on acupuncture at the Hegu acupoint revealed that the acupuncture-induced signal increases and decreases in different brain regions, with the PAG and left lentiform nuclei showing signal elevation and the bilateral ACC and occipital lobe showing signal reduction. The analgesic effects of acupuncture might be the result of the interactions between multiple functional areas. An fMRI study on acupuncture in patients with sciatica revealed significantly enhanced functional activity in the PAG, implying that the analgesic effect of acupuncture was related to its activation of the PAG, which inhibited the transduction of pain signals. Additionally, other studies found that the analgesic effects of acupuncture may be achieved by enhancing the connection between the PAG and the posterior cingulate cortex, regulating the functional connectivity of the DMN, and intervening in the connection between the PAG and the insula.

The thalamus plays a crucial role in acupuncture-induced analgesia, as it is not only a pain sensory center, but also a pain regulatory center. The thalamic nucleus submedius, together with the ventrolateral orbital cortex and the PAG, may constitute a regulatory pain pathway. This pathway serves as the coordination center for acupuncture-induced analgesia, and participates in modulating nociceptive input at the level of the spinal cord and trigeminal nerve by activating the brainstem descending inhibitory system. Research has shown that pain stimuli can activate multiple brain areas, including the thalamus, whereas acupuncture can attenuate these activation signals to varying extents. A study on electrical stimulation-induced analgesia revealed alterations in the functional connectivity of the thalamus with various pain-related areas, suggesting that the thalamus plays a key role in the analgesic mechanisms of acupuncture.

Studies have found that the amygdala exhibits deactivation after acupuncture-induced analgesia, whereas it exhibits activation after pain stimuli. Therefore, it was inferred that the amygdala is also involved in the analgesic effects of acupuncture, altering the cognitive and perceptual level of pain by regulating the balance of the autonomic nervous system. An fMRI study involving only healthy volunteers revealed extensive functional connectivity between the amygdala and the brain regions involved in pain perception and regulation. Furthermore, acupuncture was found to exert significant control over the amygdala-related brain networks. In a resting-state functional brain imaging study of the acupuncture treatment of patients with chronic low back and leg pain, functional connectivity analysis with the left amygdala as the seed region showed enhanced functional connectivity in the thalamus, brainstem, hippocampal gyrus, cingulate gyrus, and insula, which demonstrated from a different perspective that the amygdala is a key component of the endogenous pain regulatory network. Additionally, acupuncture performed at the Zusanli and Hegu acupoints led to decreased signals in the cingulate gyrus when subjects experienced *deqi*, and increased signals in the cingulate gyrus when they perceived pain. Therefore, this technique was able to induce inhibitory effects on pain perception and other aspects.

Hsieh et al. applied low-frequency electroacupuncture stimulation to the Hegu acupoint of healthy volunteers, which led to increased activation of the hypothalamus, insula, ACC, and cerebellum. Thus, they concluded that the hypothalamus plays an important role in mediating the analgesic effects of acupuncture. Other researchers also compared the brain responses to acupuncture between patients with carpal tunnel syndrome (CTS) and healthy volunteers. They found that manual acupuncture-induced deactivation in the amygdala and greater activation in the lateral hypothalamic area. Furthermore, it was found that different stages in the treatment process led to the deactivation of different brain regions. More specifically, pre-treatment pain was accompanied by hypersensitivity in the contralateral somatosensory areas, with digit 2 or 3 representation blurring in SI, whereas successful treatment led to significantly decreased activation in the contralateral SI and primary motor cortex (M1), with greater separation of digit representation in the SI, implying that acupuncture can promote the plasticity and recovery of nerve function. Studies on fibromyalgia have found that pain intensity is related to DMN functional connectivity. After 4 weeks of acupuncture treatment alone, patients who experienced a significant reduction in pain showed significant attenuation in the connectivity between the DMN and the insula. By examining the regional homogeneity (ReHo) changes of the PM and DMN in patients with neck pain, it was found that administering single- and multi-acupoint treatments led to different effects on PM and DMN despite achieving the same clinical efficacy. These results imply that the two methods involve different central analgesic effects. More specifically, the targets of multi-acupoint treatment may be located in the medial superior frontal gyrus and SMA, in which analgesic effects are achieved by affecting the medial pain system and blocking the descending pain pathway. The analgesic effect of acupuncture can also increase the patient's adaptability to pain and reduce avoidance behaviors. Moreover, acupuncture at the Zusanli acupoint can increase the amplitude of low-frequency fluctuation (ALFF) in multiple brain areas, producing a wider range and increased amplitude compared to sham acupoints.

A number of studies have found that despite the differences in the brain areas regulated by acupuncture, its analgesic effects are primarily achieved by integrating the functions of the PM or brain areas related to emotional regulation, especially the core areas of the DMN and its antagonistic brain networks, which supports the hypothesis that acupuncture modulates the LPNN. The immediate effects of acupuncture-induced analgesia refer to effects that occur within 30 min after the insertion of the needle(s), whereas pain relief or increased pain threshold that occurs after 30 min are known as the follow-up effects (also called the long-term or sequelae effects) of acupuncture-induced analgesia. The immediate effects of acupuncture-induced analgesia are primarily due to spinal cord mechanisms, whereas its follow-up effects are primarily due to negative-feedback pain modulatory systems above the level of the brainstem. In a study on the temporal changes in resting-state functional brain activity induced by acupuncture at the Zusanli acupoint (a key analgesic acupoint), the highest number of brain regions with significantly increased ALFF occurred 10 and 25 min after and gradually decreased at 45 and 60 min after the removal of the needle. This finding suggests that post-acupuncture effects have a significant impact on resting-state brain network activities, with key time points occurring at 10 and 25 min after the removal of the needle.

7.2.3.2 Acupuncture Treatment for Low Back Pain

Baliki et al. were the first to indicate that patients with chronic back pain exhibited reduced activation in the mPFC, medial thalamic nucleus, and ACC at rest compared to healthy subjects, which led to extensive functional changes throughout the brain and disrupted the normal state of the DMN, thereby leading to cognitive and behavioral abnormalities.

Acupuncture is a safe, effective, and simple method for the treatment and diagnosis of low back pain. Li et al. evaluated the pre- and post-treatment changes in the DMN of patients with chronic low back pain. They found that patients with chronic pain showed lower connectivity within the DMN than healthy controls, in areas including the dorsolateral prefrontal cortex (dlPFC), mPFC, ACC, and precuneus, and that acupuncture treatment essentially restored the levels of functional connectivity in these regions to almost those of the control group. Therefore, they concluded that the therapeutic efficacy of acupuncture is achieved through the modulation of the DMN. Another study on the application of acupuncture at the Weizhong acupoint for the treatment of lower back pain found that the functional brain areas exhibiting increased and decreased ReHo included the PFC, insula, right precuneus, right hippocampus, and temporal, cingulate, and parietal cortices. Moreover, a significant increase was observed in the functional connectivity between the thalamus and parahippocampal gyrus when subjects experienced back pain. Electroacupuncture performed at the Dachangshu and Weizhong acupoints in healthy subjects involved the pain center and the DMN. During electroacupuncture, the number of strong functional connections decreased, but a small number of new connections were formed, which may be implicated in the analgesic effects of acupuncture at the Weizhong and Dachangshu acupoints.

7.2.3.3 fMRI Research on the Neural Mechanisms of Acupuncture Treatment for CTS

Acupuncture has been gradually gaining recognition as an important non-surgical intervention for the clinical treatment of CTS. Patients with CTS exhibit significant maladaptive plasticity in the somatosensory cortex. For example, compared to healthy subjects, CTS patients show significant cortical activation after non-noxious stimulation of the fingers on the affected side. Furthermore, the boundaries between the SI representations of the second and third digits (D2/D3) were blurred, leading to closer inter-digit separation distances, which were significantly negatively correlated with the conduction delay of the sensory nerves. Based on these observations, a longitudinal study was performed to analyze the neural response patterns of CTS patients and healthy controls before and after acupuncture treatment, with the expectation that acupuncture would rectify the maladaptive central plasticity caused by CTS. The results of the longitudinal study showed that at baseline (before treatment), the boundaries between the SI representations of the second and third digits (D2/D3) were blurred, or the separation distances were reduced, while after acupuncture treatment, the D2/D3 separation distances had increased. Furthermore, the greater the D2/D3 separation distance, the milder the symptom of paresthesia in CTS patients, with the two showing a statistically significant negative correlation ($P < 0.05$). The results of that study, therefore, indicated that acupuncture, as a form of somatosensory stimulation, can promote beneficial plasticity changes in the CNS, which are manifested as more prominent cortical digit representations (Fig. 7.4).

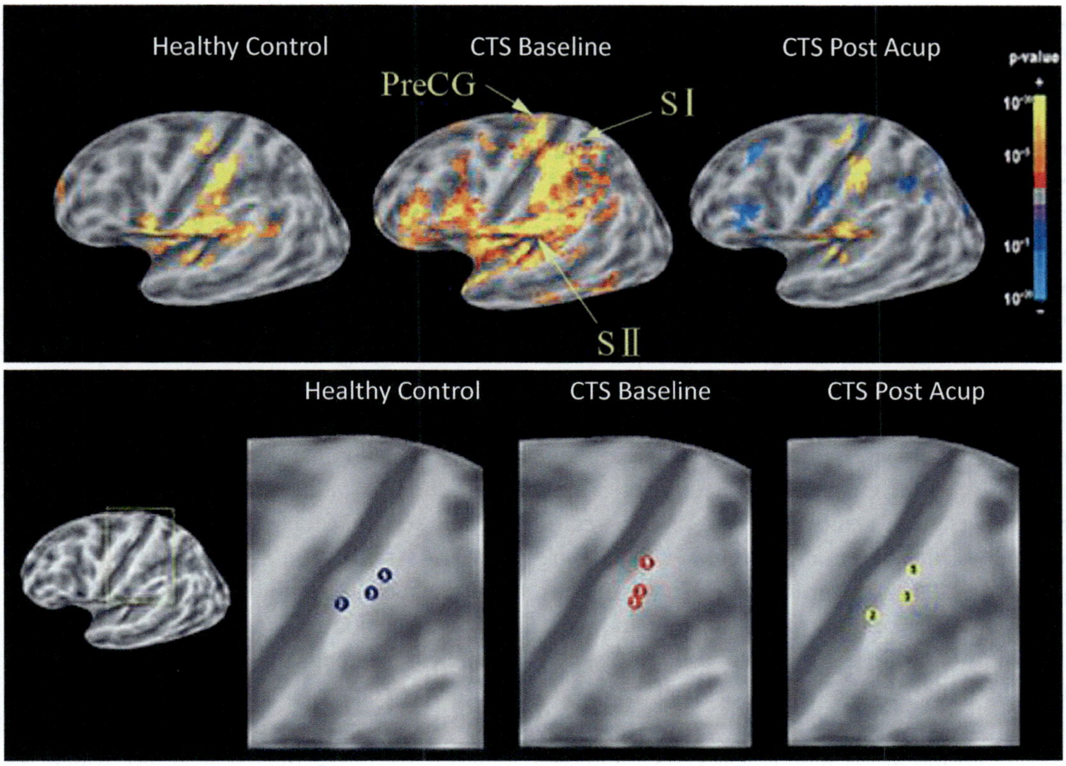

Fig. 7.4 Functional changes of the brain before and 5 weeks after acupuncture treatment: At baseline levels (before treatment), the boundaries between the representations of the second and third digits (D2/D3) in the primary somatosensory cortex are blurred, or the inter-digit separation distances are reduced. At 5 weeks after acupuncture treatment, the separation distances between the cortical representations of the second and third digits are increased. CTS patients with larger D2/D3 separation distances experienced milder symptoms of paresthesia, with a statistically significant negative correlation between the two

7.2.4 Acupuncture Treatment for Depression

Depression is a globally prevalent mental health condition with an incidence that rises continually each year. Pharmaceutical therapy is currently the primary approach for the treatment of depression. The disadvantages of the clinical use of antidepressants, however, include slow onset and numerous side effects. The use of acupuncture to treat depression offers advantages such as good therapeutic efficacy and a virtual lack of side effects, and this approach has been included in the latest clinical practice guidelines of the American College of Physicians. Studies involving structural and functional brain MRIs have shown that the core symptoms of depression, including low mood and volitional deficits, are significantly related to abnormal neural activities in the amygdala, striatum, cingulate cortex, and PFC. Therefore, the neural activity and functional connectivity of these brain areas can serve as biomarkers for the diagnosis and prognosis of depression.

Scalp acupuncture for the treatment of depression primarily involves acupoints along the Governor Vessel, such as the Baihui, Yintang, and Sishencong acupoints, in order to invigorate the brain, awaken the spirit, soothe the liver, resolve stagnation, and regulate emotions. Clinical studies have found no significant differences in the therapeutic efficacy between scalp acupuncture and fluoxetine in the treatment of depression, although the single-drug therapy for depression led to significantly higher side effects than acupuncture treatment. As for fMRI research on the use of scalp acupuncture to treat depression, researchers have explored the brain areas activated by acupuncture at the Baihui acupoint in patients with depression and its regulatory effects on DMN. They found that compared to sham acupoints, needling the Baihui acupoint could regulate multiple functional areas of the brain in patients with depression, including the cingulate cortex, insula, hippocampus and cerebellum, as well as modulate their DMN, thereby triggering depression-related consistent responses specific to the cerebello-cerebral and cortico-limbic networks.

The long-term clinical use of acupuncture has demonstrated effectiveness in treating depression with auricular acupuncture. At the turn of the twenty-first century, Zhu Bing and Rong Peijing from the Institute of Acupuncture and Moxibustion of the Chinese Academy of Chinese Medical Sciences first developed a transcutaneous auricular vagus nerve stimulator (taVNS), which is based on the connection between auricular acupoints and the vagus nerve (Fig. 7.5). Since then, controlled clinical trials have demonstrated that the taVNS is effective in the treatment of mild to moderate depression. Therefore, given its easy implementation, low cost, and minimal side effects, the taVNS can be used as an alternative method of therapy for depression. Fang et al. found that the taVNS produced modulatory effects on the nucleus tractus solitarius (NTS)-limbic lobe network (Fig. 7.6), and that 4 weeks of taVNS therapy significantly modulated the functional connectivity of the DMN in patients with major depressive disorder (MDD) (Fig. 7.7). taVNS therapy also produced regulatory effects on the right amygdala-left dlPFC network, which is implicated in emotional and cognitive functions. Moreover, the activation level of the anterior insula during the first stimulation period was significantly associated with clinical improvements at the end of the 4-week treatment, implying that insular fMRI activity can serve as a cortical imaging marker for the early prediction of taVNS efficacy.

It is believed that the stimulatory signals produced by abdominal acupuncture can penetrate the abdominal wall to act directly on the enteric nervous system, excite the neurons of the enteric nervous system, and regulate the production, secretion, and utilization of certain neuropeptides in the human body. The application of abdominal acupuncture in patients with depression showed significant enhancement in the amygdala-cingulate cortex and striatum-PFC functional connectivity in the treatment group, which was significantly correlated with changes in depression scale scores.

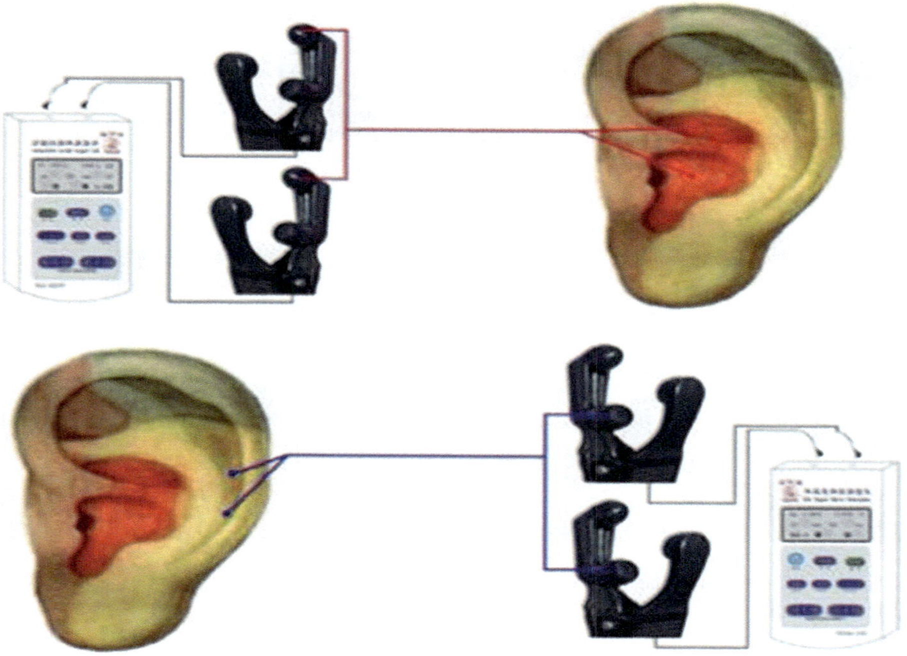

Fig. 7.5 Modulatory effects of taVNS on the NTS-limbic lobe network: Red represents the vagus nerve area of the auricular acupoints at the auricular concha. Yellow represents the control area at the superior scapha

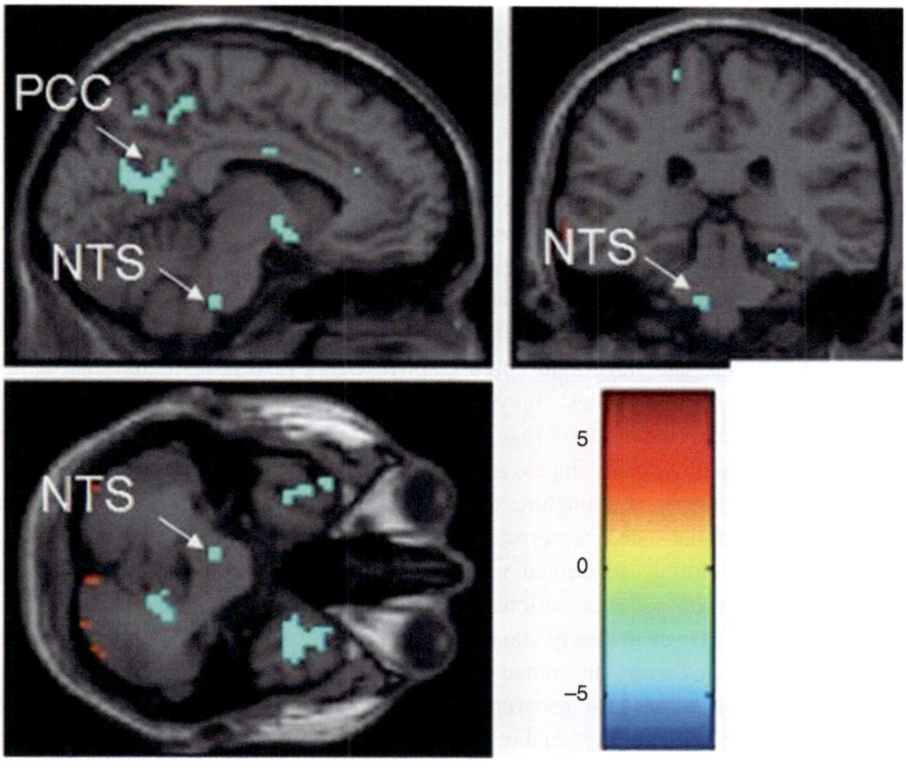

Fig. 7.6 Modulation of DMN functional connectivity in MDD: Auricular acupuncture stimulation produced negative activation in the nucleus tractus solitarius (NTS) and posterior cingulate cortex (PCC), revealing the pathway for stimulating the auricular acupoint-vagus nerve-NTS-limbic lobe network

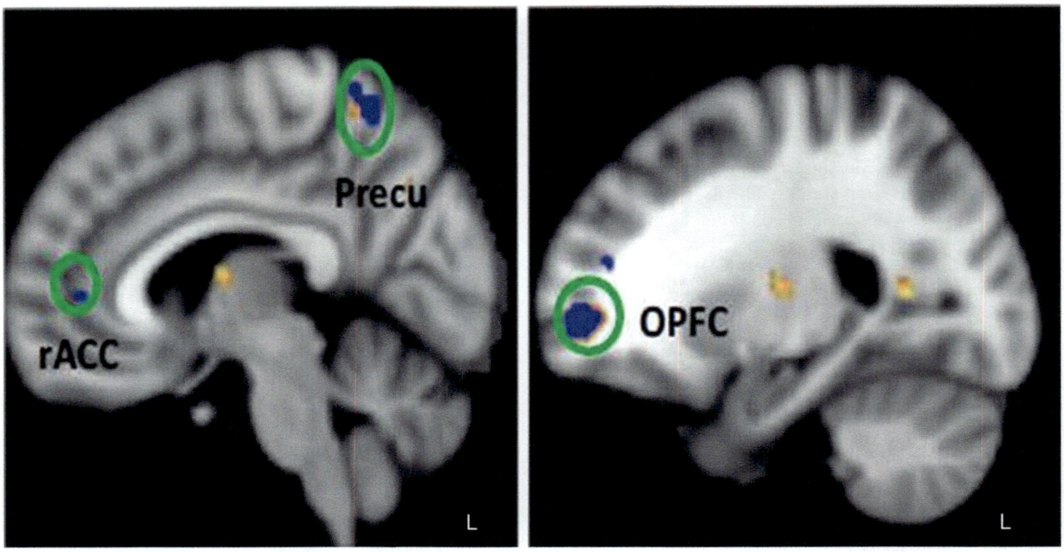

Fig. 7.7 Changes in functional connectivity between the DMN and multiple brain areas (blue) after 4 weeks of treatment with auricular concha vagus nerve stimulation in patients with depression: Increased functional connectivity of the DMN with the precuneus and orbital gyrus was negatively correlated with the reduction in the Hamilton Depression Rating Scale scores (yellow)

7.2.5 Acupuncture Treatment for Facial Palsy

Peripheral facial palsy is primarily characterized by the motor dysfunction of certain facial expression muscles, and acupuncture has been shown to be an effective treatment for this condition. In a task-based fMRI study on acupuncture in patients with facial palsy compared to healthy volunteers, significant differences were found in the brain responses of the visual areas, sensorimotor areas, and cerebellum among patients at different pathological stages (early-stage, late-stage, and cured groups). Based on these differences, it was inferred that acupuncture exerted different regulatory effects at different pathological stages, and the responses of the brain to acupuncture are closely related to its functional state. Furthermore, acupuncture can affect multiple functional network areas in the brain, with patients exhibiting weak functional connectivity at the early stages, which gradually strengthens over the course of disease recovery. Patients who have recovered from facial palsy undergo cortical functional reorganization, and acupuncture can induce DMN alternations to achieve emotional regulation.

7.2.6 Acupuncture Treatment for AD

AD is a neurodegenerative disease characterized by progressive cognitive and memory impairments, and is the most common type of senile dementia. Common acupoints used in the acupuncture treatment of AD include the Siguan acupoints (bilateral Hegu and Taichong acupoints), which serve to soothe the liver, regulate the circulation of *qi*, calm the spirit, stabilize the mind, open up the orifices, and awaken the spirit. Using resting-state and task-based fMRI, Wang et al. evaluated the brain activation effects of acupuncture at the Siguan acupoints in patients with AD and mild cognitive impairment (MCI). fMRI data were acquired from the AD, MCI, and control groups before, during, and after acupuncture, followed by comparative analysis. The results showed that the immediate acupuncture effects at the Siguan acupoints included the activation of the bilateral cerebellar hemispheres, fusiform gyrus, middle temporal gyrus, parahippocampal gyrus, superior frontal gyrus, inferior frontal gyrus, inferior parietal lobule, and bilateral thalamus. These activation

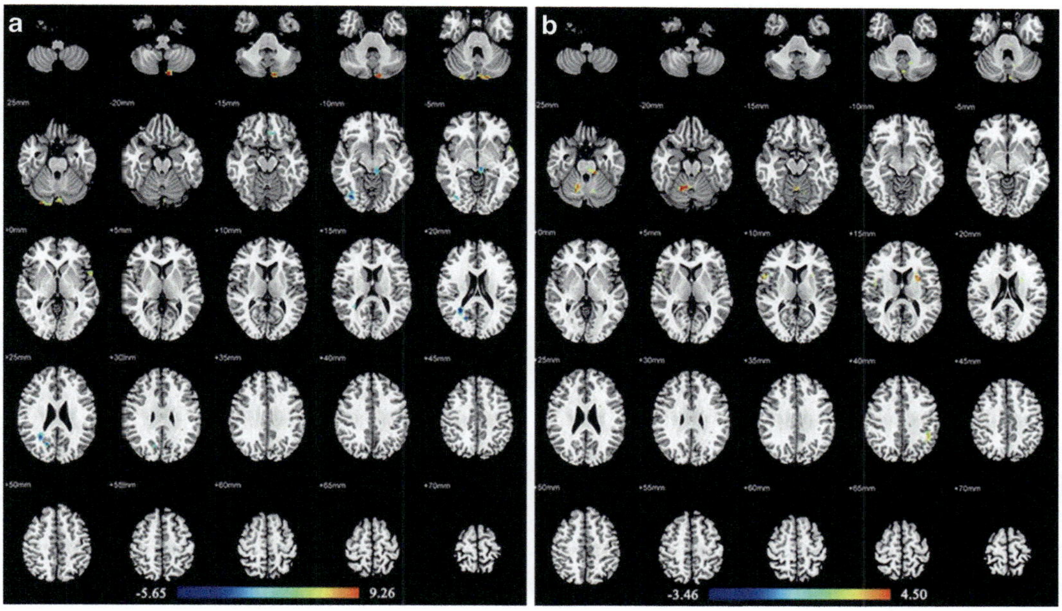

Fig. 7.8 Different brain activation patterns elicited by needling the true Siguan acupoints (**a**) and sham acupoints (**b**) in AD patients: Activations elicited by true acupuncture are primarily at the bilateral cerebellum, right inferior frontal gyrus, middle temporal gyrus, left globus pallidus, central operculum, prefrontal lobe, superior parietal gyrus, and supramarginal gyrus; deactivations are at the right cuneus, globus pallidus, inferior occipital gyrus, left straight gyrus, cerebellum, and putamen. Activations elicited by sham acupuncture are primarily at the bilateral cerebellum, right central operculum, and left inferior parietal lobule, while no deactivations are observed

areas are typically implicated in AD, and are closely associated with cognition and memory, meaning that acupuncture can stimulate or activate these diseased areas in patients with AD, including the hippocampal memory network and DMN. These findings, therefore, have provided preliminary evidence for the cognitive regulatory mechanisms of acupuncture in AD. Shan et al. obtained task-based fMRI scans to evaluate the specificity of brain responses to acupuncture at the Siguan acupoints in patients with AD and MCI. In their study, they first compared the different brain activation patterns induced by immediate acupuncture effects between true and sham acupoints. Their results revealed that compared to sham acupoints, true acupoints elicited extensive activation in cognition-related brain areas of patients with cognitive impairment, which included cognitive areas (frontotemporal lobe, supramarginal gyrus, etc.), somatosensory areas (superior parietal gyrus, etc.), and the cerebellum (Fig. 7.8). Additionally, they compared the differences in brain activation elicited by needling at the Siguan acupoints between patients with cognitive impairment and healthy controls. They found that the Siguan acupoints led to the deactivation of certain brain areas (cognitive and visual areas, basal ganglia, and cerebellum) in AD and MCI patients but produced extensive activations in the healthy controls. These findings indicate the specific modulatory effects elicited by needling at the Siguan acupoints in patients with cognitive impairment, thereby providing preliminary objective evidence for its therapeutic efficacy.

7.2.7 Acupuncture Treatment for Functional Dyspepsia (FD)

FD is the most prevalent type of digestive disease, and has shown good response to acupuncture treatment. Zeng et al. studied the central mechanisms of acupuncture treatment for FD at three levels. First, they utilized MRI and diffusion tensor imaging (DTI) to identify potential target brain areas involved in the central mechanism of acupuncture treatment for FD, from both a structural and functional perspective. Second, they performed fMRI scans to compare the effects of the classic acupoints for FD treatment (single Weishu acupoint, single Weimu acupoint, and combined Weishu-Weimu acupoints) on functional brain activity in FD patients, in order to evaluate the central mechanisms of acupuncture treatment for FD. Finally, they used PET/computed tomography (CT) and fMRI to observe the differences in CNS responses under different treatment durations and different physical states in response to the acupuncture treatment, which allowed them to evaluate part of the central mechanism involved in the effects of the treatment course and physical state on gastric regulation by acupuncture.

7.2.7.1 Research on the Pathological Alterations of Brain Function in FD Patients

The results of resting-state fMRIs showed that when compared to healthy controls, FD patients exhibited increased or decreased ReHo in multiple brain areas, of which, the increase in ACC ReHo was positively correlated with symptom severity, whereas the decrease in thalamic ReHo was negatively correlated with symptom severity. Furthermore, FD patients showed differences in the resting-state functional connectivity of the ACC, insula, and thalamus, as well as significantly reduced gray matter density in the right insula, right precentral gyrus, and left midcingulate cortex (MCC). When scores for the Self-Rating Anxiety Scale (SAS) and Self-Rating Depression Scale (SDS) were included as covariates, FD patients showed a significant increase in the fractional anisotropy (FA) values of the corona radiata.

7.2.7.2 Research on the Central Mechanism of Acupuncture Treatment for FD

The Weishu-Weimu acupoint combination (Zhongwan-Zusanli combination) is a classic acupuncture treatment for gastrointestinal diseases. It has been shown that acupuncture-induced regulation of the ACC, insula, and key limbic areas is an important central mechanism underlying the acupuncture treatment of FD.

7.2.7.3 Research on the Factors Influencing the Gastrointestinal Regulatory Effects of Acupuncture

Acupuncture effects can be influenced by various factors, including the duration of the treatment course, different acupuncture techniques, and the patient's physical state. With regards to the immediate effects of acupuncture at the Zusanli acupoint, on fMRI, FD patients showed deactivations in the right supramarginal gyrus, right OFC, right ACC, right mPFC, and left superior occipital gyrus when compared with healthy controls. After a long course of acupuncture treatment, FD patients showed widespread reduction in all limbic-cerebral areas with abnormally elevated glucose metabolism. After a short course of acupuncture treatment, the hypermetabolic regions detected in FD patients included the inferior occipital gyrus, middle occipital gyrus, precuneus, right middle temporal gyrus, and right medial frontal gyrus; while the hypometabolic regions included the cerebellum, left lentiform nucleus, brainstem, and postcentral gyrus. Compared to 5 sessions of acupuncture treatment, 20 sessions resulted in a more widespread reduction in all hypermetabolic regions, and more significantly modulated the functional activities of the disease-related areas, such as the insula, ACC, and thalamus. This implies that under different physical states, acupuncture performed at the same acupoint will elicit different brain functional responses; therefore, physical state has a significant impact on acupuncture effects. Additionally, Fang et al. found that performing manual acupuncture at body acupoints for 1 month alleviated symptoms of dyspepsia in FD patients, while also improving their mental state and quality of life. This may be associated with the regulation of the brain-gut axis, whereby abnormalities in brain functions related to the body's internal environment are normalized, causing an increase in the frequency and propagation speed of gastric peristaltic waves and the secretion of gastrin.

7.2.8 Acupuncture Treatment for Crohn's Disease (CD)

CD is a type of inflammatory bowel disease characterized by a chronic and recurrent nature. Based on many years of clinical practice, needling and moxibustion have been shown to be safe and effective treatments for CD. Using MRI, researchers have revealed the structural differences in gray matter between CD patients and healthy subjects. More specifically, they observed the increased gray matter volume of the putamen, globus pallidus, thalamus, hippocampal gyrus, PAG, PPC, and precuneus, and the decreased gray matter volume of the bilateral ACC, insula, dmPFC, postcentral gyrus, superior temporal gyrus, right MCC, left SMA, precentral gyrus, superior frontal gyrus, middle frontal gyrus, middle temporal gyrus, inferior temporal gyrus, and inferior parietal cortex. The gray matter volume of the right ACC, dorsomedial PFC (dmPFC), and left insula was significantly negatively correlated with disease duration. Furthermore, there were significant decreases in the cortical thickness of the bilateral orbitofrontal cortex (OFC), inferior parietal cortex, superior temporal gyrus, upper part of the left middle frontal gyrus, pars triangularis of the inferior frontal gyrus, middle temporal gyrus, right PCC and fusiform gyrus, bilateral superior frontal gyrus, left insula, ventral part of the ACC, postcentral gyrus, and right precentral gyrus. The cortical thickness of the left insula and OFC was significantly negatively correlated with disease duration. Further studies identified differences in functional brain activity between CD patients and healthy subjects. More specifically, CD patients with abdominal pain showed decreased ReHo values in the insula, MCC, and SMA, as well as increased ReHo values in the temporal pole, whereas CD patients without abdominal pain showed decreased ReHo values in the hippocampus/parahippocampus and increased ReHo values in the dmPFC. The ReHo values of the insula and MCC are significantly negatively correlated with the Visual Analogue Scale (VAS) scores for abdominal pain.

Following herb-partitioned moxibustion, brain areas involved in regulating the resting-state brain function of CD patients that exhibited significantly elevated ReHo values included the bilateral MCC, globus pallidus, putamen, inferior frontal gyrus, SMA, occipital lobe, cerebellum, brainstem, left PCC, parahippocampal gyrus, paracentral lobule, angular gyrus, fusiform gyrus, right insula, precentral gyrus, and postcentral gyrus; while brains areas with reduced ReHo values included the bilateral middle temporal gyrus, lingual gyrus, left medial superior frontal gyrus, inferior temporal gyrus, temporal pole, right OFC, middle frontal gyrus, and caudate nucleus. Following electroacupuncture, the brain areas involved in regulating the resting-state brain function of CD patients that exhibited significantly elevated ReHo values included bilateral MCC, thalamus, hippocampal gyrus, inferior frontal gyrus, precentral gyrus, paracentral lobule, superior temporal gyrus, left parahippocampus, globus pallidus, cerebellum, right insula, putamen, postcentral gyrus, SMA, lingual gyrus, and brainstem, and the brain areas with reduced ReHo values included the bilateral ACC, OFC, inferior temporal gyrus, temporal pole, occipital lobe, left superior parietal cortex, angular gyrus, cuneus, right middle frontal gyrus, and caudate nucleus. In the moxibustion group, ReHo changes in the medial superior frontal gyrus, middle frontal gyrus and superior temporal pole were significantly positively correlated with Crohn's Disease Activity Index (CDAI) scores, while ReHo changes of the MCC, precentral gyrus, postcentral gyrus, SMA, and PCC were significantly negatively correlated with CDAI scores. In the electroacupuncture group, ReHo changes of the ACC, middle frontal gyrus, and superior temporal pole were significantly positively correlated with CDAI scores, and ReHo changes in the MCC, thalamus, insula, hippocampal gyrus, precentral gyrus, postcentral gyrus, and SMA were significantly negatively correlated with CDAI scores. Brain regions with common responses for both moxibustion and electroacupuncture in regulating the resting-state brain function of CD patients included the left MCC, superior temporal pole, right precentral gyrus, postcentral gyrus, SMA, and middle frontal gyrus. Brain regions with differential responses between moxibustion and electroacupuncture in regulating the resting-state brain function of CD patients included the left medial superior frontal gyrus and PCC for moxibustion, and the bilateral thalamus, left hippocampal gyrus, right insula, and ACC for electroacupuncture.

The following conclusions can be drawn from the above study: (1) compared to healthy subjects, remissive CD patients showed significant differences in the gray matter structure and functional activity of multiple brain regions involved in the regulation of pain, emotion, cognition, and homeostasis, which can partly be explained by the higher levels of anxiety and depression experienced by patients; however, relatively specific functional brain activities were detected in remissive CD patients with and without abdominal pain; (2) herb-partitioned moxibustion and electroacupuncture can regulate abnormal resting-state functional brain activities in remissive CD patients, with the two techniques eliciting common and differential responses in different brain regions. The universal feature of CNS responses shared between the two is the global regulation of the entire brain in the treatment of remissive CD patients. The unique feature of the CNS responses of electroacupuncture treatment is the global regulation of the homeostatic afferent processing network, whereas that of moxibustion is the global regulation of the DMN.

7.3 Research Applications of PET Imaging in the Brain Mechanisms of Acupuncture

The application of PET in functional brain imaging enables the direct observation of real-time activities in the living body in response to specific stimuli, while maintaining the integrity of its physiological state. Therefore, this technique coincides with the holistic approach of Chinese medicine, offering a non-invasive, objective, intuitive, and practical method for studying the effects of acupuncture.

Fruitful research has been conducted by adopting functional brain imaging techniques in the field of acupuncture, with promising results obtained by studying the relationship between different acupoints (e.g., Zusanli, Taichong, Quchi, etc.) and the brain, as well as the mechanisms of acupuncture treatments for various diseases, including depression, VD, and AD. As a functional imaging technique with excellent properties, PET/CT has been used to explore the rules of selecting acupoints along meridians and has provided new ideas for investigating the central mechanisms of acupuncture. With the recent widespread application of functional brain imaging in the field of acupuncture, substantial progress has been made in acupoint specificity, acupoint combination, and acupuncture techniques, with a growing number of studies turning toward the mechanisms of selecting acupoints along the meridians.

7.3.1 Applications of PET Imaging in Experimental Acupuncture Research

By performing PET imaging, Lai et al. observed the central activation effects of needling the Shenmen acupoint in rat models of AD. Their results showed that the acupuncture treatment led to improvements in memory in the model group compared to the pre-treatment levels, along with higher glucose metabolism activity in the frontal lobe, hippocampus, thalamus, hypothalamus, and temporal lobe. This implies that needling the Shenmen acupoint produced certain CNS effects and improved the metabolic activity of AD-related brain areas, while also suggesting that acupuncture does not activate a single specific brain area, but multiple disease-related brain areas or a central network system (Fig. 7.9). Lu et al. used PET imaging to evaluate the central activation effects and underlying mechanisms of needling the Zusanli acupoint in rats with AD. They found that compared to the model

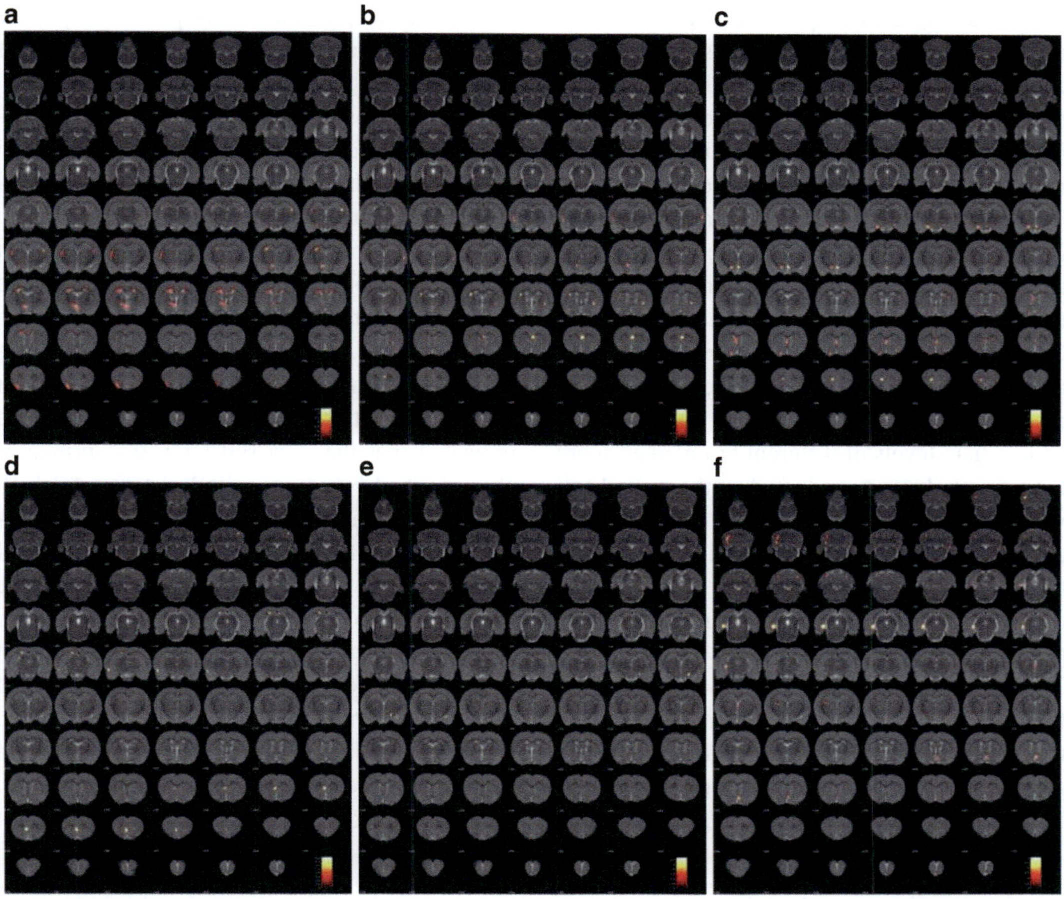

Fig. 7.9 Central activation maps of acupuncture at the Shenmen acupoint: Brain activation maps of the AD group versus the control group on day 1 and day 30, which show significantly reduced glucose metabolism in the hippocampus, dorsal thalamus, striatum, piriform cortex, and sensory cortex (**a**, **b**). Brain activation maps of the AD+HT7 group versus the AD group, which show increased glucose metabolism in the hippocampus, orbital cortex, cerebellum, piriform nucleus, retrosplenial cortex, sensory cortex, and olfactory cortex after 20 treatments (**c**, **d**). Brain activation maps of the AD+Sham group versus the AD+HT7 group, which show increased glucose metabolism in the hippocampus, dorsal thalamus, olfactory cortex, cerebellum, pontine, and dentate gyrus after treatment (**e**, **f**)

group, the brain activation areas in the acupuncture group were concentrated primarily in the limbic system, temporal lobe, right amygdala, and hippocampus, and compared to the sham acupuncture group, the brain activation areas in the acupuncture group mainly included the amygdala and temporal lobe. Therefore, it was proposed that needling the Zusanli acupoint would increase the volume of cerebral perfusion and the glucose metabolism levels of specific brain areas, thereby producing positive effects on the cognitive abilities of AD patients. By performing electroacupuncture at the Yifeng and Tinggong acupoints in healthy guinea pigs, researchers were able to observe the effects of this intervention on the glucose metabolism levels in the auditory cortex. Their results showed significantly higher glucose metabolism levels in the auditory cortex of the electroacupuncture group, suggesting that these acupoints can improve the regional energy metabolism of neurons in the auditory cortex and enhance their physiological activity. Other researchers have observed the effects of electroacupuncture at the

Ganshu and Qimen acupoints on PET functional imaging of rat models of liver *qi* stagnation. The electroacupuncture group showed glucose hypometabolism in the left frontal lobe, parietal lobe, paracentral lobule, supracallosal gyrus, thalamus, and hypothalamus, as well as glucose hypermetabolism in the left frontal lobe, parietal lobe, basal ganglia, temporal lobe, right frontal lobe, and subthalamus. These findings indicate that electroacupuncture at the Ganshu and Qimen acupoints can regulate the glucose metabolism levels of brain areas that closely associated with emotions. Based on the glucose metabolism levels of different brain areas, a preliminary study was conducted on the central activation effects of acupuncture at the source acupoints of the liver and kidney meridians in rats with primary hypertension. The results of that study showed that acupuncture performed at the Taichong acupoint, Taixi acupoint, or Taichong + Taixi acupoints led to significant differences in brain activation areas and glucose metabolism levels. A comparison of these three groups with the sham acupuncture group also showed significant differences in glucose metabolism. Therefore, acupuncture at the Taichong and Taixi acupoints may be one of the central mechanisms for the effective lowering of blood pressure.

7.3.2 Applications of PET/CT in Clinical Acupuncture Research

7.3.2.1 PET/CT Imaging Research on the Brain Responses to Acupuncture under Normal Physiological Conditions

Application of PET in Clinical Research on Single-Point Acupuncture

There is a wide range of clinical applications for single-point acupuncture, and acupoints with significant and specific therapeutic effects include the Hegu, Waiguan, Sanyinjiao, and Zusanli acupoints. By combining the results of PET functional brain imaging with the therapeutic effects of clinical acupuncture, it is possible to more clearly elucidate the brain mechanisms of acupuncture.

Observations of PET imaging findings following acupuncture at the Waiguan acupoint revealed activations at the bilateral parietal lobe, occipital lobe, cuneus, and other areas, implying that there is an association between the Waiguan acupoint and related brain areas, thus validating the hypothesis that acupoint specificity is related to brain function. Additionally, preliminary findings on the PET imaging characteristics of different needling sensations during Waiguan acupuncture indicated that the *deqi* sensation was primarily characterized by soreness and distention, which was accompanied by increased glucose metabolism in the left frontal lobe and superior temporal gyrus. Gong et al. performed PET imaging of the brain in healthy women during acupuncture at the right Sanyinjiao acupoint, and observed increased glucose metabolism in the bilateral SMA and dlPFC, and contralateral medial PFC, pre-SMA, ACC, SI, and motor cortex. They also observed decreased glucose metabolism in the hippocampus, occipital lobe, lingual gyrus, and parahippocampal gyrus. These findings suggest that the effects of Sanyinjiao are related to brain activation, which can serve as objective evidence for research on acupuncture. Furthermore, the PET imaging findings of acupuncture at the right Zusanli acupoint in healthy subjects showed significantly elevated glucose metabolism levels in subcortical structures associated with the autonomic nervous system, such as the hypothalamus, head of the caudate nucleus, and brainstem. Most of these regions are involved in the regulation of visceral organs, which is consistent with the effects of the Zusanli acupoint. Lai et al. examined the effects of true and sham acupuncture at the Waiguan acupoint on PET brain functional imaging, and their results demonstrated significant differences in the brain areas activated between the two groups. Compared to the sham acupuncture group, the true acupuncture group showed activations primarily in the insula, temporal lobe, and left cerebellum. In the study by Hsieh et al., PET was performed to observe the central, analgesia-related brain areas activated by acupuncture at the Hegu acupoint. They found that compared to acupuncture at a non-analgesic acupoint, brain regions that were specifically activated included the hypothalamus, which extended to the midbrain, insula, ACC, and cerebellum. Therefore, they speculated that the hypothalamus is a key target region activated by analgesic acupoints, and one of the possible factors mediating the analgesic effects of acupuncture, thereby providing robust evidence for research on the central mechanisms of acupuncture-induced analgesia.

PET Imaging Research on the Brain Responses to Multi-Point Acupuncture under Normal Physiological Conditions

Observations on the effects of an acupuncture prescription (combination of the Tanzhong, Zhongwan, Qihai, Xuehai, Waiguan, and Zusanli acupoints) of healthy elderly individuals revealed significantly elevated glucose metabolism in the bilateral frontal and left temporal lobes of the treatment group compared to the sham group. These findings indicate that acupuncture at this acupoint combination can enhance the glucose metabolism of cognition-related brain areas in healthy elderly individuals with significant specificity. Furthermore, Park et al. observed the central activation effects of simultaneous acupuncture at two specific acupoints (Taichong and Neiting). They found elevated glucose metabolism in the left insula, bilateral thalamus, superior frontal region of the right frontal lobe, and inferior frontal region of the left frontal lobe, as well as reduced glucose metabolism in the cingulate cortex and parahippocampal gyrus of the left limbic lobe. In another PET study by An et al., electroacupuncture applied at the Quchi and Hegu acupoints in healthy volunteers led to changes in rCBF and glucose metabolism. More specifically, increased cerebral perfusion was observed in the superior parietal, right superior frontal, left middle frontal, and middle parietal gyri. These results show that CBF and glucose metabolism in the frontal regions increased to varying extents following acupuncture, while producing consistent functional changes, thus suggesting that acupuncture at specific acupoints can promote the level of synergistic functions in target brain areas.

7.3.2.2 PET/CT Imaging Research on the Brain Responses to Acupuncture under Pathological Conditions

Vascular Dementia

VD is primarily characterized by the decline or impairment of memory, cognition, language, personality, behavior, attention, and other mental faculties, which can adversely affect the patient's work life and social activity. VD not only brings about long-term suffering and severely impacts the patient's quality of life, but also creates a heavy burden on family, society, and the country. In the treatment of VD, PET findings revealed that the addition of the Baihui acupoint to conventional body acupuncture led to greater increases in the glucose metabolism of the frontal lobe, parietal lobe, occipital lobe, thalamus, lentiform nucleus, and cerebellum of the unaffected side, as well as the frontal lobe, thalamus, caudate nucleus, and cerebellum of the affected side compared to the conventional acupuncture group. This may be one of the mechanisms by which acupuncture at the Baihui acupoint alleviates VD-related symptoms. Huang et al. observed the effects of needling the Baihui, Shuigou, and Shenmen acupoints on the functional metabolism of the lentiform nucleus, which is a brain area specific to VD. The treatment group showed significantly enhanced glucose metabolism in the lentiform nucleus of the unaffected side, whereas the control group did not show any changes in the bilateral lentiform nuclei. Furthermore, electroacupuncture treatment of VD patients at the Sishencong, Baihui, Shenting, and bilateral Fengchi head acupoints increased the glucose metabolism of the frontal, parietal, and occipital lobes to varying extents, which was also correlated with changes in the cognitive efficacy index and activities of daily living index. Additionally, VD patients treated with conventional body acupuncture showed significant increases in the glucose metabolism of the bilateral frontal lobe and thalamus, as well as the unaffected temporal lobe and lentiform nucleus, which were accompanied by improvements in dementia symptoms. A study examining the effects of the "Yiqi Tiaoxue, Fuben Peiyuan" (i.e., "*Qi*-Reinforcing and Blood-Regulating," "Foundation-Strengthening and Vitality-Cultivating") acupuncture prescription on the central metabolism of VD patients found that the treatment led to significant increases in the unaffected temporal lobe, hippocampus, and cingulate gyrus, as well as the bilateral frontal lobe, thalamus, and caudate nucleus compared to before treatment. Significant differences were also detected when compared with the sham non-meridian, non-acupoint group. Thus, the results of this study have also demonstrated the specificity of acupoints, and the central effects of acupuncture.

Ischemic Stroke

Ischemic stroke, also known as cerebral infarction, has been shown to benefit from the promotion of cerebral metabolism and effective energy utilization induced by acupuncture, which can alleviate the ischemic state of the brain tissues and facilitate the recovery of nerve function.

PET imaging was performed to observe the central activation effects of acupuncture at the Waiguan acupoint in stroke patients with lesions restricted to the left basal ganglia. The results indicated that compared to the sham group, the treatment group showed activations at the left cerebellum, cerebellar tonsils, bilateral superior temporal gyrus, and right inferior frontal gyrus, implying that needling the Waiguan acupoint can induce regional increases in the glucose metabolism of specific brain areas. Yong et al. compared the pre- and post-intervention PET images of post-stroke patients who received needling at the Waiguan acupoint, sham needling, sham-acupoint needling, or non-needling. Compared with the non-needling group, the needling group exhibited significant activation of Brodmann Area (BA) 30, while compared with the sham needling group, the needling group exhibited significant activation of BA 13, 19, and 47. No significant activation was found in the comparison among other groups; therefore, needling the Waiguan acupoint should regulate cerebral functional areas related to the chronic stage of ischemic stroke, which may be associated with its effects in post-stroke recovery. Fang et al. performed electroacupuncture at the Baihui and Qubin acupoints in patients after ischemic stroke, which led to significant increases or decreases in the glucose metabolism of bilateral motor-related brain regions. They concluded, therefore, that electroacupuncture can exert beneficial regulatory and facilitatory effects on cerebral motor functions. In a PET study examining the effects of the Xingnao Kaiqiao needling technique in patients after acute cerebral infarction, the results showed significant improvements in whole-brain metabolism, as well as metabolism in the central cerebral infract and peri-infarct edema zones, which exhibited significant activation, and specific effects when compared to non-meridian, non-acupoint needling (Fig. 7.10).

Other Neurological Diseases

Encouraging progress has been made in research on the application of PET/CT imaging techniques to the acupuncture treatment of AD, PD, migraine, and other neurological disorders. PET imaging findings of AD patients before and after treatment with needling at the bilateral Hegu and Taichong acupoints revealed significantly increased glucose metabolism in the frontal and temporal lobes after treatment, along with significant improvement in cognition-related symptom scores. In a study by Huang et al., PD patients were treated using acupuncture combined with Western medicine. After 5 weeks of treatment, the patients showed significantly elevated glucose metabolism in the parietal lobe, temporal lobe, occipital lobe, hypothalamus, and cerebellum of the mildly affected hemisphere, and in the parietal and occipital lobes of the severely affected hemisphere, whereas patients treated with Western medicine alone did not exhibit significant changes after treatment. These findings, therefore, demonstrate the clinical efficacy of acupuncture treatment in PD. Additionally, Jie et al. observed the effects of acupuncture at the Fengchi, Yanglingquan, and Waiguan acupoint combination on the cerebral glucose metabolism

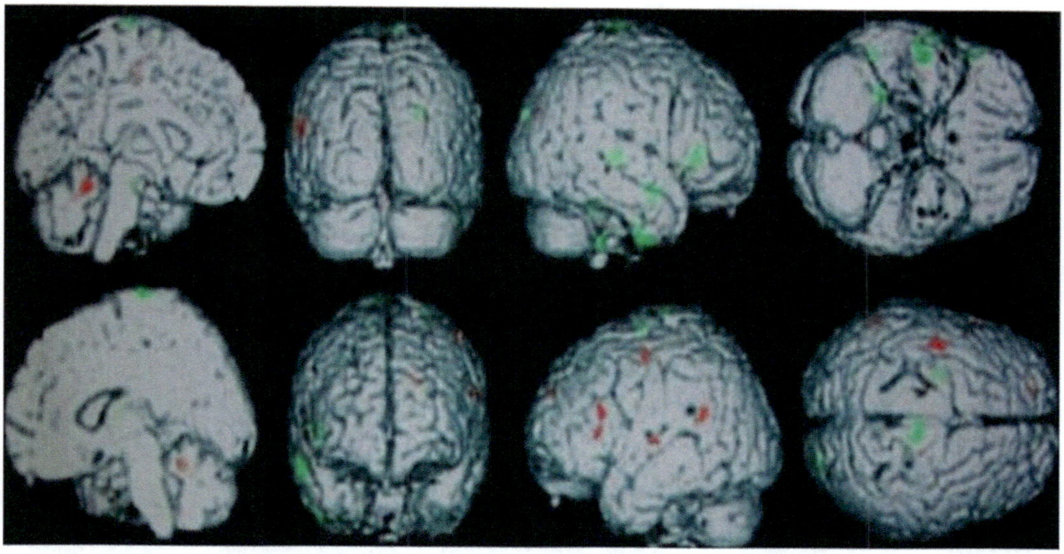

Fig. 7.10 Changes in brain glucose metabolism 3 weeks after electroacupuncture at the Baihui and Qubin acupoints: Red represents brain areas with increased glucose metabolism; green represents brain areas with decreased glucose metabolism

of patients with migraine. They found that the acupuncture group exhibited increased cerebral glucose metabolism in the middle temporal cortex (MTC), OFC, insula, middle frontal gyrus, angular gyrus, PCC, precuneus, and MCC; whereas the parahippocampal gyrus, hippocampus, fusiform gyrus, postcentral gyrus, and cerebellum showed decreased glucose metabolism. Therefore, these brain areas may be related to the functional specificity of acupoints related to the treatment of migraine (Fig. 7.11).

PET/CT imaging was utilized to observe the effects of short- and long-course acupuncture treatment on the functional brain activity of FD patients. The results revealed that long-course acupuncture in FD patients led to extensive reductions in all limbic-cerebral regions with abnormally elevated glucose metabolism, which included the bilateral insula (BA13), ACC (BA24, BA32), MCC (BA31, BA32), PCC (BA29, BA30), thalamus, parahippocampal gyrus (BA35, BA19), left IFG (BA3), and cuneus (BA7). After short-course acupuncture treatment, FD patients showed increased glucose metabolism in the IOG, MOG, precuneus, right MTG, and right medial frontal gyrus, as well as decreased metabolism in the cerebellum, left lentiform nucleus, brainstem, and postcentral gyrus. Compared to short-course acupuncture, long-course acupuncture led to more extensive reductions in various brain regions with abnormally elevated glucose metabolism in FD patients, and more significantly regulated the functional activities of the insula, ACC, thalamus, and other disease-related brain areas (Fig. 7.12).

7.3.3 Summary

To summarize the research findings above, under normal physiological conditions, PET/CT imaging studies on acupuncture focused primarily on unilateral or bilateral acupuncture, the number of acupoints, the location and distribution of acupoints, and other aspects. Most studies have shown that under normal physiological conditions, acupuncture can activate a variety of brain regions that are associated with the functions of the acupoints examined, thus validating the specificity of acupoint effects. Moreover, this further demonstrates the holistic action of acupoints, and

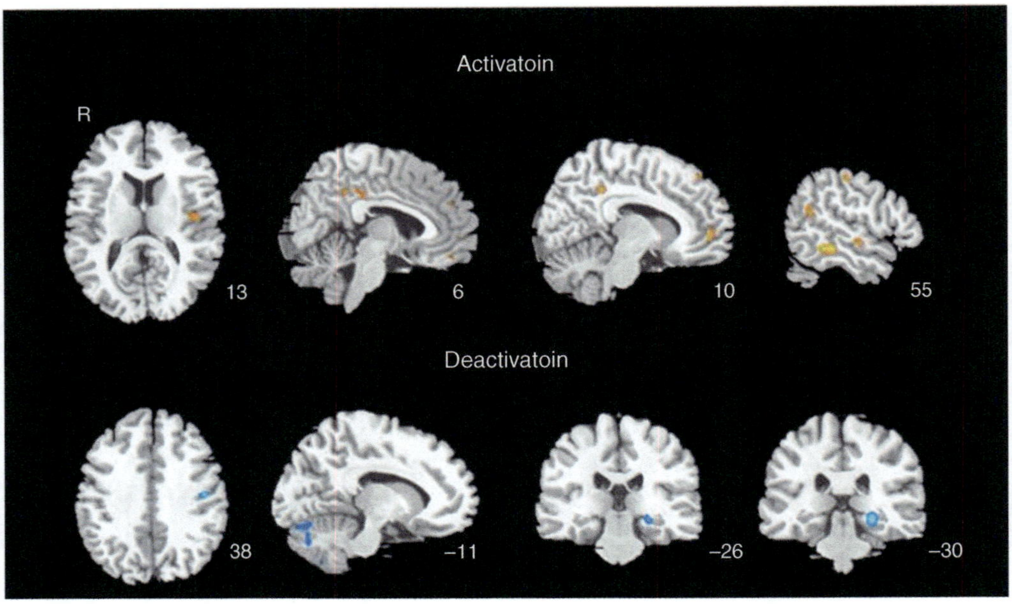

Fig. 7.11 PET imaging of acupuncture at the Waiguan, Yanglingquan, and Fengchi acupoints in the treatment of migraine: Compared to the control group, the treatment group showed increased glucose metabolism in the middle temporal cortex (MTC), orbitofrontal cortex (OFC), insula, middle frontal gyrus, angular gyrus, posterior cingulate cortex (PCC), precuneus, and middle cingulate cortex (MCC), and decreased glucose metabolism in the parahippocampal gyrus, hippocampus, fusiform gyrus, postcentral gyrus, and cerebellum (reproduced with permission from [50])

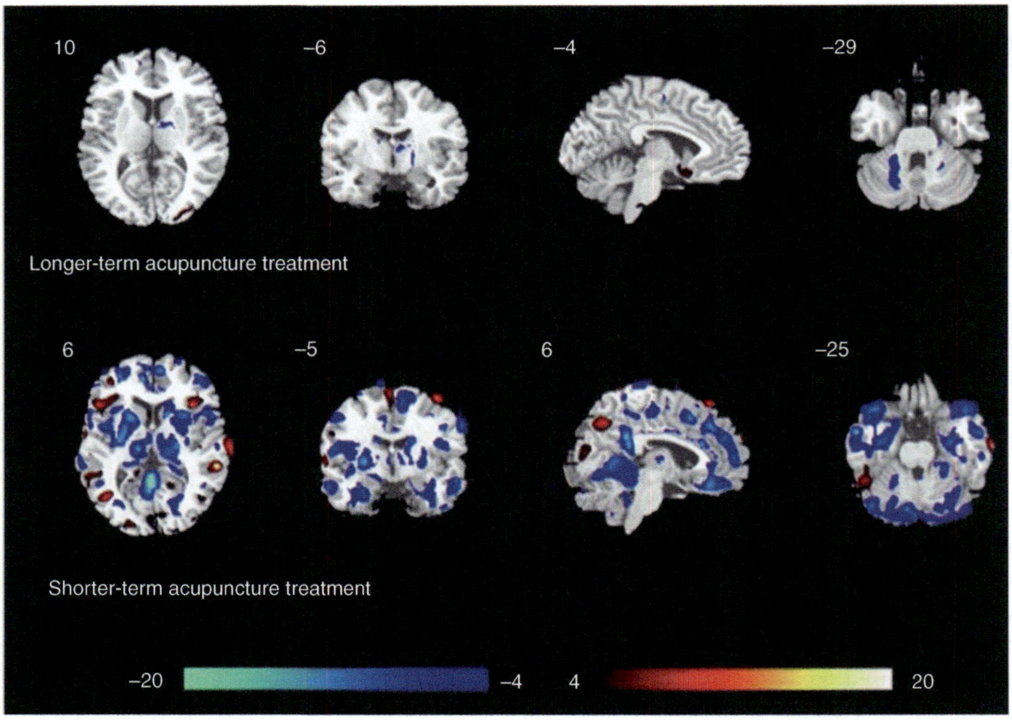

Fig. 7.12 Functional brain imaging of patients with functional dyspepsia after different lengths of treatment courses: Red represents regions with increased metabolism; blue represents regions with decreased metabolism

their bidirectional regulatory effects. Under pathological conditions, research on the brain mechanisms of acupuncture has focused primarily on cerebrovascular diseases, such as AD, VD, and ischemic stroke, followed by diseases related to the digestive system and pain. Current studies have shown the good therapeutic efficacy of acupuncture in various neurological diseases, and that its mechanisms may involve the modulation of metabolic levels in impaired or dysfunctional brain areas, or the regulation of healthy brain metabolic functions to promote the recovery of damaged areas. The results of experimental and clinical research on acupuncture have both validated the specificity of acupoints, as well as the multi-target, multi-level holistic therapeutic efficacy and comprehensive effects of acupuncture treatment. Regardless of whether it is under normal physiological or pathological conditions, performing acupuncture at different acupoints can elicit significant differences in the PET imaging of activated functional brain areas. Furthermore, the acupuncture effects of a specific acupoint are not only achieved through the activation of a single brain area, but that of multiple functionally connected brain areas.

The combination of PET/CT imaging with acupuncture has led to increased research on the mechanisms of acupuncture at the global, dynamic, and central level, while providing a pathway to visualize these underlying mechanisms. However, existing studies are still limited by low reproducibility, with a variety of factors (e.g., specific implementation of PET/CT techniques, complexity of brain functions, rationality of experimental design) giving rise to differences in the final results. Therefore, in the future, uniform practices and standards for acupuncture will need to be adopted, experimental protocols will need to be continuously optimized, and large-sample randomized controlled clinical trials will need to be performed, to more comprehensively elucidate the mechanisms underlying the effects of acupuncture and provide high-quality, objective evidence for clinical practice.

7.4 Research Applications of PET/MR in the Brain Mechanisms of Acupuncture

As a natural rehabilitative therapy with a long history of use and clinical application in China, acupuncture has been widely utilized in the treatment of many neurological diseases, such as depression, AD, epilepsy, PD, and stroke. PET/MR can be used to display both changes in brain function and alterations in brain metabolism, allowing for the comprehensive exploration of brain pathophysiological mechanisms caused by diseases at the molecular metabolic and functional levels. PET/MR is a non-invasive method for fully examining the brain mechanisms of acupuncture treatment. Current PET/MR studies have mainly utilized separate PET and fMRI scanners to investigate the brain mechanisms of acupuncture and acupuncture-induced analgesia.

7.4.1 Advances in Neuroimaging Research on the Brain Mechanisms of Acupuncture

The *deqi* sensation in acupuncture is a widely recognized needling sensation that is considered to be a predictor and precondition for the effectiveness of acupuncture. Given the importance of *deqi* in evaluating the effectiveness of acupuncture, there has been growing interest in studying the CNS mechanisms of *deqi* in recent years, as thus far, the mechanisms of action for *deqi* are not well understood. The main clinical features of *deqi* are pain, soreness, and dull pain. Studies that combined PET with fMRI have found that compared with superficial needling, needling that elicited *deqi* was related to increased glucose metabolism in the hypothalamus and cerebellar vermis. According to PET studies, *deqi* in acupuncture led to increased glucose metabolism in BA6, 8, 19, 21, 28, 33, 35, 37, and 47, the parahippocampal gyrus, lentiform nucleus, locus coeruleus, and red nucleus. As for fMRI studies, *deqi* elicited by classical acupuncture activated the ACC, insula, cerebellum, superior frontal gyrus, medial frontal gyrus, inferior frontal gyrus, and amygdala, which are all areas that are also activated by acute and chronic pain, suggesting that *deqi* acts by regulating or even restoring the PM to its normal state. *Deqi* can also activate the hypothalamus, nucleus accumbens, and other structures involved in the descending anti-injury pathway. During acupuncture stimulation, the fMRI findings of subjects who perceived pain without *deqi* or *deqi* (mixed sensations) with severe pain showed changes in brain activation patterns predominantly involving the activation of the ACC, caudate nucleus, putamen, anterior thalamus, and posterior insula, which are brain areas related to pain perception. Therefore, the activation of these regions was interpreted as the mechanisms of pain rather than *deqi*. The combination of fMRI and PET/CT can more fully elucidate the central mechanisms of *deqi* in acupuncture.

Although acupuncture has been used to achieve analgesia for more than 2000 years, its scientific validation remains incomplete, and the potential mechanisms underlying it are still poorly understood. The subjective experience of pain involves neural networks related to the sensory discrimination of stimuli, as well as those related to affective and cognitive responses. The affective component of pain is associated with a neural network that includes the amygdala, insula, ACC, and medial frontal cortex. From the perspective of functional brain networks, not only can *deqi* achieve analgesic effects by modulating the DMN and somatosensory functional network, it can also regulate the spatiotemporal range of large spontaneous activities in the interoceptive autonomous network, thereby promoting the endogenous pain modulation circuit and homeostatic control mechanisms. PET imaging before and after acupuncture in patients with chronic pain revealed the asymmetric hypometabolism of the thalamus. fMRI showed that when the commonly used analgesic acupoint, Hegu (LI4), was stimulated, significant hypoactivation was detected in the limbic system, nucleus accumbens, amygdala, hippocampus, parahippocampus, hypothalamus, and ventral tegmental area. Additionally, there is growing evidence suggesting the critical importance of endogenous opioids in the experience of pain and analgesia, as it is now generally accepted that endogenous opioids are one of the key mediating mechanisms in acupuncture-induced analgesia. ^{11}C-diprenorphine is a radiolabeled opioid agonist PET tracer, which can be used for the in vivo characterization and presentation of opioid receptors. In a combined fMRI and ^{11}C-diprenorphine PET study on acupuncture analgesia performed on 22 subjects, blood-oxygen-level-dependent (BOLD) signal changes were detected in the right OFC, brainstem, thalamus, insula, amygdala, ACC, and medial PFC. Increased activation was found in the OFC, whereas decreased activation was found in the left insula and bilateral brainstem during acupuncture. Moreover, ^{11}C-diprenorphine PET during acupuncture led to decreased metabolism in the right OFC, left medial PFC, right thalamus, and right insula, as well as increased metabolism in the bilateral insula, right medial PFC/ACC, left OFC, and right brainstem. The PET and fMRI findings above indicate that the majority of brain areas affected by acupuncture-induced analgesia do not overlap in terms of function and metabolism, with only the right OFC showing both functional and metabolic changes. This suggests that the right OFC may be an important area involved in the regulation of endogenous opioid concentration during the process of acupuncture-induced analgesia, whereas the functional signal changes of other areas may have been mediated by other neurotransmitters. This also implies that acupuncture-induced analgesia is at least partially mediated by the opioid system. These functionally and metabolically abnormal brain areas constitute the origins of the descending projections to the hypothalamus and PAG, while the PAG is considered a critical region in the descending pain inhibition system. Therefore, it was speculated that functional and metabolic abnormalities in the right OFC may indicate the activation of the descending pain inhibition system. Furthermore, no changes in functional activation or metabolism were detected in the placebo acupuncture group, which shows that there are indeed brain mechanisms that are elicited specifically by acupuncture-induced analgesia. The combination of fMRI activation with ^{11}C-diprenorphine PET metabolic changes can reflect the acupuncture-induced alterations in neural activity driven by endogenous opioids. Therefore, the results above can help us to identify the regions in which BOLD signal changes are related to the release of endogenous opioids or to mediation by other neurotransmitter systems.

Current PET/MR research involving acupuncture is still in its nascent stages, although PET/MR is the most comprehensive multimodal imaging method available for studying the brain mechanisms of acupuncture. It allows the non-invasive observation of functional and metabolic changes in the brain following acupuncture, while also providing robust evidence based on molecular imaging to address issues such as the validity of acupoints and acupoint specificity of therapeutic effects, thereby facilitating a complete understanding of the neurophysiological mechanisms of acupuncture treatment.

7.4.2 Advantages of Multimodal Imaging Techniques in Research on the Brain Mechanisms of Acupuncture

Acupuncture is an ancient method that can be used to treat a series of diseases, but its specific mechanisms remain unclear. Randomized controlled trials have demonstrated that true acupuncture is more effective than sham acupuncture. Furthermore, several studies have shown that deep brain structures respond differently to true than to sham acupuncture, implying that acupuncture does indeed have an effect on the brain. This suggests that acupuncture treatment involves its own unique physiological mechanisms, and does not simply produce placebo effects. The effects of acupuncture on the brain may arise from the physiological mechanisms of different secretory responses in peripheral and central neurons caused by stimulating the afferent fibers from muscle tissues. Acupuncture can clearly generate complex changes related to pain transmission and perception, though these changes are not yet fully understood. The traditional view is that there are still uncertainties about the specificity of acupoints, and whether it is necessary for the acupuncture needle to be inserted at a specific acupoint in order to maximize its effects, which are issues that require further validation. Furthermore, some have proposed that the difference in responses elicited by the exact position of acupoints is not significant, whereas differences can be found in terms of needling depth, presence or absence of stimuli, and importance of *deqi*. Thus, it has been suggested that to a large extent, acupuncture is a complex placebo or that needle insertion alone is sufficient to achieve therapeutic effects, which are unrelated to the selection of acupoint position or needling depth. These problems have led to confusion about the true nature of the brain mechanisms underlying acupuncture, which urgently require further investigation and verification at the level of brain function and metabolism.

Previous neuroimaging studies on the brain mechanisms of acupuncture have focused primarily on a single imaging modality (i.e., fMRI or PET), and only a few studies have performed PET and fMRI on separate scanners to elucidate the mechanisms underlying the changes in brain function and metabolism in acupuncture-induced analgesia. However, the biggest problem with such studies is the non-simultaneous acquisition of data, which does not allow the objective description of the relationship between the function and metabolism of brain areas affected by acupuncture-induced analgesia. With the advent of integrated PET/MR, it is now possible to simultaneously acquire brain functional and metabolic information before, during, and after acupuncture treatment, which will facilitate the comprehensive observation of functional and metabolic changes of the brain throughout the process of acupuncture. Additionally, integrated PET/MR research can help us to explore the differences in acupuncture interventions and acupuncture-induced pain effects on brain function, thereby determining the potential mechanisms of acupuncture treatment in chronic pain. Moreover, there are currently no reports on cerebral perfusion and metabolic changes after acupuncture. Integrated PET/MR can simultaneously acquire cerebral perfusion and metabolic information, which is useful for exploring the relationship between the two in the brain mechanisms of acupuncture.

At present, the most commonly used PET tracer is ^{18}F-FDG, which can reflect glucose metabolism, and previous studies have focused largely on this tracer. Nevertheless, there are other targeted PET tracers that can reflect different neural pathways, enabling the in vivo exploration of the release and distribution of different neurotransmitters related to these targeted tracers, as well as their corresponding neural pathway mechanisms, before and after acupuncture treatment. Based on these explorations, the comprehensive and objective elucidation of the brain mechanisms underlying acupuncture treatment can be performed, which will further promote the application of acupuncture in different diseases. Integrated PET/MR combines the structural, functional, and metabolic information of the brain, and therefore has a wide range of prospective applications in research on the brain mechanisms of acupuncture treatment. The application of multimodal imaging based on integrated PET/MR is bound to be of great significance to research on the brain mechanisms of acupuncture, and will have a profound impact on the entire field of acupuncture treatment.

In summary, integrated PET/MR offers a two-in-one multimodal imaging method for studying the brain mechanisms of acupuncture. The implementation of this technique to examine the long-term effects of acupuncture treatment on brain function and metabolism will be useful for achieving a better understanding of the brain mechanisms of acupuncture, and will most certainly commence a new chapter.

Suggested Readings

An YS, Moon SK, Min IK, et al. Changes in regional cerebral blood flow and glucose metabolism following electroacupuncture at LI 4 and LI 11 in normal volunteers. J Altern Complement Med. 2009;15(10):1075–81.

Asghar AU, Green G, Lythgoe MF, et al. Acupuncture needling sensation: the neural correlates of deqi using fMRI. Brain Res. 2010;22(1315):111–8.

Bai L, Tian J, Zhong C, et al. Acupuncture modulates temporal neural responses in wide brain networks: evidence from fMRI study. Mol Pain. 2010;6:73.

Baliki MN, Geha PY, Apkarian AV, et al. Beyond feeling: chronic pain hurts the brain, disrupting the default-mode network dynamics. J Neurosci. 2008;28(6):1398–403.

Bao C, Liu P, Wu H, et al. Different brain responses to electro-acupuncture and moxibustion treatment in patients with Crohn's disease. Sci Rep. 2016;6:36636.

Deng D, Liao H, Duan G, et al. Modulation of the default mode network in first-episode, drug-Naive major depressive disorder via acupuncture at baihui (GV20) acupoint. Front Hum Neurosci. 2016;10:230.

Dougherty DD, Kong J, Webb M, et al. A combined [^{11}C] diprenorphine PET study and fMRI study of acupuncture analgesia. Behav Brain Res. 2008;193(1):63–8.

Fang J, Hui KS. Kathleen, Nixon Erika, et al. Deqi and sharp pain during acupuncture at Taichong elicits opposite functional brain network effects—an fMRI study. Chinese Imag J Integrat Trad West Med. 2012;10(1):4–9.

Fang J, Jin Z, Wang Y, et al. The salient characteristics of the central effects of acupuncture needling: limbic-paralimbic-neocortical network modulation. Hum Brain Mapp. 2009;30(4):1196–206.

Fang J, Rong P, Hong Y, et al. Transcutaneous vagus nerve stimulation modulates default mode network in major depressive disorder. Biol Psychiatry. 2016;79(4):266–73.

Fang Z, Ning J, Xiong C, et al. Effects of electroacupuncture at head points on the function of cerebral motor areas in stroke patients: a PET study. Evid Based Complement Alternat Med. 2012;2012(4):902413.

Gong P, Zhang M, Jiang L. Research on effect of acupuncture at Sanyinjiao on brain function by means of positron emission tomographic imaging. Chin J Integr Tradit West Med. 2006;26(2):119–22.

Guo Q, Liu Q, Yang F, et al. Advances in the application of PET techniques in acupuncture research. Chinese Acupunct Moxibust. 2019;39(3):337–41.

Hou X, Chen W, Chen J, et al. Default mode network ReHo of patients with neck pain treated with acupuncture at an acupoint combination. Magn Reson Imaging. 2014;6:436–40.

Hsieh JC, Tu CH, Chen FP, et al. Activation of the hypothalamus characterizes the acupuncture stimulation at the analgesic point in human: a positron emission tomography study. Neurosci Lett. 2001;307(2):105–8.

Huang W, Pach D, Napadow V, et al. Characterizing acupuncture stimuli using brain imaging with FMRI-a systematic review and meta-analysis of the literature. PLoS One. 2012;7(4):e32960.

Huang Y, Chen J, Lai XS, et al. Effects of needling in Baihui (DU20), Shuigou (DU26) and Shenmen (HT7) on glucose metabolism in the lentiform nucleus in patients with vascular dementia. Acad J First Med Coll PLA. 2005;25(11):1405–7.

Hui K, Liu J, Makris N, et al. Acupuncture modulates the limbic system and subcortical gray structures of the human brain: evidence from fMRI studies in normal subjects. Hum Brain Mapp. 2000;7(5):251–3.

Hui K, Liu J, Marina O, et al. The integrated response of the human cerebro-cerebellar and limbic systems to acupuncture stimulation at ST 36 as evidenced by fMRI. NeuroImage. 2005;27(3):479–96.

Jiang J, Liu G, Shi S, et al. Musical electroacupuncture may be a better choice than electro-acupuncture in a mouse model of Alzheimer's disease. Neural Plast. 2016;2016:3131586.

Jie Y, Fang Z, Yue F, et al. A PET-CT study on the specificity of acupoints through acupuncture treatment in migraine patients. BMC Complement Altern Med. 2012;12(1) 123.

Kalia LV, Lang AE. Parkinson's disease. Lancet. 2015;386(9996):896–912.

Kaptchuk TJ. Acupuncture: theory, efficacy, and practice. Ann Intern Med. 2002;136(5):374–83.

Kong J, Tu PC, Zyloney C, et al. Intrinsic functional connectivity of the periaque-ductal gray, a resting fMRI study. Behav Brain Res. 2010;211(2):215–9.

Lai X, Huang Y, Tang A, et al. Effect of acupuncture at the Baihui acupoint on brain tomography under pathological conditions. J Guangzhou Univ Trad Chinese Med. 2008;25(5):410–3.

Lai X, Ren J, Lu Y, et al. Effects of acupuncture at HT7 on glucose metabolism in a rat model of Alzheimer's disease: an ^{18}F-FDG-PET study. Acupunct Med. 2016;34(3):215–22.

Lai X, Zhang G, Huang Y, et al. A cerebral functional imaging study by positron emission tomography in healthy volunteers receiving true or sham acupuncture needling. Neurosci Lett. 2009;452(2):194–9.

Li C, Yang J, Sun J, et al. Brain responses to acupuncture are probably dependent on the brain functional status. Evid Based Complement Alternat Med. 2013;2013:175278.

Li J, Zhang JH, Yi T, et al. Acupuncture treatment of chronic low back pain reverses an abnormal brain default mode network in correlation with clinical pain relief. Acupunct Med. 2014;32(2):102–8.

Li S, Rong P, Gao G, et al. Effects of electroacupuncture at the auricular concha on the hippocampal Raf/ERK/RSK/CREB signaling pathway in a rat model of depression. Acupunct Res. 2019;44(8):554–9.

Liang P, Wang Z, Qian T, et al. Acupuncture stimulation of taichong (Liv3) and hegu (LI4) modulates the default mode network activity in Alzheimer's disease. Am J Alzheimers Dis Other Dement. 2014;29(8):739–48.

Liu B, Chen J, Wang J, et al. Altered small-world efficiency of brain functional networks in acupuncture at ST36: a functional MRI study. PLoS One. 2012;7(6):e39342.

Liu R, Fang J, Rong P, et al. Effects of electroacupuncture at auricular concha region on the depressive status of unpredictable chronic mild stress rat models. Evid Based Complement Alternat Med. 2013;2013:789674.

Liu Y, Guo Y, Liu N, et al. Effects of "Xiusanzhen" on the expression of inflammatory factors in a mouse model of Parkinson's disease. Liaon J Trad Chinese Med. 2018;20(11):63–6.

Lu Y, Huang Y, Tang C, et al. Brain areas involved in the acupuncture treatment of AD model rats: a PET study. BMC Complement Altern Med. 2014;14(1):1–8.

Maeda Y, Kettner N, Lee J, et al. Acupuncture evoked response in contralateral somatosensory cortex reflects peripheral nerve pathology of carpal tunnel syndrome. Med Acupunct. 2013;25(4):275–84.

Mi Z, Gao J. Research advances in the pathogenic mechanism and acupuncture treatment of depression. J Clin Med Pract. 2019;23(8):123–7.

Park MS, Sunwoo YY, Jang KS, et al. Changes in brain FDG metabolism inducedby acupuncture in healthy volunteers. Acta Radiol. 2010;51(8):947–52.

Rong P, Fang J, Yu Y, et al. Overview of the neuromodulation technique based on acupuncture brain science. Sci Technol Rev. 2017;35(11):77–84.

Shan Y, Wang J, Wang Z, et al. Neuronal specificity of acupuncture in Alzheimer's disease and mild cognitive impairment patients: a functional MRI study. Evid Based Complement Alternat Med. 2018;2018:1–10.

Shan Y, Wang Z, Zhao Z, et al. An fMRI study of neuronal specificity in acupuncture: the multiacupoint siguan and its sham point. Evid Based Complement Alternat Med. 2014;2014:103491.

Shao G, Chen Y, Yan B, et al. PET/CT functional brain imaging of acupuncture at the Weizhong (BL40) and Zusanli (ST36) acupoints. Chinese J Nucl Med. 2006;26(1):54–6.

Sun P, Chu H. Li Pei, et al. Post-stroke depression treated with acupuncture therapy of dredging the Governor Vessel and regulating mentality: a randomized controlled trial. Chinese Acupunct Moxibust. 2013;33(1):3–7.

Tian L, Wang J, Sun R, et al. Research advances on the mechanisms of scalp acupuncture for the treatment of ischemic stroke. Acupunct Res. 2016;41(1):87–9.

Wu X, Zheng X, Guo X, et al. Research advances on the effects of acupuncture treatment on 5-HT, its receptors and HPA-related hormones in rats with insomnia. Chin Arch Tradit Chin Med. 2018;36(1):127–9.

Xu N, Fang J. Acupuncture imaging. People's Med Publ House. 2018;25(85):193–255.

Yang J, Yang MX, Zeng F, et al. Visualized characterization for cerebral response of acupuncture deqi: Paradox underway. Evid Based Complement Alternat Med. 2013;2013:894750.

Yong H, Tang C, Wang S, et al. Acupuncture regulates the glucose metabolism in cerebral functional regions in chronic stage ischemic stroke patients—a PET-CT cerebral functional imaging study. BMC Neurosci. 2012;13(1):75.

Yu J, Chu J, Gao L, et al. Effects of grain-sized moxibustion on the learning and memory abilities, and amyloid deposition of transgenic Alzheimer's disease mice. Acupunct Res. 2014;39(1):58–62,82.

Zeng F, Qin W, Ma TT. Influence of acupuncture treatment on cerebral activity in functional dyspepsia patients and its relationship with efficacy. Am J Gastroenterol. 2012;107(8):1236–47.

Zhang G, Huang Y, Tang C, et al. Characteristics of PET cerebral functional imaging during "Deqi" of acupuncture in healthy volunteers. Acupunct Res. 2011;36(1):46–51.

Zhang M, Xv GH, Wang WX, et al. Electroacupuncture improves cognitive- deficits and activates PPAR-γ in a rat model of Alzheimer's disease. Acupunct Med. 2017;35(1):44–51.

Zhou C, Cao H, Yu L, et al. Changes in the pain center and default mode network induced by electroacupuncture at the Weizhong and Dachangshu acupoints: a task-based fMRI study. Natl Med J China. 2016;7:531–4.

Zhu Y, Chen Y, Yu T, et al. Effect of "qi-tonifying, blood-regulating, and constitution-strengthening" acupuncture on cerebral glucose metabolism in healthy elderly persons. Shanghai J Acupunct Moxibust. 2011;30(8):571–3.

8 Research Applications of Positron Emission Tomography/Magnetic Resonance (PET/MR) Imaging in Alzheimer's Disease (AD)

Shaozhen Yan, Min Liu, Zhigang Qi, and Jie Lu

Alzheimer's disease (AD) is the most common type of neurodegenerative disease and is primarily characterized by progressive cognitive dysfunction and behavioral impairment. It accounts for approximately 50–75% of senile dementia cases. Mild cognitive impairment (MCI) is an intermediate state of cognition, somewhere between normal aging and dementia, and has a high risk of conversion to AD or other types of dementia, with approximately 10–15% of MCI cases converting to AD each year. With the steady increase in life expectancy, the incidence of AD has grown each year, and the number of patients with AD worldwide is projected to reach 130 million by 2050, which will place an immense burden on social development and home care. However, the pathogenesis of AD remains poorly understood, and currently, there is no effective pharmaceutical treatment. Therefore, AD continues to be a key focus of and challenge to research in the field of global medicine. The characteristic pathological changes observed in AD involve senile plaques that are formed by the extracellular deposition of β-amyloid (Aβ), intracellular neurofibrillary tangles (NFTs) that are formed of hyperphosphorylated tau protein, and extensive neuronal loss. The primary imaging techniques currently utilized in AD research include MRI and PET. Structural MRI can show the atrophy of the medial temporal lobe (MTL), which is now considered to be a diagnostic marker of AD, while functional MRI (fMRI) is a valuable tool for exploring the functional changes of the brain and the neurobiological mechanisms of AD. PET, however, is an important imaging technique for the detection of AD-specific brain metabolism and the in vivo assessment of pathological proteins. In this chapter, we will summarize the advances in research regarding the application of fMRI, PET, and PET/MR in the study of AD.

S. Yan · M. Liu · Z. Qi · J. Lu (✉)
Department of Radiology and Nuclear Medicine, Xuanwu Hospital, Capital Medical University, Beijing, China

8.1 Research Applications of MRI in AD

The rapid development of imaging technology has driven the continual advancement of functional brain MRI techniques. Due to their non-invasiveness, high reproducibility, flexible and diverse scan methods, and relatively high spatial and temporal resolution, these techniques have been widely used in the clinical and scientific research of AD. Brain MRI techniques consist primarily of brain structural imaging, diffusion tensor imaging (DTI) for mapping white matter tracts, arterial spin labelling (ASL) for measuring cerebral hemodynamics, magnetic resonance spectroscopy (MRS) for reflecting cerebral metabolism and chemical substances, and blood oxygenation level-dependent (BOLD) imaging

J. Lu, G. Zhao (eds.), *PET/MR: Functional and Molecular Imaging of Neurological Diseases and Neurosciences*, https://doi.org/10.1007/978-981-19-9902-4_8

for reflecting brain functional changes. Since functional changes of the brain occur earlier than structural atrophy in patients with AD, functional brain imaging is of crucial clinical and scientific significance to the research on early diagnosis and pathogenesis of AD.

8.1.1 Research Applications of Structural MRI in AD

Structural MRI can reveal the scope and degree of brain atrophy, thereby reflecting the cumulative neuronal damage, and is directly associated with the clinical symptoms of patients with AD. This MRI technique is widely used in clinical settings, as it involves simple operating procedures while providing highly robust and reproducible structural information of the brain. Voxel-based morphometry (VBM) is an advanced technique of neuroimaging analysis that not only allows the evaluation of anatomical differences of the brain as a whole but is also less affected by subjective human factors and has a higher accuracy and efficiency. Moreover, VBM can facilitate the comparison of different studies and has been widely utilized in AD research. It can also reduce the bias caused by region of interest (ROI) selection and inter-observer or inter-operator variability. In longitudinal studies, VBM helps to circumvent the shortcomings of cross-sectional studies, such as the effects of individual differences in brain size and short observation periods.

In 2011, the National Institute on Aging—Alzheimer's Association incorporated structural MRI into the diagnostic criteria for AD, listing MTL atrophy as one of the imaging biomarkers for AD diagnosis. Studies have shown that patients with AD exhibit a significant loss of cerebral gray matter, with prominent volume reductions in the hippocampus and entorhinal cortex. Furthermore, disease progression is accompanied by deterioration caused by progressive atrophy of the hippocampus (Fig. 8.1) and entorhinal cortex. A large number of studies have also demonstrated that hippocampal atrophy is a highly sensitive and specific diagnostic marker for AD. Hippocampal atrophy occurs approximately 5 years after the onset of the clinical symptoms of dementia, and significant reductions in hippocampal volume can be observed at the time of AD diagnosis. Based on a meta-analysis of structural MRI data involving 700 patients with mild to moderate AD, it was found that compared to age-matched controls, the hippocampal volume loss in patients with AD was approximately 23–24%, while that of patients with MCI was 15–20%. The reduction of the hippocampal volume in patients with AD involved nearly all hippocampal subregions but occurred predominantly in the cornu ammonis (CA) 1 area, whereas hippocampal atrophy in patients with MCI was generally limited to CA1, with some studies reporting the involvement of CA3/dentate gyrus (DG), CA4/DG, or the subiculum. The hippocampal volume can be used to discriminate between AD and MCI with relatively high

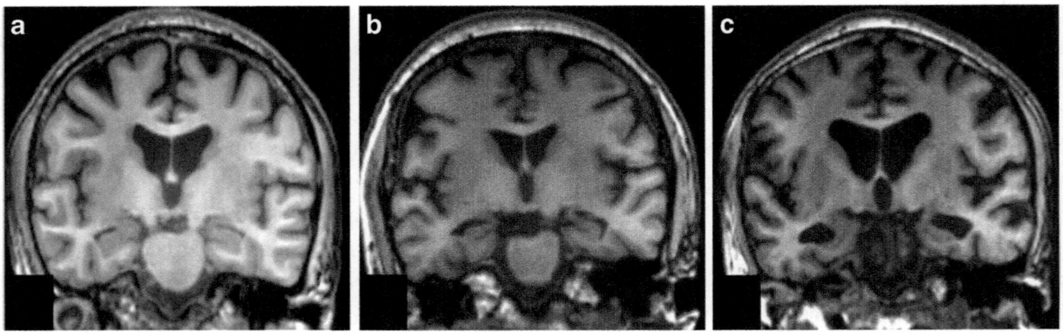

Fig. 8.1 Structural changes in the hippocampus of patients with AD and MCI: A healthy 63-year-old female subject, MMSE 29, MoCA 28, CDR 0, and no hippocampal atrophy (**a**); a 60-year-old male patient with MCI, MMSE 27, MoCA 27, CDR 0.5, and mild hippocampal atrophy (**b**); and a 64-year-old male patient with AD, MMSE 20, MoCA 15, CDR 2, and significant hippocampal atrophy (**c**)

accuracies (86.8% and 73.5%, respectively). One study found that the accuracy of using the volume of the hippocampal subregions to discriminate between amnestic MCI and normal controls (NCs) was 92%, which was significantly higher than the discriminative ability of hippocampal volume. Since the entorhinal cortex is the first region to exhibit pathological changes in AD, the thickness and volume of this region have been found to be lower in AD and MCI patients than in control subjects. The combination of hippocampal and entorhinal cortical volumes for the two-way classification of AD, MCI, and NC has a significantly higher accuracy than individual hippocampal and entorhinal cortical indicators, with the specificity and sensitivity of the optimal cut-off point exceeding 80%. These findings indicate that composite indicators can significantly improve the diagnostic accuracy for AD and MCI.

Given that several decades may pass before the onset of AD symptoms, it is difficult to clearly elucidate the evolution of AD pathologies based on a simple cross-sectional description of morphological changes of the brain. Therefore, it is necessary to ensure that long-term follow-up examinations of patients with AD are performed at multiple time points. Some studies have reported a follow-up time of up to 9 years to verify the conversion from MCI to AD. VBM can be used to evaluate the patterns of gray matter loss in patients with MCI; those that convert to AD tend to exhibit more extensive gray matter loss than those that do not, with abnormal patterns similar to those of patients with AD, whereas the gray matter densities of those that do not convert to AD are similar to those of control patients. A follow-up study found that the NC group had the largest hippocampal and entorhinal cortical volumes, while those with MCI that converted to AD had the smallest, and those with stable MCI were somewhere in the middle. Furthermore, compared to patients with MCI that did not convert, those who converted showed an average decrease of 9% in the left and 13% in the right hippocampal volumes.

In addition to neurogenerative disorders, hippocampal volume is also affected by sex and apolipoprotein E (ApoE) ε4 carrier status. Being a carrier of the ApoE ε4 gene is one of the greatest genetic risk factors for AD. Based on one longitudinal study, those with MCI that converted to AD who also carried the ApoE ε4 allele showed more rapid hippocampal atrophy than patients with stable MCI. Furthermore: AD and MCI patients who were ApoE ε4 carriers had lower hippocampal volume than non-carriers; female ApoE ε4 carriers with AD had a lower volume than non-carriers, and male ApoE ε4 carriers showed no significant difference in volume compared to non-carriers. Moreover, female ApoE ε4 carriers with MCI had more severe reductions in the hippocampal volume than male carriers. Therefore, hippocampal atrophy is clearly more severe in ApoE ε4 carriers than non-carriers, and in women than in men, demonstrating the relationship between sex, ApoE ε4, and hippocampal volume.

Structural MRI studies allow the early detection of gray matter damage, particularly hippocampal atrophy of the MTL in patients with AD, which can serve as a simple and effective means for the early diagnosis of AD and an accurate prediction of disease progression.

8.1.2 Research Applications of DTI in AD

DTI primarily involves measuring the diffusion of water molecules in different directions within brain tissues, to reflect the microstructural changes of the white matter. This technique can be used for the quantitative analysis of the white matter and has unique advantages in assessing its structural integrity. There are two main parameters in DTI: (1) fractional anisotropy (FA), which represents the difference in diffusion in all directions and reflects the structural integrity of the white matter; and (2) mean diffusion (MD), which reflects the average diffusivity of water molecules in all directions, primarily reflecting the extent to which the diffusion of water molecules is restricted in the brain. The combination of these two parameters allows for the accurate assessment of white matter integrity. Tissue damage can lead to changes in the diffusion of water molecules within the damaged tissue, which decreases the FA value and increases the MD value. Therefore, measuring FA and MD allows for the quantitative determination of tissue damage.

Previous research on AD has focused primarily on cerebral gray matter; however, an increasing number of recent studies have revealed the presence of white matter abnormalities in early-stage AD. The retrogenesis hypothesis posits that late-myelinating, small-diameter white matter fibers, such as the commissural fibers (e.g., corpus callosum, anterior commissure, and posterior commissure), are damaged earlier than early-myelinating, large-diameter white matter tracts, such as the primary motor tracts. The results of a DTI study of the corpus callosum indicated that patients with MCI had decreased FA values in the body of the corpus callosum, but no abnormalities in the genu or splenium. Furthermore, during the progression from MCI to AD, the destruction of white matter began in the commissural fibers and extended to the projection and association fibers. Taken together, these findings support the retrogenesis hypothesis. Additionally, based on tractography studies, patients with AD had decreased FA values in the right anterior cingulate cortex (ACC), left posterior cingulate cortex (PCC), and left corpus callosum, and increased MD values in the right uncinate fasciculus, left splenium of the corpus callosum, and bilateral superior corona radiata, while the motor-related internal capsule and vision-related optic radiation were relatively intact (Fig. 8.2). Compared to patients with MCI, those with AD showed significantly lower FA and higher MD values in the bilateral parahippocampal gyrus, bilateral inferior fronto-occipital fasciculus, and bilateral PCC. Patients with MCI exhibited decreased FA values in the corpus callosum, fornix, and right cingulate gyrus, and increased MD values in the subgenual ACC and fornix white matter, demonstrating that DTI can objectively reflect white matter damage in patients with AD and MCI, serving as imaging evidence for relevant white matter degenerative changes. Recent studies

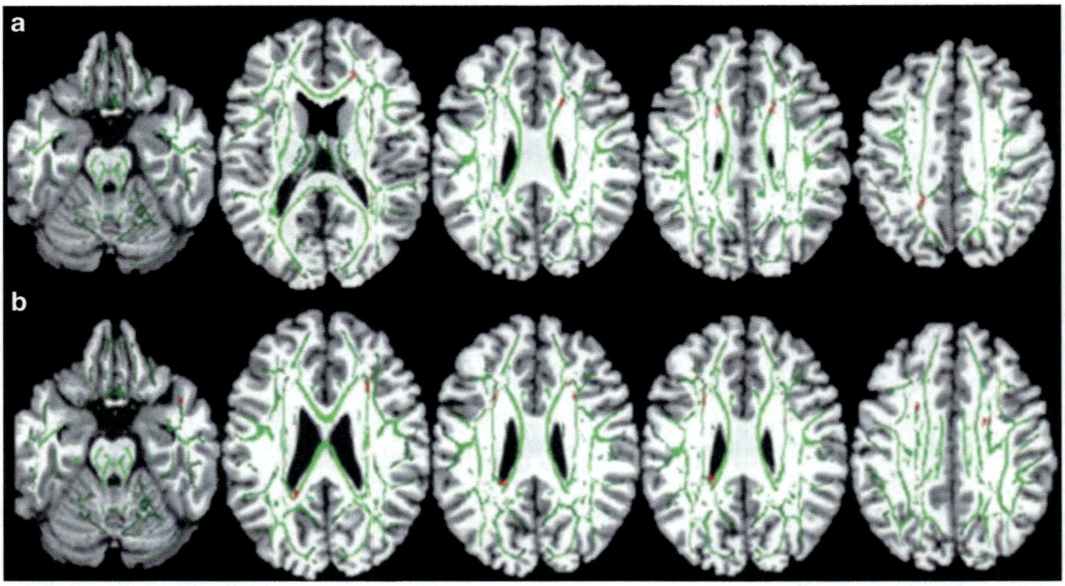

Fig. 8.2 White matter tract changes in patients with AD: White matter tractography in patients with AD revealed decreased FA values in the right anterior cingulate cortex, left posterior cingulate cortex, and left corpus callosum (red) (**a**), and increased MD values in the right uncinate fasciculus, left splenium of the corpus callosum, and bilateral superior corona radiata (red) (**b**). Mean FA and MD tract skeleton (green) overlaid on the T1WI MNI template

have found that DTI is associated with pathological Aβ and tau protein in AD. More specifically, the Aβ(+) group had higher FA values than the Aβ(−) group in the right superior longitudinal fasciculus, right inferior longitudinal fasciculus, genu and body of the corpus callosum, left corona radiata, and left fornix, while FA values were positively correlated with Aβ deposition. The Aβ(+) group also had lower MD values than the Aβ(−) group in the right frontal lobe, and MD values were weakly negatively corelated with Aβ deposition (correlation coefficient, −0.392). Additionally, tau deposition in the anterior temporal lobe was an indicator for the loss of white matter integrity in patients with AD, suggesting that DTI can serve as an important imaging marker for predicting and monitoring tau progression in patients with AD. It was previously thought that gray matter was critical to cognitive function; however, recently, the focus has gradually shifted toward the relationship between white matter and cognitive function, with many arguing that the impact of white matter on cognitive function is comparable to that of the cerebral cortex. In patients with AD, the decreased FA values of the right cingulate gyrus, left corpus callosum, and inferior temporal gyrus are positively correlated with Mini Mental State Examination (MMSE) scores, while elevated MD values in the cingulate gyrus and fornix can reflect the impairment of contextual memory, thus implying that the cognitive decline in patients with AD is intricately linked with white matter damage. A genetic association analysis of AD risk loci and hippocampal FA values revealed that the single nucleotide polymorphism (SNP) rs2203712 of the CELF1 gene was significantly associated with hippocampal FA values, implying that the combination of DTI parameters with CLEF1 and its gene network analysis can provide new insights into the pathophysiological mechanism of AD and may become a potential therapeutic target. In summary, DTI enables the early detection of white matter damage in patients with AD and provides a new avenue for further investigation into the pathological changes associated with AD.

8.1.3 Research Applications of ASL in AD

ASL is a new, non-invasive, MRI-based cerebral perfusion imaging technique. The principle behind this technique is to apply an inversion pulse upstream of the imaging plane in order to invert, and therefore label, the spin of water protons in arterial blood. Then, subtraction is performed between the images acquired before and after labelling to obtain the perfusion parameter maps, which provide the quantitative parameter of cerebral hemodynamics, i.e. cerebral blood flow (CBF). This parameter reflects the flow and distribution of blood in brain tissue at a given moment, which can be used to evaluate neurovascular function.

CBF can be measured using radionuclide cerebral perfusion imaging (e.g., $^{15}O\text{-}H_2O$ PET imaging) or dynamic contrast-enhanced MRI. However, $^{15}O\text{-}H_2O$ has a relatively short half-life, and therefore, limited clinical application, and dynamic contrast-enhanced MRI requires the injection of contrast agents. ASL, on the other hand, does not require the injection of exogenous contrast agents, is non-invasive, does not involve ionizing radiation, and has good reproducibility, which has promoted its widespread utilization in AD research. Studies performed on a healthy population have demonstrated a good correlation between whole-brain CBF and glucose metabolism, although with varying levels of correlation in different brain areas. More specifically, the correlation was strongest in the caudate nucleus and putamen, and weakest in the MTL. However, these findings could be attributed to the differences in physiological states during data acquisition, as the two imaging modalities were performed asynchronously. Patients with MCI exhibited reduced CBF in the bilateral temporo-parietal lobes, posterior midcingulate cortex, and insula, with the posterior cingulate cortex and medial parietal lobe showing the most significant reductions. Patients with AD primarily exhibited reduced CBF in the temporal, parietal, and occipital lobes; PCC; and precuneus (Fig. 8.3). The scope of CBF reduction gradually broadened as the disease progressed,

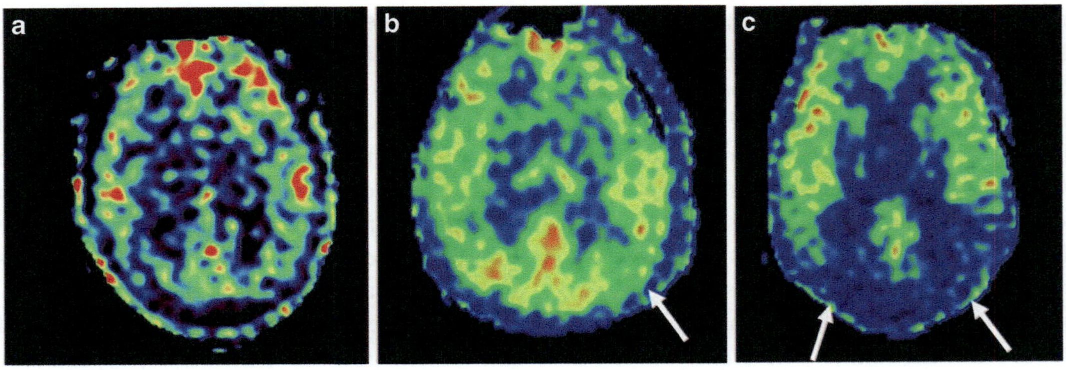

Fig. 8.3 CBF images of healthy elderly subjects, and patients with MCI and AD: A healthy 67-year-old female, MMSE 29, CDR 0, transverse T1WI MRI shows no abnormal brain structures, and ASL shows no CBF decrease (**a**), a 70-year-old male patient with MCI, MMSE 23, CDR 0.5; transverse T1WI MRI shows no abnormal brain structure, and ASL shows CBF decrease in the right parietal lobe (white arrow) (**b**), and a 70-year-old female with AD, MMSE 20, CDR 1; transverse T1WI MRI shows left parietal lobe atrophy, and ASL shows CBF decreases in bilateral parietal lobes (white arrows) (**c**)

with patients with AD showing more significant decreases in CBF values than patients with MCI, when comparing the same areas of the brain. Although the majority of ASL studies have reported decreased CBF in AD, some have proposed that regional CBF increases, believed to be caused by neurocompensatory responses, can be detected in early-stage AD. These hyperperfusions may represent different manifestations of the various stages of AD in which patients with MCI may present with hyperperfusion in the bilateral frontal lobes and right inferior temporal gyrus, which is gradually followed by decompensation, manifesting as hypoperfusion. CBF can also facilitate the diagnosis of AD. Using the parietal lobe and hippocampus as ROIs, the accuracy of discriminating AD from subjective cognitive decline was 89.0%, while using the parietal and occipital lobes as ROIs, the accuracy of discriminating AD from MCI was 83.8%. The combination of CBF with the Entorhinal Cortical Atrophy (ERICA) score significantly improved the diagnostic performance for AD, with a predictive probability of 95.7%. Neuropsychological scales, such as the Montreal Cognitive Assessment (MoCA) and the MMSE, are frequently used to assist in the diagnosis of AD. Other studies have found that CBF decreases in the parietal lobe and PCC, as measured using ASL in AD and MCI patients, were positively correlated with MoCA and MMSE scores. Therefore, by utilizing ASL, a confirmed diagnosis can be attained in the early or even prodromal stages of AD, rather than after the onset of symptoms, which will contribute to slowing down disease progression to the greatest possible extent.

Despite the differences in their clinical presentations, there are substantial overlaps among the different types of dementia, which has increased the difficulty of diagnosing dementia and its various subtypes. ASL studies have revealed differences in the perfusion patterns of AD, frontotemporal dementia, and Lewy body dementia. AD presented with decreased CBF in the supratentorial region, with especially prominent reductions in the posterior areas of the cerebrum. Patients with Lewy body dementia had the lowest CBF values but showed no change in the CBF of the temporal lobes. In patients with frontotemporal dementia, the lowest CBF values were found in the frontal lobe, whereas for patients with AD, the lowest CBF values were found in the temporal lobes. Based on these findings, it is evident that the differences in ASL perfusion patterns exhibited by these three types of dementia can facilitate their differential diagnosis. ASL is also a useful method for differentiating between AD and vascular dementia.

Comparisons of the perfusion differences between patients with post-stroke dementia and patients with AD with healthy controls revealed that the gray-white matter CBF ratio in patients with post-stroke dementia was lower than that of healthy controls, whereas patients with AD showed reduced perfusion in the parietal lobe without a decrease in the gray-white matter CBF ratio. Thus, CBF decreases in patients with AD were mainly distributed in the cerebral gray matter, whereas those in patients with vascular dementia were distributed in both gray and white matter, although predominantly in the white matter. The distinct patterns of CBF changes in AD and vascular dementia suggest that ASL scans may be a useful for discriminating the two. Despite the continuously ongoing clinical drug trials for AD, there is a lack of effective treatment methods, and the main purpose of drug therapy is to improve the patient's cognitive function or at least maintain a stable condition and delay disease progression. Early treatment is critical to the prognosis and outcome of patients with AD, while ASL provides an intuitive approach for observing the changes in a patient's condition before and after treatment. By utilizing ASL to measure the CBF in early-stage patients with AD before and six months after treatment with cholinesterase inhibitors, it was found that these patients showed increased white matter CBF in the PCC and prefrontal cortex, and did not exhibit cognitive decline. Another study evaluating the therapeutic efficacy of acupuncture at the Siguan acupoints of patients with AD revealed increased cerebral perfusion in originally hypoperfused brain areas (left precuneus and left PCC), as well as other areas such as the left cortical areas around the calcarine fissure; lingual gyrus; fusiform gyrus; hippocampus; and frontal, occipital, and temporal lobes. Furthermore, the acupuncture group showed increased CBF in the frontal lobes and insula compared to the sham acupuncture group (Fig. 8.4). These results indicate that ASL can detect the changes in cerebral perfusion induced by drug therapy in early-stage AD and can therefore be used to evaluate the prognosis of AD treatments.

With the continuous innovation and improvement of ASL, one hope is that this imaging technique will be able to accurately reflect functional changes in the brains of patients with AD, elucidate the role of vascular factors in AD, and serve as a biomarker for AD, thereby providing valuable imaging information for the early diagnosis, differential diagnosis, monitoring of therapeutic efficacy, and other aspects of research on the pathological mechanisms of AD.

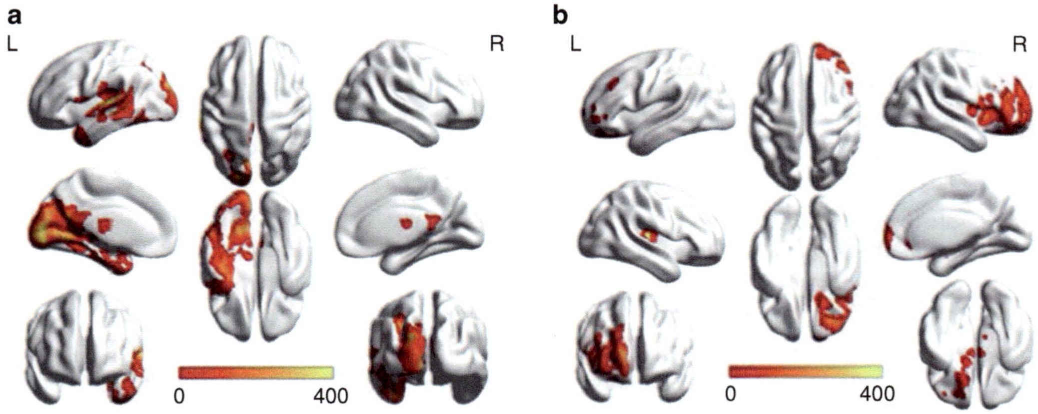

Fig. 8.4 Cerebral perfusion changes in patients with AD following acupuncture at the Siguan acupoints: Six months after receiving acupuncture at the Siguan acupoints, patients with AD showed increased CBF in originally hypoperfused areas (left precuneus and left PCC), as well as the left cortical areas around the calcarine fissure; lingual gyrus; fusiform gyrus; hippocampus; and frontal, occipital, and temporal lobes (**a**). Patients with AD in the acupuncture group showed increased CBF in the frontal lobe and insula compared to the sham acupuncture group during follow-up at 6 months (**b**)

8.1.4 Research Applications of MRS in AD

Proton MRS is a non-invasive imaging technique that can be used for the in vivo examination of energy metabolism and chemical concentration changes in tissues, and the analysis of diseases before the appearance of anatomical and morphological abnormalities. This technique is now extensively utilized in the quantitative and semi-quantitative in vivo evaluation of metabolite concentrations in AD brain tissues.

MRS studies on AD primarily involve the measurement of the peak heights and ratios of various metabolites in various ROIs of the brain. Among them, N-acetylaspartate (NAA), which is primarily found in neuronal mitochondria, can serve as an endogenous marker of neurons and axons, and a specific indicator for neuronal activity. Choline (Cho) is associated with phospholipid metabolism in the cell membrane and can be an indicator of cell membrane damage. Elevated creatine (Cr) levels signify impairments in energy production, and Cr is therefore used as an internal reference in many MRS studies as its concentration is relatively constant across a variety of pathological and physiological conditions. Myo-inositol (mI) can only be found in living glial cells and can therefore serve as a marker of glial cells in brain tissue, with elevated mI levels indicating the occurrence of glial cell proliferation. Glutamate (Glu) and glutamine complex (Glx) are involved in the glutamate–glutamine cycle between neurons and glial cells in the human body, while abnormal glutamate metabolism signifies the disrupted functional integrity of neurons and glial cells.

As abnormalities of cerebral metabolism in patients with AD occur earlier than morphological changes, MRS can be utilized for the early diagnosis of AD. One study indicated that the whole-brain distribution patterns of MRS in patients with AD involve significantly decreased NAA levels in the PCC and bilateral hippocampus, as well as significantly decreased Cho/Cr, NAA/Cr, and mI/Cr levels in the PCC, superior temporal gyrus, prefrontal cortex, and caudate nucleus. Patients with amnestic MCI exhibit decreased Glu levels in the PCC as well as decreased NAA levels, increased mI levels, and no Glu abnormalities in the cingulate gyrus and hippocampus. The NAA/mI ratio of the PCC discriminated between patients with MCI that converted to AD and those that did not, with an accuracy (area under the curve, AUC) of 0.779. The combination of NAA/mI ratio and parahippocampal volume could predict the outcome of AD 2 years before the appearance of clinical symptoms (AUC = 0.910). MRS studies examining the effects of ApoE ε4 on the NAA/Cr and Cho/Cr ratios of the left hippocampus found that ApoE ε4 carriers had a significantly lower NAA/Cr ratio in the left hippocampus than non-carriers, suggesting a more prominent decrease in the neuronal activity or density of the hippocampus in ApoE ε4 carriers. Therefore, ApoE ε4 can specifically regulate the metabolic activities of the left frontal lobe and hippocampus in patients with amnestic MCI and AD. Furthermore, MRS can also serve as a non-invasive imaging marker of Aβ. In elderly subjects with normal cognition, the mI/Cr (r = 0.17, p = 0.003) and Cho/Cr (r = 0.13, p = 0.022) ratios of the PCC were found to be positively correlated with whole-brain Aβ deposition. The longitudinal follow-up MRS of the PCC/precuneus revealed that in patients with MCI, mI/Cr increased by 2.3% and NAA/mI decreased by 2.0% each year, while in the Aβ(+) group, mI/Cr increased by 2.93% and NAA/mI decreased by 3.55% each year. These findings indicate that Aβ levels in the cerebrospinal fluid (CSF) can affect changes in mI/Cr and NAA/mI ratios. Additionally, MRS can be used to evaluate the efficacy of AD treatments and related drug therapies. Henigsberg et al. performed MRS on 12 patients with mild to moderate AD after 26 weeks of treatment with donepezil and found a significant increase in the NAA/Cr ratio and a significant decrease in the mI/Cr ratio of the dorsolateral prefrontal cortex. These findings suggest that donepezil can prevent functional deterioration of the neurons in the dorsolateral prefrontal cortex, and that MRS is useful for the evaluation of drug therapies. MRS can provide information on cerebral metabolic, pathological, and biochemical changes in a safe and non-invasive manner, thereby enabling the exploration of clinical manifestations and pathogenic mechanisms in patients with AD. MRS, therefore, is of crucial theoretical significance and clinical value.

8.1.5 Research Applications of fMRI in AD

fMRI involves the use of BOLD imaging to measure the hemodynamic changes accompanying the changes in cerebral activity, thereby indirectly reflecting neuronal activity. There are several advantages of this technique, including being non-invasive, lacking ionizing radiation, and having a high temporal resolution. It can display the functional activities of specific brain areas, playing an indispensable role in the accurate localization of functional areas of the brain and the presentation of cognitive networks within the brain. Therefore, fMRI is now a key imaging technique in cognitive neuroscience and clinical medical research, and has been widely utilized in AD research.

fMRI can be divided into task-based and resting-state studies according to whether subjects are given specific tasks during the scan. Early fMRI studies predominantly involved task-based fMRI, which examined the task-related increases and decreases of neural activity, and localized functional areas of the brain based on the changes in regional signal intensity. Task-related fMRI can be used to study memory-related activation patterns in patients with AD, and such tasks include verbal (e.g., picture naming and semantic association) or non-verbal stimuli (e.g., scene and picture encoding), of which episodic memory tasks are the most common. When performing encoding tasks, patients with MCI show decreased activation of the right hippocampus and PCC, leading to a decline in immediate memory and memory recall. The hippocampus is a key area for memory tasks that is primarily responsible for encoding new information, while the PCC is responsible for encoding previously learned items. Therefore, patients with MCI may have functional impairments in the hippocampus and PCC. Since task-based fMRI requires subjects to perform different tasks during the MRI scan, compliance is often poor among cognitively impaired patients with AD. In contrast, resting-state fMRI scans are easy to perform and only require the subject to lie still, eliminating the effects of variations in task performance on the study findings. Therefore, resting-state fMRI is becoming increasingly more popular in AD research.

The default mode network (DMN) is a network that remains active in the absence of external tasks. It was first discovered when PET was used to measure the ratio of oxygen consumption to oxygen supply in the healthy human brain at rest, which revealed that areas of the brain such as the medial prefrontal lobe, PCC, and precuneus were more active during the resting state and less active in the presence of external tasks. Therefore, the network composed of these areas of the brain was known as the DMN. A consistent finding from resting-state fMRI in patients with AD is the reduced functional connectivity of the DMN, especially of the PCC/precuneus, hippocampus/parahippocampus, and DMN with other areas of the brain. Patients with amnestic MCI showed decreased functional activity in the DMN, including the bilateral precuneus/PCC, right inferior parietal lobule, and left fusiform gyrus, as well as increased functional activity in the left prefrontal cortex, inferior parietal lobe, and medial temporal gyrus, suggesting that increased frontal and parietal activity may compensate for damage to the DMN (Fig. 8.5). Dynamic changes can be observed in the DMN connectivity of patients with AD; more specifically, in the early stages of AD, the connectivity of the posterior DMN begins to decrease, whereas that of the anterior and ventral DMN is enhanced, and as the disease progresses, the connectivity of the entire network decreases. This implies that DMN abnormalities can serve as an imaging biomarker for the diagnosis and monitoring of patients with AD. Apart from the studies above that have focused on the DMN, the majority of previous studies have proposed that the cerebellum is not affected in early-stage AD, although more recent studies have found that patients with

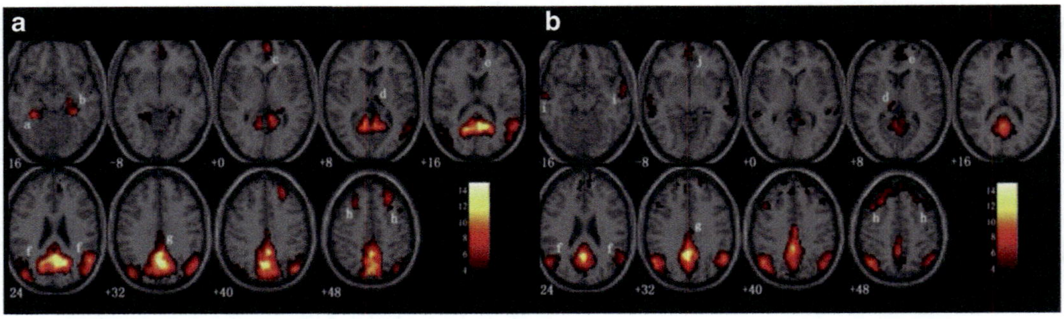

Fig. 8.5 Default mode network (DMN): The DMN of healthy elderly subjects consists of the medial prefrontal cortex, anterior cingulate cortex, posterior cingulate cortex, precuneus, and bilateral inferior parietal lobe (**a**). Lower functional activity of the DMN is detected in patients with amnestic MCI (**b**)

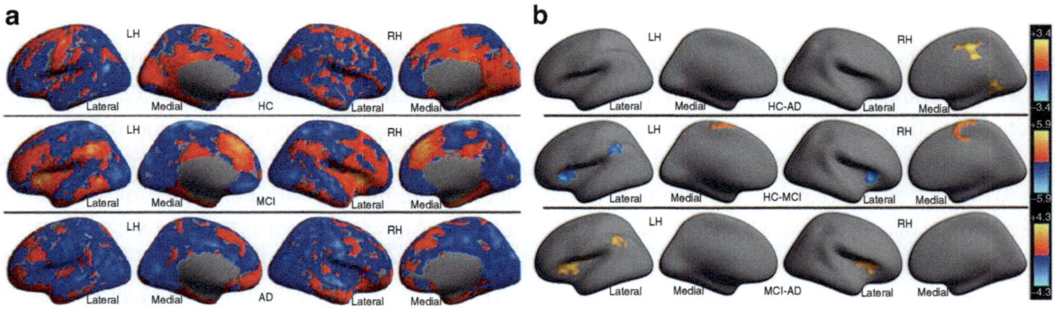

Fig. 8.6 Functional connectivity of the cerebellar limbic network (**a**) and inter group differences (**b**) in healthy controls (HCs), patients with MCI, and those with AD. Compared with HCs, patients with AD showed weaker functional connectivity in the right mid-cingulate cortex and lingual gyrus with the cerebellar limbic network and stronger functional connectivity in the left temporal pole with the cerebellar limbic network. Compared to patients with MCI, those with AD showed weaker functional connectivity in the bilateral orbitofrontal cortex extending to the anterior insula, and left inferior parietal lobule with the cerebellar limbic network. Compared to HC, patients with MCI showed weaker functional connectivity in the bilateral paracentral lobules and mid-cingulate cortex with the cerebellar limbic network, and enhanced functional connectivity of the bilateral posterior orbitofrontal cortex extending to the anterior insula, left inferior parietal lobule, and right fusiform gyrus with the cerebellar limbic network

AD and MCI exhibit reduced cerebellar limbic network activity (Fig. 8.6a). Compared with healthy controls, patients with AD show reduced functional connectivity in the right mid-cingulate cortex and lingual gyrus with the cerebellar limbic network, and enhanced functional connectivity in the left temporal pole with the cerebellar limbic network. Compared to patients with MCI, those with AD showed reduced functional connectivity of the bilateral posterior orbitofrontal cortex extending to the anterior insula and left inferior parietal lobule with the cerebellar limbic network. Compared to healthy controls, patients with MCI showed reduced functional connectivity of the bilateral paracentral lobules and mid-cingulate cortex with the cerebellar limbic network, and enhanced functional connectivity of the bilateral posterior orbitofrontal cortex extending to the anterior insula, left inferior parietal lobule, and right fusiform gyrus with the cerebellar limbic network (Fig. 8.6b). These findings signify the presence of functional cerebellar deficits in the early stages of AD and can serve as imaging evidence for future studies on cerebellar function in patients with AD.

Other common research methods include regional homogeneity (ReHo), which can be used to detect the correlation of regional activities in the whole brain, and amplitude of low-frequency fluctuation (ALFF). He et al. showed that patients with AD had reduced ReHo values in the PCC and precuneus, whereas patients with MCI had significantly increased ReHo values in the left inferior parietal lobule, which may be a compensatory change. Moreover, ReHo values can be used to discriminate patients with AD from those with MCI and healthy controls with an accuracy of 85%. ALFF is a method for observing spontaneous neuronal activity based on the amplitude of changes in BOLD signals relative to the baseline functional brain activity. Patients with AD had lower ALFF values compared to healthy controls in the bilateral PCC, PCC, precuneus, inferior parietal lobule, and multiple temporal areas, and higher ALFF values in the bilateral hippocampus, parahippocampal gyrus, middle temporal gyrus, and inferior temporal gyrus. However, other studies did not find elevated ALFF values in patients with mild AD. The differences in these results can be attributed to the different stages of AD. It is worth noting that significant alterations in ALFF activity can already be detected in early MCI that is independent of age, sex, and brain atrophy, therefore suggesting that ALFF abnormalities could serve as a potential biomarker for the early diagnosis of AD. Nevertheless, resting-state fMRI is susceptible to a variety of factors, and further investigation is needed to understand the neural basis of resting-state fMRI.

ApoE ε4 is a key genetic risk factor for developing AD that can also accelerate disease progression, brain atrophy, and pathological protein deposition. Patel et al. compared the DMN functional connectivity and white matter FA values between 14 ApoE ε4 carriers and 22 non-carriers, and found that ApoE ε4 carriers had reduced DMN functional connectivity, although there were no differences in cognitive function or white matter FA between the two groups, implying that functional changes preceded structural abnormalities in white matter among individuals at high risk for AD. A study on functional connectivity which used the hippocampus as the seed region found the asymmetric right lateralization of the hippocampal functional network in healthy subjects, whereas patients with AD showed a smaller hippocampal functional network with attenuated right lateralization. Furthermore, patients with AD exhibit disrupted functional connectivity of the right hippocampus with the medial prefrontal lobe, ventral ACC, right inferior temporal cortex, bilateral precuneus, and PCC. Of these, the medial prefrontal lobe, ventral ACC, and PCC are part of the DMN, which further supports the view that DMN dysfunction is present in patients with AD. Further fMRI analyses of hippocampal subregions have demonstrated the decreased functional connectivity of hippocampal subregions compared to healthy controls, mainly with the medial prefrontal lobe, superior frontal gyrus, precuneus, and PCC. Moreover, the functional connectivity of the right CA1-right precuneus had a significant positive correlation with MMSE scores, reflecting clinical cognitive levels in early-stage AD (Fig. 8.7). A longitudinal study showed that the functional connectivity of the hippocampal subregions can help to discriminate between AD and MCI patients (sensitivity and specificity, 83.3%), with a higher discriminative ability than functional connectivity based on using the entire hippocampus as the seed region. Therefore, fMRI analysis based on the activation levels of the hippocampal subregions can provide valuable imaging information for AD research. Additionally, resting-state fMRI can be used to evaluate the functional changes of the brain in patients with AD after acupuncture treatment. In fact, the enhanced functional connectivity of the hippocampus-medial prefrontal lobe in patients with AD after acupuncture may be the mechanism underlying the therapeutic efficacy of acupuncture at the Siguan acupoints (Fig. 8.8).

Multimodal imaging studies can help us to achieve a deeper understanding of the pathophysiological mechanism of AD from multiple perspectives, including structure, perfusion, and function, which will provide valuable information for early diagnosis of AD as well as evaluation of treatment prognosis.

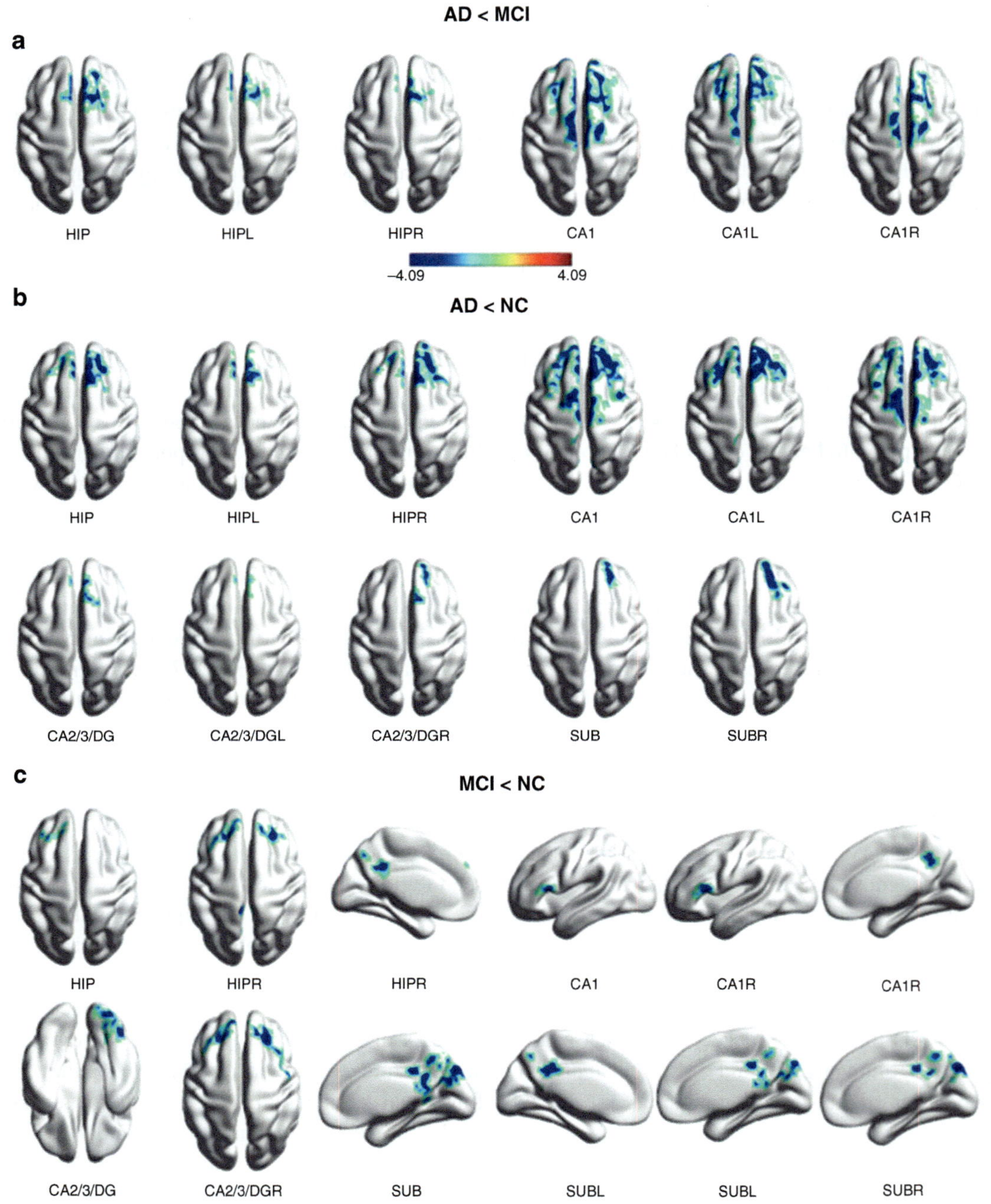

Fig. 8.7 Alterations in the functional connectivity of hippocampal subregions in patients with AD and MCI: Compared to healthy controls (HC), patients with AD showed reduced functional connectivity in all hippocampal subregions, mainly with the frontal cortex (**a**). Compared to patients with MCI, those with AD only showed reduced functional connectivity between CA1 and the frontal lobe (**b**). Compared to HC, patients with MCI showed reduced functional connectivity in all hippocampal subregions, mainly with the frontal lobe, and posterior cingulate cortex/precuneus (**c**) (Reproduced with permission from [38])

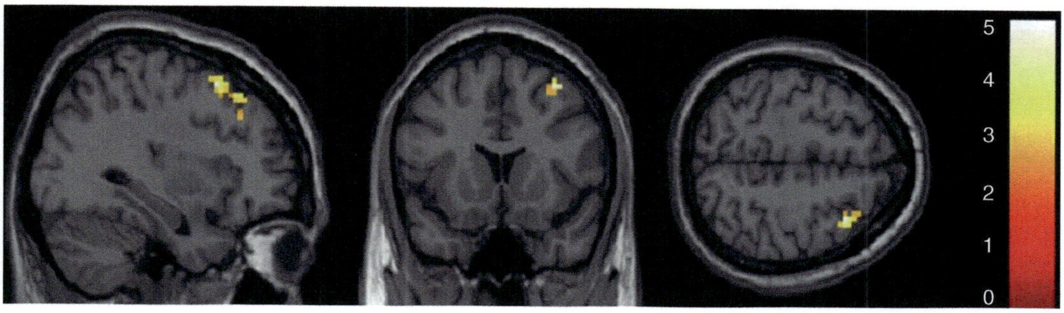

Fig. 8.8 Alterations in hippocampal functional connectivity in the AD group following acupuncture treatment: Enhanced functional connectivity (yellow) in the right medial prefrontal lobe-left hippocampus in patients with AD following acupuncture treatment

8.2 Research Applications of PET Imaging in AD

PET is an indispensable element of *in vivo* functional imaging techniques at the molecular level that can qualitatively and quantitatively evaluate the functional metabolic levels of tissues and organs based on the distribution characteristics of radiotracers in the body. Owing to its high sensitivity and specificity, PET plays a crucial role in the early diagnosis, differential diagnosis, disease evaluation, and outcome prediction of AD. Current PET imaging studies on AD mainly target glucose metabolism, Aβ, tau protein, and the cholinergic system.

8.2.1 Research Applications of ^{18}F-Fluorodeoxyglucose (FDG) PET Imaging in AD

^{18}F-FDG PET imaging measures the glucose uptake of neurons and glial cells. It is highly sensitive at detecting synaptic dysfunction and can identify glucose hypometabolism before the occurrence of cell death and brain tissue atrophy, which makes it more sensitive at diagnosing early-stage AD than structural MRI. ^{18}F-FDG imaging allows the differentiation among different types of neurodegeneration based on the hypometabolism of specific brain areas. Cerebral glucose metabolism is fairly evenly distributed in healthy subjects (Fig. 8.9a). In contrast, patients with MCI first present with hypometabolism in the MTL (Fig. 8.9b); typical patients with AD present with significant hypometabolism of the parietal lobe, temporal lobe, and PCC, followed by that of the frontal lobe (Fig. 8.9c); patients with frontotemporal dementia present with hypometabolism in the frontal lobe and anterior temporal lobe; whereas patients with dementia with Lewy bodies present with hypometabolism of the occipital lobe. However, the clinical application of ^{18}F-FDG PET is limited by the qualitative assessment of images, in which visual scoring is determined to a large extent by the observer's experience. The delineation of standard ROIs and voxel-based analysis can improve the identification of early-stage AD by ^{18}F-FDG PET. The ApoE ε4 allele is a high-risk genetic factor for the onset of AD. In a longitudinal study examining the relationship between ApoE ε4 and brain metabolism, the longitudinal analysis of ^{18}F-FDG PET images from 48 ApoE ε4 carriers and non-carriers with MCI showed that compared to ApoE ε4 non-carriers, ApoE ε4 carriers showed a more rapid decrease of glucose metabolism in the superior frontal lobe, lateral temporal lobe, MTL, caudate nucleus, thalamus, PCC, and amygdala, which indicates that the ApoE ε4 allele can accelerate the decrease in cerebral glucose metabolism (Fig. 8.10).

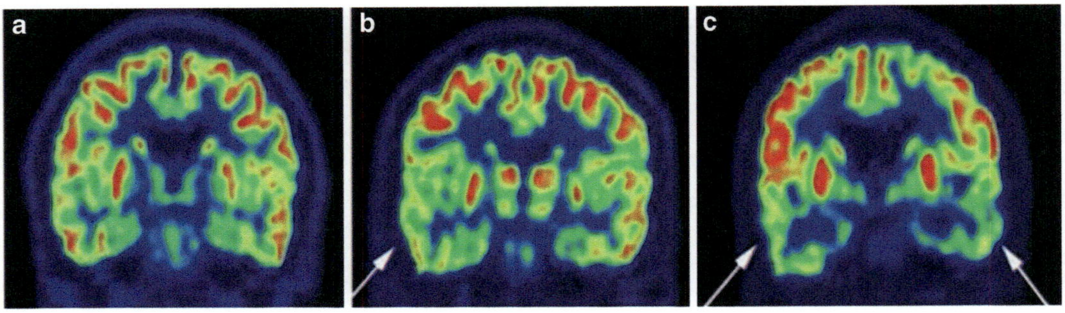

Fig. 8.9 ^{18}F-FDG PET imaging of cognitively normal subjects, patients with MCI, and those with AD: A 60-year-old, cognitively normal male subject showing no glucose hypometabolism on ^{18}F-FDG PET imaging (**a**). A 62-year-old female patient with MCI showing glucose hypometabolism in the right temporal lobe (white arrow) on ^{18}F-FDG PET imaging (**b**). A 59-year-old male patient with AD showing glucose hypometabolism in the bilateral temporal lobes (white arrows) on ^{18}F-FDG PET imaging (**c**)

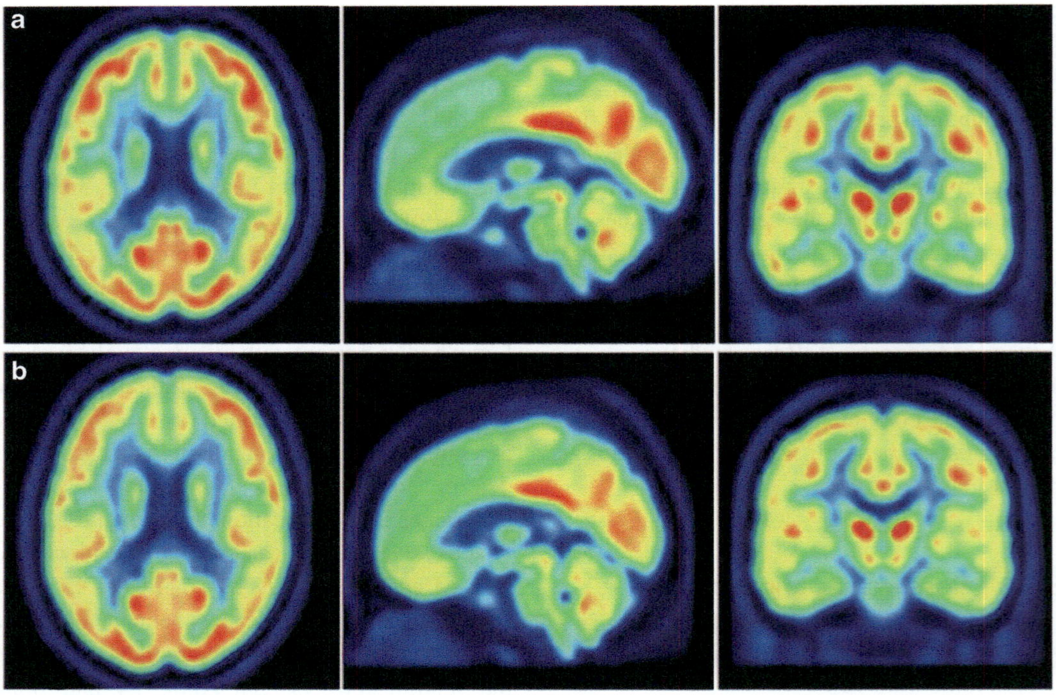

Fig. 8.10 Longitudinal ^{18}F-FDG PET imaging of patients with MCI: ^{18}F-FDG PET imaging of ApoE ε4 non-carriers at baseline and after 72 months (**a**) shows non-significant decreases in cerebral glucose metabolism. ^{18}F-FDG PET imaging of ApoE ε4 carriers at baseline and after 72 months (**b**) shows more rapid decreases in the glucose metabolism of the frontal lobe, lateral temporal lobe, medial temporal lobe, caudate nucleus, thalamus, posterior cingulate cortex, and amygdala than ApoE ε4 carriers

8.2.2 Research Applications of Aβ PET Imaging in AD

Aβ is derived from the active amyloid precursor protein (APP) found on cell membranes. APP mutations, together with mutations of presenilin-1 (PSEN1) and presenilin-2 (PSEN2), can cause the increased extracellular release of Aβ, which will accumulate to form oligomers and fibers, eventually forming plaques. Brain Aβ deposition can be detected in early-stage AD, with a large number of studies identifying Aβ deposition in the brains of cognitively normal elderly subjects. The Aβ hypothesis posits that Aβ formation is the chief component of AD that can trigger a series of pathogenic processes, including inflammation, tau protein deposition to form NFTs, synaptic dysfunction, cell death, and finally dementia.

The Aβ PET tracer to be employed in clinical settings was ^{11}C-Pittsburgh compound B (PiB or 2-[4′-(methylamino)phenyl]-6-hydroxybenzothiazole), which binds to fibrillar Aβ deposition with high selectivity, exhibits good agreement with pathological results, and has a rapid clearance rate in normal brain tissues, which popularized its application in early clinical studies. Compared to cognitively normal subjects, patients with AD show increased cortical ^{11}C-PiB uptake, and the uptake concentration in descending order was the frontal lobe, parietal lobe, temporal lobe, and occipital lobe; although high uptake was also detected in the striatum, it was not associated with clinical symptoms. According to the 2018 National Institute on Aging and the Alzheimer's Association Research Framework for Alzheimer's Disease, biomarkers can be used independently of clinical symptoms for the assessment of AD. Thus, positive CSF Aβ or PET findings of cortical Aβ deposition can be used to confirm the presence of AD pathological changes, whereas negative findings for Aβ can be used to exclude AD pathological changes. A ^{11}C-PiB PET imaging study found that the percentages of PiB-positive subjects in the healthy elderly, MCI, and AD group were 22, 61, and 97%, respectively.

The short half-life of ^{11}C (t1/2 = 20.4 min) has prevented its use in institutions without cyclotrons, and its high associated cost is a barrier to its routine application in clinical examinations. In contrast, the second-generation ^{18}F-labelled Aβ tracers have a longer half-life than those labelled with ^{11}C, and those that have been approved by the US Food and Drug Administration (FDA) or European Medicines Agency for clinical use include ^{18}F-florbetapir, ^{18}F-florbetaben, ^{18}F-flutemetamol, and ^{18}F-NAV4694. ^{18}F-florbetapir (also known as ^{18}F-AV-45) is currently the most commonly used Aβ tracer, with some studies suggesting that its sensitivity and specificity to Aβ deposition are 92% and 100%, respectively. ^{18}F-AV-45 uptake is absent in the cerebral cortex of healthy elderly subjects, with only a small amount of non-specific uptake detected in the white matter (Fig. 8.11a). In patients with MCI, ^{18}F-AV-45 uptake can be detected in the right frontal lobe and right parietal operculum (Fig. 8.11b), while in patients with AD, ^{18}F-AV-45 can be detected in almost the entire cerebral cortex (Fig. 8.11c). A

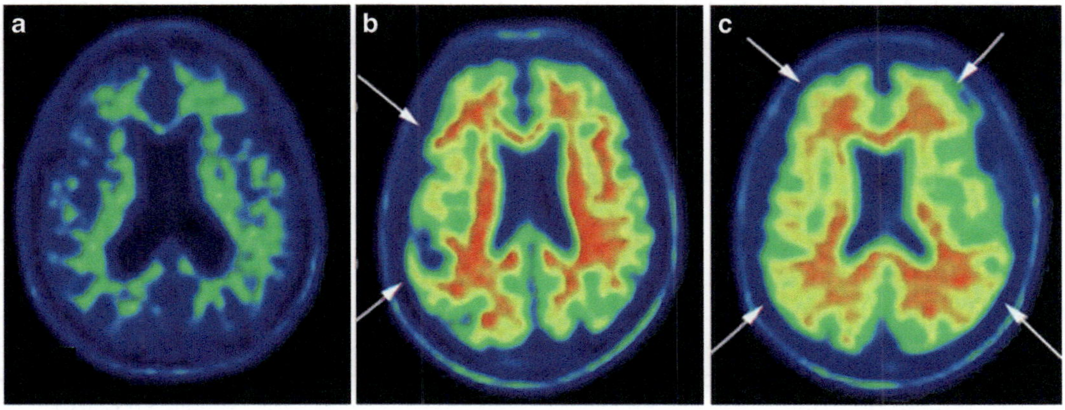

Fig. 8.11 ^{18}F-AV45 PET imaging of healthy elderly subjects, patients with MCI, and those with AD: A healthy 65-year-old male subject, whose ^{18}F-AV45 PET findings show no cortical Aβ deposition, with only a small amount of non-specific Aβ deposition in white matter (**a**). A 63-year-old male MCI patient, whose ^{18}F-AV45 PET findings indicate Aβ deposition in the right frontal lobe and right parietal operculum (white arrows) (**b**). A 65-year-old female AD patient, whose ^{18}F-AV45 findings indicate Aβ deposition in almost the entire cerebral cortex (white arrows) (**c**)

^{18}F-AV-45 PET imaging study on healthy elderly, MCI, and AD subjects found significant differences among the standardized uptake value ratios (SUVR) of the three groups, with the SUVR of healthy elderly subjects showing a linear association with age, while that of MCI and patients with AD showing no association with age. Another ^{18}F-AV-45 PET imaging study on healthy elderly subjects demonstrated that subjects with greater Aβ deposition experienced more rapid deterioration in their episodic memory performance. Fig. 8.11 presents the ^{18}F-AV-45 PET imaging findings of NC, patients with MCI, and those with AD, which shows that healthy elderly subjects.

In studies examining the correlation of Aβ deposition of different brain regions with glucose metabolism and clinical cognitive scores, researchers compared the ^{11}C-PiB PET and ^{18}F-FDG PET images of patients with AD and found ^{11}C-PiB uptake in all brain areas was correlated with deficient ^{18}F-FDG PET uptake. Furthermore, the glucose metabolism of most brain areas in patients with AD was highly correlated with cognitive scores, but ^{11}C-PiB uptake was not significantly correlated with any cognitive scores, and the two were also not significantly correlated among cognitively normal subjects. These findings suggest that Aβ deposition is unable to reflect the cognitive levels of patients with AD, and involve different pathophysiological mechanisms of glucose hypometabolism. In addition, subjects with subjective cognitive impairment showed negative correlations in the ^{11}C-PiB uptake of the hippocampus, medial orbitofrontal lobe/ACC, PCC/precuneus, and temporo-parietal lobe with the level of atrophy, but this correlation was absent in the MCI and AD groups. Another study reported that ^{11}C-PiB uptake in the hippocampus and inferior temporal lobe of healthy elderly subjects was associated with atrophy, but this correlation was absent in patients with amnestic MCI and AD. Based on the correlation analyses of Aβ with cerebral glucose metabolism and atrophy, it is evident that Aβ imaging can predict neurodegenerative changes in early-stage AD, but the amount of Aβ deposition was not correlated with the severity of neurodegeneration in the MCI and AD populations.

8.2.3 Research Applications of Tau Protein PET Imaging in AD

Tau proteins are a major component of normal mature neuronal microtubule-associated proteins and consist of six subtypes. Normal tau proteins bind with axonal tubulin to promote the assembly of tubulin into microtubules and maintain the stability of microtubules. In different neurodegenerative diseases, the different subtypes of tau proteins can be aggregated in specific ways and become abnormally hyperphosphorylated, thus forming insoluble fibrillar deposits within cells. In AD, all six subtypes of tau proteins are hyperphosphorylated and deposited to form paired helical filaments (PHFs), which are entangled with straight filaments to form NFTs. The progressive spread of NFTs in the brain follows a specific order, which was divided by Braak into six stages: in the early stages, deposition occurs in the limbic system, including the entorhinal cortex and hippocampus (Braak stages I–III), and may be asymptomatic, while after Braak stage IV, the amount and extent of NFT deposition is highly correlated with cognitive function. In AD, 40% of abnormally phosphorylated tau (p-tau) is not deposited as NFTs in the cytoplasm, which can compete with normal tau protein to bind with tubulin, and inhibit the assembly of microtubules, thereby forming NFTs. Since the concentration of p-tau is substantially lower than that of Aβ in patients with AD, while tau and Aβ are both β-sheet proteins, a good tau tracer must have a high selectivity for tau proteins (i.e., significantly higher binding with tau than with Aβ), high affinity for p-tau, and low non-specific binding. These requirements imply that it is significantly more challenging to create tau tracers than Aβ tracers.

Tau protein tracers are divided into non-selective and selective tracers. The PET tracer, ^{18}F-FDDNP, was initially used for Aβ imaging, but was later discovered to bind non-selectively to both extracellular Aβ and intracellular NFTs, which restricted its application in AD imaging. Selective tau imaging agents are divided into first generation and second generation. First-generation imaging agents, such as ^{18}F-THK523, are quinoline derivatives, which have a high affinity for tau proteins that is 12 times that for Aβ. In vitro studies have found that it can bind selectively with tau PHFs, but not with tau proteins in diseases other than AD, including α-synuclein found in Lewy bodies in PD. In terms of in vivo imaging, ^{18}F-THK523 showed high uptake in the temporal lobe, parietal lobe, orbitofrontal lobe, and hippocampus of patients with AD, but also showed high retention in white matter, which made it difficult to interpret the imaging findings visually, and has limited its application in clinical settings. Subsequent improvements in PET tracers led to the creation of ^{18}F-THK5105, ^{18}F-THK5117, and ^{18}F-THK5351, which have faster hemodynamics, lower white matter retention, and higher signal-to-noise ratio. In addition, novel benzimidazole-pyridine derivatives, such as ^{18}F-807 and ^{18}F-808, have a higher binding affinity to tau PHFs that is 25 times higher than that with Aβ. Among them, ^{18}F-807, also known as ^{18}F-AV-1451 or ^{18}F-flortaucipir, is currently the only tau PET tracer approved by the US FDA. This tracer targets cortical regions that are highly consistent with the anatomical distribution of tau PHFs, has low white matter retention, and its cerebral retention is highly correlated with disease severity. However, it exhibits off-target binding in the choroid plexus, basal ganglia, thalamus, and substantia nigra. Studies have found that the two benzimidazole derivatives, astemizole and lansoprazole, have a higher affinity for tau proteins than for Aβ. Based on which, a tau tracer, ^{11}C-PBB3, was developed, which can bind with high selectivity to tau proteins, and be applied in imaging studies on AD and other tauopathies. Second-generation selective tau tracers were optimized to reduce off-target binding. For example, structural modifications were made to ^{18}F-AV-1451 to produce ^{18}F-RO-948 and ^{18}F-PI-2620, which had a higher specificity than that of first-generation tracers and virtually no off-target binding.

Tau proteins undergo a different spreading process to amyloids in the brain. Cho et al. performed Aβ PET (^{18}F-AV-45) and tau PET (^{18}F-AV-1451) imaging on 195 subjects (53 AD, 52 amnestic MCI, 23 non-amnestic MCI, and 67 HC), in order to analyze the spreading process of Aβ and tau deposition based on the deposition amount in ROIs and frequency of deposition. They found that tau deposition was most frequently observed in the entorhinal cortex (49.2%) and parahippocampal gyrus (39.0%), followed by the fusiform gyrus, inferior temporal gyrus, amygdala, middle temporal gyrus, superior parietal lobe, and PCC, whereas the frequency of tau deposition was lowest in the ACC and primary cortical regions (precentral gyrus, middle occipital gyrus, paracentral gyrus, and postcentral gyrus). Thus, tau deposition began from the entorhinal cortex of the limbic system and spread to anatomically and functionally connected regions in the MTL (PCC and inferior temporal gyrus), rather than spreading to adjacent regions. This study has also confirmed the tau spreading hypothesis, which posits that tau proteins can spread to anatomically and functionally related regions through white matter and synaptic connections. Conversely, the frequency of Aβ deposition, in descending order, was the frontotemporal lobe, middle and inferior temporal gyrus, middle frontal lobe, and superior frontal lobe, from which Aβ was spread to the entire cortex, with the MTL showing the lowest frequency (i.e., parahippocampal gyrus, entorhinal cortex, amygdala, and hippocampus). Furthermore, the study also found that the frequency of gray matter volume reduction, in descending order, was the hippocampus, amygdala, entorhinal cortex, and parahippocampal gyrus, with other cortical regions showing relatively low frequencies, and the lowest frequencies occurring in the ACC and postcentral gyrus. This order is almost in complete agreement with that of tau protein deposition, which suggests that tau protein deposition is closely associated with neurodegeneration. In addition, tau PET imaging can sensitively capture the early and late changes in AD. Multimodal analysis, including ^{11}C-PiB, ^{18}F-FDG, ^{18}F-AV-1451 and MRI, was performed on 96 patients with typical AD and atypical AD (cognitive impairments primarily involving domains other than episodic memory), which revealed that the correlation was highest between the SUVRs of ^{18}F-AV-1451 and ^{18}F-FDG in the same brain region, followed by that between ^{18}F-AV-1451 uptake and MRI-based cortical thickness, while that between ^{11}C-PiB and cortical thickness was the lowest. The results of this study showed that the cerebral deposition of abnormal tau proteins in AD is more closely related to the metabolic environment of the corresponding regions, and that the relationship between tau proteins and cortical thickness is affected by age and other clinical indicators.

A cross-sectional study revealed sex differences in the tau deposition of ApoE ε4 carriers. More specifically, quantitative ^{18}F-AV-1451 PET analysis was performed on 108 patients with MCI, which showed interaction effects between gender and ApoE ε4 in the entorhinal cortex, amygdala, parahippocampal gyrus, PCC, and occipital lobe, with female ApoE ε4 carriers showing greater tau deposition than male carriers (Fig. 8.12). In addition, CSF total tau (t-tau) and p-tau showed significant interactions effects between gender and ApoE ε4, which were not affected by Aβ deposition to a certain extent. On the basis of these studies, Yan et al. combined ^{18}F-AV-1451 PET with structural MRI to analyze the effects of gender and ApoE ε4 on tau deposition and brain atrophy, which revealed that female ApoE ε4 carriers (FACs) with AD formed a special group that had significantly higher tau deposition in the MTL, middle temporal gyrus, and other regions compared to other AD groups (non-FACs, male ApoE ε4 carriers, and male ApoE ε4 non-carriers) (Fig. 8.13). Moreover, no significant differences in tau deposition were detected among the groups. These findings indicate that greater attention should be given to elderly female ApoE ε4 carriers in the prevention and treatment of AD. These results have also provided strong evidence to clarify the interaction effects of gender and ApoE ε4 on tau deposition in the AD spectrum, as well as the relationship between tau proteins and brain atrophy.

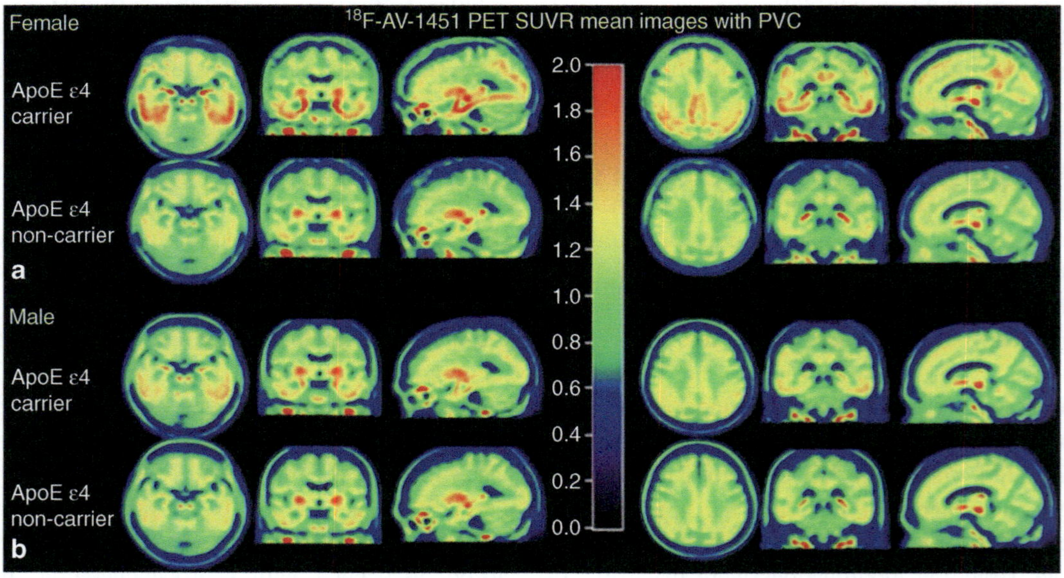

Fig. 8.12 ^{18}F-AV-1451 PET imaging of patients with MCI: Female ApoE ε4 carriers showed greater tau deposition than female ApoE ε4 non-carriers (**a**) and male ApoE ε4 carriers, whereas tau deposition did not differ between male ApoE ε4 carriers and non-carriers (**a** and **b**) (Reproduced with permission from [29])

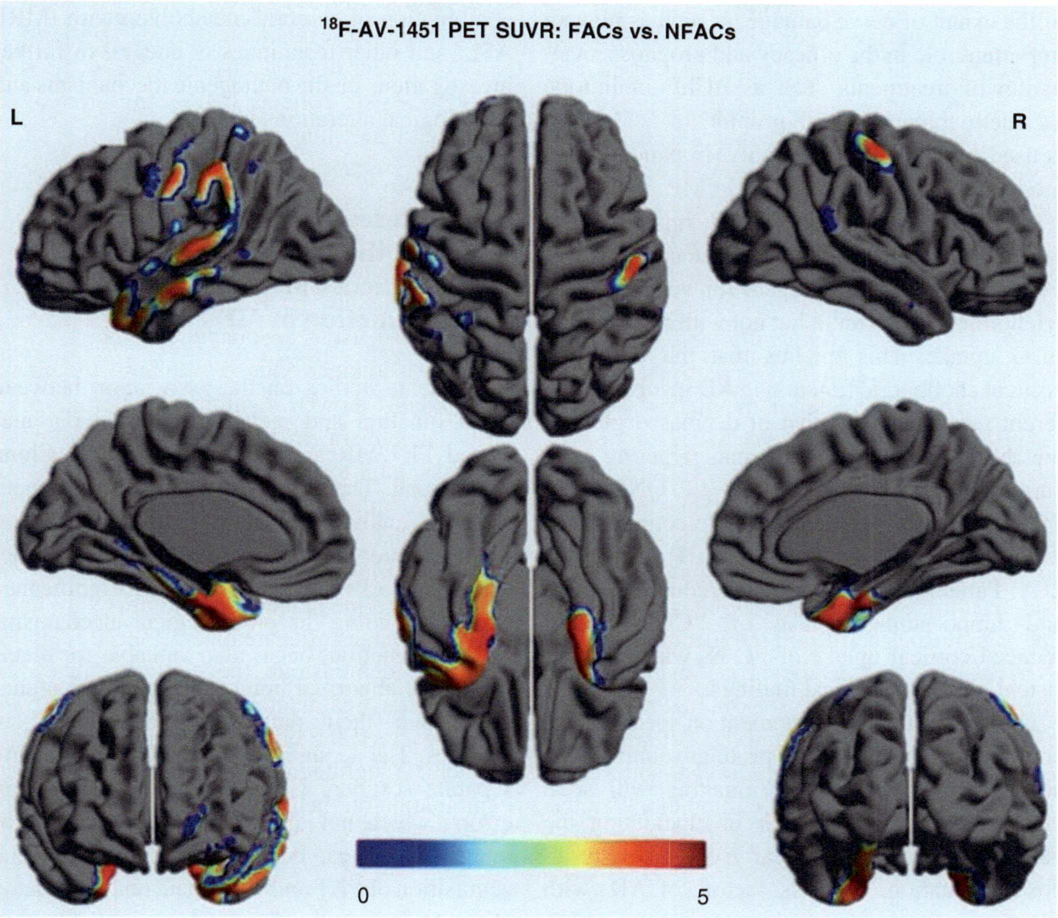

Fig. 8.13 Comparison of ^{18}F-AV-1451 PET between female ApoE ε4 carriers with AD and other AD groups: Female ApoE ε4 carriers (FACs) showed significantly higher tau deposition in the medial temporal lobe, middle temporal gyrus, and other brain areas compared to other groups (non-FACs, male ApoE ε4 carriers, and male ApoE ε4 non-carriers)

8.2.4 Research Applications of Cholinergic PET Imaging in AD

The cholinergic system is inextricably linked with cognitive function. In particular, the majority of efferent cholinergic fibers projecting from the nucleus basalis of Meynert (NBM) to the cortex and amygdala constitute the main pathways that can affect cognition. AD pathologies can cause the destruction or loss of cholinergic neurons, leading to the disruption of acetylcholine synthesis. Studies involving the post-mortem examination of brain tissues from patients with AD have demonstrated deficits of choline acetyltransferase and acetylcholinesterase (AChE) in the cerebral cortex, hippocampus, and amygdala, with the most severe reduction occurring in the NBM.

Cholinergic PET imaging is currently less commonly applied in AD than Aβ and tau imaging, and is mainly divided into AChE and acetylcholine receptor imaging. This technique can be employed in the evaluation of early-stage AD pathologies, differentiation of AD from other neurodegenerative diseases, dynamic monitoring of the extent of nerve damage, as well as play an important role in the efficacy and prognosis evaluation of treatments such as AChE inhibitors. ^{11}C-methylpiperidin-4-yl propionate (^{11}C-PMP) is used to detect AChE activity. In patients with moderate to severe AD, ^{11}C-PMP uptake is reduced in the neocortex and hippocampus, which is associated with the reduced uptake of ^{123}I-IBVM (an imaging agent for vesicular acetylcholine transporters), but not with reduced ^{18}F-FDG uptake. This implies that the decreased cortical cholinergic function in AD involves a different mechanisms to that of decreased glucose metabolism. PET imaging agents targeting muscarinic receptors including ^{11}C-QNB and ^{11}C-NMPB, while those targeting nicotinic receptors include ^{11}C-nicotine (^{11}C-N) and ^{18}F-2FA. Patients with AD exhibit reduced cortical and hippocampal uptake of ^{11}C-QNB, and reduced cortical uptake of ^{11}C-N, which is consistent with pathological findings.

As research and development on specific tracers for AD pathological proteins continue to advance, multi-tracer PET imaging will soon become a crucial approach in elucidating the pathogenic mechanisms, early diagnosis, prognosis evaluation, and risk factors of AD, with broad prospects for clinical and scientific applications.

8.3 Research Applications of PET/MR in AD

Functional research of the brain has always been a topic of widespread concern, as imaging is an indispensable method in understanding and exploring brain functions. fMRI can provide information on brain function, perfusion changes, and other aspects, while ^{18}F-FDG PET is an important means by which to examine neuronal function. Imaging equipment has undergone rapid technological development in recent years, and the most advanced technique so far is simultaneous scanning with integrated PET/MR for the "one-stop" acquisition of imaging information on brain anatomy, function, blood flow, and metabolism. Thus, the "functional-functional" combination of cerebral metabolism with fMRI, ASL, and other techniques is integral to further investigations on the pathogenic mechanisms and pathological alterations in AD.

8.3.1 Research Applications of the Relationship Between Glucose Metabolism and Brain Function in AD

At present, studies on the association between brain function and metabolism based on integrated PET/MR are relatively scarce in China and abroad. The ability to simultaneously measure and analyze the characteristic relationship between cerebral glucose metabolism and functional networks is not only of great significance to understanding the physiological mechanisms of brain function, but is also valuable for elucidating the abnormal brain metabolism, dysfunctions, and their pathogenic mechanisms in diseases. The acquisition of PET and MRI using separate scanners is susceptible to registration errors, which not only affects the accuracy of imaging findings, but also does not allow the acquisition of PET and fMRI data under the same physiological state, thus making it difficult to clarify the intrinsic relationship between brain metabolism and functional changes. Integrated PET/MR enables the acquisition of cerebral glucose metabolism and functional information under the same physiological state, which offers the possibility of examining the relationship between metabolism and neural activity.

Functional ^{18}F-FDG PET/MR using integrated PET/MR was performed to explore the relationship between functional connectivity and glucose metabolism of 22 healthy subjects in the eyes-open (11 subjects) and eyes-closed (11 subjects) states. Increased regional activity was detected in the visual system and salience network (cingulate cortex and insula) during the eyes-open state compared to the eyes-closed state, and this pattern of increased glucose metabolism was consistent with the spatial pattern of functional connectivity. These findings provide direct evidence for the relationship between glucose metabolism and neuronal activity, that is, the biological basis for brain functional connectivity is the glucose metabolism of local neurons. On the basis of resting-state fMRI, the PCC was used as a seed region to calculate the brain areas involved in the DMN, which mainly consisted of the medial prefrontal lobe, insula, inferior parietal lobule, and hippocampus (Fig. 8.14a); while hypermetabolic brain areas in the resting state mainly included the PCC/precuneus, medial prefrontal lobe, middle frontal gyrus, transverse temporal gyrus, and putamen (Fig. 8.14b). The spatial distribution of the DMN based on resting-state fMRI was basically consistent with that of PET-based hypermetabolic regions, with the right PCC of the DMN showing the highest correlation between glucose uptake and functional connectivity. In another study using integrated PET/MR to examine the correlations between ^{18}F-FDG PET and different fMRI parameters during the resting state in 26 subjects, significant spatial correlations were found between the distribution of glucose metabolism with the ReHo, fractional ALFF (fALFF), and degree of centrality (DC) measured simultaneously using fMRI. The spatial distribution of glucose uptake in the limbic network had the weakest spatial correlation with DC among the anatomical and functional networks (correlation coefficient, 0.11), whereas the fALFF and ReHo of the DMN had the strongest correlation with the spatial distribution of glucose uptake (correlation coefficients, 0.89 and 0.89, respectively). The heterogeneity in the relationship between resting-state fMRI parameters and PET among different brain networks may reflect the different activity levels of these networks during the resting state, which may have led to differences in time scale when combining the two techniques, thus suggesting that there may be variations in the degree of neurometabolic coupling for different brain networks. These results provide a basis for studying the alterations in the coupling between brain metabolism and functional connectivity under pathological conditions. Marchitelli et al. recently utilized integrated PET/MR to evaluate the correlation between ^{18}F-FDG PET and resting-state fMRI under the same physiological state in amnestic MCI/AD patients. The relationship between ^{18}F-FDG PET and fMRI parameters (ReHo, fALFF, and independent component analysis) revealed abnormal changes in the PCC and precuneus of amnestic MCI/AD patients, with patients showing lower correlations between ^{18}F-FDG PET and fMRI parameters than healthy elderly subjects. This implies that amnestic MCI/AD patients have weaker neuroenergetic coupling between glucose utilization and the rapid transmission of neural information. In general terms, brain connectivity and brain network theory posits that the integrity of normal brain function must usually be established based on the coordination of multiple connected brain areas. Patients with AD, however, suffer from regional

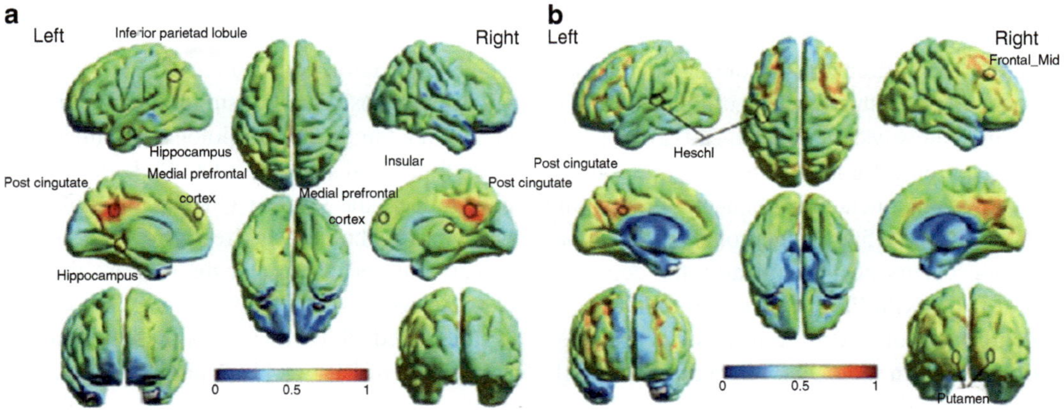

Fig. 8.14 Spatial distribution maps of resting-state fMRI DMN and PET glucose uptake: Spatial distribution maps of resting-state fMRI DMN (**a**) and PET glucose uptake (**b**)

pathological changes, which result in abnormal functional connectivity between brain areas, i.e., "disconnections," eventually leading to functional impairments. An integrated PET/MR study on 40 patients with mild AD, 21 patients with MCI, and 26 HC found that patients with AD had decreased functional connectivity in the hippocampus and precuneus, but showed hypermetabolism in the hippocampus and hypometabolism in the precuneus (AD < MCI < HC), which validates the "disconnection" hypothesis of AD. Further analysis was performed on the relationship between functional connectivity and glucose metabolism in patients with AD at the level of hippocampal subregions, which revealed that the functional connectivity between the left CA2/3DG and right medial prefrontal lobe was significantly negatively correlated with glucose metabolism, thus suggesting that the left CA2/3/DG is the dominant subregion involved in hippocampal disconnection. Therefore, integrated PET/MR has provided a new and advantageous method for studying the pathophysiological mechanisms of AD.

Based on molecular studies, it was found that the distribution of pathological proteins in the brains of patients with AD was dependent on the directionality of signaling pathways. At the level of fMRI brain networks, undirected functional connectivity (temporal synchronization between spatially-distant brain areas) only measures the strength of connections without direction, whereas directed functional connectivity (effective connectivity) measures whether there are interactions between brain areas, as well as the direction and strength of these interactions, which can reflect the direction of transmission in signaling pathways. Riedl et al. (2015) proposed a novel approach for measuring effective connectivity known as metabolic connectivity mapping (MCM). Since 75% of neuronal energy consumption occurs postsynaptically, the combination of fMRI with PET can be used to obtain the directionality of signal transmission between brain regions. In their study, integrated PET/MR was performed on 24 healthy subjects in the eyes-open and eyes-closed conditions for MCM analysis. Their results revealed the bidirectional flow of information between the primary and higher-order visual cortices, and top-down signaling in the frontoparietal network, while additional top-down modulation from the salience network was detected only in the eyes-open condition. As a novel method that can be used to infer the direction of functional connectivity between brain regions based on neuroenergetics, MCM allows the comprehensive analysis of multimodal information in order to study the cerebral mechanisms of signal processing. By analyzing the integrated ^{18}F-FDG PET/fMRI data of 35 patients with early-stage AD and 18 healthy subjects, two distinct effective connectivity subnetworks were found in the DMN of the healthy subjects: one involving bidirectional connectivity between the hippocampus and medial prefrontal cortex, and another involving predominantly input signals into the medial parietal cortex. Patients with AD, however, had reduced input into the medial parietal cortex, and loss of input from the hippocampus into the medial prefrontal cortex. This suggests that specific disruptions of effective connectivity can be identified in the DMN of patients with AD, which can help to explain molecular theories about the upstream and downstream spreading of neuropathology in AD.

8.3.2 Research Applications of the Relationship Between Glucose Metabolism and Cerebral Perfusion in AD

Regional cerebral perfusion is closely associated with the glucose metabolism of neural activities, and is an important physiological indicator of brain functional state. ^{18}F-FDG PET imaging not only reflects the level of glucose metabolism in brain tissues, but also indirectly reveals the state of cerebral perfusion, and the two are theoretically related.

Integrated PET/MR allows the simultaneous acquisition of ^{18}F-FDG PET and ASL in order to obtain information on both glucose metabolism and cerebral perfusion. A study on healthy subjects found that the CBF data acquired using

ASL showed good agreement with classic methods of CBF quantification, and hence is one of the key techniques for CBF quantification. No abnormalities were found in the CBF and ^{18}F-FDG uptake of cognitively normal subjects (Fig. 8.15a). In contrast, patients with MCI showed decreased CBF in the right temporal lobe and decreased ^{18}F-FDG uptake in the bilateral temporal lobes (Fig. 8.15b), with ^{18}F-FDG uptake covering a greater extent of reduction than CBF. Patients with AD showed decreased CBF and ^{18}F-FDG uptake in the bilateral parietal lobes, with overlaps in abnormal brain areas between the two techniques (Fig. 8.15c). As the disease progressed, the extent of reductions in CBF and ^{18}F-FDG uptake continued to expand. In an integrated PET/MR study involving 45 patients with AD, 20 patients with MCI, and 11 healthy elderly subjects, voxel-wise analysis of variance, ROI analysis, and independent component analysis were performed on the ^{18}F-FDG PET and ASL images. The results revealed a high degree of overlap between regions of hypoperfusion and hypometabolism in the precuneus, parietal cortex, temporal cortex, and occipital cortex of patients with AD, but with ASL showing a smaller extent of abnormal brain regions. In patients with MCI, ^{18}F-FDG PET imaging showed hypometabolism in the bilateral inferior parietal lobule, superior temporal

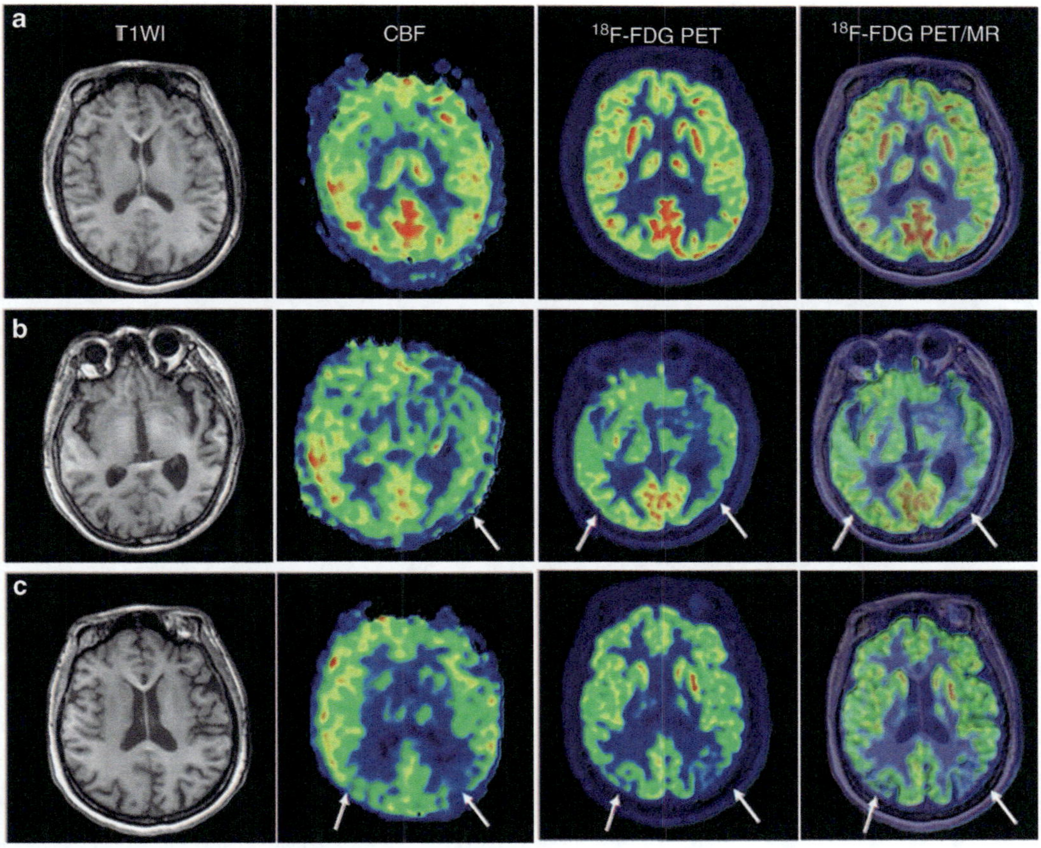

Fig. 8.15 A cognitively normal, 67-year-old, healthy female subject underwent integrated ^{18}F-FDG PET/MR; T1WI shows no significant atrophy in brain structures; CBF imaging shows no abnormal reductions in CBF; and ^{18}F-FDG PET shows no abnormal ^{18}F-FDG uptake (**a**). A 69-year-old male patient with MCI; T1WI shows enlargement of the left posterior horn of the lateral ventricle; CBF imaging shows CBF reduction in the left temporal lobe; and ^{18}F-FDG PET showed reduced ^{18}F-FDG uptake in the left temporal lobe (**b**). A 69-year-old female patient with AD; no significant atrophy observed in brain structures; bilateral parietal lobes (white arrows) show reduced CBF and ^{18}F-FDG uptake, with overlapping brain areas between the two abnormal presentations (**c**)

gyrus, precuneus, PCC, middle temporal gyrus, and right dorsolateral prefrontal cortex, whereas ASL revealed no hypoperfused regions, which suggests that ^{18}F-FDG PET is more sensitive than ASL at detecting preclinical AD. In resting-state fMRI, reductions in functional connectivity can be interpreted as weakened coherence in neural activities. Given that cerebral perfusion is the physiological basis of neuronal BOLD signals, impairments in cerebral perfusion may cause abnormal functional connectivity between brain regions. In an integrated PET/MR study on 24 healthy subjects aiming to examine the relationship among cerebral perfusion, glucose metabolism, and neuronal activity, similarities were found in the spatial distributions of the three indicators, with glucose metabolism showing a higher correlation with fMRI metrics than with CBF, of which, ReHo showed the highest correlation. These findings imply that integrated PET/MR is able to provide reliable information for the potential mechanisms underlying cerebral activity (Fig. 8.16). In another integrated PET/MR study involving 42 patients with AD and 27 HC, resting-state fMRI data were analyzed to evaluate brain functional connectivity, CBF data acquired through ASL were used to evaluate cerebral hemodynamic parameters, and glucose metabolism measured through ^{18}F-FDG PET was employed to assess neuronal activity. Patients with AD exhibited consistent reductions in glucose metabolism, fMRI functional connectivity, and CBF in the precuneus. After controlling for glucose metabolism levels, the functional connectivity of the precuneus was positively associated with CBF in patients with AD, which implies that the decrease in its functional connectivity is

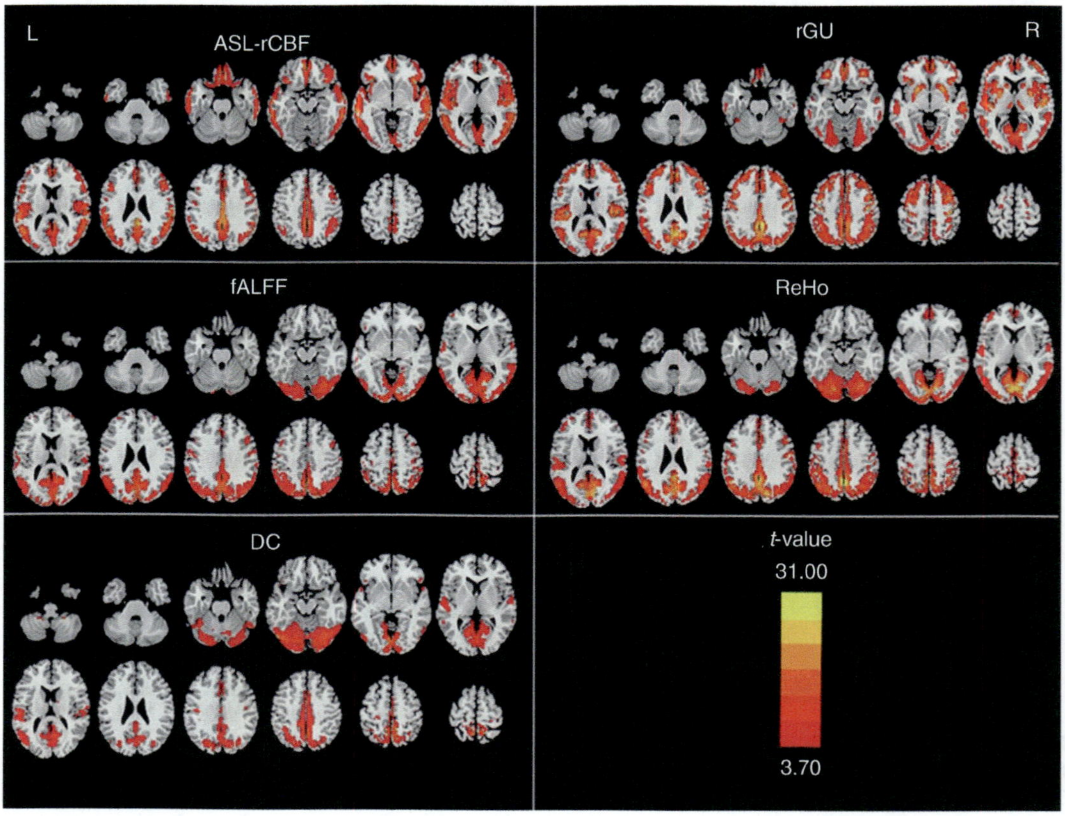

Fig. 8.16 Integrated PET/MR of healthy subjects showing similarities in the spatial distributions of relative glucose uptake (rGU), cerebral blood flow (CBF), fractional amplitude of low-frequency fluctuations (fALFF), regional homogeneity (ReHo), and degree of centrality (DC)

related to ASL-derived hypoperfusion, and is independent from glucose hypometabolism. These findings suggest that impaired hemodynamic processes can contribute to deficits of brain functional connectivity in patients with AD.

In future, integrated PET/MR is expected to simultaneously acquire information on brain function, cerebral perfusion, and glucose metabolism through a single scan. Therefore, this technique will offer unique advantages in elucidating the pathophysiological basis and pathogenic mechanisms of abnormal brain metabolism, CBF and brain function in AD, thereby serving as a more convenient, effective, and accurate imaging method for the diagnosis and differential diagnosis of AD.

Suggested Readings

Agosta F, Pievani M, Geroldi C, et al. Resting state fMRI in Alzheimer's disease: beyond the default mode network. Neurobiol Aging. 2012;33:1564–78.

Aiello M, Salvatore E, Cachia A, et al. Relationship between simultaneously acquired resting-state regional cerebral glucose metabolism and functional MRI: a PET/MR hybrid scanner study. Neuroimage. 2015;113:111–21.

Alsop DC, Detre JA, Grossman M. Assessment of cerebral blood flow in Alzheimer's disease by spin-labeled magnetic resonance imaging. Ann Neurol. 2000;47:93–100.

Binnewijzend MA, Benedictus MR, Kuijer JP, et al. Cerebral perfusion in the predementia stages of Alzheimer's disease. Eur Radiol. 2016;26:506–14.

Binnewijzend MA, Kuijer JP, Benedictus MR, et al. Cerebral blood flow measured with 3D pseudocontinuous arterial spin-labeling MR imaging in Alzheimer disease and mild cognitive impairment: a marker for disease severity. Radiology. 2013;267:221–30.

Cho H, Choi JY, Hwang MS, et al. In vivo cortical spreading pattern of tau and amyloid in the Alzheimer disease spectrum. Ann Neurol. 2016;80(2):247–58.

Clark CM, Pontecorvo MJ, Beach TG, et al. Cerebral PET with florbetapir compared with neuropathology at autopsy for detection of neuritic amyloid-beta plaques: a prospective cohort study. Lancet Neurol. 2012;11(8):669–78.

Dai W, Lopez OL, Carmichael OT, et al. Mild cognitive impairment and Alzheimer disease: patterns of altered cerebral blood flow at MR imaging. Radiology. 2009;250:856–66.

Franzmeier N, Rubinski A, Neitzel J, et al. Functional connectivity associated with tau levels in ageing, Alzheimer's, and small vessel disease. Brain. 2019;142:1093–107.

Gardini S, Venneri A, Sambataro F, et al. Increased functional connectivity in the default mode network in mild cognitive impairment: a maladaptive compensatory mechanism associated with poor semantic memory performance. J Alzheimers Dis. 2015;45:457–70.

Gottler J, Preibisch C, Riederer I, et al. Reduced blood oxygenation level dependent connectivity is related to hypoperfusion in Alzheimer's disease. J Cereb Blood Flow Metab. 2019;39:1314–25.

Han SD, Houston WS, Jak AJ, et al. Verbal paired-associate learning by APOE genotype in non-demented older adults: fMRI evidence of a right hemispheric compensatory response. Neurobiol Aging. 2007;28:238–47.

Hoenig MC, Bischof GN, Seemiller J, et al. Networks of tau distribution in Alzheimer's disease. Brain. 2018;141:568–81.

Im HK, Nebes R, Snitz B, et al. Regional amyloid burden and intrinsic connectivity networks in cognitively normal elderly subjects. Brain. 2014;137:3327–38.

Jack CR, Bennett DA, Blennow K, et al. NIA-AA research framework: toward a biological definition of Alzheimer's disease. Alzheimers Dement. 2018;14(4):535–62.

Kantarci K, Lowe V, Przybelski SA, et al. Magnetic resonance spectroscopy, beta-amyloid load, and cognition in a population-based sample of cognitively normal older adults. Neurology. 2011;77:951–8.

Kuhl DE, Koeppe RA, Minoshima S, et al. In vivo mapping of cerebral acetylcholinesterase activity in aging and Alzheimer's disease. Neurology. 1999;52(4):691–9.

Lacalle-Aurioles M, Mateos-Perez JM, Guzman-De-Villoria JA, et al. Cerebral blood flow is an earlier indicator of perfusion abnormalities than cerebral blood volume in Alzheimer's disease. J Cereb Blood Flow Metab. 2014;34:654–9.

Liu M, Paranjpe MD, Zhou X, Duy PQ, Goyal MS, Benzinger TLS, Lu J, Wang R, Zhou Y. Sex modulates the ApoE epsilon4 effect on brain tau deposition measured by (18)F-AV-1451 PET in individuals with mild cognitive impairment. Theranostics. 2019;9(17):4959–70.

Marchitelli R, Aiello M, Cachia A, et al. Simultaneous resting-state FDG-PET/fMRI in Alzheimer disease: relationship between glucose metabolism and intrinsic activity. Neuroimage. 2018;176:246.

Mitolo M, Stanzani-Maserati M, Capellari S, et al. Predicting conversion from mild cognitive impairment to Alzheimer's disease using brain (1)H-MRS and volumetric changes: a two-year retrospective follow-up study. Neuroimage Clin. 2019;23:101843.

Nowrangi MA, Lyketsos CG, Leoutsakos JM, et al. Longitudinal, region-specific course of diffusion tensor imaging measures in mild cognitive impairment and Alzheimer's disease. Alzheimers Dement. 2013;9:519–28.

Paranjpe MD, Chen X, Liu M, et al. The effect of ApoE epsilon4 on longitudinal brain region-specific glucose metabolism in patients with mild cognitive impairment: a FDG-PET study. Neuroimage Clin. 2019;22:101795.

Riederer I, Bohn KP, Preibisch C, et al. Alzheimer disease and mild cognitive impairment: integrated pulsed arterial spin-labeling MRI and (18)F-FDG PET. Radiology. 2018;288:198–206.

Riedl V, Bienkowska K, Strobel C, et al. Local activity determines functional connectivity in the resting human brain: a simultaneous FDG-PET/fMRI study. J Neurosci. 2014;34:6260–6.

Rzezga A, Becker JA, Van Dijk KR, et al. Neuronal dysfunction and disconnection of cortical hubs in non-demented subjects with elevated amyloid burden. Brain. 2011;134:1635–46.

Scherr M, Utz L, Tahmasian M, et al. Effective connectivity in the default mode network is distinctively disrupted in Alzheimer's disease-a simultaneous resting-state FDG-PET/fMRI study. Hum Brain Mapp. 2021;42:4134–43.

Sorg C, Riedl V, Muhlau M, et al. Selective changes of resting-state networks in individuals at risk for Alzheimer's disease. Proc Natl Acad Sci U S A. 2007;104:18760–5.

Su L, Blamire AM, Watson R, et al. Whole-brain patterns of (1)H-magnetic resonance spectroscopy imaging in Alzheimer's disease and dementia with Lewy bodies. Transl Psychiatry. 2016;6:e877.

Tahmasian M, Pasquini L, Scherr M, et al. The lower hippocampus global connectivity, the higher its local metabolism in Alzheimer disease. Neurology. 2015;84:1956–63.

Thomas B, Sheelakumari R, Kannath S, et al. Regional cerebral blood flow in the posterior cingulate and precuneus and the entorhinal cortical atrophy score differentiate mild cognitive impairment and dementia due to Alzheimer Disease. AJNR Am J Neuroradiol. 2019;40:1658–64.

Villemagne VL, Fodero-Tavoletti MT, Masters CL, et al. Tau imaging: early progress and future directions. Lancet Neurol. 2015;14(1):114–24.

Voevodskaya O, Poulakis K, Sundgren P, et al. Brain myoinositol as a potential marker of amyloid-related pathology: a longitudinal study. Neurology. 2019;92:e395–405.

Wang H, Tan L, Wang HF, et al. Magnetic resonance spectroscopy in Alzheimer's disease: systematic review and meta-analysis. J Alzheimers Dis. 2015;46:1049–70.

Yan S, Qi Z, An Y, et al. Detecting perfusion deficit in Alzheimer's disease and mild cognitive impairment patiets by resting-state fMRI. J Magn Reson Imaging. 2019;49(4):1099–104.

Yan S, Zheng C, Cui B, et al. Multiparametric imaging hippocampal neurodegeneration and functional connectivity with simultaneous PET-MRI in Alzheimer's disease. Eur J Nucl Med Mol Imaging. 2020;47(10):2440–52.

Yan S, Zheng C, Manish DP, Li J, et al. Association of sex and APOE ε4 with brain tau deposition and atrophy in older adults with Alzheimer's disease. Theranostics. 2020;10(23):10563–72.

Zhang HY, Wang SJ, Liu B, et al. Resting brain connectivity: changes during the progress of Alzheimer disease. Radiology. 2010;256:598–606.

Zhou J, Greicius MD, Gennatas ED, et al. Divergent network connectivity changes in behavioural variant frontotemporal dementia and Alzheimer's disease. Brain. 2010;133:1352–67.

Research Applications of Positron Emission Tomography/Magnetic Resonance (PET/MR) Imaging in Parkinson's Disease (PD)

9

Tianbin Song, Yanhui Yang, Tao Wu, and Chuantao Zuo

PD is a common neurodegenerative disease affecting the elderly, with a prevalence of 15–328/100,000 people, approximately 1.7% of those over 65 years of age, and an incidence of 10–21/100,000 people each year. The etiology and pathogenesis of PD remain poorly understood, and it is currently believed to be caused by a combination of genetic and environmental factors. Typical pathological changes that occur in PD include the degeneration of dopaminergic neurons in the substantia nigra and the appearance of Lewy bodies within neurons. Lewy bodies are eosinophilic inclusions formed by the abnormal aggregation of alpha (α)-synuclein. The most common clinical presentation of PD is progressive motor dysfunction, with major motor symptoms including bradykinesia, resting tremor, muscle rigidity, and postural instability, accompanied by a wide range of non-motor symptoms, such as olfactory dysfunction, depression, constipation, sleep disorders, and cognitive impairment. Partial improvements in clinical symptoms can be achieved through pharmacological (primarily levodopa) and surgical (primarily deep brain stimulation, DBS) treatments, but to date, there has been no cure for PD. At present, the diagnosis of PD is primarily dependent on clinical examinations, and its diagnostic criteria are based on the presence of two or more core motor symptoms, bradykinesia plus resting tremor, and/or muscle rigidity. Owing to the lack of objective diagnostic methods, the rate of early diagnosis for PD is relatively low; therefore, the main challenge of imaging in the research of PD is the development of imaging markers for the early and differential diagnosis of PD. Additionally, the neural mechanisms underlying the clinical symptoms of PD remain unclear, which may be further elucidated with the help of imaging studies, thereby facilitating the development of effective treatment methods and targets.

T. Song · Y. Yang ·
Department of Radiology and Nuclear Medicine, Xuanwu Hospital, Capital Medical University, Beijing, China

T. Wu
Department of Neurology, Xuanwu Hospital, Capital Medical University, Beijing, China

C. Zuo (✉)
Department of Nuclear Medicine/PET Center, Huashan Hospital, Fudan University, Shanghai, China
e-mail: zuochuantao@fudan.edu.cn

9.1 Research Applications of MRI in PD

The brain MRI techniques utilized in PD primarily include voxel-based morphometry (VBM), susceptibility-weighted imaging (SWI), quantitative susceptibility mapping (QSM), diffusion tensor imaging (DTI), arterial spin labeling (ASL), and blood-oxygen-level dependent (BOLD)

J. Lu, G. Zhao (eds.), *PET/MR: Functional and Molecular Imaging of Neurological Diseases and Neurosciences*, https://doi.org/10.1007/978-981-19-9902-4_9

imaging, which can serve as markers for the diagnosis, differential diagnosis, and monitoring of disease progression in PD.

9.1.1 Research Applications of Structural MRI in PD

9.1.1.1 Research Applications of VBM Analysis in PD

VBM is the objective, automated analysis of brain morphology with the Statistical Parametric Mapping (SPM) software, using voxels as the basic unit. It involves the quantitative computation and analysis of gray and white matter volume changes in each voxel on the MR image, thereby enabling the evaluation of whole-brain anatomical changes. The advantages of VBM include strong objectivity, good reproducibility, ease of use, and readiness for clinical promotion. Using VBM, patients with PD were found to have more significant volume reductions in the frontal cortex, temporal cortex, and anterior cingulate cortex (ACC), while reduced gray matter volume in the frontal cortex was associated with abnormal executive function (Fig. 9.1). Furthermore, studies have found that PD patients with olfactory dysfunction exhibited gray matter atrophy of the right piriform cortex and increased gray matter volume of the left orbitofrontal cortex (OFC). In mid- to advanced-stage PD, the level of atrophy in the right side of the amygdala was positively correlated to the olfactory dysfunction score. In early-stage PD, the atrophy of the piriform cortex and OFC was positively correlated with olfactory dysfunction scores, while the atrophy of the OFC increased in severity as olfactory function decreased. Taken together, these findings suggest that morphological changes in the olfactory areas may serve as a sensitive indicator for the early diagnosis of PD.

9.1.1.2 Research Applications of SWI and QSM in PD

SWI exploits the differences in the susceptibility of various tissues to produce image contrast. Due to the significant level of iron deposition in the substantia nigra (SN), this region can be clearly displayed using SWI sequences. In healthy patients, SWI reveals a hyperintense area shaped like a swallow tail in the dorsolateral region of the SN pars compacta, known as the "swallow tail sign." This hyperintense region is absent in patients with PD, which is known as the "absent swallow tail sign." It has been reported that the absent swallow tail sign can confirm a diagnosis of PD with relatively high sensitivity (>88%), but with large variations in specificity (37–95%).

QSM is a novel technique developed based on SWI. It utilizes a special reconstruction method to reconstruct magnetic susceptibility images and can quantify iron content based on susceptibility values, with its results generally expressed as parts per million (ppm). QSM has been shown to have a high direct correlation with iron content, and can therefore be used to quantify the susceptibility characteristics of tissues. Therefore, the iron content in the brain can be accurately assessed by calculating the inherent susceptibility of the brain tissues themselves. Currently accepted findings from QSM studies indicate that patients with PD have significantly higher iron deposition in the SN than healthy controls (Fig. 9.2) and that the extent of the increase in the deposition is positively associated with the Hoehn and Yahr (H-Y) stages of PD. These results suggest that increased iron deposition in the SN may be useful for the diagnosis and disease assessment of PD.

9.1.1.3 Research Applications of DTI in PD

DTI can be used for the non-invasive tracing of white matter tracts and to reflect their anatomical connectivity, enabling the visualization of the anatomical direction, trajectory, and commissures of white matter fibers, as well as abnormal manifestations such as sparseness, compression, disruption, and damage. By utilizing different parameters such as mean diffusivity (MD) and fractional anisotropy (FA), DTI can reflect the integrity of nerve fibers in a quantitative manner. MD describes the degree of diffusion exhibited by the water molecules within each voxel and is an indicator of the size of diffusion barriers, such as cell membranes or myelin sheaths. FA describes the anisotropy and integrity of white matter and other tissues and can be affected by factors such as changes in the structural microen-

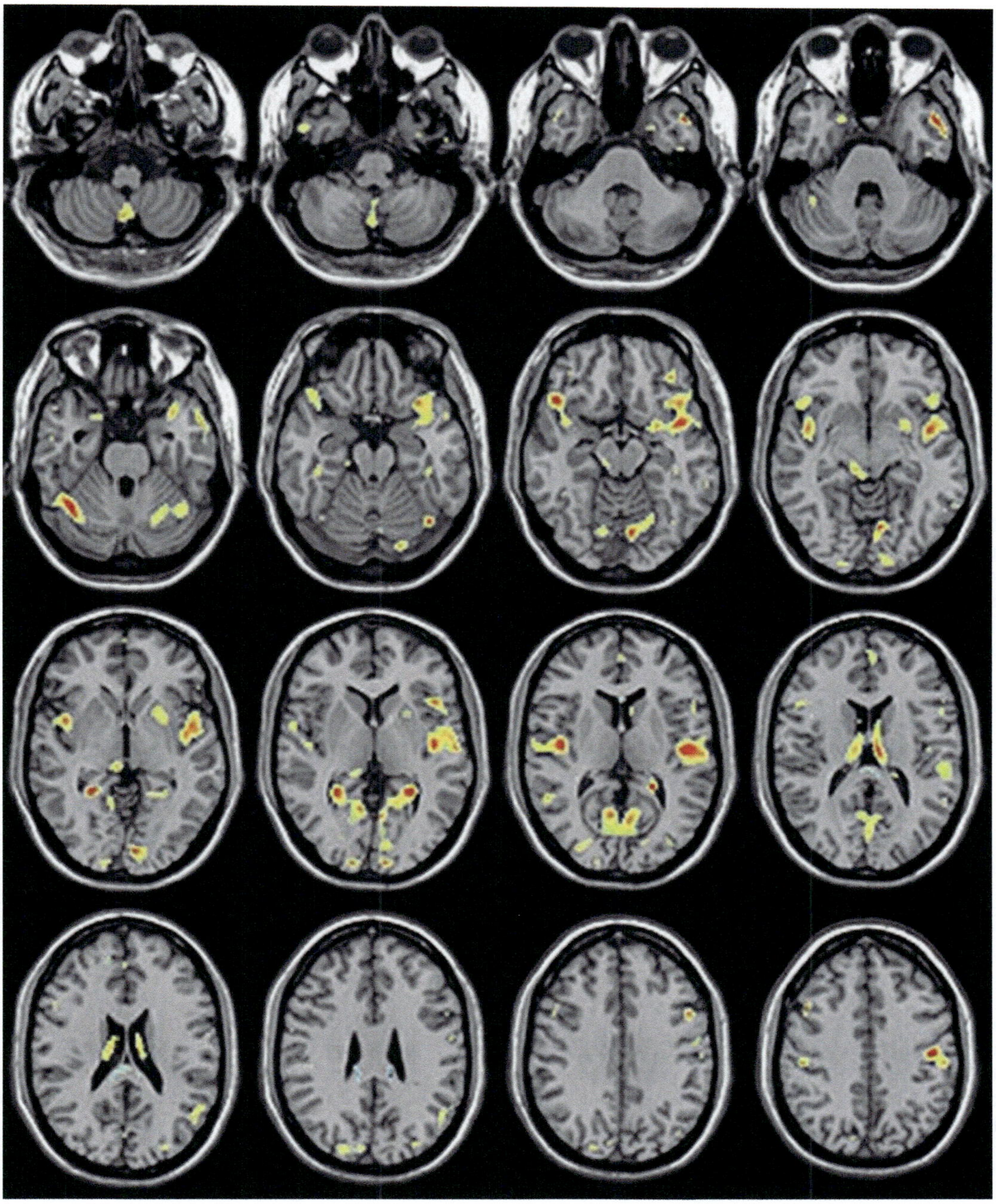

Fig. 9.1 Differences in brain volume between patients with PD and healthy controls. VBM analysis shows significant atrophy in the brain volume of PD patients, primarily involving the left putamen, bilateral precentral gyrus, bilateral temporal lobes, bilateral cerebellar hemispheres, and bilateral occipital lobes. Volume increases were detected in some regions, primarily in the splenium of the corpus callosum and cingulate gyrus. Yellow and red represent areas with volume decreases; blue and green represent areas with volume increases

vironment of tissues and decreases in the number of myelinated fibers. Studies have shown that compared to healthy controls, patients with PD had significantly lower FA values in the bilateral uncinate, posterior cingulate, and superior longitudinal fasciculi, as well as increased MD values in the bilateral posterior cingulate and right superior longitudinal fasciculi, thus revealing the major white matter fiber bundles which are impaired in patients with PD. Additionally,

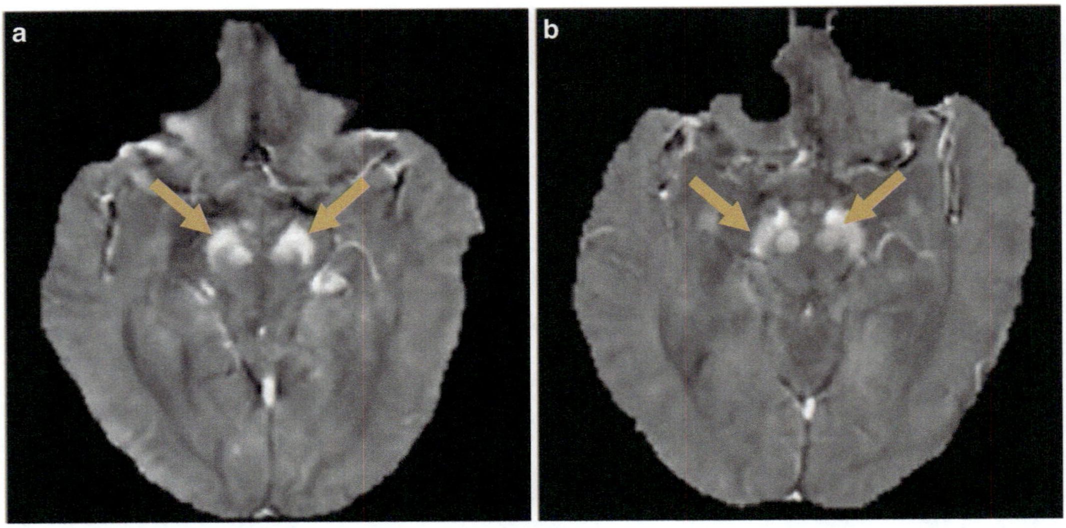

Fig. 9.2 Differences in nigral iron deposition between patients with PD and healthy controls. The QSM value of the substantia nigra (115 ppm) in PD patients (**a**) is significantly higher than that (86 ppm) of healthy controls (**b**), suggesting that the iron deposition in the substantia nigra of the PD group is significantly higher than that of the healthy control group. Arrows: iron deposition in the substantia nigra

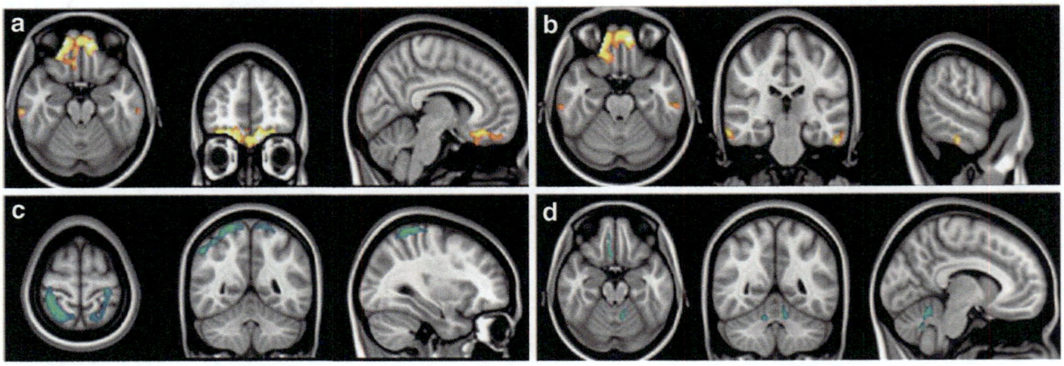

Fig. 9.3 Different areas of the brain for use as DTI parameters between patients with PD and healthy controls. Increased MD values in the bilateral orbitofrontal cortex (**a**), increased MD values in the gray matter of the bilateral inferior temporal gyrus (**b**), decreased MD values in the bilateral parietal lobes and left precentral (**c**), and decreased FA values in the bilateral cerebellum and right gyrus rectus of patients with PD (**d**). Yellow indicates an increase in value, while blue and green indicate a decrease

patients with PD showed abnormal changes in FA and MD values compared to healthy controls in the bilateral OFC, cerebellum, inferior temporal gyrus, parietal cortex, and left precentral gyrus (Fig. 9.3). In PD patients with olfactory dysfunction, the FA value of the left cerebellar white matter was positively correlated, whereas the MD value of the right cerebellar white matter was negatively correlated, with their odor detection threshold. These results imply that abnormal structural changes in the cerebellum may be related to olfactory dysfunction in patients with PD.

9.1.2 Research Applications of ASL in PD

ASL involves the use of radiofrequency pulses to label water molecules in blood, serving as an endogenous contrast agent, thereby achieving non-invasive perfusion MRI and providing a better reflection of cerebral perfusion function. Studies involving ASL have found that patients with PD showed reduced cerebral blood flow (CBF) in the right cerebellar peduncles, left middle and inferior frontal gyri, and left caudate nucleus. Another study found that these patients showed not only reductions in the absolute values of whole-brain perfusion but also significant reductions in the absolute values of perfusion in the subcortical basal ganglia and thalamus. However, relative to their respective average whole-brain perfusion levels, the patients showed elevated regional CBF (rCBF) in the bilateral basal ganglia and thalamus. These findings imply that the general reduction in whole-brain perfusion may be accompanied by the re-distribution of CBF. Additionally, studies have also reported that CBF in the left middle frontal gyrus and left caudate nucleus of patients with PD are positively correlated with their non-motor neuropsychological scores as measured by the Mini-Mental State Examination (MMSE), and Montreal Cognitive Assessment (MoCA), indicating that reductions in CBF may be associated with cognitive decline in PD.

9.1.3 Research Applications of BOLD-fMRI in PD

BOLD-fMRI is the most widely-used fMRI technique in PD research and consists of task-based fMRI and resting-state fMRI (RS-fMRI). The advantage of task-based fMRI is that the tasks can be designed to target specific symptoms in each patient. Since movement dysfunction is the core symptom of PD, the majority of task-based fMRI studies involve motor tasks, including external triggers, voluntary movement, motor imagery and execution, motor learning, response inhibition, complex movement, and simple movement. Other tasks, such as cognitive-task, dual-task (e.g., performing motor and cognitive tasks simultaneously), or even multi-task fMRI, have also been implemented. Compared to task-based fMRI, one of the greatest advantages of RS-fMRI is its simple experimental design, which can remain consistent across different studies, is favorable for large-sample studies, and has the potential for clinical applications. Nearly all of the various RS-fMRI methods used for analyzing regional brain activity and network connectivity have been utilized in PD research. A recent meta-analysis found that the resting-state regional brain activity of patients with PD is primarily characterized by the reduced amplitude of low-frequency fluctuations (ALFF) in the left putamen. Extensive neural network involvement can be observed in patients with PD, and clinical symptoms are closely associated with impairments in specific brain network functions. Of the networks, the SN-striatal-thalamic-cortical circuit plays a vital role in the generation and progression of motor symptoms in PD. Therefore, a large number of studies have utilized functional connectivity to explain the neural mechanisms of PD. fMRI has been widely used to study the neural mechanisms underlying the clinical symptoms, prodromal stage, and neuromodulation of PD, as well as to establish imaging biomarkers.

9.1.3.1 Research on Basal Ganglia Circuitry in PD

The abnormal regulation of the basal ganglia circuit is an important contributing factor to the clinical symptoms of PD. The basal ganglia-thalamic-cortical circuits are of great significance to understanding the functions of the basal ganglia and uncovering the pathophysiological basis of movement disorders, especially PD. The basal ganglia consist of the striatum (caudate nucleus and putamen), globus pallidus (GP), SN, and subthalamic nucleus (STN). A number of basal ganglia-thalamic-cortical circuits have been discovered, which include the motor, oculomotor, associative, limbic, and orbitofrontal circuits. The most widely-used model in PD research is the direct-indirect pathway of basal ganglia motor circuitry. That is, excitatory impulses from the motor and somatosensory cortices are transmitted via the putamen to the basal ganglia, while efferent impulses can project either directly from the striatum to the internal GP (GPi) and SN pars reticulata (SNr; direct pathway), or via the external GP (GPe) and STN to the GPi/SNr (indirect pathway). The GPi/SNr then transmits the impulses via the thalamus to the cerebral cortex to regulate movement. The direct pathway exerts a facilitatory effect on movement, whereas the indirect pathway exerts an inhibitory effect, and the balance between these two pathways is critical to maintaining normal movement. Both pathways are regulated by dopamine, which excites the direct pathway and inhibits the indirect pathway, thereby achieving a balance between them. The lack of dopamine in patients with PD strengthens the inhibitory effect of the striatum on the GPe, while lessening that on the STN, causing the over-excitation of the GPi/SNr, which then over-inhibits the thalamus-cortex and brainstem motor centers, in turn giving rise to the typical clinical presentation of PD. Subsequent studies discovered a type of "hyper-direct" (cortical-STN-GPi/SNr) pathway, in which excitatory cortical impulses are directly transmitted to the STN without passing through the striatum. Although current models of basal ganglia circuitry explain some of the clinical symptoms of PD, such as difficulty initiating movement, there are still a number of symptoms that are not yet fully explained, such as tremors and increased muscle tone, or the many other non-motor symptoms. Therefore, further improvements are needed for existing models of basal ganglia circuitry. fMRI has been widely utilized in research on the basal ganglia circuitry in PD. fMRI studies have found significantly attenuated functional connectivity between the posterior putamen and cortical or brainstem motor areas in patients with PD, which is expected given that the striatum is a key node in the direct and indirect pathways of basal ganglia motor circuitry. It was also found that the degree of attenuation was associated with the severity of motor symptoms. Furthermore, the STN is a key region in the indirect and "hyper-direct" pathways, and fMRI studies have revealed significantly enhanced functional connectivity between the STN and cortical motor areas in patients with PD. These findings demonstrate that important causes of motor dysfunction in patients with PD are the attenuated functional connectivity in the direct pathway of the basal ganglia, and the enhanced functional connectivity in the indirect and "hyper-direct" pathways, which subsequently decrease the facilitatory effects and increase the inhibitory effects on the cortical motor areas.

9.1.3.2 Research on the Neural Mechanisms of Clinical Symptoms in PD

The clinical symptoms of PD consist of both motor and non-motor symptoms. Our as yet incomplete understanding of the neural mechanisms underlying the clinical symptoms of PD has hindered the development of effective treatment methods and therapeutic targets. Therefore, using fMRI to study the common motor and non-motor symptoms of PD will help elucidate the relationship between pathological changes and clinical presentations.

(1) Motor symptoms: Bradykinesia refers to the slowness of movement and decreased movement amplitude or speed, and is the most important cause of movement dysfunction in patients with PD. Bradykinesia in PD is unlike the movement disorders caused by other neurological diseases (e.g., stroke), as it is primarily due to abnormalities in central motor control mechanisms caused by impairments of the dopaminergic system. Certain characteristic manifestations can be observed in PD-related bradykinesia, including a more intense involvement of movement initiation compared to movement execution, difficulties with spontaneous movement but relative ease of performing externally triggered movement, and deficits in motor automaticity. The neural mechanisms of bradykinesia are still poorly understood, and imaging studies involving bradykinesia have mostly utilized task-based fMRI. A meta-analysis of task-based fMRI in PD found that patients with PD had decreased activation of the posterior putamen and that the extent of the decrease was associated with the severity of motor symptoms. Another typical manifestation of spontaneous movement in patients with PD is the hypoactivation of the

supplementary motor area (SMA) and weaker functional connectivity between the striatum and cortical motor areas, such as the primary motor cortex, premotor cortex, and SMA (Fig. 9.4). The SMA is an important signal receptor area in the basal ganglia motor circuitry, and its predominant role in motor control includes motor planning and initiation. Treatment with levodopa (L-Dopa) can improve bradykinesia in patients with PD, while also normalizing SMA activity and network functional connectivity. Taken together, these findings indicate that impairments of the striatal-SMA pathway caused by damage to the SN dopaminergic system is a major cause of bradykinesia in PD. The enhanced functional connectivity of the cerebellar-cortical and other circuits may be a reflection of the reorganization and compensation of neural circuits under pathological conditions.

Motor automaticity deficit, one of the causes of bradykinesia, refers to the ability to correctly execute certain motor skills without attention directed toward the details of the movement, as the result of long-term training. The majority of PD-related bradykinesia symptoms are due to deficits in motor automaticity, and present as the slowing or decreased amplitude of daily motor behaviors, such as difficulty initiating movement, reduced arm swing, freezing of gait (FOG), and micrographia. According to fMRI studies of healthy subjects, decreased neural activity in the cortex (especially the prefrontal lobe), increased activity in the posterior putamen (motor striatum), and enhanced functional connectivity with cortical motor areas can be seen during the process of motor automaticity. These observations demonstrate that motor automaticity is accompanied by increased neural network efficiency and that the posterior putamen plays a critical role in the generation and storage of automatic programs. In patients with PD, the typical imaging findings of motor automaticity deficits include attenuated functional connectivity in the striatal-cortical motor pathway, hypoactivation of the posterior putamen, and hyperactivation of the prefrontal cortex (PFC). These findings imply that the neural mechanisms of motor automaticity

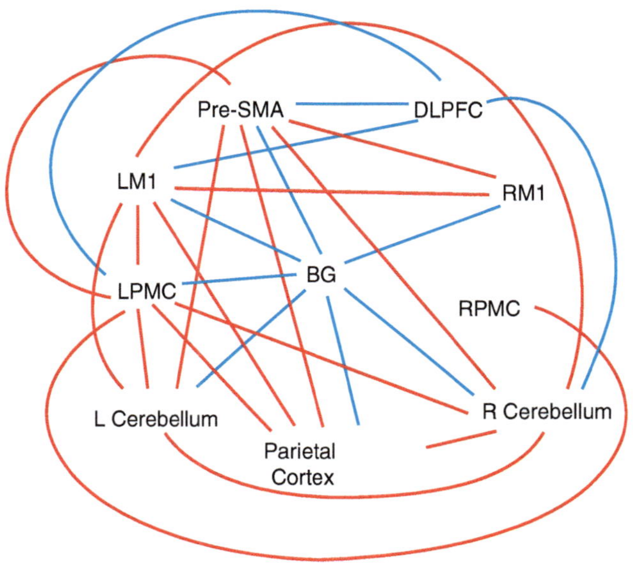

Fig. 9.4 Neural network connectivity changes related to bradykinesia in patients with PD. Cool/warm colors represent the enhancement/attenuation of functional connectivity in patients with PD compared with healthy controls. *BG* basal ganglia; *DLPFC* dorsolateral prefrontal cortex; *Pre-SMA* pre-supplementary motor area; *LM1* left primary motor cortex; *RM1* right primary motor cortex; *LPMC* left premotor cortex; *RPMC* right premotor cortex; *L Cerebellum* left cerebellum; *R Cerebellum* right cerebellum

deficits in PD primarily involve reduced motor network efficiency and the inability of the posterior putamen to generate automatic programs and store automatic motor skills acquired before disease onset, causing patients to lose their original automatic skills and have difficulty learning and storing new motor skills, leading to movement disorders. To compensate for these deficits, patients must devote a significant amount of attentional control to perform daily activities, which is one of the factors contributing to patients with PD being so prone to fatigue.

FOG is a temporary, episodic gait disturbance, often characterized by initiation hesitation, inability to step forward, and sudden difficulty with walking. It is a common pathological gait observed in patients with PD, and a manifestation of bradykinesia that is frequently seen in clinical settings. FOG mostly occurs as sudden episodes, and is therefore a major cause of falls and disability in patients, restricting their freedom of movement and seriously affecting their activities of daily living and quality of life. However, the efficacies of pharmacological and surgical treatments are thus far unsatisfactory. The pathophysiological mechanisms of FOG are still poorly understood, and it is believed that cognitive impairment, especially executive dysfunction, may play a crucial role in the development of FOG. Imaging studies on patients with PD-FOG revealed atrophy in the parietal cortex, temporal cortex, occipital cortex, dorsolateral PFC, thalamus, caudate nucleus, brainstem, and other regions, as well as impairments in the regional activity or functional connectivity of the motor, executive-attention, visual, and other networks. In particular, impairments in local structure, brain function, and network connectivity were observed in the basal ganglia, pontine nuclei, PFC, and SMA, while the degree of impairment was associated with the severity of FOG symptoms. These imaging studies have provided a theoretical basis for the selection of therapeutic targets, and the abovementioned brain areas are commonly used as targets in neuromodulation therapy for FOG, including deep brain stimulation (DBS) and transcranial magnetic stimulation (TMS).

Tremor is another major motor symptom of PD, which is characterized by a distinctive resting tremor, i.e., a tremor that becomes more prominent when the patient is at rest and lessens during voluntary movement. PD tremor usually first appears unilaterally on the distal end of the upper extremity, but as the disease progresses, it may begin to affect the head, lower extremities, and so on. Since tremors can interfere with fMRI signals, the majority of fMRI studies are conducted on patients with no or mild tremors, which has led to the scarcity of fMRI studies related to PD tremors. Simultaneous electromyography (EMG) and electroencephalography (EEG) recordings during fMRI scans can help with filtering tremor-induced interference in fMRI signals and analyzing the relationship between tremor generation and amplitude and fMRI data. Tremor generation is related to the basal ganglia motor circuitry, and tremor amplitude to the connectivity of the cerebellar-thalamic circuit. The results of this study suggest that the pathology of the basal ganglia circuitry is the basis for PD tremor generation, but also that functional impairments in the cerebellar-thalamic circuit must be present to produce clinical symptoms of tremor. A subsequent study further verified the crucial role of the cerebellum in the pathogenesis of PD tremors. However, the application of continuous θ-burst TMS at the cerebellum did not improve PD tremors. Therefore, further investigations are needed to understand the role of the cerebellar-thalamic circuit in the pathophysiological mechanisms of PD tremors.

(2) Non-motor symptoms: In addition to motor symptoms, patients with PD also present with a wide range of non-motor symptoms, such as cognitive impairment, psychiatric symptoms, hyposmia, sleep disorders, etc. Some of these non-motor symptoms, such as hyposmia and sleep disorders, occur earlier than typical motor symptoms, i.e., in the prodromal stage. Therefore, the neural mechanisms of non-motor symptoms in PD is a research topic garnering keen interest in China and abroad because of the great

significance for the development of effective treatments and early diagnosis.

Cognitive impairment is a common clinical symptom in PD, and mild cognitive impairment (MCI) can appear during the prodromal stage in some patients. Approximately 24% of patients with PD exhibit cognitive impairment at disease onset. Furthermore, half of all patients experience continuous cognitive decline within 3 years of onset, and the cumulative prevalence of PD dementia (PDD) can be as high as 80% at 20 years after disease onset. The symptoms of cognitive impairment in PD are heterogenous, primarily involving attention and executive function, memory, psychomotor speed, and visuospatial abilities. Based on the differences in clinical presentations, treatment response, and prognosis, these cognitive impairments can be divided into two overlapping cognitive syndromes: frontostriatal dysfunction (predominantly related to dopaminergic imbalance) and posterior cortical syndrome (unrelated to dopamine deficiency). Posterior cortical syndrome may be related to gray matter α-synuclein pathologies and(or) AD-type pathologies, and patients with this syndrome are more likely to develop dementia.

fMRI studies have primarily focused on the default mode network (DMN), which encompasses the precuneus/PCC, medial PFC, inferior parietal lobule, medial, and lateral temporal cortices, and hippocampus. Complex network analysis revealed that the network characteristics of PD-MCI involved enhanced local connectivity and weakened distant connectivity. As cognitive function gradually declined, the decrease in network connectivity and abnormalities in network patterns became more prominent, with significant alterations in the DMN of PD patients with cognitive impairment. Furthermore, attenuated functional connectivity was also observed between the PCC and the bilateral PFC, left parieto-occipital cortex, and right temporal gyrus. Based on independent component analysis (ICA), PD-MCI patients were found to have weaker connectivity in the dorsal attention network with the right anterior insula and adjacent frontal areas, whereas the posterior cortical areas showed enhanced connectivity with the DMN. Brain network alterations were more prominent in PDD than in PD-MCI, showing increasing exacerbation of abnormal connectivity in the ventral PFC, parietal cortex, temporal cortex, and basal ganglia network with the progression of cognitive impairment. These changes were also accompanied by decreased functional connectivity of the medial PFC and PCC and increased functional connectivity of the left and right hippocampus.

Psychiatric symptoms are also common nonmotor symptoms of PD, some of which are induced by dopamine therapy, such as impulse control disorder (ICD), whereas others are caused by the pathophysiological changes of the disease itself. Common examples of the latter include apathy, anxiety, and depression, which can appear in various stages of PD, even before the onset of motor symptoms. Depression in PD is related to the limbic system, and the degree of atrophy in the temporal cortex, especially the amygdala and hippocampus, is correlated with the severity of depression. fMRI studies have also revealed that amygdala hyperactivation is associated with the severity of depression. Furthermore, attenuation has been observed in the functional connectivity of the amygdala with the frontoparietal and limbic systems. The amygdala plays a vital role in the integration of external stimuli and the generation of emotional responses, while abnormal amygdala hyperactivation may reflect the excessive and uncontrolled emotional processes in patients with PD depression. Imaging studies have also revealed that PD depression and anxiety are accompanied by structural and functional changes in the OFC, dorsolateral and ventromedial PFC, ACC, and thalamus, as well as abnormal functional connectivity in the cortical-limbic system.

PD patients with apathy exhibit atrophy of the precuneus, inferior parietal lobule, OFC and dorsal ACC, as well as increased resting-state functional activity in the OFC and ACC. Impaired OFC function may cause abnormal top-down control, which can lead to excessive avoidance behaviors. The dorsal ACC is involved in emotional self-control, problem-solving, error detection, and adaptive response, while its abnormal functioning may be a key factor in the cognitive and affective components of apathy. Additionally, patients with PD apathy have reduced activity in the SMA, which primarily controls motor planning and initiation, thus its hypoactivation may contribute to the lack of initiative in patients with apathy.

ICD refers to a group of abnormal behaviors that are driven by a strong urge, and performed in the absence of self-control or consideration for consequences, and may be detrimental to oneself or others. Examples of these include pathological gambling, compulsive shopping, hypersexuality, compulsive eating, kleptomania, etc. The incidence of ICD among patients with PD is 5.9–13.7%. ICD primarily involves the limbic system and ventral striatum, which are key areas in decision-making and reward behaviors. Molecular imaging studies have found increased dopamine uptake in the ventral striatum. At present, there are only a handful of fMRI studies on PD-ICD, which have revealed increased functional connectivity between the DMN and salience network, as well as decreased functional connectivity among the striatum, limbic system, and cortical motor areas in PD-ICD.

Hyposmia is not only one of the most common non-motor symptoms in PD (prevalence 50–90%), but also one of the earliest symptoms. The olfactory bulb is involved in early-stage α-synuclein pathology, which implies that hyposmia can serve as a marker for the early diagnosis of PD. PD hyposmia is accompanied by reductions in olfactory bulb volume and depth of olfactory fossa, as well as atrophy of the piriform cortex and PFC. Furthermore, PD patients with hyposmia showed significantly reduced striatal dopamine transporter (DAT) uptake than those without hyposmia. Additionally, fMRI studies found that PD patients with hyposmia had significantly lower regional homogeneity (ReHo) in olfaction-related brain areas (amygdala, olfactory gyrus, parahippocampal gyrus, and insula), as well as weaker functional connectivity within the limbic/paralimbic regions and the amygdala.

(3) Research on the neural mechanisms of prodromal PD: The pathogenesis of PD is a process that unfolds from the prodromal stage to the clinical stage. The clinical stage begins when typical symptoms of motor dysfunction occur once the pathological changes involve the basal ganglia. Before this, however, there is prodromal stage that lasts for several years, perhaps even for more than a decade. The abnormal aggregation of α-synuclein first appears in the peripheral nerves, such as the sympathetic nerves, parasympathetic nerves, and gastrointestinal tract, then gradually spreads to the brainstem, midbrain, basal ganglia, and cortex. According to Braak staging, the aggregation of α-synuclein in the brainstem will lead to the appearance of non-motor symptoms, including rapid eye movement sleep behavior disorder (RBD), hyposmia, and constipation, which are the initial symptoms of PD. As there are no effective means by which to cure this disease in the clinical stage, it is only possible to delay or even prevent the onset of PD through early diagnosis and timely intervention during the prodromal stage. However, the neural mechanisms of the prodromal stage remain poorly understood, and there is a lack of methods for the early diagnosis and identification of warning signs in the prodromal stage. Therefore, prodromal biomarkers have come under the spotlight of research in China and abroad, primarily focusing on high-risk populations with RDB, olfactory dysfunction, and other symptoms, or those carrying pathogenic mutations for PD.

Patients with RBD have a high conversion rate to PD, with approximately two-third of patients with PD exhibiting RBD before motor symptoms, about 30% of RBD patients developing PD within 3 years, and 50–75% of RBD patients developing PD within 10 years. Therefore, RBD is an ideal research target when studying the pathophysiological changes of prodromal PD, and developing early diagnostic markers. Based on molecular imaging studies, RBD patients were found to have abnormalities in multiple systems, including the dopaminergic, cholinergic, serotonergic, and sympathetic nervous systems. Neuromelanin MRI and diffusion MRI revealed that RBD patients showed atrophy and hypointensities in the SN and locus coeruleus, as well as decreased FA in the SN. Furthermore, fMRI studies found that RBD patients shared similar patterns of attenuated connectivity in the basal ganglia circuitry with early-stage patients with PD, and these abnormalities could discriminate RBD patients from healthy controls (sensitivity 96%, specificity 74%). These findings demonstrate that RBD and patients with PD exhibit similar neuropathophysiological changes, which can serve as a theoretical basis for explaining the high conversion rate of RBD to PD. Additionally, fMRI performed on asymptomatic carriers of PD pathogenic mutations also revealed abnormal connectivity in the basal ganglia circuitry, which includes weaker connectivity of the posterior putamen-cortical motor areas, accompanied by enhanced connectivity of the anterior putamen- and cerebellar-cortical circuits. Taken together, these studies confirm the presence of abnormal functional connectivity in the basal ganglia circuitry prior to clinical PD, which could serve as an imaging marker for the early diagnosis and warning of PD. However, existing imaging studies are limited by their small sample sizes and short follow-up duration, and large-sample, long-term studies are still needed to establish imaging markers for the early warning and diagnosis of PD.

(4) Research on PD imaging markers: A number of studies have attempted to use fMRI as a tool to assist the diagnosis of PD, reporting sensitivities and specificities of up to 90–95% when discriminating between patients with PD and healthy individuals (Fig. 9.5).

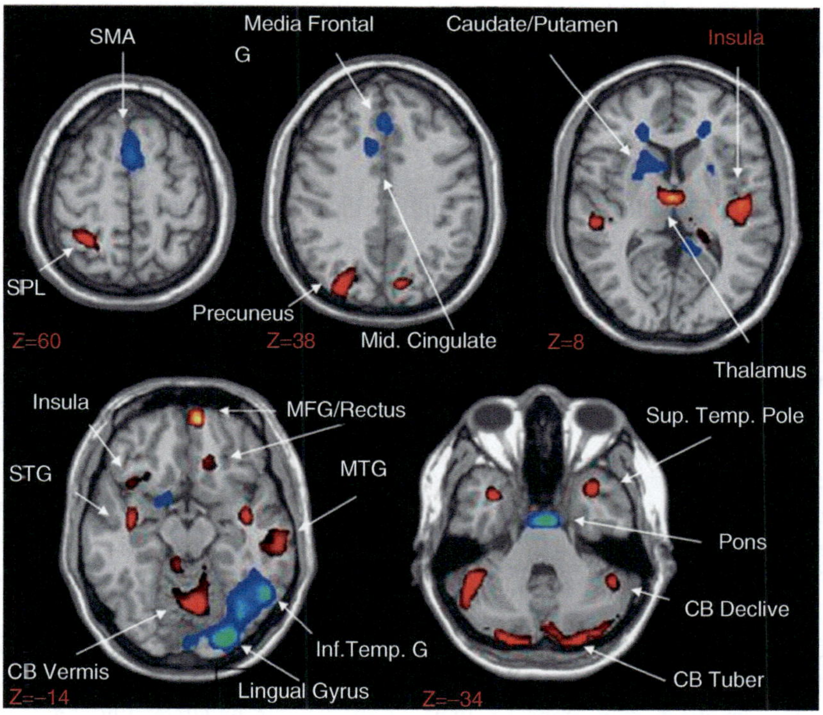

Fig. 9.5 PD-related spatial covariance pattern. The Parkinson's disease-related spatial covariance pattern (PDRP), established based on fMRI and pattern recognition methods, has an accuracy of up to 95% when discerning PD patients from healthy controls. Cool/warm colors represent regions with decreased/increased brain activity in patients with PD compared to healthy controls. *SPL* superior parietal lobule; *Media Frontal G* medial frontal gyrus; *Mid. Cingulate* middle cingulate cortex; *Caudate/Putamen* caudate nucleus/putamen; *STG* superior temporal gyrus; *MFG/Rectus* middle frontal gyrus/gyrus rectus; *MTG* middle temporal gyrus; *CB Vermis* cerebellar vermis; *Inf. Temp. G* inferior temporal gyrus; *Lingual Gyrus* lingual gyrus; *Sup. Temp. Pole* superior temporal pole; *CB Declive* cerebellar declive; *CB Tuber* cerebellar tuber

However, it is still difficult to draw conclusions due to the limited number of studies and the small sample sizes of most studies. Moreover, these findings are limited to the group level, and cannot be used for the diagnosis and differential diagnosis at the individual level. Furthermore, the low signal-to-noise ratio of fMRI may limit the usefulness of this technique as an imaging marker for PD. Thus, in addition to further improving scanning and analysis methods, combining fMRI with other MRI techniques may also help to improve diagnostic accuracy.

There is a lack of markers for the objective monitoring of disease progression in PD, which is also a popular topic of imaging research. At present, only a small number of fMRI studies have been reported in this field. A 3-year follow-up study found that patients with PD showed continuous decreases in the network functional connectivity of the motor and occipital cortices as the disease progressed. Other studies have also demonstrated reductions in the local activity of the temporal and occipital lobes with disease progression, and alterations in network connectivity were most significant in the early clinical stage, primarily involving the gradual attenuation of functional connectivity in the precuneus/PCC, right parietal cortex, left inferior occipital gyrus and left lingual gyrus, as well as between the occipital and temporal cortices, as the disease progressed.

(5) Research on neuromodulatory mechanisms: Pharmacological or surgical neuromodulation therapy can improve the clinical symptoms of PD, but these treatments can produce certain adverse reactions, which have restricted their clinical application. Therefore, clarifying the neuromodulatory mechanisms involved may improve their therapeutic efficacy, and reduce adverse reactions. The majority of fMRI studies have focused on the neural mechanisms of L-Dopa treatment, and found that the administration of L-Dopa can achieve the relative normalization of abnormalities in local brain activity or network connectivity. After 5–10 years of L-Dopa treatment, about half of the patients will develop levodopa-induced dyskinesia (LID), which is a common complication that has limited the long-term clinical application of L-Dopa. The pathogenic mechanisms of LID remain poorly understood, while the significant dyskinesia in LID patients makes it difficult to perform imaging scans and hence there are very few imaging studies in this area. In an fMRI study where LID patients were given a single dose of L-Dopa and scanned until symptoms of dyskinesia appeared, the results suggested that compared to PD patients without LID after L-Dopa treatment, patients with LID showed significantly increased activity in the SMA, primary motor cortex and putamen, as well as enhanced functional connectivity among these regions. This shows that these motor areas are a key factor contributing to the oversensitivity to L-Dopa treatment, which can explain the pattern of dynamic network changes leading to the occurrence of LID.

DBS is the most commonly utilized surgical method for the treatment of PD, but its neuromodulatory mechanisms remain unclear. Although current stimulation electrodes have been shown to be safe for fMRI studies using 1.5 Tesla (T) MRI scanners, the majority of research institutions still have reservations about safety concerns. Thus, there is a dearth of fMRI studies on DBS treatment in PD, which all involve small sample sizes or individual case reports. A study on brain network changes before and after STN-DBS treatment found that STN-DBS improved the effective connectivity of the cortex-striatum and thalamus-cortex.

fMRI has been extensively applied in PD research. The findings obtained will help to improve our understanding on the changes in basal ganglia circuitry, neural mechanisms of motor/non-motor symptoms, neural mechanisms of the prodromal stage, and neuromodulatory mechanisms in PD, which will facilitate the development of novel therapeutic methods and targets, thus highlighting the unique advantages of fMRI in studying the neurophysiological mechanisms of PD. Additionally, fMRI may also serve as an imaging marker to assist the diagnosis or evaluate the progression of PD, but this awaits the validation of further investigations.

9.2 Research Applications of PET Imaging in PD

9.2.1 PD and Atypical Parkinsonian Syndromes

PD accounts for 75% of parkinsonian syndromes, while other forms of atypical parkinsonian syndromes include multiple system atrophy (MSA), progressive supranuclear palsy (PSP), and corticobasal degeneration (CBD), which share many clinical presentations with PD, thus causing difficulties in early differential diagnosis. Essential tremor (ET) is also easily confused with early-stage PD, but the two conditions involve completely different treatments and prognoses.

MSA is a rare and fatal neurodegenerative disease, at the onset of which there can be differences in the timing of involvement in the extrapyramidal, pyramidal, and autonomic nervous systems, resulting in variable clinical presentations. However, as the disease progresses, all patients will eventually develop pathological impairments and clinical manifestations in multiple anatomical structures of the central nervous system, therefore the name MSA. MSA encompasses a variety of clinical presentations, including parkinsonism, cerebellar symptoms, and autonomic nervous system dysfunction, from which MSA can be divided into the parkinsonism subtype (MSA-P), which predominantly involves parkinsonian symptoms and the cerebellar subtype (MSA-C), which primarily involves cerebellar symptoms. The diversity of clinical presentations, especially in the early stages, has meant that MSA lacks specificity in its clinical presentations and is prone to misdiagnosis. Furthermore, the pathogenesis of MSA is still poorly understood. It is generally considered to be a sporadic disease, but researchers have recently discovered a genetic predisposition to MSA. The basic pathological features of MSA include neuronal degeneration, neuronal loss, and glial cell proliferation of the intermediolateral cell column of the spinal cord, pons transverse fibers, basal pontine nuclei, medulla oblongata, middle cerebellar peduncle, cerebellar hemisphere, SN, GP, and putamen, as well as the degeneration of specific white matter fibers. A pathologically significant feature of MSA is the appearance of glial cytoplasmic inclusions (GCIs) composed of α-synuclein in the cytoplasm of oligodendrocytes.

PSP is a relatively common form of atypical parkinsonian syndrome. Its age of onset is generally 50–70 years, with an average disease duration of 5–9 years, and its characteristic clinical presentations include postural instability, axial dystonia, vertical supranuclear ophthalmoplegia, pseudobulbar palsy, and dementia. However, recent findings from case reports based on pathological diagnosis have revealed substantial variability in the clinical presentations of PSP, with classical PSP (Richardson's syndrome) accounting for two-third of cases, and the remaining cases chiefly presenting with parkinsonism, pure hypokinesia with FOG, corticobasal syndrome (CBS), non-fluent variant of primary progressive aphasia, frontotemporal dysfunction and cerebellar ataxia, which can easily be misdiagnosed. Pathological diagnosis remains the gold standard of PSP diagnosis, and there is a lack of objective biomarkers in clinical practice, nor are there objective biological indicators for the prenatal diagnosis of PSP. The etiology of PSP is still poorly understood, and it is currently believed to be a type of tauopathy. PSP may involve cortical and subcortical structures, and its clinical manifestations are related to impairments in the dopaminergic, GABAergic, cholinergic and noradrenergic pathways. The major brain areas affected by PSP pathology include the STN, GP, superior colliculus, pretectum, periaqueductal grey, SN, pontine nuclei, and frontal lobe (especially the cortical motor areas), which exhibit neuronal loss, gliosis, and abnormal protein deposition.

CBD was initially regarded as a specific clinical pathological entity, known as "corticodentatonigral degeneration with neuronal achromasia." This condition is defined on the basis of clinical and pathological features, with the former primarily hyperphosphorylated tau proteins in neurons and glial cells, as well as the presence of transactive response DNA binding protein 43 (TDP-43). CBD is primarily manifested as symptoms of motor and cognitive impairment derived from the asymmetric pathologies of the frontoparietal cortex and basal ganglia. The age of onset for CBD is 45–77.2 years (mean: 63.7 years) and its disease duration is 2.2–12.5 years (mean: 6.6 years). The majority of patients do not share a similar family history. PET is a functional imaging technique with broad application prospect for exploring the diagnosis, disease duration, treatment monitoring, and pathological molecular mechanisms of PD and parkinsonian syndromes (MSA, PSP, CBD, etc.) With respect to the molecular pathological mechanisms of these diseases, PET imaging has primarily focused on metabolic imaging, receptor and protein imaging, inflammation imaging, and hypoxia imaging. In recent years, the implementation of SPM in the brain network analysis of metabolic imaging has conferred significant advantages to the differential diagnosis of PD and parkinsonian syndromes. Through the use of various imaging agents, receptor and protein imaging can reflect the different molecular pathological characteristics involved when studying different diseases, such as dopaminergic abnormalities and α-synuclein deposition. Furthermore, with the continuous development of PET/MR, multi-modal imaging that combines function with structure will play a greater role in future research.

9.2.2 PET Imaging Methods and their Clinical Value

9.2.2.1 PET Imaging of the Nigrostriatal Dopaminergic Neurotransmission System

In current clinical diagnosis and research of PD, the most commonly utilized method of PET imaging is dopaminergic neurotransmission imaging. The principle behind this imaging technique is that L-Dopa is converted under the action of aromatic amino-acid decarboxylase (AADC) to dopamine, which is then transported stored in synaptic vesicles by the vesicular monoamine transporter 2 (VMAT2), and ultimately released from the vesicles into the synaptic cleft. Once the dopamine released into the synaptic cleft binds with and activates the dopamine receptors on the postsynaptic membrane, part of it is degraded, and part of it is reabsorbed via presynaptic DAT reuptake. The evaluation of AADC, VMAT2, and DAT function comes under presynaptic dopaminergic imaging, whereas the evaluation of dopamine receptor function comes under postsynaptic dopaminergic imaging, and commonly used imaging agents are shown in Fig. 9.6.

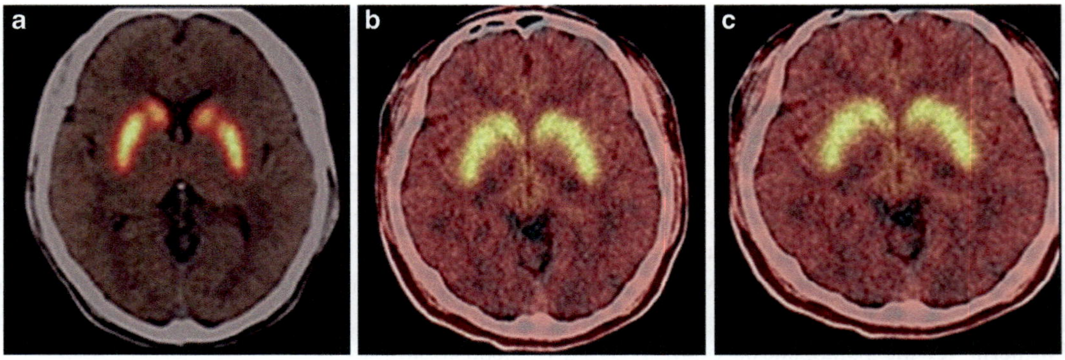

Fig. 9.6 Nigrostriatal dopaminergic neurotransmission in healthy subjects. From left to right: transverse DAT imaging with ^{11}C-CFT (**a**), VMAT2 vesicle imaging with ^{18}F-DTBZ (**b**), and dopaminergic neurotransmitter imaging with ^{18}F-DOPA (**c**)

^{18}F-DOPA PET imaging primarily reflects the density of striatal dopaminergic terminals and AADC activity. Patients with PD exhibit reduced striatal uptake, and their uptake levels give an indication of the number of residual SN dopaminergic neurons. However, in the early stages of the disease, the compensatory upregulation of AADC activity may cause the severity of neurodegeneration to be underestimated. ^{11}C-CFT, ^{18}F-FP-CIT, and other DAT imaging agents are only taken up by the dendrites and axon terminals of dopaminergic neurons, and can therefore also represent the integrity of nigrostriatal projections. DAT PET imaging findings are similar to those of ^{18}F-DOPA, showing a sensitivity of about 90% in the early diagnosis of PD. However, in contrast to ^{18}F-DOPA, the compensatory downregulation of DAT levels in the early stages may overestimate the severity of neurodegeneration. The results of ^{18}F-DTBZ VMAT2 imaging are somewhere between the two former techniques and are currently considered to be the most reliable reflection of dopaminergic neuron survival. For all presynaptic dopaminergic imaging in PD, the findings indicate that in the early stages, there is an asymmetric reduction in striatal uptake, with the posterior putamen contralateral to the affected limb showing the most significant reduction, but with the ipsilateral (i.e., contralateral to the unaffected limb) posterior putamen also showing a slight decrease, thus implying that this finding may be useful for early diagnosis; in mid- to advanced-stage PD, significant reductions in uptake can be observed in the bilateral putamen, as well as some reduction in the caudate nucleus. Patients with ET have normal DAT imaging findings, which can be used to differentiate ET from PD, whereas patients with MSA and PSP may present with abnormal findings in presynaptic dopaminergic imaging, and are therefore more difficult to be differentiated from PD. Raclopride (RAC) imaging of dopamine D_2 receptors indicates that in early-stage PD, there is increased upregulation of striatal dopamine receptors, which then returns to normal levels, whereas the distribution of dopamine receptors in MSA and PSP remains consistently low. Thus, this point of difference can be used to discriminate PD from atypical parkinsonian syndromes, but not between MSA and PSP.

PET imaging of the nigrostriatal dopaminergic neurotransmission system is a sensitive approach for detecting the loss of dopaminergic neurons in symptomatic and high-risk patients with parkinsonism. Normal striatal DAT distribution can be used to exclude dopamine deficiency syndrome and is associated with a good prognosis. Furthermore, the 2015 Movement Disorder Society guidelines for PD state that dopaminergic neuroimaging can help to discriminate between patients with PD and non-PD presentations, such as patients with ET. However, the guidelines also point out that dopaminergic neuroimaging cannot be used as a criterion for the differential diagnosis between PD and atypical parkinsonian syndromes.

9.2.2.2 PET Imaging of Brain Glucose Metabolism

The glucose utilization of the brain in the resting state can reflect the status local synaptic activity and biochemical homeostasis, while abnormalities in the latter can alter whole-brain functional connectivity in a disease-specific manner. Thus, characteristic manifestations can be identified in patients with PD. Given the recent advances in algorithms for image analysis, the value of glucose metabolism imaging in clinical applications has increased significantly.

Previous studies using SPM to analyze whole-brain metabolism found that patients with PD exhibited increased metabolism in the bilateral thalamus, lentiform nucleus, and cerebellum. Moreover, by calculating the relative glucose metabolic rates, the results further demonstrated that the metabolism of these regions increased, while that of the bilateral parietal cortex decreased as the disease continued to worsen. The metabolic changes in the brain areas above can be explained by alterations in the motor cortico-basal-thalamic-motor cortical loop in PD. After PD onset, the decrease in nigrostriatal dopamine levels will attenuate the direct inhibitory effects of the direct pathway on the GPi, whereas in the indirect pathway, STN over-excitation will enhance the excitatory effects on the GPi. The joint effect of these two pathways will cause the GPi to exert excessive inhibitory effects, which in turn will reduce the excitation by the motor thalamic nuclei on the corresponding cortical areas, thereby causing patients with PD to develop bradykinesia, muscle rigidity, and other motor symptoms. Additionally, the hypermetabolism of the lentiform nucleus may have been induced by the increased afferent impulses from the STN, which will also increase the metabolism of the thalamus as it receives increased inhibitory impulses from the lentiform nucleus. Another explanation for thalamic hypermetabolism is the excessive afferent excitatory impulses from the pontine nuclei, thalamic intralaminar nuclei, and motor cortex. The hypometabolism of the parietal cortex is due to the decrease in excitatory impulses received by the premotor cortex from the thalamus.

PDRP is a recently discovered imaging marker of PD based on ^{18}F-FDG PET images. It is a special brain metabolic network resulting from abnormalities in the basal-thalamic-cortical circuit and its related functional/anatomical pathways. This abnormal brain metabolic network is disease-specific, largely characterized by the relative hypermetabolism of the GP, thalamus, pons, and cerebellum, and the relative hypometabolism of the premotor cortex, SMA, and posterior parietal cortex. Studies have shown that PDRP can not only be utilized in the early diagnosis of PD, but is also very useful in discriminating idiopathic PC from parkinsonism-plus syndrome, and can even be applied to the objective evaluation of therapeutic efficacy after DBS. Despite the disparities in the methods utilized by the different studies to perform resting-state imaging, PDRP has been confirmed in multiple, independent patient cohorts both in China and abroad.

PET imaging of glucose metabolism can be applied to the early diagnosis of PD, and abnormal PDRP values can be detected approximately 2 years before the onset of motor symptoms. This implies that abnormal functional network activities may be a characteristic of premotor PD, reflecting the decompensation of brain metabolic functions prior to the appearance of motor symptoms, and can therefore serve as an effective means for the early diagnosis or even premotor diagnosis of PD. RBD refers to the loss of normal skeletal muscle relaxation during REM sleep, leading to violent movements, increased motor activity, and increased dreaming. Among which, 90% of cases can be detected through polysomnography. RBD is considered a prodromal symptom of PD, and patients may convert to PD, MSA, DLB, or other neurodegenerative diseases (Fig. 9.7). There are promising prospects for the application of abnormal changes in the brain glucose metabolism of RBD patients in the prediction of disease conversion.

PDRP is not only an effective method for the early diagnosis or even the premotor diagnosis of PD, but can also reflect disease severity. In a study observing the changes over the longitudinal follow-up of brain metabolism in 15 PD patients

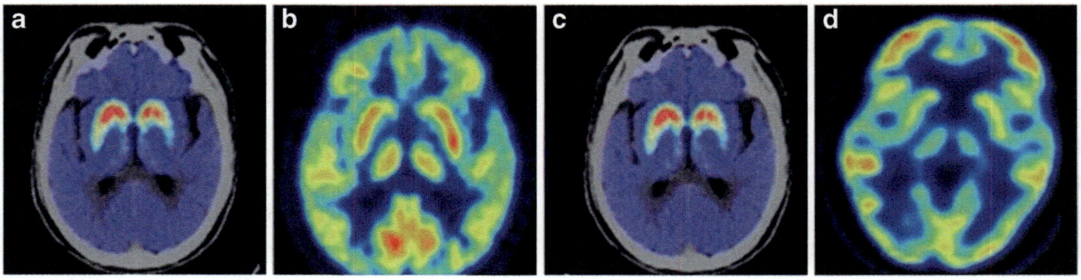

Fig. 9.7 DAT and FDG PET findings of patients with PD and MSA. A 64-year-old male patient with PD, whose chief complaint was involuntary tremors of the right limbs for more than 1 year. Transverse PET showed reduced DAT distribution in the bilateral putamen, with significant reductions in the left, and increased glucose metabolism of the bilateral putamen (**a**, **b**). A 56-year-old female patient with MSA whose chief complaint was movement instability for more than 2 years, that had deteriorated for more than 2 months. PET findings revealed reduced DAT distribution and decreased glucose metabolism in the bilateral putamen (**c**, **d**)

with hemi-motor symptoms, the results showed a steady increase of putamen metabolic rate in the cerebral hemispheres during the pre-symptomatic stage (contralateral to the asymptomatic limb), and abnormal PDRP values occurred about 2 years before the appearance of motor symptoms. This suggests that abnormal functional network activity is a feature of premotor PD, reflecting the compensation of brain glucose metabolism prior to motor symptoms. The study also found that as PD progressed, increased glucose metabolism was observed in the STN, GPi, dorsal pons, and motor cortex, whereas decreased glucose metabolism was detected in the PFC and parietal cortex. Moreover, PDRP values increased with increasing PD disease duration and were positively correlated with the decrease in striatal DAT and increase in motor scores. These findings suggest that PDRP can be utilized for the objective evaluation of PD severity and monitoring of therapeutic efficacy. Therefore, it is expected to be applied in the objective assessment of novel treatment methods for PD.

9.2.2.3 Comparison of Brain PET Image Analysis Methods

Based on the practical implementation of image analysis, it is possible to maximize the extraction of useful information from ^{18}F-FDG PET images for the diagnosis and differential diagnosis of PD, thereby further expanding the impact and decision-making power of PET in clinical settings. In traditional ROI methods, the ROI is delineated in order to calculate the radioactivity count within the selected region, and statistical analysis is performed on the values obtained after comparison with the radioactivity of the reference region, providing the final results. Despite the intuitiveness and convenience of ROI methods, they are strongly subjective, have poor reproducibility, and tend to overlook small regions of voxel differences between PET images.

The general three-compartment model is a modified kinetic model, based on the Sokoloff model, that takes into account the dephosphorylation process. The three-compartment model of ^{18}F-FDG consists of plasma, brain tissue, and tissue ^{18}F-FDG, whereas ^{18}F-FDG-6-PO_4 is not involved in further metabolic processes. At equilibrium, the glucose utilization rate is a constant. Assuming that there is no glycogen synthesis or breakdown, the rate of glucose phosphorylation will be equal to the rate of glycolysis, and the rate of any step in the glycolytic process is equal to the rate of the overall process. Thus, the rate of glucose metabolism can be calculated based on the concentration of ^{18}F-FDG-6-PO_4 in a retained and equilibrium state. The quantification of glucose metabolism is relatively cumbersome in clinical and scientific research, as it involves the continuous sampling of arterial blood to determine the amount of radiotracer and its metabolites in the blood. Furthermore, it also requires the dynamic imaging of the brain region in question, and finally obtaining the glucose metabolic rate of each brain region based on the quantitative formula of glucose metabolism. Therefore, quantitative methods of glucose metabolism are not commonly implemented in clinical and scientific studies.

Due to the drawbacks of ROI methods and the tediousness of quantitative analyses for glucose metabolism, SPM software swiftly replaced manual ROI methods and is now the internationally recognized approach in functional brain imaging research, with preliminary applications in SPECT and PET functional brain imaging studies in China.

SPM is a software that can combine the subject's PET images with statistical methods. Based on the statistical comparisons of voxel-wise differences in the PET images, parametric statistical models are assumed at each voxel, and a general linear model is used to describe the changes in the PET images at the voxel level, followed by the generation of a statistical parametric table. SPM analysis enables the comparative analysis of patients' brain ^{18}F-FDG with those of age- and gender-matched controls, in order to determine regions of glucose hypermetabolism or hypometabolism relative to healthy controls. These regions can then be compared with disease-specific functional brain templates, which is of great significance for confirming the diagnosis of specific diseases, including the diagnosis and differential diagnosis of PD and parkinsonian syndromes.

SPM analysis is a method of univariate analysis that can only achieve the direct comparison of imaging data between patients and healthy controls at the voxel level but cannot determine the interconnectivity among different brain regions. In contrast, principal component analysis (PCA) is a multivariate method of spatial covariance analysis that can evaluate the functional interactions among different brain regions, so as to determine the presence of abnormalities at the network level, while also establishing and validating disease-specific brain metabolic network patterns. Therefore, this approach can make up for the shortcomings of previous univariate analyses that directly compared the imaging data of patients and healthy controls, and is especially suitable for neurodegenerative diseases involving neural circuits. Furthermore, with the advancement of voxel-based algorithms, PCA can further achieve the computation of pattern expression values for each individual through the objective quantification of glucose metabolism at the voxel level.

Recent improvements in traditional PCA, with respect to its discriminant ability for ^{18}F-FDG PET micro-signals, have further enhanced the value of implementing brain metabolic patterns in predictive diagnosis at the prodromal stage and carry crucial significance. Unlike traditional PCA, deep learning is characterized by the following features: (1) it allows a larger number of features or components, and therefore discriminate, extract and classify complex disease- and non-specific factors in image analysis and network building; (2) it emphasizes the hierarchical depth of the analytical model, usually utilizing 5, 6, or even 10 layers of hidden nodes; and (3) it has prominent and excellent feature learning abilities. By relying on the advantages above, deep learning can achieve the deep mining of ^{18}F-FDG PET data, based on which brain metabolic network patterns related to parkinsonian syndromes can be established. Thus, theoretically speaking, deep learning will be equipped with a higher sensitivity for diagnosing early-stage diseases, higher disease-related specificity, and the ability to maximize the exclusion of interferences from non-disease-related factors.

9.2.2.4 Establishment of a Normative Database for Brain ^{18}F-FDG PET Imaging

Brain ^{18}F-FDG PET imaging is currently still utilized by physicians to perform imaging diagnosis through visual analysis based on their personal experiences. Although the emergence of the standardized uptake value (SUV) has provided a basis for diagnosis, there remains the need for a more unified set of diagnostic criteria. Therefore, it is necessary to accumulate a large number of normative ^{18}F-FDG PET images through multi-center collaboration, followed by normalization and SUV measurement for each brain area, in order to establish a normative database of glucose metabolism in different brain areas based on ^{18}F-FDG PET. This database will provide an objective reference and diagnostic criteria for the PET imaging diagnosis of PD and other neurodegenerative diseases, avoid the errors caused by visual observation, and satisfy the requirements for communication and remote consultation among different medical institutions, thereby laying a foundation for the establishment and exchange of neural functional network databases.

The research team at the PET Center of Huashan Hospital affiliated with Fudan University grouped the brain PET images of 255 healthy subjects by age and applied a data-driven normalization algorithm for image and data processing and analysis. Based on this, they established a normative database of brain glucose metabolism for this PET Center, which showed a decreasing trend in the glucose metabolism of all brain areas with increasing age. Using this algorithm, the research team found that age had the least impact when the right paracentral lobule and right cerebellum were used as the reference regions. Additionally, the normative database of glucose metabolism for different brain regions can facilitate the differentiation between healthy and non-healthy subjects, while the establishment of databases specific to different neurodegenerative diseases will enable the more intuitive and objective diagnosis of these diseases.

9.2.3 Differential Diagnosis

9.2.3.1 PET Imaging Techniques for MSA

^{18}F-DOPA PET imaging has demonstrated significantly reduced uptake in the striatum and red nucleus of MSA patients. Unlike PD, MSA does not exhibit compensatory increases (upregulation effects) in striatal ^{18}F-DOPA uptake in the early stages of the disease. VMAT2 PET imaging revealed that MSA patients had a reduced distribution of dopaminergic vesicles in the striatum. Based on DAT PET imaging, MSA patients showed abnormal presynaptic dopaminergic imaging findings in the striatum, which was difficult to differentiate from those of patients with PD. Dopamine D_2 receptor imaging showed decreased postsynaptic dopamine receptors in the striatum of MSA patients. Unlike patients with PD, MSA patients did not exhibit compensatory upregulation of striatal postsynaptic dopamine receptor distribution during the early stages of the disease.

9.2.3.2 PET Imaging Techniques for PSP

VMAT2 PET imaging of PSP patients revealed a decrease in the distribution of striatal dopaminergic vesicles. Given that DAT imaging is only observed in the dendrites and axonal terminals of dopaminergic neurons, it can reflect the integrity of nigrostriatal neural projections. Based on DAT imaging in PSP, patients were found to have abnormal presynaptic dopaminergic imaging findings, which were difficult to differentiate from those of patients with PD. The PET imaging of tau proteins (e.g., ^{18}F-AV1451) revealed that PSP patients had higher ^{18}F-AV1451 uptake than healthy controls in the GP, putamen, caudate nucleus, thalamic nuclei, midbrain, and cerebellar nuclei. Moreover, the different locations of abnormal depositions can help to discriminate between AD and PSP.

9.2.3.3 PET/CT Imaging Techniques for CBD

VMAT2 and dopamine D_2 receptor PET imaging shows normal or slightly decreased levels of striatal dopaminergic vesicles and dopamine receptors among CBD patients. However, these findings are primarily based on case reports and await further investigations. Since DAT imaging is only observed in the dendrites and axonal terminals of dopaminergic neurons, it can reflect the integrity of nigrostriatal neural projections. CBS patients exhibit decreased striatal DAT distribution, with a more prominent DAT imaging only observed in the dendrites and axonal terminals of dopaminergic neurons, it can reflect the integrity of nigrostriatal neural projections. DAT imaging is only observed in the dendrites and axonal terminals of dopaminergic neurons, it can reflect the integrity of nigrostriatal neural projections. Patients with CBS exhibit a decrease in striatal DAT distribution, with a more prominent asymmetry in striatal DAT reduction than patients with PD (Fig. 9.8). Tau protein imaging can assist in discriminating between CBD and AD. Furthermore, PET imaging of microglial cells revealed that CBD patients showed active microglial proliferation in the caudate nucleus, putamen, SN, pons, pre-/postcentral gyrus, and frontal cortex.

9.2.3.4 Key Elements of Differential Diagnosis Based on PET Imaging

The differential diagnosis of parkinsonian syndromes primarily involves the discrimination of PD from atypical parkinsonian syndromes, as well as from other diseases with motor dysfunction.

(1) Parkinsonian syndromes: ^{18}F-FDG PET imaging has been shown to have superior differential diagnostic performance than PET imaging of the nigrostriatal dopaminergic neurotransmission system. Studies have found that PD and atypical parkinsonian syndromes exhibited different characteristics of brain glucose metabolism. PD was primarily characterized by the hypometabolism of the

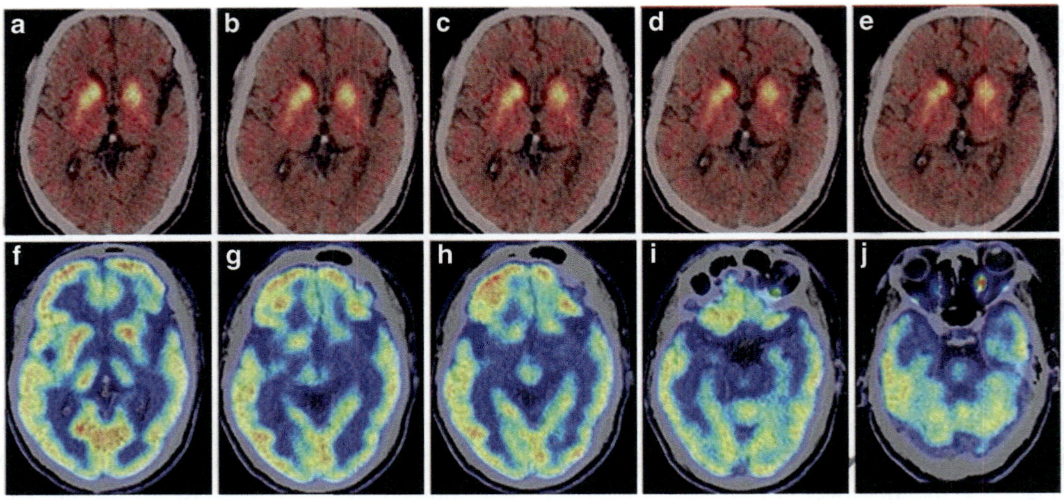

Fig. 9.8 DAT and FDG PET imaging in CBD. A 60-year-old male patient with CBD who transverse PET imaging revealed decreased DAT distribution in the bilateral caudate nucleus and putamen (**a**–**e**), as well as decreased glucose metabolism in the left basal ganglia, left thalamus, midbrain, and pons (**f**–**j**)

parieto-occipital and frontal cortices; MSA by the hypometabolism of the bilateral putamen and cerebellum; PSP by the hypometabolism of the PFC, caudate nucleus, and midbrain; and CBD by the asymmetric hypometabolism of the cortex and putamen. However, the accuracy of these qualitative diagnostic methods is suboptimal. In recent years, disease-related brain metabolic patterns based on ^{18}F-FDG PET imaging can achieve higher diagnostic accuracy. This approach enables quantitative analysis based on the computation of pattern expression values, thus achieving the diagnosis and differential diagnosis of PD at the individual level, as well as the monitoring of disease progression and clinical therapeutic efficacy. The PDRP is characterized by hypermetabolism of the GP/putamen, thalamus, pons, and cerebellum, as well as hypometabolism of the premotor area and posterior parietal cortex. The MSA-related brain metabolic pattern is characterized by hypometabolism of the bilateral putamen and cerebellum. The PSP-related brain metabolic pattern is characterized by hypometabolism of the bilateral medial PFC, ventrolateral PFC, orbitofrontal cortex, caudate nucleus, medial thalamus, and midbrain.

Disease-related brain metabolic network patterns based on ^{18}F-FDG PET imaging are very valuable in differential diagnosis. By performing ^{18}F-FDG PET imaging for two of the most common parkinsonian syndromes (i.e., MSA and PSP), it is possible to obtain the respective brain metabolic network patterns of these two diseases, that is, the MSA-related brain metabolic network pattern (MSARP) and the PSP-related brain metabolic network pattern (PSPRP). The MSARP is characterized by the decreased glucose metabolism of the bilateral putamen and cerebellum; whereas the PSPRP is characterized by the decreased glucose metabolism of the bilateral medial PFC, ventrolateral PFC, caudate nucleus, medial thalamus, and upper brain stem. Thus, an automated differential diagnosis program developed on the basis of these disease-related brain metabolic network pattern will be able to calculate the probabilities that a patient is suffering from these three diseases at the individual level, and therefore provide a final diagnosis. Studies have shown that the sensitivity, specificity, positive predictive value, and negative predictive value of this method for the diagnosis of PD was 84, 97, 98, and 82%, respectively, while also demonstrating a comparably excellent diagnostic performance for MSA (sensitivity: 85%, specificity: 96%, positive predictive value: 97%, and negative predictive value: 83%) and PSP (sensitivity: 88%, specificity: 94%, positive predictive value: 91%, and negative predictive value: 92%). Therefore, differential diagnosis based on brain metabolic network patterns may serve as a useful tool for discriminating and confirming the diagnosis of patients enrolled in clinical trials. At present, it is believed that patients who are difficult to diagnose based on clinical symptoms can undergo nigrostriatal dopaminergic functional imaging to facilitate the differential diagnosis between typical and atypical parkinsonian syndromes, followed by further ^{18}F-FDG PET imaging to identify the different types of parkinsonian syndromes (e.g., idiopathic PD, MSA, PSP, CBD, etc.).

(2) Huntington's disease (HD) is an autosomal-dominant heritable neurodegenerative disease, primarily characterized by the slow progression of deteriorating involuntary movements, psychiatric symptoms, and cognitive impairment. The age of onset is generally 30–50 years, and most cases have a positive family history. HD is caused by an abnormal increase in the copies of trinucleotide (cytosine-adenine-guanine, CAG) repeats, and the pathogenic gene is located on the short arm of chromosome 4. The primary pathological changes in HD are found in the striatum and cerebral cortex, manifesting as extensive neuronal degeneration and loss. The dopamine D_1 and D_2 receptors of the striatum are the first to be affected, with PET imaging showing reduced binding between the imaging agent and receptors, as well as the correlation between the extent of reduction and clinical severity. D_2 receptor imaging is also associated with the copy number of CAG repeats, while the cortical D_2 receptor binding with the imaging agent has been shown to decrease with disease progression The findings of ^{18}F-FDG PET imaging have primarily revealed decreased glucose metabolism in the striatum and cerebral cortex, especially the frontal lobe, which can be detected even in the early stages of the disease. As with PD, the HD-related brain metabolic pattern can be acquired through special post-processing, which is characterized by the glucose hypometabolism of the caudate nucleus, putamen, and cingulate gyrus, as well as the hypermetabolism of the medial thalamus, cerebellum, motor cortex and occipital cortex. A prospective study on HD gene mutation carriers demonstrated that this pattern can be detected before the appearance of clinical symptoms, and showed high expression values, which decreased as the disease progressed, while the reduction in thalamic metabolic activity was associated with the appearance of clinical symptoms.

(3) ET: ET, also known as idiopathic tremor, is an autosomal-dominant hereditary disease with tremor as its only clinical presentation. This disease has a slow progression or shows no progression for long periods of time. ET patients present with normal DAT imaging findings, which can be used to differentiate it from parkinsonian syndromes.

9.3 Research Applications of PET/MR in PD

The predominant pathogenic mechanism of PD is the selective and progressive loss of dopaminergic neurons in the SN. PET tracers that are currently utilized in the clinical diagnosis of PD include ^{18}F-FDG and PET tracers for the synaptic function of dopaminergic neurons. ^{18}F-FDG PET can faithfully reflect the PDRP of patients with PD. Brain PET imaging of dopaminergic synaptic function includes presynaptic and postsynaptic functional imaging. The former primarily involves molecular probes targeting DAT (tracer: ^{11}C-CFT) and VMAT2 (tracer: ^{18}F-AV133). Integrated PET/MR allows the one-stop acquisition of multi-modal imaging information, including brain metabolism, structure, function, and blood flow, from patients with PD. Thus, combined imaging with different PET targeted tracers and MRI sequences will enable more in-depth explorations on the relationship between impaired dopaminergic neuronal function in PD and abnormal changes in CBF, iron deposition, brain function, and brain structure. This will facilitate a more comprehensive elucidation of PD pathogenesis, and enable the better discrimination of PD from other neurodegenerative diseases with parkinsonism (e.g., MSA, PSP, etc.).

9.3.1 Association between MRI Brain Structure and PET Glucose Metabolic Patterns in PD

9.3.1.1 Research Applications of the Relationship between Brain Volume Changes and Abnormal Glucose Metabolism in PD

Patients with PD often present with PD-MCI, and the prevalence of PDD in the long term can be as high as 80%, while the decline in cognitive function has a direct impact on the patient's quality of life. To patients with PD-MCI, the identification of relatively specific molecular imaging markers to monitor cognitive function is of critical significance. Previous studies have utilized PET/MR to examine the relationship between the brain structure and metabolism of PD patients with and without cognitive impairment, which revealed that PD patients with cognitive impairment showed extensive reductions in gray matter volume and decreased glucose metabolism. However, in both PD-MCI and PDD patients, the extent of decrease in cortical glucose metabolism did not coincide entirely with the atrophy level of the corresponding cortical area, with some areas showing a greater extent of cortical hypometabolism than cortical atrophy, and other areas showing a lower extent of cortical hypometabolism than cortical atrophy. In PD-MCI patients, local atrophy was observed in the temporal, parietal, and frontal cortices, whereas hypometabolism was found in the temporo-occipital cortex, temporo-parietal junction, and frontal cortex, which suggests that cortical hypometabolism occurs earlier than the atrophy of the corresponding cortical areas in these patients. Furthermore, PD-MCI patients showed a greater extent of glucose hypometabolism than cortical atrophy in the bilateral angular gyrus, inferior parietal lobule, superior frontal gyrus, right middle orbitofrontal gyrus, middle frontal gyrus, middle temporal gyrus, and lingual gyrus, whereas the extent of cortical atrophy exceeded that of glucose hypometabolism in the motor cortex and SMA. These findings indicate that in PD patients with cognitive impairment, cerebral glucose metabolism can better reflect their cognitive function than atrophic changes, while PD-related cortical hypometabolism and atrophy may be continuous stages in the development of cognitive impairment. PDD patients demonstrated a greater extent of hypometabolism than atrophy in the occipital, parietal and frontal cortices, but a smaller extent of hypometabolism than atrophy in the central motor area, SMA, right temporal cortex, left hippocampus, bilateral putamen, GP, and left thalamus. Compared to PD patients without dementia, PDD patients showed decreased glucose metabolism in the bilateral medial frontal and right parietal cortices. Moreover, studies have also found that PDD patients had decreased glucose metabolism in the occipital cortex, as well as significant atrophy in the hippocampus and frontal cortex compared to PD patients without dementia. These results suggest that the progression of dementia in patients with PD may be related to extensive metabolic reductions in the occipital cortex, and atrophy in the hippocampus and frontal cortex. Further investigations are needed on the association between cortical metabolic changes and structural alterations in patients with PD. Since integrated PET/MR allows the simultaneous acquisition of brain metabolic and structural information, it is currently the best approach for studying the pathogenic mechanisms underlying cognitive impairment in PD.

9.3.1.2 Research Applications of the Relationship between Neuromelanin Reduction and Specific DAT Tracer Uptake in PD

The onset of PD is caused by the decrease in SN dopaminergic neurons, and therefore the reduction of neuromelanin content in the SN can reflect the extent of damage to SN dopaminergic neurons. However, the relationship between neuromelanin content and the integrity of striatal dopaminergic neurons is still poorly understood. It is currently possible to combine neuromelanin-sensitive MRI (NM-MRI) with specific PET tracers targeting DAT and the presynaptic function of dopaminergic neurons, in order to elucidate the relationship among the three. By utilizing the ^{18}F-AV133 PET targeted tracer in integrated PET/MR, it is possible to comprehensively present the extent of neuromelanin reduction and the impairment of dopaminergic neuron presynaptic function in the SN region (Fig. 9.9). Additionally, NM-MRI can be combined with DAT PET imaging to assess the association between SN neuromelanin level and striatal DAT reduction. The results indicated that patients with PD had a lower neuromelanin content in the ventral than the dorsal SN, but no significant association was found between the decrease in SN neuromelanin content and the decrease in striatal DAT. However, for the clinically defined most affected side of these patients with PD, a significant relationship was observed between the neuromelanin reduction of the ventral SN and DAT reduction in the

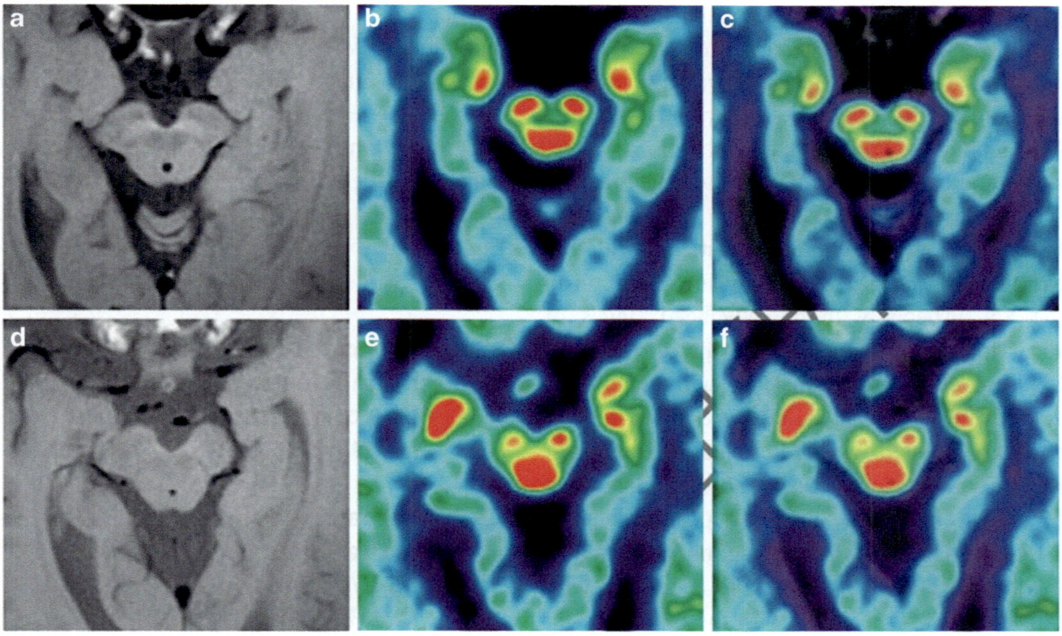

Fig. 9.9 Integrated ^{18}F-AV133 PET/neuromelanin-sensitive MRI of healthy subjects and patients with PD. Healthy subjects (**a**–**c**); patients with PD (**d**–**f**). In healthy subjects, transverse neuromelanin-sensitive MRI (NM-MRI) shows normal neuromelanin hyperintensities in the bilateral substantia nigra, with no signal decrease or morphological changes (**a**); transverse ^{18}F-AV133 PET imaging (**b**), and fused ^{18}F-AV133 PET/MR (**c**) show good ^{18}F-AV133 uptake in the bilateral substantia nigra. In patients with PD, transverse NM-MRI (**d**) shows a decrease in the scope of hyperintense signals, which is more prominent on the right; transverse ^{18}F-AV133 PET imaging (**e**), and fused ^{18}F-AV133 PET/MR (**f**) show reduced ^{18}F-AV133 uptake in the bilateral substantia nigra, which is more prominent on the right

corresponding striatal region receiving projections from the ventral SN.

9.3.1.3 Research Applications of the Relationship among Brain Iron Deposition, Glucose Metabolism, and Impaired Dopaminergic Neuronal Function in PD

Iron is involved in a number of normal biochemical processes of brain tissues, including neuronal development, enzyme function, DNA synthesis, oxidative phosphorylation, neurotransmitter synthesis, and mitochondrial respiration. Brain iron deposition is a part of normal brain aging, but excessive iron deposition is often believed to be the cause of various neurodegenerative diseases, such as PD, AD, and HD. The main hypothesis is that excessive iron deposition will increase the generation of free radicals, which will promote oxidative stress and neuronal death of iron-overloaded cells. The quantitative susceptibility mapping (QSM) sequence is currently the only MRI technique that can quantify brain iron deposition and can therefore be used to reflect excessive brain iron deposition in patients with PD. Studies have found that patients with PD exhibited significantly higher iron deposition in the SN, especially in the advanced stages of PD. This finding demonstrates that the level of SN iron deposition is consistent with the clinical course of PD and that the level of SN iron deposition is associated with the clinical symptoms of PD to some extent. Furthermore, studies have found differences in SN iron deposition among different PD subtypes (tremor-dominant PD, bradykinesia/rigidity-dominant PD, and PD with mixed motor symptoms), with the bradykinesia/rigidity-dominant subtype demonstrating the most significant levels of excessive iron deposition in the SN. It is presently still unclear whether there is an association between excessive iron deposition and dopaminergic neuronal impairments. Integrated PET/MR allows us to better explore the relationship between SN iron deposition and glucose metabolism in patients with PD. Both monomeric and aggregated β-amyloid can bind with iron, leading to the accumulation of iron in β-amyloid plaques and the conversion of Fe^{3+} into Fe^{2+}. Previous studies have utilized ^{11}C-PIB PET to compare the deposition of β-amyloid plaques in the cerebral cortex of patients with PD with and without dementia. Their results revealed no significant difference in the cortical deposition of β-amyloid plaques between the two groups, which suggests that the onset of dementia symptoms in PD may be related to the unique biological processes of PD itself. There is a link between increased brain iron deposition and AD-related cognitive decline, with previous studies finding that β-amyloid deposition and iron deposition may be associated to some extent with the cognitive abilities of healthy elderly subjects. The relationship between dopaminergic neuronal impairment and iron deposition remains poorly understood. Thus, integrated PET/MR involving PET tracers for the presynaptic function of dopaminergic neurons (e.g., ^{18}F-AV133) can serve as a direct multimodal imaging technique to examine the relationship between iron brain deposition and dopaminergic neuronal impairment in PD (Fig. 9.10).

9.3.2 Association between MRI Brain Function and PET Glucose Metabolic Patterns in PD

9.3.2.1 Research Applications of the Relationship between RS-fMRI and Glucose Metabolism

According to existing RS-fMRI studies, unmedicated patients with PD showed reduced functional connectivity between the head of the caudate nucleus and DMN, the body of the caudate nucleus and frontoparietal network (FPN), as well as the tail of the caudate nucleus and visual network. As for medicated patients with PD, improvements were observed in the func-

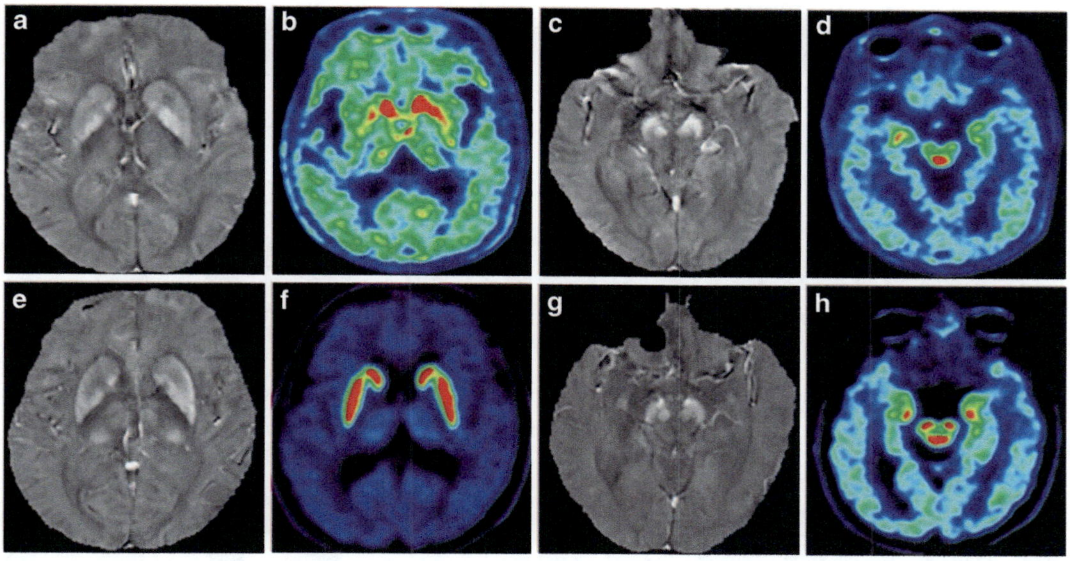

Fig. 9.10 Integrated ^{18}F-AV133 PET/MR in patients with PD and healthy controls. Patients with PD (**a**–**d**); healthy subjects (**e**–**h**). Transverse QSM imaging of PD patients shows the status of iron deposition in the putamen (**a**). Transverse ^{18}F-AV133 PET imaging shows the asymmetric reduction of ^{18}F-AV133 uptake in the bilateral putamen, which is more prominent in the posterior portion (**b**). Transverse QSM imaging shows that the level of iron deposition (115 ppm) is higher than that of the healthy controls (86 ppm) (**c**). Transverse ^{18}F-AV133 PET imaging shows reduced ^{18}F-AV133 uptake in the substantia nigra (**d**). Transverse QSM of healthy subjects shows the status of iron deposition in the putamen (**e**). Transverse ^{18}F-AV133 PET imaging shows the symmetric distribution of ^{18}F-AV133 uptake in the bilateral putamen (**f**). Transverse QSM imaging shows the iron deposition in the substantia nigra of healthy subjects (**g**). Transverse ^{18}F-AV133 PET imaging shows the symmetric uptake of ^{18}F-AV133 in the substantia nigra (**h**)

tional connectivity of the network connecting the medial PFC and head of the caudate nucleus, as well as the network connecting the dorsolateral PFC and the body of the caudate nucleus. The PDRP can be observed in patients with PD, but the relationship between the RM-fMRI and PET glucose metabolic patterns of patients with PD is currently unclear. Integrated PET/MR is able to address the problem of temporal synchronization between PET and MRI, as it can simultaneously acquire PET and fMRI from patients with PD. Thus, it is suited to studying the interactions between RS-fMRI and ^{18}F-FDG PET glucose metabolism among patients with PD and is currently the most ideal imaging technique available for investigating the relationship between brain structure and function in PD (Fig. 9.11). Nevertheless, current integrated PET/MR research on PD is still in its early stages and awaits further exploration.

9.3.2.2 Research Applications of the Relationship between ASL CBF and Glucose Metabolism in PD

Integrated PET/MR allows the simultaneous acquisition of ^{18}F-FDG PET and ASL quantitative data. Thus, it is an ideal technique for the simultaneous acquisition of cerebral perfusion and glucose metabolic characteristics in PD, and for examining the association between the two. In previous studies combining pseudo-continuous ASL (pCASL) with ^{18}F-FDG PET imaging for the integrated assessment of CBF and brain metabolism in patients with PD, decreased CBF was observed in the bilateral temporal cortex, insula, posterior parietal cortex, inferior parietal lobule, lateral occipital cortex, and PFC, whereas increased CBF was observed in the cerebellum, pons, right thalamus GP, sensorimotor cortex, central lobule, and SMA. At the same time,

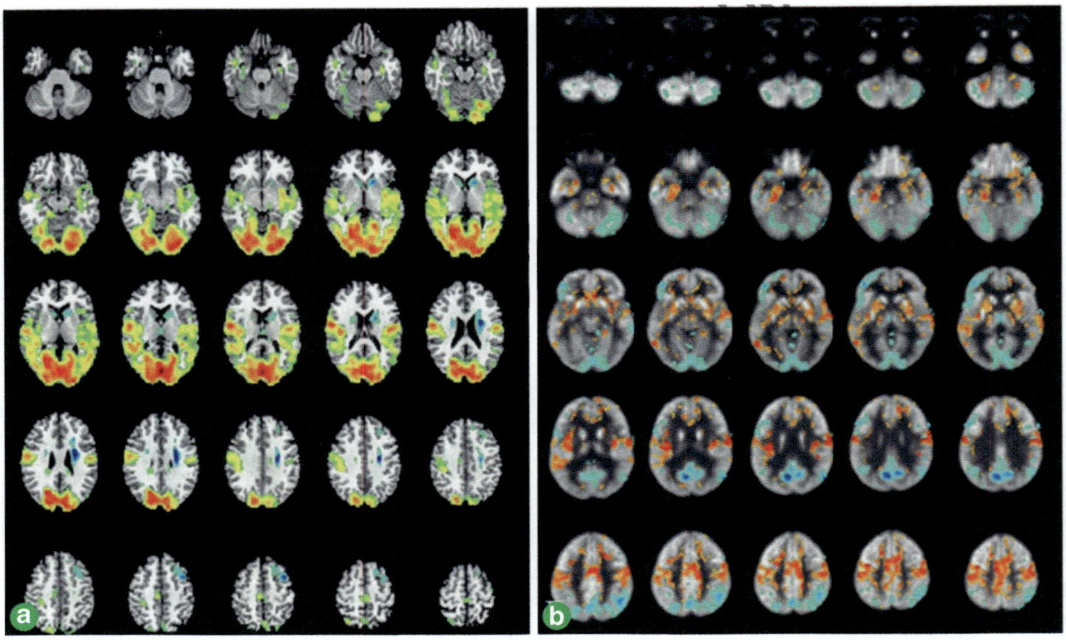

Fig. 9.11 Simultaneous RS-fMRI and PET performed using integrated PET/MR in patients with PD. Differences in functional connectivity between healthy controls and PD patients with the left motor cortex as the seed region. Warm color areas indicate healthy controls had higher levels than PD patients; cool color areas indicate healthy controls had lower levels than patients with PD (**a**). Increases and decreases in the glucose metabolic patterns of patients with PD compared to healthy controls. Warm color areas indicate patients with PD had higher levels than healthy controls; cool color areas indicate patients with PD had lower levels than healthy controls (**b**)

patients with PD exhibited decreased glucose metabolism of the bilateral temporal cortex, posterior parietal cortex, inferior parietal lobule, occipital cortex, PFC and SMA, as well as increased glucose metabolism in the cerebellum, pons, thalamus, GP, sensorimotor cortex, limbic association cortex, and central lobule (Fig. 9.12). Thus, patients with PD showed partial overlaps between the areas with altered CBF and brain metabolism, which suggests that there is some association between the changes in CBF and brain glucose metabolic patterns in patients with PD.

9.3.3 Research Applications in the Differential Diagnosis and Treatment of PD

9.3.3.1 Differential Diagnosis of PD and Other Parkinsonian Syndromes

The main parkinsonian syndromes include PD, PSP, and MSA. MSA responds poorly to levodopa treatment and is accompanied by pyramidal signs, cerebellar dysfunction, and autonomic dysfunction. As certain clinical symptoms of MSA overlap with those of PD, it is clinically difficult to differentiate between PD and MSA in the early stages. By combining DTI with ^{18}F-FDG PET imaging, MSA-P patients were shown to have elevated MD and reduced glucose metabolism in the posterior putamen compared to patients with PD. This suggests that there is an association between microstructural damage and decreased glucose metabolism of the putamen in patients with MSA-P. Histopathological studies have also shown that MSA patients had increased iron concentration in neuronal ribosomes, which gave rise to neurodegeneration. SWI can accurately detect hypointense signals corresponding to increased iron deposition, and higher iron deposition can lead to decreased SWI signals in the putamen. Compared with patients with PD, MSA-P patients exhibit significant SWI hypointensities in the dorsolateral or posterior putamen, which implies that iron-mediated oxidative stress is more severe in MSA patients, and may have been the cause of reduced glucose metabolism.

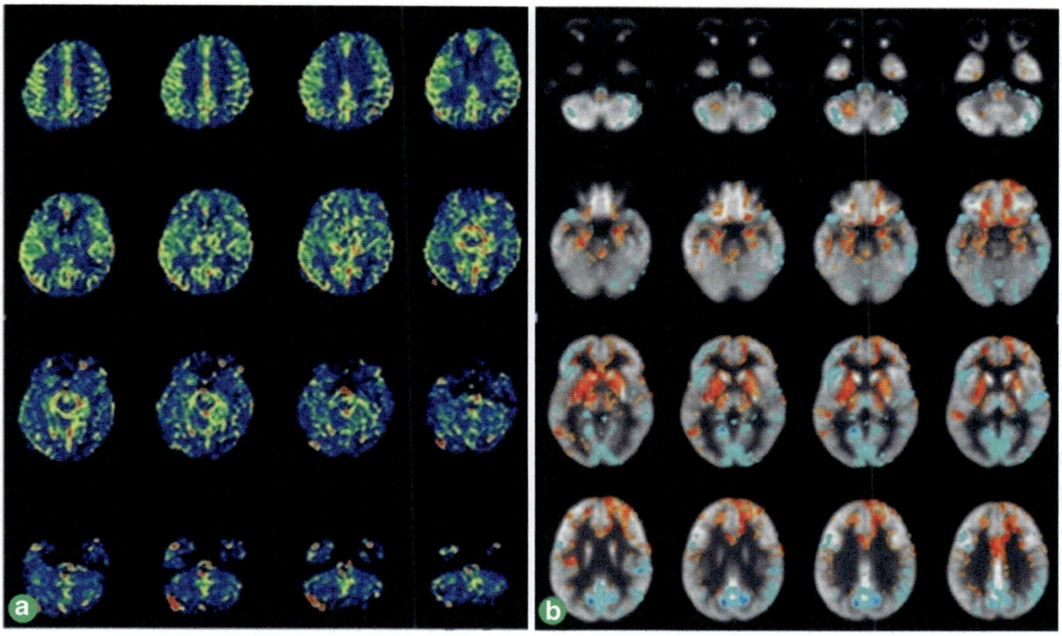

Fig. 9.12 Simultaneous ASL and PET performed using integrated PET/MR in patients with PD. ASL-derived CBF maps of patients with PD showing decreased CBF of the bilateral temporal cortex, insula, posterior parietal cortex, inferior parietal lobule, lateral occipital cortex, and prefrontal cortex (**a**). Patients with PD show increased glucose metabolism of the cerebellum, pons, thalamus, globus pallidus, sensorimotor cortex, limbic association cortex, and central lobule (**b**)

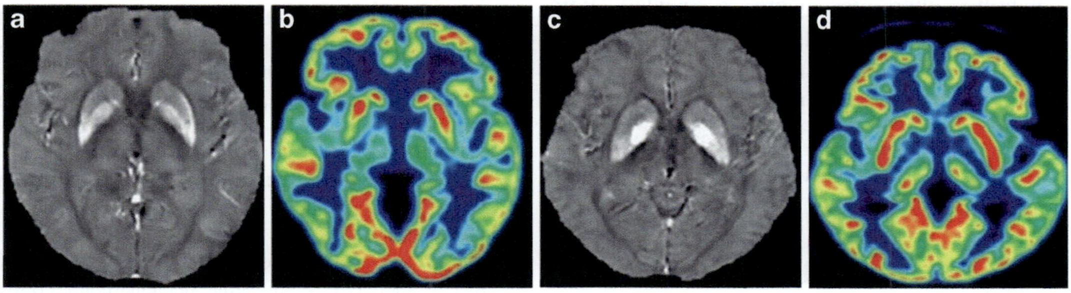

Fig. 9.13 Integrated ^{18}F-FDG PET/MR of MSA-P and patients with PD. Transverse QSM imaging of MSA-P patient showing significantly increased iron deposition in the bilateral posterior putamen (**a**). Transverse ^{18}F-FDG PET imaging showing decreased ^{18}F-FDG uptake in the bilateral posterior putamen, which is more prominent on the right (**b**). Transverse QSM imaging of PD patient showing the status of iron deposition in the bilateral putamen (**c**). Transverse ^{18}F-FDG PET imaging showing significantly increased ^{18}F-FDG uptake in the bilateral putamen (**d**)

Significantly elevated iron deposition in the posterior putamen combined with significantly reduced glucose metabolism can be used to differentiate between MSA and PD (Fig. 9.13). Since integrated PET/MR can simultaneously acquire ^{18}F-FDG PET and CBF maps to combine the images from two imaging modalities, it is a useful technique for differentiating among the three parkinsonian syndromes, i.e., PD, PSP, and MSA. Patients with PD exhibit higher glucose metabolism and perfusion than MSA and PSP patients in the caudate nucleus, putamen, midbrain, pons and cerebellum. Cerebellar SUV_{mean} and CBF_{mean} can be used to discriminate between PD and MSA (area under the curve, AUC: 0.892 and 0.792, respectively); while midbrain SUV_{mean}

and caudate nucleus CBF_{mean} can be used to differentiate between PD and PSP (AUC: 0.896 and 0.903, respectively). In the future, integrated PET/MR is expected to enable the simultaneous acquisition of information on dopaminergic neuronal function and cerebral perfusion, which will serve as a simpler, more efficient, and feasible method for the diagnosis and differential diagnosis of parkinsonian syndromes.

9.3.3.2 Efficacy Evaluation in PD

STN ablation with MR-guided focused ultrasound (MRgFUS) is a potential treatment for PD. Previous studies have utilized integrated ^{18}F-FDG PET imaging to examine the pre- and post-operative glucose metabolism of 8 patients with PD who underwent MRgFUS STN ablation. Their results revealed that after STN ablation, the glucose metabolism of the cerebellum, STN, GPi, motor cortex, and cingulate gyrus was lower than pre-operative levels, whereas the glucose metabolism of the posterior parietal and occipital cortices was higher than pre-operative levels. MRgFUS also led to a significant decrease in the PDRP expression of patients with PD, and these metabolic alterations were associated with improvements in clinical symptoms as measured by the motor scores of the Unified Parkinson's Disease Rating Scale (UPDRS). These findings suggest that integrated PET/MR is an excellent technique for studying the mechanisms related to surgical treatment in PD.

9.3.3.3 Basic Research and Drug Testing in PD

Integrated PET/MR has an enormous potential for application in the basic research of and pharmaceutical treatment testing for PD. This technique can assist clinicians with understanding the specific mechanisms of action involved in dopaminergic drugs in the brains of patients with PD, while also enabling the visualization of research on dopamine receptor antagonism and hemodynamic changes in the nigrostriatal region. At present, novel PET tracers, such as those for DAT and α-synuclein, can be combined with MRI-based structural and functional information, in order to uncover new research directions in the pathogenic mechanisms of PD.

The ability of integrated PET/MR to simultaneously acquire multi-modal imaging information, such as brain function, structure, and metabolism, from patients with PD will facilitate a more comprehensive understanding on the pathophysiological mechanisms underlying the pathogenesis of PD, thereby contributing to the early diagnosis and differential diagnosis of PD. Additionally, integrated PET/MR is currently the most ideal imaging tool for PD assessment, providing objective and comprehensive evidence based on molecular imaging for elucidating the mechanisms underlying the pharmacological and surgical treatments of PD.

Suggested Reading

An H, Zeng X, Niu T, et al. Quantifying iron deposition within the substantianigra of Parkinson's disease by quantitative susceptibility mapping. J Neurol Sci. 2018;386:46–52.

Asanuma K, Tang C, Ma Y, et al. Network modulation in the treatment of Parkinson's disease. Brain. 2006;129(Pt 10):2667–78.

Baggio HC, Sala-Llonch R, Segura B, et al. Functional brain networks and cognitive deficits in Parkinson's disease. Hum Brain Mapp. 2014;35(9):4620–34.

Baudrexel S, Seifried C, Penndorf B, et al. The value of putaminal diffusion imaging versus 18-fluorodeoxyglucose positron emission tomography for the differential diagnosis of the Parkinson variant of multiple system atrophy. Mov Disord. 2014;29(3):380–7.

Baudrexel S, Witte T, Seifried C, et al. Resting state fMRI reveals increased subthalamic nucleus-motor cortex connectivity in Parkinson's disease. Neuroimage. 2011;55(4):1728–38.

Berg D, Postuma RB, Adler CH, et al. MDS research criteria for prodromal Parkinson's disease. Mov Disord. 2015;30(12):1600–11.

Fling BW, Cohen RG, Mancini M, et al. Asymmetric pedunculopontine network connectivity in parkinsonian patients with freezing of gait. Brain. 2013;136(8):2405–18.

Gao L, Wu T. The study of brain functional connectivity in Parkinson's disease. Transl Neurodegener. 2016;28(5):18.

González-Redondo R, García-García D, Clavero P, et al. Grey matter hypometabolism and atrophy in Parkinson's disease with cognitive impairment: a two-step process. Brain. 2014;137(Pt 8):2356–67.

Haslinger B, Erhard P, Kämpfe N, et al. Event-related functional magnetic resonance imaging in Parkinson's disease before and after levodopa. Brain. 2001;124(3):558–70.

Helmich RC, Janssen MJ, Oyen WJ, et al. Pallidal dysfunction drives a cerebellothalamic circuit into Parkinson tremor. Ann Neurol. 2011;69(2):269–81.

Helmich RC, Thaler A, Van Nuenen BF, et al. Reorganization of corticostriatal circuits in healthy G2019S LRRK2 carriers. Neurology. 2015;84(4):399–406.

Herz DM, Eickhoff SB, Lkkegaard A, et al. Functional neuroimaging of motor control in Parkinsonls disease: a meta-analysis. Hum Brain Mapp. 2014;35(7):3227–37.

Herz DM, Haagensen BN, Christensen MS, et al. Abnormal dopaminergic modulation of striato-cortical networks underlies levodopa induced dyskinesias in humans. Brain. 2015;138(6):1658–66.

Huang P, Xuan M, Gu Q, et al. Abnormal amygdala function in Parkinson's disease patients and its relationship to depression. J Affect Disord. 2015;183:263–8.

Jokinen P, Scheinin N, Aalto S, et al. [(11)C]PIB-, [(18)F]FDG-PET and MRI imaging in patients with Parkinson's disease with and without dementia. Parkinsonism Relat Disord. 2010;16(10):666–70.

Lehéricy S, Benali H, Van de Moortele P, et al. Distinct basal ganglia territories are engaged in early and advanced motor sequence learning. Proc Natl Acad Sci U S A. 2005;102(35):12566–71.

Lehéricy S, Vaillancourt DE, Seppi K, et al. The role of high-field magnetic resonance imaging in parkinsonian disorders: pushing the boundaries forward. Mov Disord. 2017;32(4):510–25.

Li L, Wu P, Wu J, et al. The value of dopamine transporter PET imaging in the differential diagnosis of Parkinson's disease and progressive supranuclear palsy. Chin J Clin Neurosci. 2018;26(3):262–8.

Manza P, Zhang S, Li CSR, et al. Resting-state functional connectivity of the striatum in early-stage Parkinson's disease: cognitive decline and motor symptomatology. Hum Brain Mapp. 2016;37(2):648–62.

Martín-Bastida A, Lao-Kaim NP, Roussakis A, et al. Relationship between neuromelanin and dopamine terminals within the Parkinson's nigrostriatal system. Brain. 2019;142(7):2023–36.

Neurology Group of the Chinese Society of Nuclear Medicine. Expert consensus on the operation and clinical application of dopamine transporter brain PET imaging technology. Chin J Nucl Med Mol Imaging. 2020;40(5):298–302.

Rodriguez-Rojas R, Pineda-Pardo JA, Martinez-Fernandez R, et al. Functional impact of subthalamotomy by magnetic resonance-guided focused ultrasound in Parkinson's disease: a hybrid PET/MR study of resting-state brain metabolism. Eur J Nucl Med Mol Imaging. 2020;47(2):425–36.

Rolinski M, Griffanti L, Piccini P, et al. Basal ganglia dysfunction in idiopathic REM sleep behaviour disorder parallels that in early Parkinson's disease. Brain. 2016;139(8):2224–34.

Skidmore FM, Yang M, Baxter L, et al. Apathy, depression, and motor symptoms have distinct and separable resting activity patterns in idiopathic Parkinson disease. Neuroimage. 2013;81:484–95.

Su M, Wang S, Fang W, et al. Alterations in the limbic/paralimbic cortices of Parkinson's disease patients with hyposmia under resting-state functional MRI by regional homogeneity and functional connectivity analysis. Parkinsonism Relat Disord. 2015;21(7):698–703.

Sun X, Liu F, Ruan W, et al. Correlation and differential diagnostic value of ^{18}F-FDG imaging and ASL cerebral perfusion imaging acquired by synchronous PET/MR in Parkinsonism. Chin J Nucl Med Mol Imaging. 2019;38(6):337–43.

Tessitore A, de Micco R, Giordano A, et al. Intrinsic brain connectivity predicts impulse control disorders in patients with Parkinson's disease. Mov Disord. 2017;32(12):1710–9.

Teune LK, Renken RJ, de Jong BM, et al. Parkinson's disease-related perfusion and glucose metabolic brain patterns identified with PCASL-MRI and FDG-PET imaging. NeuroImage Clin. 2014;5:240–4.

Van Bergen JMG, Li X, Quevenco FC, et al. Simultaneous quantitative susceptibility mapping and Flutemetamol-PET suggests local correlation of iron and β-amyloid as an indicator of cognitive performance at high age. Neuroimage. 2018;174:308–16.

Wang Y, Wu P, Zuo C, et al. Influence of different PET reconstruction algorithms on Parkinson's disease-related pattern expression. Chin Comput Med Imaging. 2013;19(6):549–52.

Wang J, Zuo CT, Jiang YP, et al. F-18-FP-CIT PET imaging and SPM analysis of dopamine transporters in Parkinson's disease in various Hoehn & Yahr stages. J Neurol. 2007;254(2):185–90.

Wu T, Hallett M. A functional MRI study of automatic movements in patients with Parkinson's disease. Brain. 2005;128(10):2250–9.

Wu T, Hallett M. The Cerebellum in Parkinson's Disease. Brain. 2013;136(3):696–709.

Wu P, Lin C, Zhang H, et al. Establishing a Parkinson's disease brain metabolic network pattern based on ^{18}F-FDG PET imaging. Chin J Nucl Med Mol Imaging. 2013;33(4):275–8.

Wu T, Long X, Zang Y, et al. Regional homogeneity changes in patients with Parkinson's disease. Hum Brain Mapp. 2009;30(5):1502–10.

Wu T, Ma Y, Zheng Z, et al. Parkinson's disease-related spatial covariance pattern identified with resting-state functional MRI. J Cereb Blood Flow Metab. 2015;35(11):1764–70.

Wu T, Wang L, Hallett M, et al. Effective connectivity of brain networks during self-initiated movement in Parkinson's disease. Neuroimage. 2011;55(1):204–15.

Yoon RG, Kim SJ, Kim HS, et al. The utility of susceptibility-weighted imaging for differentiating Parkinsonism-predominant multiple system atrophy from Parkinson's disease: correlation with 18F-flurodeoxyglucose positron-emission tomography. Neurosci Lett. 2015;584:296–301.

Zuo C, Ge J, Jiang C, et al. Re-examining the value of ^{18}F-FDG PET brain imaging in the diagnosis and differential diagnosis of Parkinson's disease. Chin J Nucl Med Mol Imaging. 2019;38(6):321–4.

Zuo C, Guan Y. The value of single-case statistical parametric mapping analysis of ^{18}F-FDG PET imaging in the differential diagnosis of parkinsonian syndromes. Chin J Nucl Med Mol Imaging. 2019;38(6):331–6.

10 Research Applications of Positron Emission Tomography/Magnetic Resonance (PET/MR) Imaging in Epilepsy

Chao Zhang, Kun Shang, Jingjuan Wang, Yufeng Zang, and Jie Lu

Epilepsy is a neurological condition involving recurrent seizures that are induced by abnormal neuronal discharges in the brain. According to statistics, there are approximately 6.5 million individuals with epilepsy worldwide. The high disability and fatality rates, numerous complications, and high medical costs associated with epilepsy place a heavy burden on families and society. Over the past few decades, there has been a gradual deepening in our understanding of epilepsy, which has in turn brought about a series of transformations in the diagnosis and classification of this condition. Nevertheless, the pathogenesis of epilepsy remains poorly understood. Recent advances in neuroimaging have led to the emergence of new PET and MRI techniques, including structural MRI (sMRI), magnetic resonance spectroscopy (MRS), diffusion tensor imaging (DTI), perfusion-weighted imaging (PWI), and functional MRI (fMRI). These techniques have promoted the rapid development of research on epilepsy, encompassing areas such as surgical planning, cognitive function in patients with epilepsy, and the pathophysiological mechanisms of epilepsy. The findings of this research have contributed to a deeper understanding of epilepsy, and have broadened the indications for the surgical treatment of patients with epilepsy.

C. Zhang · K. Shang · J. Wang · J. Lu (✉)
Department of Radiology and Nuclear Medicine, Xuanwu Hospital, Capital Medical University, Beijing, China

Y. Zang
Center for Cognition and Brain Disorders, The Affiliated Hospital of Hangzhou Normal University, Hangzhou, China

10.1 Research Applications of MRI in Epilepsy

Multi-sequence, multi-directional imaging can be obtained using MRI, providing a far higher soft-tissue resolution and therefore more diagnostic information than computed tomography (CT). Therefore, MRI can be used to detect hippocampal sclerosis (HS), cortical dysplasia, secondary cortical damage, and other microstructural alterations that cannot be seen on CT images. In turn, MRI plays a crucial role in the etiological diagnosis, pre-surgical localization, and post-surgical assessment of epilepsy, and is currently the preferred imaging modality for the pre-surgical localization and assessment of patients with refractory epilepsy.

10.1.1 Research Applications of sMRI in Refractory Epilepsy

Voxel-based morphometry (VBM) has been extensively utilized for the analysis of imaging data in epilepsy research. VBM utilizes three-dimensional (3D) volumetric T1-weighted

J. Lu, G. Zhao (eds.), *PET/MR: Functional and Molecular Imaging of Neurological Diseases and Neurosciences*, https://doi.org/10.1007/978-981-19-9902-4_10

imaging to achieve a higher gray/white matter contrast and to perform arbitrary plane reconstruction. HS is one of the most commonly missed diagnoses on MRI scans, and the individualized, automated segmentation of brain structures via VBM can be used to quantify hippocampal volume, thereby facilitating the diagnosis of HS. Current studies have demonstrated that temporal lobe epilepsy (TLE) is not a focal disease, but rather a network-based disease involving a number of cortical and subcortical structures that jointly drive its pathogenesis. By utilizing VBM, it has been found that varying degrees of volumetric atrophy in the ipsilateral thalamus and entire cerebral cortex (Fig. 10.1) were found with HS in patients with TLE. Apart from commonly implemented structural imaging at 1 mm resolution, the manual segmentation of higher-resolution structural images of the hippocampus allows a more accurate depiction of the hippocampal subregions, which further enhances the accuracy of localization. The development of fully automated software implies that manual delineation can be replaced with the fully automated segmentation of the hippocampal subregions, producing results concordant with pathological findings, while also improving efficiency through batch processing.

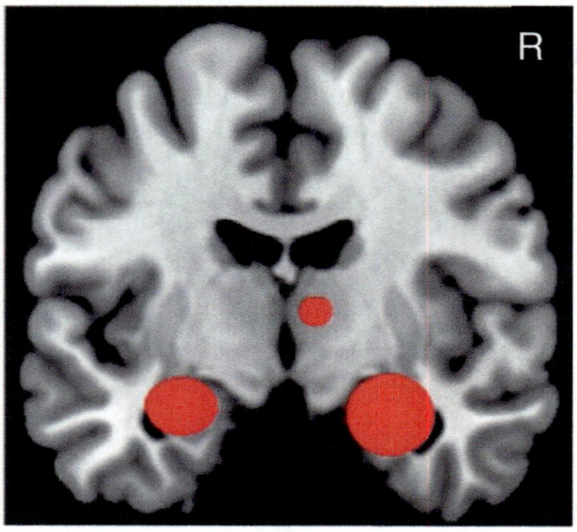

Fig. 10.1 Hippocampal and ipsilateral thalamic atrophy in patients with right TLE. Voxel-based morphometry (VBM) analysis revealed in the comparison between patients with right medial temporal lobe epilepsy (TLE) and healthy controls that in addition to bilateral hippocampal atrophy, atrophy can also be observed in the thalamus ipsilateral to the epileptogenic focus. Red indicates volume reduction

The thalamus, a critical anatomical structure in TLE with HS as well as other types of MRI-negative epilepsy, is an important node in the pathogenesis of epilepsy. The first regions to be affected are the interconnected parts of the mediodorsal thalamic nuclei and temporal lobe, and then the cerebral cortex. Post-mortem studies have demonstrated that patients with TLE had significantly reduced neuronal densities in the mediodorsal thalamic nuclei ipsilateral to hippocampal lesions. Furthermore, TLE patients, both with and without medial temporal lobe (MTL) sclerosis, exhibited bilateral thalamic atrophy, although those with MTL sclerosis showed more severe atrophy. The variability in the topological structure of the hippocampus in patients with medial TLE may be one of the factors determining whether the condition can be controlled following surgery. Some researchers have also classified medial TLE based on the level of atrophy in the subregional microstructure of the hippocampus, amygdala, and entorhinal cortex, and post-surgical follow-ups revealed that different TLE subtypes had different post-surgical prognoses; therefore, the pre-surgical structural classification of medial TLE was a good predictor of the post-surgical outcome. These results suggest that pre-surgical morphological alterations in microstructure may serve as a marker to predict surgical efficacy. Additionally, other studies have reported that extracortical atrophy in TLE patients is associated with post-surgical relapse, which is possibly caused by the cumulative excitotoxicity of the cerebral cortex from chronic, recurrent seizures.

Post-processing techniques of brain sMRIs can be utilized to identify hippocampal lesions and whole-brain abnormalities that cannot be detected with conventional MRI, making them useful techniques for both pre-surgical localization and the evaluation of surgical efficacy, although further research is needed to verify individualized analysis.

10.1.2 Research Applications of DTI in Refractory Epilepsy

By comparing the Brownian motion of water molecules in brain tissues, DTI can be used to non-invasively evaluate the integrity of axons and the myelin sheath. Abnormal neuronal discharges occur in the cerebral cortex during epileptic seizures and given that white matter fibers form the basic framework for the propagation of epileptic discharges, changes in the structural connectivity of white matter are of crucial significance to the pre-surgical assessment and surgical localization of patients with epilepsy. DTI primarily involves the evaluation of white matter alterations based on parameters such as fractional anisotropy (FA) and mean diffusivity (MD). FA describes the proportion of the total diffusion tensor occupied by the anisotropic component and is the most frequently used quantitative indicator for evaluating the integrity of the white matter structure. As such, a decreased FA signifies axonal degeneration and myelin degradation. MD is the diffusivity of water molecules in organs and tissues and is found by averaging the sum of diffusion tensors in all directions. An increased MD indicates a decrease in the intracellular levels of water molecules, while an increase in the extracellular levels of water molecules signifies neuronal degeneration.

In patients with TLE, DTI revealed reduced FA values for white matter on the affected side, primarily involving the fornix and the parahippocampal, uncinate, and cingulate fasciculi, while also extending into extratemporal regions, including the anterior and posterior longitudinal fasciculus, internal and external capsules, corpus callosum, and deep gray matter nuclei (e.g., hypothalamus, putamen, etc.) (Fig. 10.2). Wieshmann et al. found, using DTI, that during the interictal period, the hippocampus on the affected side exhibited significantly elevated MD values and significantly reduced FA values. Since the FA of water molecule diffusion in the hippocampus is less prominent than that in white matter, the MD value is more valuable for the detection and localization of hippocampal lesions. The extensive involvement of cerebral white matter networks, as demonstrated by DTI, also confirms that TLE can cause abnormalities in the structural network of the whole brain. Furthermore, the involvement of extratemporal structures may be one of the important factors contributing to post-surgical relapse.

In addition to pre-surgical localization in epilepsy, DTI can also be used to assess the post-surgical recovery of brain function. A follow-up study on patients who underwent anterior temporal lobectomy found that the increased FA values of the ipsilateral external capsule, posterior limb

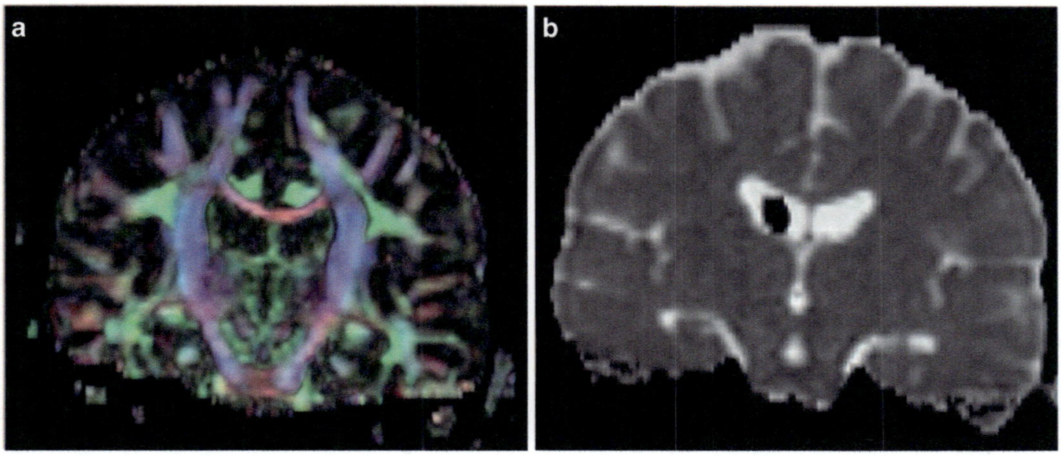

Fig. 10.2 DTI shows changes in white matter parameters of patients with TLE. Left temporal lobe (affected side) shows reduced FA values—left hippocampus: 0.58, right hippocampus: 0.62 (**a**). Left temporal lobe (affected side) shows elevated MD values—left hippocampus: 1.2, right hippocampus: 0.88 (**b**)

of the internal capsule, and optic radiation were associated with post-surgical language recovery. DTI studies on extratemporal neocortical epilepsy are relatively scarce.

DTI cannot be utilized to resolve the orientation of multiple fibers in a single voxel; therefore, new techniques based on probability density functions, such as q-ball imaging, high angular resolution diffusion imaging, and diffusion spectrum imaging, gradually began to emerge. High angular resolution diffusion imaging was used to construct structural connectivity networks, which were in turn correlated with functional networks specific to the time and frequency domains of intracranial video electroencephalography (VEEG), in order to quantify the coupling between structure and function. The results revealed significantly enhanced structure-function coupling during the transition from the pre-ictal to the ictal period, and that short-range structural connections are the primary cause of increased coupling. Therefore, research based on structure-function coupling contributes to the development of new therapies for epilepsy. Additionally, another study using diffusion spectrum imaging to examine the relationship between the cortex and subcortical nuclei in TLE patients found varying degrees of alterations in global connectivity (GC), node structure, and local connectivity.

The advancement of diffusion-based techniques for white matter imaging facilitates a more accurate and precise preoperative localization of epileptogenic foci and plays an important role in further investigating the pathogenesis of epilepsy.

10.1.3 Research Applications of MRS in Refractory Epilepsy

MRS can be utilized for the non-invasive detection of metabolic markers in the brain, therefore providing characteristic indicators that reflect neurometabolism and introducing a new approach of epilepsy research from a metabolic perspective. ^{1}H-MRS plays a crucial role in the detection of metabolic changes in patients with epilepsy. N-acetyl aspartate (NAA) is only synthesized in neuronal mitochondria, whereas creatine (Cr) levels are relatively high in glial cells. Therefore, a decrease in the NAA peak signifies neuronal loss or hypoplasia, whereas an increase in Cr indicates the presence of gliosis. As such, a large number of studies have used the NAA/Cr ratio as an indicator of the function of neuron-glia units, finding that this parameter reflects dysfunctional neuron-glia units rather than neuronal loss, and is therefore useful for determining brain tissue atrophy. Studies have confirmed that MRS has a higher sensitivity than hippocampal structural changes in the lateralization of medial TLE, as well as a greater specificity for detecting epileptogenic foci. The majority of studies utilized the NAA/[choline (Cho) + Cr] ratio as the diagnostic criterion for localization. Additionally, most studies involving single-voxel MRS have reported that the minimum value of NAA/(Cho + Cr) within the normal range is 0.72, and values lower than 0.05 are considered abnormal, which signifies the presence of HS (Fig. 10.3) and suggests neuronal loss and/or dysfunction. Furthermore, elevated Cho and Cr levels indicate the presence of reactive gliosis. Since abnormal hippocampal discharges on the affected side can be transmitted via the hippocampal or posterior commissure to the contralateral hippocampus to form mirror foci, chronic epileptic seizures can also lead to metabolic abnormalities in the contralateral hippocampus, although to a lesser degree than the affected side. In MRI-negative TLE patients, the decrease in NAA/Cr and NAA/Cr + Cho can facilitate localization and is a relatively sensitive indicator for the quantitative diagnosis of epilepsy. Some studies have reported that the NAA peak in MRS imaging is negatively correlated with the frequency of epileptic seizures, that is, the NAA peak value exhibited a trend of gradual decrease with increasing frequency of epileptic seizures. Moreover, in the absence of abnormalities in conventional MRI and VEEG, abnormal changes can still be detected using MRS. Abnormal ^{1}H-MRS findings in the hippocampus have significant value in predicting surgical efficacy, with abnormal hippocampal MRS indicating poor post-surgical

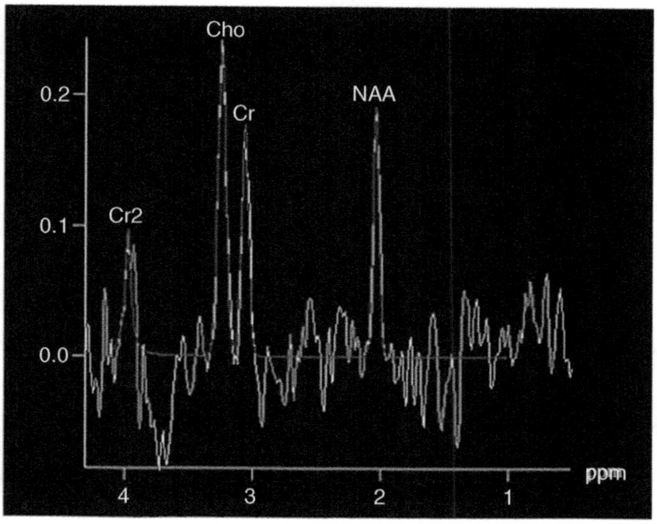

Fig. 10.3 MRS of hippocampal sclerosis. MRS of the hippocampal body showing a significantly decreased NAA peak and a slightly increased Cho peak

outcomes in patients. Other metabolites, such as γ-aminobutyric acid (GABA) and glutamate, which serve as inhibitory or excitatory neurotransmitters in the brain, may also be useful in localizing epileptogenic foci or monitoring the response of epileptic patients to drug treatment. However, further research is needed in this area. MRS can be used for the non-invasive in vivo measurement of brain metabolism (Fig. 10.3), and indirectly reflecting pathological changes within epileptic foci.

10.1.4 Research Applications of ASL in Refractory Epilepsy

ASL has several advantages over other perfusion imaging techniques, including non-invasiveness, absence of ionizing radiation, no risk of allergic reactions, low cost, simple and fast procedures, and ease of acquisition, among others. Therefore, this technique has been implemented in the lateralization and localization of epilepsy diagnoses, as well as for dynamic follow-up evaluations.

The mechanisms underlying the hyperperfusion induced by epileptic activity are currently still poorly understood. The cerebral blood flow (CBF) in the epileptogenic zone during the ictal period is typically elevated, owing to the pathological activity of the neurons, which may be related to the transient loss of self-regulatory function in the peripheral vascular system, or the regional release of glutamate and other excitatory neurotransmitters due to increased neuronal firing. During the interictal period, the epileptogenic zone tends to exhibit lower function and activity, resulting in reduced CBF (Fig. 10.4).

A controlled study, in which ASL was performed to measure the CBF of 12 patients with refractory TLE, revealed that patients had asymmetrical CBF in the bilateral temporal lobes and that the CBF in the epileptic side was lower than that of the contralateral side. Another study explored the correlation between CBF and brain glucose metabolism in 10 patients with medial TLE, using the simultaneous acquisition of ASL and PET imaging data during the interictal period, and quantitative analysis on regional CBF (rCBF). The results showed significantly reduced CBF in the affected side compared to the contralateral side, whereas comparisons between the two techniques indicated no significant difference in the mean CBF of the temporal lobe as measured using ASL and PET. Taken together, these findings have laid the foundation for research on the clinical applications of ASL in epilepsy.

A significant advantage of ASL is that it can be combined with sMRI to provide a reliable and informative imaging evaluation for mesial temporal sclerosis and neocortical epilepsy. According to ASL studies, patients with TLE

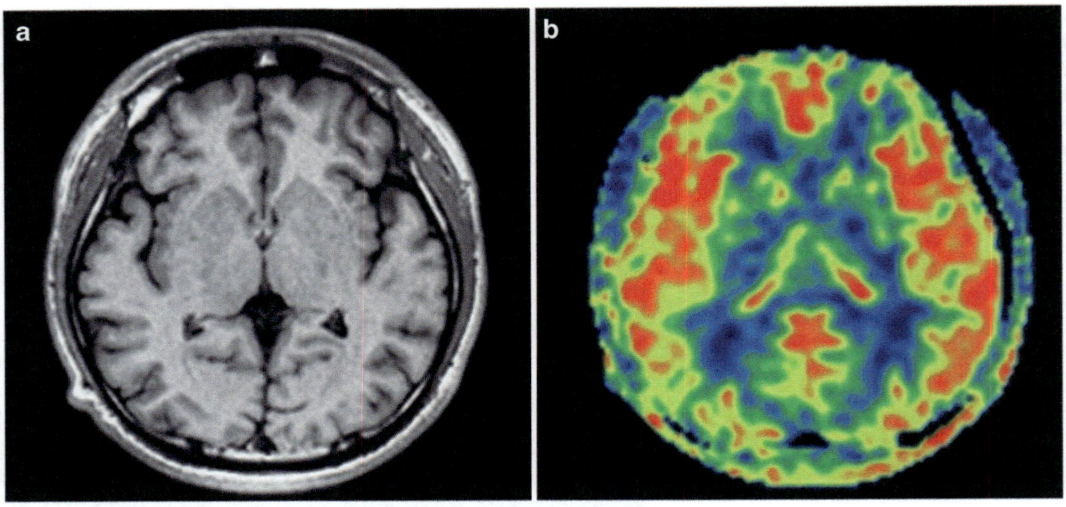

Fig. 10.4 ASL of patients with hippocampal sclerosis. Transverse T_1-weighted MRI shows no significant abnormalities (**a**); however, ASL shows reduced perfusion in the right occipital lobe compared to the contralateral side (**b**)

exhibit reductions in the CBF reductions of multiple brain areas, including the bilateral hippocampus, parahippocampal gyrus, frontal lobe, thalamus, and cingulate gyrus, among others. They also found that the extent of the reduction in the CBF of the affected temporal lobe is higher than that of the contralateral side, demonstrating a sensitivity of 76% and specificity of 78.3% in the differential diagnosis of TLE. ASL studies on patients with idiopathic generalized epilepsy (IGE) revealed reductions in the CBF of multiple brain areas, including the frontal and temporal lobes, the thalamus, and the basal ganglia. Moreover, a number of ASL-based epilepsy studies have all observed reductions in CBF in multiple brain areas in patients with epilepsy, with significantly more brain areas exhibiting CBF changes than those with abnormalities detected by morphometry.

Monitoring with subdural and/or deep brain electrodes is the generally accepted gold standard for the localization of epileptogenic foci; however, it is highly invasive, operationally challenging, and extremely costly, which has restricted its clinical application. Therefore, with the rapid advancement of imaging technology in recent years, techniques such as PET, SPECT, and fMRI have now become the most commonly adopted methods for the pre-surgical localization and examination of refractory epilepsy. A comparative study was performed between ASL and ^{18}F-fluorodeoxyglucose (FDG) PET with respect to the localization of epileptogenic foci in patients with refractory neocortical epilepsy, which revealed that ASL showed a good agreement with ^{18}F-FDG PET (κ = 0.84) and can therefore be implemented in the pre-surgical localization of epileptogenic foci in patients with refractory neocortical epilepsy. Using the bilateral hippocampal head, amygdala, and MTL of TLE patients (with and without MTL atrophy) as regions of interest (ROIs), a team of Chinese researchers applied ASL to measure the rCBF of these regions and calculate their asymmetry indices (AI). Their results revealed statistically significant differences in rCBF and AI between epilepsy patients with and without MTL atrophy, which can assist the pre-surgical localization of epileptogenic foci. These findings, therefore, suggest that ASL can be combined with other imaging techniques to improve the accuracy of the lateralization and localization of epileptogenic foci.

Another advantage of utilizing ASL to assess cerebral perfusion in epilepsy is that it can be performed during the preictal, ictal, and postictal periods. In the first study to utilize 3.0 Tesla (T) MR ASL for the dynamic observation of CBF changes in the epileptogenic foci, ASL scan performed immediately after seizure onset showed increased CBF in the right parieto-occipital cortex, whereas ASL repeated 1 week later revealed hypoperfusion in the same region. This study has demonstrated that ASL can be utilized for the routine dynamic examination of CBF changes in patients with epilepsy. The results of a Chinese study including 48 patients with medial TLE, in which ASL was performed to study the correlation between temporal CBF and disease duration, showed that CBF was negatively correlated with disease duration; that is, a longer onset time was accompanied by lower temporal CBF in the affected side.

The basic and clinical studies above all demonstrated that ASL can present changes in whole-brain perfusion and limited perfusion parameters in patients with epilepsy. Furthermore, it can serve as a valuable reference for the lateralization and localization of epileptogenic foci, and provide new imaging evidence for understanding the pathophysiological mechanisms of epilepsy.

10.1.5 Research Applications of Blood-Oxygen-Level-Dependent (BOLD) Imaging in Refractory Epilepsy

10.1.5.1 Research Applications of Task-Based fMRI in Epilepsy

In the clinical diagnosis and treatment of epilepsy, surgical planning, which includes the pre-surgical localization and post-surgical functional assessment of brain areas such as the primary motor cortex, supplementary motor cortex, and language areas, is primarily performed using task-based fMRI. Task-based fMRI, whether 1.5 or 3 T, has significant clinical value in displaying somatosensory- and perception-related brain activation areas, as well as the pre-surgical localization of the Broca's and Wernicke's language areas. Task-based fMRI revealed that brain activation levels during the execution of motor tasks were higher than that during language tasks, and the changes in motor area activation were less affected by factors of magnetic field strength. Furthermore, higher activation rates were produced when the same language task was performed in a 3.0 T than a 1.5 T scanner.

The lateralization of language dominance is a crucial component of pre-surgical assessment in TLE. Although the Wada test is considered the gold standard for language lateralization in clinical settings, it is an invasive test with a certain level of operational risk, which has therefore restricted its widespread clinical application. Studies have found that fMRI shows a good agreement with the Wada test in the determination of language laterality, with the benefit of being non-invasive, having good reproducibility, and providing more comprehensive spatial localization information. Post-surgical memory decline is a common complication in TLE. fMRI studies involving memory tasks demonstrated that patients without frontal lobe activation during pre-surgical memory tasks showed a significant decline in post-surgical memory function, whereas those with pre-surgical frontal lobe activation showed relatively well-preserved post-surgical memory function. These findings imply that memory not only depends on functional changes in the hippocampus alone but also involves a memory circuit composed of multiple brain structures, in which the frontal lobe plays a crucial role. Additionally, task-based fMRI has also revealed that when performing task encoding, left TLE patients with stronger left hippocampal activation showed better verbal memory, whereas right TLE patients with stronger right hippocampal activation showed better visual memory. Therefore, the involvement of different hippocampal hemispheres is related to the different patterns of memory deficits.

A task-based fMRI study involving patients with juvenile myoclonic epilepsy found that as the difficulty of cognitive tasks increased, the strength of the functional coupling between the motor cortex and cognitive areas in the frontal and parietal lobes increased as well, facilitating the interregional spread of epileptic discharges. These results suggest that changes in the functional connectivity (FC) of patients with juvenile myoclonic epilepsy may be the underlying basis for the occurrence of motor symptoms induced by emotional or cognitive abnormalities. Moreover, EEG studies have also confirmed that cognitive tasks had the strongest effect on inducing epileptiform discharges or myoclonic seizures.

There are several drawbacks to task-based fMRI. It requires the patient to perform tasks according to specific experimental design requirements, which implies that the reliability of fMRI findings depends on the patient's ability to complete these tasks. This poses a significant challenge to patients with neurological dysfunction, which may lead to heterogeneity in task execution, thereby affecting the accuracy and reproducibility of the fMRI findings. Furthermore, the patient may be required to repeat the task a number of times in order to obtain the desired activation maps, which increases their scan time. Another drawback of task-based fMRI is the need to design different tasks (e.g., motor or language tasks) for the evaluation of different clinical functions, which is relatively complicated when it is implemented in clinical settings. These factors have, to some extent, hindered the widespread clinical application of task-based fMRI in epilepsy.

10.1.5.2 Applications of RS-fMRI in Epilepsy

Compared to task-based fMRI, RS-fMRI involves simpler and more convenient to perform and has therefore been more widely adopted in clinical research. TLE is the most common form of refractory epilepsy, and also the most commonly treated with surgery. The main goal of surgery is to control epileptic seizures. The precise and accurate localization of epileptogenic foci determines whether a patient is indicated for surgery, as well as the success or failure of surgical treatment. Approximately 30% of patients with refractory TLE are unable to receive surgical treatment due to the ambiguous localization of epileptogenic foci. MRI is considered to be the optimal approach for the non-invasive localization of epileptogenic foci. High-resolution sMRI plays a key role in the detection of epileptogenic foci, but some patients may present with contradictory MRI and VEEG or EEG findings, making it difficult to determine whether the abnormal brain signals detected using MRI are epileptogenic foci or structural changes secondary to epilepsy. Moreover, epileptic foci cannot be displayed using sMRI in 30–40% of patients, which is yet another limitation of sMRI in the pre-surgical assessment of epilepsy. The current opinion is that TLE is a disease that generally involves brain areas beyond the temporal lobe and is related to abnormalities in the brain network. In a series of RS-fMRI studies conducted on LE, it was found that in patients with unilateral TLE, the epileptogenic side of the MTL showed increased amplitude of low-frequency fluctuation (ALFF), and the extent of increase was positively correlated with the number of ipsilateral spikes as recorded by EEG-fMRI. Therefore, it was speculated that ALFF could serve as an indicator of TLE spiking, and in turn be indirectly applied to TLE lateralization. Studies on regional homogeneity (ReHo) have also found increased ReHo values in epileptogenic foci in the medial TLE. In FC studies based on RS-fMRI, TLE epileptogenic foci showed decreased FC with the ipsilateral hemisphere, and increased FC with the unaffected (contralateral) hemisphere, suggesting that brain activity in TLE is lateralized in the resting state. RS-FC studies on unilateral TLE further confirmed the presence of laterality, manifesting as more significant changes in the FC between the hippocampus on the epileptogenic side with the ipsilateral hemisphere. The combination of machine learning with RS-fMRI can facilitate the accurate lateralization of TLE, achieving an accuracy of 83% in the predictive classification of TLE lateralization when ALFF, fractional ALFF (fALFF), ReHo, and FC matrix were selected as classification features.

TLE laterality is useful for predicting the prognosis of surgery for epilepsy. Compared to post-surgical recurrence-free group, the recurrence group showed weaker FC laterality. Brain network analysis based on independent component analysis (ICA) revealed that the alleviation of seizures in TLE after surgery may be due to the surgical disruption of abnormal FC between the frontoparietal network and the sensorimotor and salience networks on the epileptogenic side. Therefore, the weakening of abnormal internetwork connectivity blocked the main transmission pathway of epilepsy (Fig. 10.5). Furthermore, the FC between the DMN and executive control

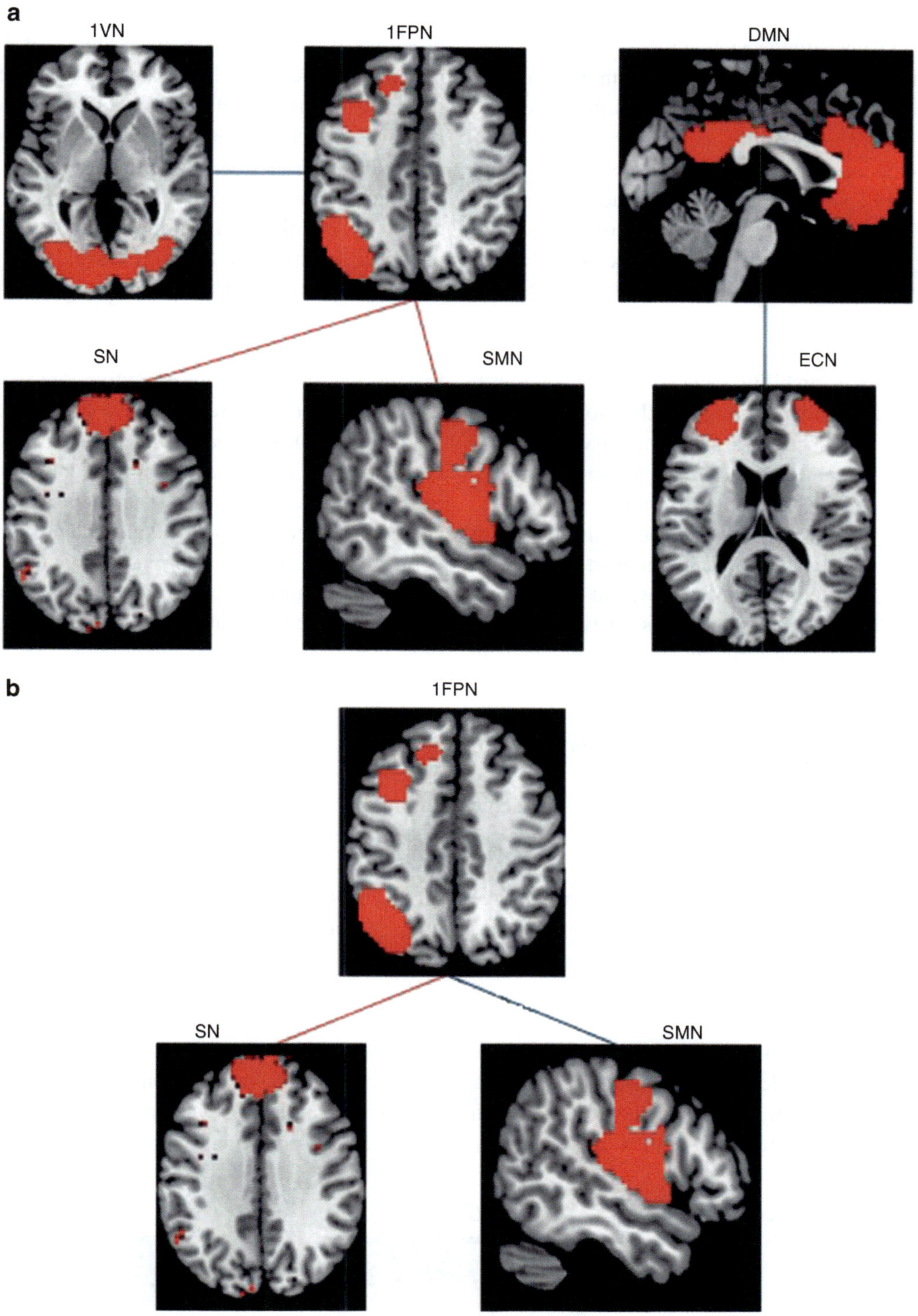

Fig. 10.5 Differences in the resting-state functional connectivity between brain networks before and after surgery in TLE. Comparison of resting-state brain network connectivity between patients with left TLE and healthy controls (**a**). Comparison of resting-state brain network connectivity before and after surgery in patients with left TLE (**b**). Red lines represent increases in FC and blue lines represent decreases in FC. *lVN* lateral visual network, *lFPN* left frontoparietal network, *SN* salience network, *SMN* sensorimotor network, *ECN* executive control network

network showed a significant positive correlation with visuospatial/executive function.

Cognitive impairment is a common complication of epilepsy that has a serious impact on the patient's quality of life, and its hazards are equivalent to, or may even exceed, those brought about by epilepsy itself. Possible mechanisms of epilepsy-induced cognitive impairment include: (1) the destruction of synaptic connections between neurons due to ictal and interictal epileptiform discharges, resulting in irreversible damage to cerebral fiber bundles; (2) changes in neuronal excitability induced by the long-term use of anti-epileptic drugs, leading to nerve damaged, (3) reduction in white matter volume; and (4) abnormal number of serotonin (5-HT) receptors and/or 5-HT receptor dysfunction.

Cognitive functions are accomplished based on the coordination of functional networks composed of different brain regions, and the destruction of normal connections between brain networks by long-term epileptic discharges may be the neural mechanism underpinning the impairment of higher-level cognitive function. The classical models related to memory changes in TLE include the functional reserve model of the hippocampus ipsilateral to the epileptogenic foci and the functional compensation model of the contralateral hippocampus. However, changes in the hippocampus alone cannot explain the variability in memory outcomes after hippocampal resection. Studies on memory function have implicated a memory circuit that is based on the coordination of multiple brain structures and is inextricably linked with the laterality of TLE. One RS-fMRI study demonstrated that TLE patients showed abnormal activity in the frontal region (including the prefrontal cortex and language areas), and this activity was closely related to the executive function and language ability of TLE patients. Furthermore, TLE patients with memory impairment exhibit decreased intra-network FC in the executive control network and abnormal prefrontal function, suggesting that the executive control network plays a pivotal role in the onset of cognitive impairment among TLE patients. Additionally, ICA revealed that the executive function of TLE patients was positively correlated with the FC between the DMN and executive control network (Fig. 10.5), implying that the abnormal FC of the executive control network is another cause for executive dysfunction.

In studies on seed-based functional/structural connectivity, TLE patients with executive dysfunction showed abnormal functional/structural connectivity between the thalamus and prefrontal cortex on the epileptogenic side, although the strength of abnormal connectivity was not correlated with executive function scores. These findings indicate that the alterations in the thalamic-prefrontal pathway may be compensatory changes in the transmission pathways of abnormal epileptic discharges (Fig. 10.6). Moreover, RS-fMRI has demonstrated that the various memory patterns in TLE involve different brain structures. More specifically, verbal memory is negatively correlated with the FC strength of the ipsilateral MTL and posterior cingulate gyrus, whereas non-verbal memory is positively correlated with the FC strength of the contralateral MTL and medial frontal cortex. Another study found that in patients with TLE, the extent of FC increase between the hippocampus on the epileptogenic side and the contralateral cerebral hemispheric structures was positively correlated with memory performance, suggesting that this

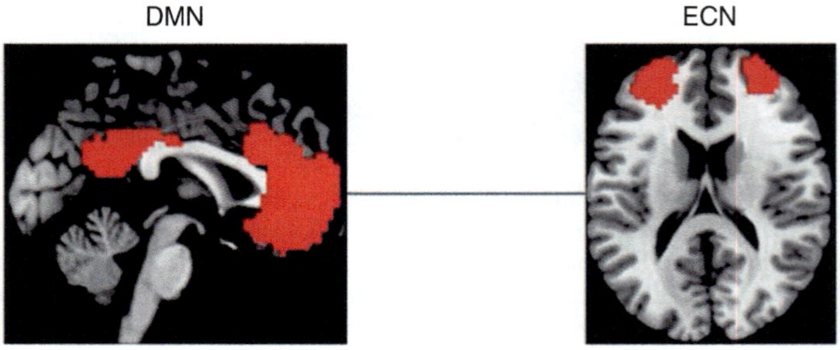

Fig. 10.6 Differences between TLE patients with and without executive control dysfunction. Projection images of the DMN and ECM onto 3D brain templates; *ECN* executive control network

increase in FC may serve as a possible compensatory pathway for maintaining memory function. Additionally, episodic memory performance in TLE was found to be closely associated with FC within the DMN, while patients with lower FCs also showed poorer memory performance. The sensorimotor network is an important network affected by epileptic discharges and is involved in a wide range of cognitive circuits. fMRI studies have shown that the FC of the sensorimotor network with the prefrontal network is essential for the maintenance of human working memory performance, while its FC with the visual network plays a crucial role in maintaining high-level visual functions.

RS-fMRI results revealed that patients suffering from epilepsy with generalized tonic-clonic seizure (GTCS) also showed suppressed DMN activity, while epileptic discharges led to FC decreases within the DMN, and patients exhibited impairments in cognitive behavior, abstract reasoning, planning, and thinking skills. Another study found that regions with RS-FC reductions within the DMN included the ventral prefrontal cortex, precuneus, posterior cingulate cortex (PCC), and inferior temporal gyrus, while these reductions were also significantly negatively associated with the patient's disease duration. Furthermore, the FC among resting-state networks, such as the decreased FC between the DMN and attentional network, may also give rise to cognitive impairments in patients with GTCS.

In TLE, the decreased ALFF of the DMN is consistent with the results of EEG-fMRI showing the "suspension" of the DMN. Patients with GTCS also exhibited reduced ReHo values in the DMN, implying that the spontaneous activity of the DMN in the resting state was suspended due to the increase in epileptic activity. During the interictal period, patients with GTCS showed an asymmetric distribution in ALFF increase, which was primarily observed in the bilateral thalamus, basal ganglia, insula, cerebellum, and anterior cingulate cortex (ACC); whereas regions with ALFF decrease primarily include the bilateral precuneus, medial prefrontal cortex and PCC. Moreover, the seizure frequency of patients with GTCS is positively associated with the ALFF of the bilateral thalamus and cerebellum and negatively associated with the medial prefrontal lobe, left precuneus, PCC, and bilateral occipital cortex. These findings indicate extensive abnormalities can be observed in the brain activities of patients with GTCS.

Differences in FC patterns have been observed between left and right TLE. Patients with left TLE show FC reductions in the bilateral hippocampus and PCC, whereas those with right TLE show FC reductions in the right hippocampus and PCC. Moreover, patients with left TLE exhibit more significant FC reductions involving more extensive brain areas, which may explain why patients with left TLE are more prone to cognitive impairment. Approximately one-third of epilepsy patients exhibit co-existing deactivations and activations. RS-fMRI studies indicate that deactivations are commonly distributed in the DMN, reflecting the fact that abnormal discharges during the interictal period can cause the "disruption and suspension" of the DMN in patients with epilepsy. The DMN function of patients with GTCS is significantly affected during the interictal period. Large-scale brain network analysis found that compared with healthy controls, patients showed increased topological properties at nodes in the middle frontal gyrus, lentiform nucleus, thalamus, and amygdala, whereas nodes in the DMN (including the PCC and inferior temporal gyrus) showed decreased topological properties, as well as reduced coupling between functional structures. Additionally, the FC within the sensorimotor network, visual network, auditory network, DMN, and dorsal attention network had all decreased by varying extents. The strength of DMN FC in patients with GTCS is closely related to the patient's age and disease duration. Decreased coupling was observed in the functional-structural networks within the DMN, and the degree of coupling was negatively correlated with the patient's disease duration. Therefore, this decoupling between the functional and structural networks may reflect the course of long-term brain damage or could serve as a potential feature for the more accurate detection of brain abnormalities in epilepsy.

In patients with GTCS, DMN activity is significantly reduced during the interictal period, and DMN activity is inhibited during epileptic discharges, which may be an important factor for the absence of seizures in these patients. Studies have suggested that the thalamus may be related to the spread of generalized spike-and-slow wave discharges in absence epilepsy, while the functional inhibition of DMN-related brain areas, including the frontal lobe and parietal lobe, may be associated with the loss of consciousness during absence seizures. Furthermore, EEG studies have demonstrated that pediatric patients with absence epilepsy showed no significant changes in the small-world properties of their brain networks during the preictal, ictal, and postictal periods. Instead, their overall network topology tended to be randomized during the postictal period, and the FC network involved in absence epilepsy underwent rapid reconstruction.

At present, fMRI techniques have been implemented in the pre-surgical planning of, as well as in research on the underlying brain mechanisms and related complications of epilepsy. However, owing to our current incomplete understanding on the pathogenic mechanisms of epilepsy, and the existing limitations of imaging methods, there is still much room for improvement with respect to the application of functional imaging in clinical practice. We believe that the continuous innovations in both the software and hardware of MRI, especially the combination of new MRI techniques with EEG and artificial intelligence, will bring about significant advances in epilepsy research and enhance the clinical value of these imaging techniques in epilepsy.

10.2 Research Applications of PET Imaging in Epilepsy

PET is a type of computed tomography imaging based on positron emission and is a non-invasive method of molecular imaging. It plays a crucial role in the clinical diagnosis and research applications of epilepsy. As a form of functional metabolic imaging, PET of the brain can reveal the metabolism, oxygen consumption, and perfusion of epileptic foci. With the continuous improvements in equipment and molecular probes, PET imaging has gradually taken its place as one of the indispensable methods in clinical practice for the localization of epileptic foci, as well as the pre- and post-surgical assessment of epilepsy.

10.2.1 PET Findings of Epilepsy

Glucose is the primary source of energy in the brain, and glucose metabolism is intimately related to neuronal activity. ^{18}F-FDG is a common tracer utilized in PET scans for epilepsy and is primarily used to evaluate the glucose metabolism of synaptic and neuronal activity in the brain. ^{18}F-FDG is transported via glucose transporters from the blood into the cell, where it is phosphorylated by hexokinase to form ^{18}F-FDG-6-phosphate. Further metabolism of ^{18}F-FDG-6-phosphate is limited, implying that this molecule is essentially trapped within the cell. A typical ^{18}F-FDG PET finding during the interictal period is the reduced radioactive uptake of the epileptogenic foci (Fig. 10.7a), and the causes for this hypometabolism include the loss of neurons, loss of neural connections, and decreased synaptic density. Hypometabolism in the epileptogenic foci may be related to the duration, frequency, and severity of epileptic seizures. During the ictal period, the elevated metabolism and blood flow of brain tissues is manifested in ^{18}F-FDG PET imaging as increased radioactive uptake in the epileptogenic foci. However, the majority of epileptic seizures occur unpredictably and persist only for a short duration, causing difficulties in conducting ictal PET imaging. In addition to the epileptogenic foci, PET imaging may sometimes reveal hypometabolism at remote brain areas, known as "diaschisis," such as the hypometabolism of the ipsilateral thalamus and contralateral cerebellum. Contralateral cerebellar hypometabolism (i.e., "crossed cerebellar diaschisis") is more commonly observed in epilepsy patients whose primary epileptogenic foci are located in the frontal or parietal lobe (Fig. 10.7b), whereas ipsilateral thalamic hypometabolism usually occurs in patients with frontal or parietal lobe

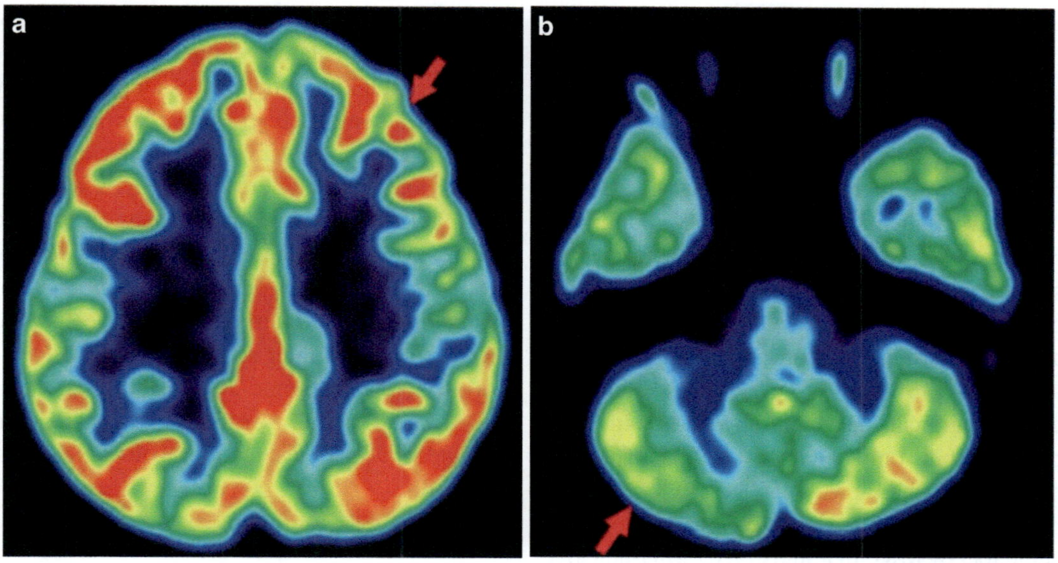

Fig. 10.7 Interictal ^{18}F-FDG PET imaging of epilepsy patients. A 26-year-old female patient who suffered from paroxysmal limb stiffness for 20 years. The patient underwent focal resection for epilepsy, and post-surgical pathology showed focal cortical dysplasia in the left frontal lobe. Pre-surgical interictal ^{18}F-FDG PET shows hypometabolism in the left frontal lobe (**a**, arrow) and right cerebellum (**b**, arrow)

epilepsy, with hypometabolism in the dorsal thalamus showing an especially close association with epileptogenic foci in the MTL. Hypometabolism may, occasionally, occur in the symmetrical area on the contralateral side, reflecting the functional inhibition of these regions under hippocampal symmetry via the corpus callosum (callosal disconnection) or fornix.

10.2.2 Research Applications of PET in the Pre-Surgical Localization of Epilepsy

The conventional treatment for epilepsy is drug therapy. However, in 20–30% of patients, epileptic seizures cannot be controlled using medication, and this condition is known as refractory epilepsy. For such patients, surgical treatment is an effective means by which to control seizures, and the key to its effectiveness is the pre-surgical assessment of epileptogenic foci. The foundation of pre-surgical evaluation is the identification of an independent epileptogenic zone, the resection of which can fully control epileptic seizures without causing any unacceptable loss of nerve function. Despite the significant improvements in the sensitivity of MRI techniques in detecting microstructural abnormalities, there is still a large proportion (~20%) of epilepsy patients in whom lesions cannot be detected using MRI. As a metabolic imaging method, ^{18}F-FDG PET can effectively make up for the deficiencies of MRI and is particularly suitable for MRI-negative epilepsy patients.

Over the past 20 years, ^{18}F-FDG PET has played a vital role in the lateralization and/or localization of MRI-negative patients with focal epilepsy. For TLE, the sensitivity of ^{18}F-FDG PET in the localization of epileptogenic foci is 85–90%. However, for extratemporal lobe epilepsy (ETLE), the localization sensitivity of ^{18}F-FDG PET is 38–55%, showing the highest sensitivity for frontal lobe epilepsy (45–90%, but generally about 55%), and a very low sensitivity for occipital lobe epilepsy. Menon et al. performed pre-surgical evaluation on 117 epilepsy patients using ^{18}F-FDG PET and found that the localization accuracy for TLE patients was 78.0%, whereas that for ETLE was only 28.6%. With respect to the ^{18}F-FDG PET lateralization of epileptic foci, lateralization error only occurred in 1–3% of patients with refractory TLE, whereas only 67% of ETLE patients showed interictal hypometabolic regions that concorded with those during the ictal period, and the hypermetabolic regions generally exhibited extensive temporal lobe involvement. Another study found that 68.8% of TLE patients benefitted from pre-surgical evaluation using ^{18}F-FDG PET, while only 23.3% of ETLE patients benefitted from this approach. Among MRI-negative patients, pre-surgical ^{18}F-FDG PET evaluation effectively altered surgical decisions in 85.4% of TLE patients, but only affected 33.3% of ETLE patients. Furthermore, ^{18}F-FDG PET can also help to enhance the detection rate of epileptogenic foci by MRI. In a study on 67 MRI-negative patients with ETLE, 68.6% of patients showed positive findings in ^{18}F-FDG PET imaging performed during the same period as MRI, while the reinterpretation of MRI findings under the guidance of ^{18}F-FDG PET led to the detection of lesions in 58.2% of patients.

^{18}F-FDG PET has a high sensitivity but low specificity for the localization of epileptogenic foci. The extent of hypermetabolism detected using interictal imaging is often larger than that of the epileptogenic foci, that is, hypometabolism can be detected in both the epileptogenic cortex and other cortical areas. Therefore, at this point, it becomes necessary to comprehensively analyze the significance of ^{18}F-FDG PET findings in conjunction with the results of VEEG. The frequent interictal epileptiform discharges (IEDs) of TLE patients alter the metabolism of extratemporal brain tissues. Furthermore, ETLE patients may also present with abnormal temporal discharges and clinical symptoms (e.g., involuntary movements) related to the temporal lobe, while frequently exhibiting functional abnormalities in brain areas remote to the epileptogenic zone, rather than those corresponding to the primary epileptogenic foci. These alterations may be related to the changes in the inhibitory effects exerted on the areas surrounding the seizure onset zone. Hartl et al. examined 63 patients with ETLE and found that cortical hypometabolism beyond the epileptogenic zone was closely related to the symptoms of epileptic seizures, often accompanied by IEDs in the corresponding cortical area. Ipsilateral temporal hypometabolism in frontal lobe epilepsy was most commonly observed among these patients. The study also found that 87.5% of ETLE patients exhibited TLE symptoms, EEG temporal IEDs and ^{18}F-FDG PET temporal hypometabolism, as opposed to only 31.0% of ETLE patients who did not exhibit temporal IEDs and temporal hypometabolism. In sum, the interpretation of pre-surgical PET findings and their significance to the localization of epileptogenic zones should be combined with EEG results, especially in MRI-negative patients, in order to avoid localization errors.

10.2.3 Research Applications of PET in the Prognostic Evaluation of Epilepsy Surgery

^{18}F-FDG PET can also be implemented in the evaluation of surgical prognosis among patients with epilepsy. TLE patients with lower temporal lobe metabolism tended to exhibit more effective post-surgical seizure control. Furthermore, thalamic metabolism was found to be an independent predictor of post-surgical outcome in TLE, whereby poor surgical prognosis was associated with contralateral thalamic hypometabolism, but not ipsilateral thalamic hypometabolism or the absence of thalamic hypometabolism. However, other studies have reported that ^{18}F-FDG PET findings were not associated with post-surgical outcomes. The variability of these results may be related to the differences in the subjects enrolled, equipment resolution, and methods of imaging analysis. In contrast, a more definite finding is that post-surgical recovery is related to the extent of hypometabolic involvement. In a long-term follow-up study of 97 patients with medial TLE (mean follow-up >6 years), Chassoux et al. demonstrated that ^{18}F-FDG PET was able to predict post-surgical outcomes. More specifically, ^{18}F-FDG PET imaging of patients who achieved complete recovery (Engel class IA) only revealed focal anteromedial temporal hypometabolism; patients with suboptimal recovery (Engel class IB–D and II) showed focal anteromedial temporal hypometabolism, together with some areas of extratemporal hypometabolism, whereas patients with the poorest recovery (Engel class III and IV) presented with bilateral hippocampal and extensive extratemporal hypometabolism. Despite these findings, further explorations are needed to identify effective predictors for whether individual patients will be seizure-free after surgical treatment. It may be possible to discover more comprehensive predictors of surgical outcome by utilizing multi-modal imaging data.

Additionally, ^{18}F-FDG PET can provide other important prognostic information. For example, in patients with unilateral TLE, bilateral temporal hypometabolism was found to be associated with memory impairment, while prefrontal hypometabolism was related to impaired executive function. Similarly, ipsilateral insular hypometabolism was found to be associated with affective and somatosensory symptoms, while hypometabolism in the bilateral lateral temporal lobes and bilateral medial frontal lobes was related to interictal aggression, which may be due to the removal of inhibitory effects from the MTL neocortex (or the medial PFC).

10.2.4 Others

In addition to ^{18}F-FDG, tracers for other metabolic pathways, receptors, and histamine can also be utilized in epilepsy imaging. For example, ^{11}C-FMZ, an imaging agent for benzodiazepine receptors, is able to bind specifically to the α subunit of the $GABA_A$ benzodiazepine receptor and is especially suitable for medial TLE patients with HS. Compared to ^{18}F-FDG, ^{11}C-FMZ shows lower cortical metabolism and clearer hippocampal imaging. 5-HT is an inhibitory neurotransmitter of the central and peripheral nervous systems that is closely connected to epileptic seizures. Imaging agents for 5-HT receptors are mostly distributed in the limbic system, hippocampus, amygdala, temporal pole, and insula; these agents are suitable for the diagnosis of epileptogenic foci in patients with TLE. Metabotropic glutamate receptor 5 (mGluR5) is a postsynaptic G-protein coupled receptor that is predominantly expressed around the postsynaptic sites of neurons and astrocytes. Imaging agents for mGluR5 are primarily utilized for the diagnosis of epileptogenic foci in patients with TLE. Compared to ^{18}F-FDG, mGluR5 tracers can more easily detect HS in patients.

With the advancement of molecular probe technology, researchers have begun to explore the relationship between ^{18}F-FDG PET metabolism and the imaging of other biomarkers in patients with epilepsy. In a study that examined the relationship between the glucose metabolism and glutamate concentration of multiple brain areas in 11 epilepsy patients, the results revealed the hypometabolism of both glucose and glutamate in the epileptogenic zones during the interictal period, but the hypermetabolism of the two during the ictal period. Moreover, correlation analysis showed that there were significant positive correlations between glucose and glutamate metabolism in both epileptogenic and non-epileptogenic zones; but no significant correlations were found between glucose metabolism and $GABA_A$ receptor binding within the scope of whole-brain gray matter. Additionally, glucose metabolism was not significantly correlated to the ReHo and ALFF as measured by RS-fMRI within the scope of whole-brain gray matter.

In summary, although ^{18}F-FDG PET can make up for the many shortcomings of localizing epileptogenic foci in MRI-negative patients, this technique has poor spatial resolution. Therefore, the combination of ^{18}F-FDG PET with MRI not only enhances the spatial resolution of localizing epileptogenic foci but also improves the detection rate of microstructural abnormalities. Therefore, the application of integrated PET/MR will usher in greater benefits to the clinical diagnosis and treatment of epilepsy.

10.3 Research Applications of PET/MR in Epilepsy

The rapid development of novel PET tracers and multimodal MRI, together with the establishment of normative brain databases, have led to substantial improvements of PET/MR in the presurgical localization and efficacy evaluation of epilepsy. The most commonly used PET tracer currently is ^{18}F-FDG, providing parameters such as glucose metabolic rate and standardized uptake value (SUV) that can be utilized in the pre-surgical localization of epilepsy. Integrated PET/MR involves the simultaneous acquisition of PET and MRI signals, in order to achieve the true synchronization of information between the two imaging modalities. This approach combines the high sensitivity of PET metabolism with the high spatial resolution of MRI, thereby offering a novel platform and perspective for the surgical resection of epileptic foci and research on epileptic networks.

10.3.1 Application of Integrated PET/MR in Epilepsy Surgery

MRI is the preferred technique for the pre-surgical localization of epileptic foci in patients with refractory epilepsy. However, no abnormalities are detected in the MRI scans of 30–40% of patients. Since ^{18}F-FDG PET has a higher sensitivity for pre-surgical localization in epilepsy, it is especially useful for the lateralization and localization of MRI-negative patients or patients with discordant MRI and ictal EEG findings. Conversely, due to the poor spatial resolution of ^{18}F-FDG PET, it has poor accuracy in anatomical localization. Therefore, ^{18}F-FDG PET/MR co-registration is now indispensable to the clinical pre-surgical evaluation of epilepsy. A number of studies have found that this approach can improve the prognosis of 86% of patients, whereas among patients in the same follow-up period who did not undergo fusion imaging, only 30–76% showed good post-surgical outcomes.

Salamon et al. demonstrated that the application of pre-surgical ^{18}F-FDG PET/MR co-registration can improve the detection rate of focal cortical dysplasia (FCD), especially in patients with FCD type I or negative MRI findings. Furthermore, it reduces the need for intracranial electrode implantation and plays a crucial role in pre-surgical non-invasive localization and accurate surgical planning. In a study on FCD type II, ^{18}F-FDG PET or MRI alone could only detect lesions in 44% or 59% of patients, respectively, whereas the integration of the two increased the detection rate to 83%. In a study on patients with MRI-negative ETLE, Ding et al. utilized ^{18}F-FDG PET/MR co-registration to guide the re-interpretation of MR images. They found that among patients whose initial MRI findings indicated subtle abnormalities or non-specific abnormalities, 58.2% were identified as epileptogenic foci after image co-registration. This change meant that the ETLE patients were more likely to receive surgical treatment, and 88% of patients had good prognosis. Their results also showed that the sensitivity of fusion imaging for detecting extratemporal hypometabolic foci was 94%, which was much higher than that of ^{18}F-FDG PET alone (68.6%). Therefore, co-registration with high-resolution MRI could improve the spatial resolution of PET imaging, and increase the likelihood of detecting epileptogenic foci. Taken together, these findings indicate that pre-surgical ^{18}F-FDG PET/MR co-registration can significantly enhance the detection of epileptogenic foci and further guide decision-making in clinical treatments, thereby improving patient prognosis.

At present, only a handful of integrated PET/MR studies have been conducted on epilepsy, and all of them have small sample sizes. Garibotto et al. were the first to report the clinical value of applying integrated PET/MR in neurological diseases, and their study included six patients with epilepsy. Based on their findings, they concluded that using integrated PET/MR for the simultaneous acquisition of PET and MRI information in a single scan session can minimize patient discomfort while maximizing clinical information. Another study compared the SUV and AI between 11 epilepsy patients and six healthy controls across 117 brain regions (96 cortical and 21 subcortical regions). Their results revealed that epilepsy patients showed hypermetabolism in the bilateral postcentral gyri and hypometabolism in the right temporal pole, while AI led to the detection of more regions with bilateral metabolic asymmetry, showing an agreement of 96.2% with SUV. Therefore, they concluded that as a novel, non-invasive imaging method, PET/MR plays a crucial role in the evaluation of epilepsy patients, and can facilitate the etiological research on the pathogenesis of epilepsy. Shin et al. performed a pilot study to assess the value of integrated PET/MR in the pre-surgical localization of refractory epilepsy. By comparing the accuracy of integrated PET/MR in pre-surgical localization with that of 3.0 T MRI and ^{18}F-FDG PET, they found that integrated PET/MR could increase the detection rate of potential epileptogenic foci. As the number of cases increased and post-surgical follow-up progressed, they found that integrated PET/MR had a relatively high sensitivity (78–82%) for detecting potential lesions, which was higher than that of MRI (71–77%) or PET (68–71%) alone. Furthermore, among the 27 patients who underwent surgical treatment, 24 entered remission after surgery, demonstrating that PET/MR is the most sensitive imaging technique for detecting epileptogenic foci and that the complete resection of epileptogenic foci can help to control epileptic seizures. As for studies on the pre-surgical localization of epileptogenic foci in children, Paldino et al. compared the diagnostic accuracy of PET/MR and PET/CT, and despite adopting different attenuation correction methods for ^{18}F-FDG PET images, there were no significant differences in the image quality obtained between the two imaging modalities. ^{18}F-FDG PET images acquired using MRI-based attenuation correction were not superior to those acquired using CT-based attenuation correction with respect to the accuracy of localizing epileptic foci in pediatric patients. However, PET/MR involves a significantly lower radiation dose than PET/CT, and can therefore be adopted as an alternative tool for pre-surgical localization in pediatric patients with epilepsy.

Increased rCBF has been observed during the ictal period, whereas rCBF is decreased during the interictal period. ASL is a non-invasive imaging method based on MR perfusion imaging that can be used to evaluate interictal cerebral perfusion. Boscolo et al. assessed the value of integrated PET/MR in the localization of 20 patients with MRI-negative epilepsy and compared the findings with the epileptogenic foci based on the comprehensive localization by a multidisciplinary clinical team. ASL perfusion information and ^{18}F-FDG PET metabolic information showed high concordance on lateralization and localization, while the addition of bilateral CBF and metabolic AI information significantly improved the detection rate of lesions and increased the diagnostic confidence of physicians. Similarly, Wang et al. utilized ^{18}F-FDG PET/MR to simultaneously acquire ASL and PET data from 12 patients with pure unilateral medial TLE. Their results showed high concordance between the regions of hypoperfusion detected using ASL and the epileptogenic foci localized using SEEG, while a significant correlation was also observed between hypoperfusion and hypometabolism. Their findings suggest that ASL can serve as a reliable, non-invasive, radiation-free pre-surgical diagnostic method. On the basis of these results, the authors of this textbook have also conducted further investigations on the pre-surgical localization of epileptogenic foci by combining CBF with metabolic information. Our study involved 20 patients with MRI-negative TLE, who underwent pre-surgical ^{18}F-FDG PET/MR for the localization of epileptogenic foci, and the findings were compared with the post-surgical pathological results. In 12 of the 20 patients, focal localization by PET and ASL was concordant with pathological results (Figs. 10.8 and 10.9); in 6 patients, ASL findings were negative but epileptogenic foci could be detected using PET; in 2 patients, no abnormalities were detected or lateralization was not possible using PET, whereas focal localization could be achieved using ASL. Analysis of the receiver operating characteristic (ROC) curves indicated that utilizing PET or ASL alone gave a sensitivity and specificity of 100 and 81.8%, or 83.3 and 54.4%, respectively, whereas the combination of the two gave a sensitivity and specificity of 100 and 90.9%, respectively. These findings have once again validated the claim that the combination of PET and ASL can significantly enhance the accuracy and specificity of focal localization in MRI-negative TLE.

In another study, PET data and ASL-derived AI were utilized to perform a comparative analysis between patients and healthy controls, which revealed that regions of metabolic and CBF asymmetry were highly concordant with patho-

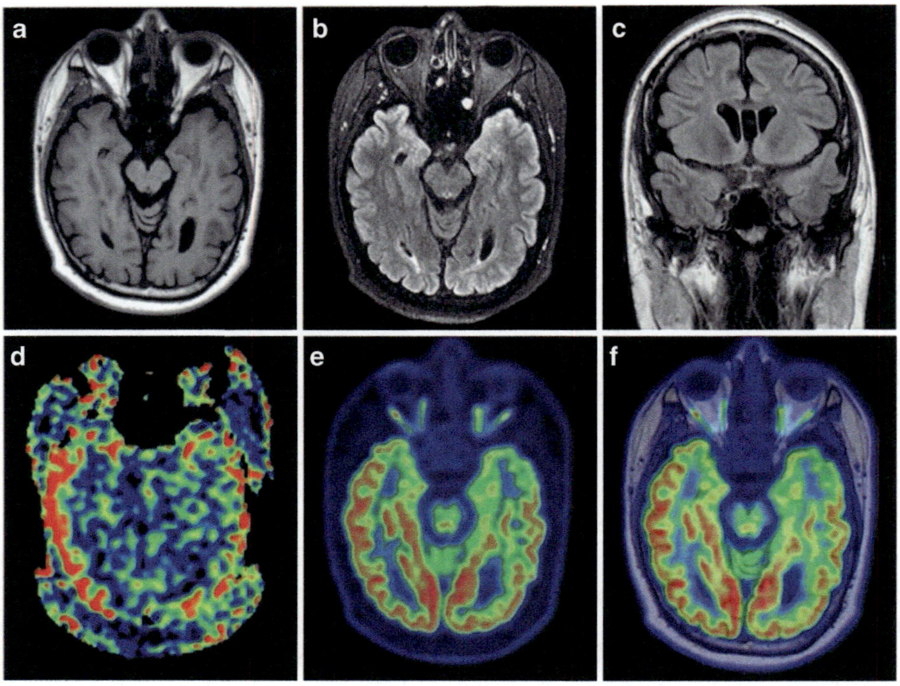

Fig. 10.8 ^{18}F-FDG PET/MR of epilepsy patient. A 17-year-old male patient suffering from recurrent seizures with loss of consciousness for more than 16 years. Transverse T_1-weighted MRI (**a**), T_2-FLAIR (**b**), and coronal T_2-FLAIR (**c**) show no significant abnormalities. ASL shows lower perfusion in the left temporal lobe compared to the right (**d**), while transverse ^{18}F-FDG PET (**e**) and integrated ^{18}F-FDG PET/MR (**f**) show lower glucose metabolism in the left temporal lobe compared to the right. Post-surgical pathology shows FDC type I of the left temporal lobe

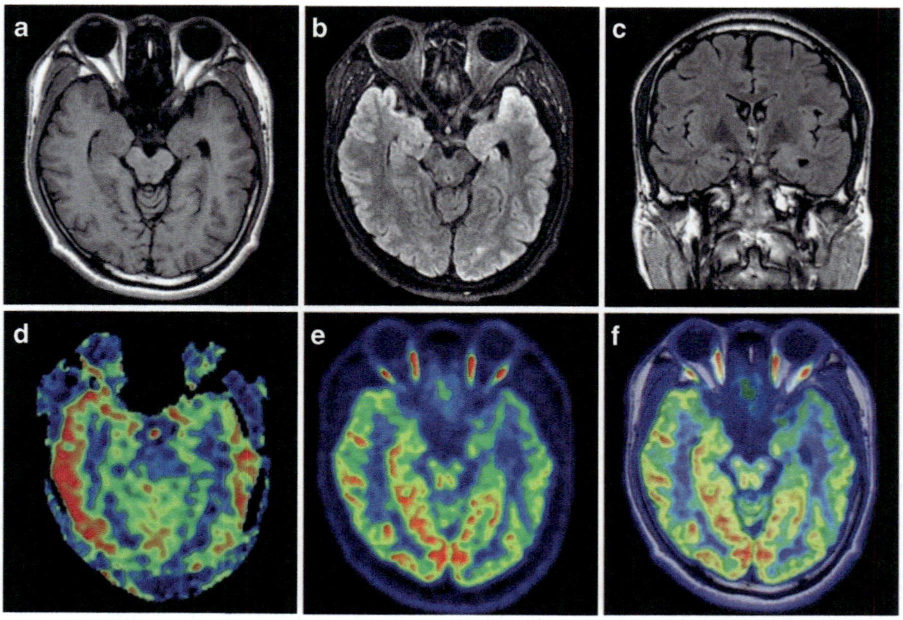

Fig. 10.9 ^{18}F-FDG PET/MR of epilepsy patient. A 23-year-old male patient suffering from epileptic seizures for 20 years. Transverse T_1-weighted MRI (**a**), T_2-FLAIR (**b**), and coronal T_2-FLAIR (**c**) show enlarged left temporal horn, and smaller left hippocampal volume compared to the right with slightly higher signal intensity. ASL shows lower perfusion in the left temporal lobe compared to the right (**d**), while transverse ^{18}F-FDG PET (**e**) and integrated ^{18}F-FDG PET/MR (**f**) show lower glucose metabolism in the left hippocampus and temporal compared to the right. Post-surgical pathology shows FCD type I of the left temporal lobe with hippocampal sclerosis type I

logical findings. The studies described above have all demonstrated that multi-parametric PET/MR is clinically valuable for the pre-surgical localization of refractory epilepsy, but further validation is still needed by increasing the number of cases.

10.3.2 Research Applications of Integrated PET/MR on the Brain Network Mechanisms of Epilepsy

Multimodal imaging can overcome the inherent deficiencies and shortcomings of single imaging techniques, allowing more comprehensive investigation of complex diseases, and has therefore come to dominate the current trend in research on disease mechanisms. In terms of epilepsy, there is now an urgent need for in-depth research on brain networks to further improve its clinical diagnosis and treatment. Integrated PET/MR permits the acquisition of information on glucose metabolism and cerebral functional activity under the same physiological and pathological states. Through the organic combination of metabolic, functional, and structural imaging, this technique offers a strong support for studying the brain network mechanisms involved in epilepsy. Some researchers have utilized PET/fMRI to examine the correlation of energy metabolism with functional indicators, namely ReHo, fALFF, and degree of centrality (DC), under normal physiological states and found significant correlations in the spatial distribution between glucose uptake and fMRI functional indicators. However, these correlations exhibited spatial heterogeneity among different anatomical regions and functional networks, with the lowest correlation observed in the limbic network and the highest observed in the DMN. Furthermore, ReHo, and fALFF showed higher correlations with PET than DC. These results have provided for the basis for studying the changes in the coupling between metabolism and functional connectivity under pathological conditions. There are currently no reports involving the use of integrated PET/MR in multimodal research on neural networks in epilepsy. The addition of metabolic information can complement and supplement the shortcomings of MRI data. Furthermore, analyzing the changes in the correlation between the two will facilitate further exploration of the pathogenic mechanisms of epilepsy, thereby providing new ideas for clinical treatment.

PET and fMRI are both important techniques in the study of functional brain networks. Researchers performed ^{18}F-FDG PET, ^{11}C-FMZ PET, and fMRI on 9 TLE patients and 8 healthy controls, to acquire their whole-brain glucose metabolism, GABA metabolism, and fMRI indicators (ALFF, ReHo, and GC). Their results revealed that glucose metabolism was significantly positively, correlated with ALFF, ReHO, and GABA metabolism, while GABA metabolism was also positively correlated with ALFF. Compared to healthy controls, TLE patients showed a decreased correlation between glucose metabolism and ALFF, increased correlation between glucose metabolism and GC, as well as decreased correlation between GABA metabolism and ALFF. These findings suggest that the correlation between metabolism and function is impaired in TLE, whereas the abnormal correlation between glutamate and ALFF may be related to the abnormal discharges distributed extensively across the brain. Therefore, elucidating this process may provide a new target for the treatment of TLE. However, this study had a small sample size, and the imaging data were acquired at different time points, implying that the different physiological and pathological states may have had certain effects on cerebral functional and metabolic information. Therefore, further validation is needed using integrated PET/MR. We have also conducted a study on the coupling mechanism between metabolism and resting-state functional activities in patients with medial TLE and HS. Integrated PET/MR was performed on 26 patients and 26 age- and gender-matched healthy controls for the simultaneous acquisition of ^{18}F-FDG PET and RS-fMRI data. We then performed between-group comparisons using parameters such as SUV ratio (SUVR), ALFF, and ReHo and analyzed the relationship of metabolic and functional parameters with prognosis. The results of our study indicated that both patients and healthy controls showed significant positive correlations between metabolic and functional parameters. However, patients exhibited a stronger coupling between metabolic and functional activities within the hippocampal network, and significant differences were observed in the degree of coupling among patients with different prognoses. This study was a preliminary exploration on the potential disruption of bioinformational coupling caused by recurrent seizures in patients with medial TLE-HS, as well as the relationship of this coupling with prognosis, providing new ideas for understanding the pathogenesis of TLE-HS and utilizing non-invasive measures to guide epilepsy surgery.

Integrated PET/MR enables one-stop brain imaging via multiple modalities. Through simultaneous acquisition and automatic image registration, it is possible to avoid the biases that may occur in post-processing image fusion at a fundamental level, while also obtaining structural, perfusion, functional, metabolic, and other information under the same physiological and pathological states. Therefore, integrated PET/MR offers unique advantages for the non-invasive and precise pre-surgical localization of epilepsy patients, as well as research on their underlying pathogenic mechanisms. First, the high resolution of MRI provides accurate anatomical images for ROI delineation, thereby overcoming the limitations of low PET resolution, improving the sensitivity and accuracy of localizing epileptogenic foci, enabling the precise determination of the extent of surgical resection for epileptogenic foci, and improving prognosis. Second, PET/MR can overcome the inherent deficiencies and shortcomings of single imaging techniques, and achieve multi-modal research on disease pathogenesis, which better facilitates the understanding of complex pathological changes in neurological diseases.

Suggested Reading

Aiello M, Salvatore E, Cachia A, et al. Relationship between simultaneously acquired resting-state regional cerebral glucose metabolism and functional MRI: a PET/MR hybrid scanner study. NeuroImage. 2015;113:111–21.

Boscolo Galazzo I, Mattoli MV, Pizzini FB, et al. Cerebral metabolism and perfusion in MR-negative individuals with refractory focal epilepsy assessed by simultaneous acquisition of ^{18}F-FDG PET and arterial spin labeling. Neuroimage Clin. 2016;11:648–57.

Chassoux F, Artiges E, Semah F, et al. ^{18}F-FDG-PET patterns of surgical success and failure in mesial temporal lobe epilepsy. Neurology. 2017;88(11):1045–53.

de Tisi J, Bell GS, Peacock JL, et al. The long-term outcome of adult epilepsy surgery, patterns of seizure remission, and relapse: a cohort study. Lancet. 2011;378(9800):1388–95.

Del Felice A, Beghi E, Boero G, et al. Early versus late remission in a cohort of patients with newly diagnosed epilepsy. Epilepsia. 2010;51(1):37–42.

Desalvo MN, Douw L, Tanaka N, et al. Altered structural connectome in temporal lobe epilepsy. Radiology. 2014;270(3):842–8.

Desarnaud S, Mellerio C, Semah F, et al. ^{18}F-FDG PET in drug-resistant epilepsy due to focal cortical dysplasia type 2: additional value of electroclinical data and coregistration with MRI. Eur J Nucl Med Mol Imaging. 2018;45(8):1449–60.

Ding YS, Chen B, Glielmi C, et al. A pilot study in epilepsy patients using simultaneous PET/MR. Am J Nucl Med Mol Imaging. 2014;4(5):459–70.

Ding Y, Zhu Y, Jiang B, et al. ^{18}F-FDG PET and high-resolution MRI co-registration for pre-surgical evaluation of patients with conventional MRI-negative refractory extratemporal lobe epilepsy. Eur J Nucl Med Mol Imaging. 2018;45(9):1567–72.

Elger CE, Helmstaedter C, Kurthen M. Chronic epilepsy and cognition. Lancet Neurol. 2004;3(11):663–72.

Garibotto V, Heinzer S, Vulliemoz S, et al. Clinical applications of hybrid PET/MRI in neuroimaging. Clin Nucl Med. 2013;38(1):e13–8.

Gross DW. Diffusion tensor imaging in temporal lobe epilepsy. Epilepsia. 2011;52(Suppl 4):32–4.

Hartl E, Rémi J, Vollmar C, et al. PET imaging in extratemporal epilepsy requires considerationof electroclinical findings. Epilepsy Res. 2016;125:72–6.

Hoeft F, Barnea-Goraly N, Haas BW, et al. More is not always better: increased fractional anisotropy of superior longitudinal fasciculus associated with poor visuospatial abilities in Williams syndrome. J Neurosci. 2007;27(44):11960–5.

Ibrahim GM, Morgan BR, Lee W, et al. Impaired development of intrinsic connectivity networks in children with medically intractable localization-related epilepsy. Hum Brain Mapp. 2014;35(11):5686–700.

Jorge DO, Hae WS, Amir HK, et al. Subsequent experience in hybrid PET-MRI for evaluation of refractory focal onset epilepsy. Seizure. 2018;61:128–34.

Kumar A, Chugani HT. The role of radionuclide imaging in epilepsy, part 1: sporadic temporal and extratemporal lobe epilepsy. J Nucl Med Technol. 2017;45(1):14–21.

Kuzniecky R, Hugg JW, Hetherington H, et al. Relative utility of 1H spectroscopic imaging and hippocampal volumetry in the lateralization of mesial temporal lobe epilepsy. Neurology. 1998;51(1):66–71.

Lee K, Salamon N. [^{18}F]fluorodeoxyglucose-positron-emission tomography and MR imaging coregistration for presurgical evaluation of medically refractory epilepsy. AJNR Am J Neuroradiol. 2009;30(10):1811–6.

Mcgill ML, Devinsky O, Kelly C, et al. Default mode network abnormalities in idiopathic generalized epilepsy. Epilepsy Behav. 2012;23(3):353–9.

Medina LS, Bernal B, Ruiz J. Role of functional MR in determining language dominance in epilepsy and nonepilepsy populations: a Bayesian analysis. Radiology. 2007;242(1):94–100.

Menon RN, Radhakrishnan A, Parameswaran R, et al. Does F-18 FDG-PET substantially alter the surgical decision-making in drug-resistant partial epilepsy? Epilepsy Behav. 2015;51:133–9.

Michael JP, Erica Y, Jeremy YJ, et al. Comparison of the diagnostic accuracy of PET/MRI to PET/CT-acquired FDG brain exams for seizure focus detection: a prospective study. Pediatr Radiol. 2017;47(11):1500–7.

Nugent AC, Martinez A, D'alfonso A, et al. The relationship between glucose metabolism, resting-state fMRI BOLD signal, and $GABA_A$-binding potential: a preliminary study in healthy subjects and those with temporal lobe epilepsy. J Cereb Blood Flow Metab. 2015;35:583–91.

Riedl V, Bienkowska K, Strobel C, et al. Local activity determines functional connectivity in the resting human brain: a simultaneous FDG-PET/fMRI study. J Neurosci 2014;34:6260–6.

Ryvlin P, Cross JH, Rheims S. Epilepsy surgery in children and adults. Lancet Neurol. 2014;13(11):1114–26.

Salamon N, Kung J, Shaw SJ, et al. FDG-PET/MRI coregistration improves detection of cortical dysplasia in patients with epilepsy. Neurology. 2008;71(20):1594–601.

Shang K, Wang J, Fan X, et al. Clinical value of hybrid TOF-PET/MR imaging based multiparametric imaging in localizing seizure focus in patients with MRI-negative temporal lobe epilepsy. AJNR Am J Neuroradiol. 2018;39(10):1791–8.

Shen L, Zhang Z, Lu G, et al. Arterial spin labelling MRI of temporal and extratemporal hypoperfusion in patients with medial temporal lobe epilepsy. Chin J Radiol. 2012;46(3):220–4.

Shen L, Zhang Z, Wang Z, et al. Cerebral perfusion resonance imaging of partial seizure and secondary generalized seizure in medial temporal lobe epilepsy. Chin J Med Imaging Tech. 2012;28(4):626–9.

Shin HW, Jewells V, Sheikh A, et al. Initial experience in hybrid PET-MRI for evaluation of refractory focal onset epilepsy. Seizure. 2015;31:1–4.

Sidhu MK, Stretton J, Winston GP, et al. A functional magnetic resonance imaging study mapping the episodic memory encoding network in temporal lobe epilepsy. Brain. 2013;136(6):1868–88.

Su L, An J, Ma Q, et al. Influence of resting-state network on lateralization of functional connectivity in mesial temporal lobe epilepsy. AJNR Am J Neuroradiol. 2015;36(8):1479–87.

Thijs RD, Surges R, O'brien TJ, et al. Epilepsy in adults. Lancet. 2019;393(10172):689–701.

Thurman DJ, Beghi E, Begley CE, et al. Standards for epidemiologic studies and surveillance of epilepsy. Epilepsia. 2011;52(Suppl 7):2–26.

Tyndall AJ, Reinhardt J, Tronnier V, et al. Presurgical motor, somatosensory and language fMRI: technical feasibility and limitations in 491 patients over 13 years. Eur Radiol. 2017;27(1):267–78.

Valentín A, Alarcón G, Barrington SF, et al. Interictal estimation of intracranial seizure onset in temporal lobe epilepsy. Clin Neurophysiol. 2014;125(2):231–8.

Vollmar C, O'muircheartaigh J, Barker GJ, et al. Motor system hyper-connectivity in juvenile myoclonic epilepsy: a cognitive functional magnetic resonance imaging study. Brain. 2011;134(6):1710–9.

Wang YH, An Y, Fan XT, et al. Comparison between simultaneously acquired arterial spin labeling and ^{18}F-FDG PET in mesial temporal lobe epilepsy assisted by a PET/MR system and SEEG. Neuroimage Clin. 2018;19:824–30.

Wang Z, Lu G, Zhang Z, et al. Altered resting state networks in epileptic patients with generalized tonic-clonic seizures. Brain Res. 2011;1374:134–41.

Wieshmann U, Symms M, Clark C, et al. Wallerian degeneration in the optic radiation after temporal lobectomy demonstrated in vivo with diffusion tensor imaging. Epilepsia. 1999;40(8):1155–8.

Yang Z, Choupan J, Reutens D, et al. Lateralization of temporal lobe epilepsy based on resting-state functional magnetic resonance imaging and machine learning. Front Neurol. 2015;6:184.

Yousry TA, Schmid UD, Alkadhi H, et al. Localization of the motor hand area to a knob on the precentral gyrus: a new landmark. Brain. 1997;120(1):141–57.

Zhang C, Yang H, Liu C, et al. Brain network alterations of mesial temporal lobe epilepsy with cognitive dysfunction following anterior temporal lobectomy. Epilepsy Behav. 2018;87:123–30.

Zhang C, Zhang H, Xu K, et al. Impaired prefrontal cortex-thalamus pathway in intractable temporal lobe epilepsy with aberrant executive control function: MRI evidence. Clin Neurophysiol. 2019;130(4):484–90.

Research Applications of Positron Emission Tomography/Magnetic Resonance (PET/MR) Imaging in Brain Tumors

11

Shuangshuang Song, Kun Guo, Zhilian Zhao, Zhigang Qi, and Jie Lu

In recent years, the incidence rate of brain tumors, for which surgical resection is the preferred treatment, has increased, and it is currently approximately 8.3–11 per 100,000 individuals. Gliomas are the most common type of primary intracranial tumors; they account for approximately 30% of all central nervous system (CNS) tumors and 70% of all primary brain tumors in adults and can be divided according to the World Health Organization (WHO) classification into low (WHO grades I and II) and high grades (WHO grades III and IV). Patients with gliomas tend to have a poor prognosis, although the prognosis is also dependent on the patient's age at onset, tumor location, surgical method, postoperative adjuvant therapy, and the molecular and genetic subtyping of the tumor(s). Low-grade gliomas typically have a more favorable prognosis than high-grade gliomas; therefore, the accurate preoperative classification of gliomas is of crucial significance to the formulation of treatment plans and prognostic prediction. There are significant limitations to using conventional MRI for the classification and diagnosis of gliomas, as this technique is based on characteristics such as contrast enhancement, space-occupying effects, edema, and necrosis. For instance, certain low-grade gliomas may exhibit contrast enhancement, whereas certain high-grade gliomas may not. Primary central nervous system lymphoma (PCNSL) is a rare subtype of non-Hodgkin's lymphoma that is highly invasive but relatively sensitive to radiotherapy and chemotherapy. The incidence rate of PCNSL, which can affect the brain parenchyma, meninges, and spinal cord, has grown among the immunocompetent population in recent years, although it is more common in the immunocompromised population. Pathologically, the vast majority of cases are classified as large B-cell lymphoma. The average age at diagnosis for PCNSL is 60 years, and it is more prevalent among women. The age of onset of PCNSL among lymphoma patients with acquired immunodeficiency syndrome (AIDS) tends to be relatively younger.

Brain metastasis is another common feature of intracranial tumors among adults, occurring in 15–40% of cancer patients. Nevertheless, improvements in methods of diagnosis and treatment, as well as advancements in neuroimaging techniques, have led to a higher detection rate of brain metastases. Lung, breast, colorectal, and genitourinary cancers, as well as melanoma, are all prone to brain metastases, although the most common route of spread is via blood-borne metastasis, which is especially common within the territory of the middle cerebral artery. Upon initial diagnosis, approximately 50% of metastases are solitary, occurring in the cerebral hemi-

S. Song · K. Guo · Z. Zhao · Z. Qi · J. Lu (✉)
Department of Radiology and Nuclear Medicine, Xuanwu Hospital, Capital Medical University, Beijing, China

J. Lu, G. Zhao (eds.), *PET/MR: Functional and Molecular Imaging of Neurological Diseases and Neurosciences*, https://doi.org/10.1007/978-981-19-9902-4_11

sphere (60%), cerebellar hemisphere (30%), and brainstem (10%). It is easier to diagnose patients with multiple metastases and a known history of tumors than diagnosing patients with an unknown history of tumors, upon the discovery of brain metastases, especially in cases of solitary brain metastases. In the latter case, therefore, a combination of imaging methods is required to achieve a correct diagnosis.

11.1 Research Applications of MRI in Brain Tumors

Since the advent of computed tomography (CT) and MRI, imaging has played an increasingly important role in guiding the surgical and radiotherapy treatment of brain tumors. Conventional MRI can be used to localize tumors, as well as display their morphology, boundaries, signal characteristics, and enhancement features. These conventional images are sufficient to aid in diagnosis or guide treatment; however, in some patients, a diagnosis cannot be confirmed based on conventional MRI alone, and additional information is needed for the differential diagnosis to facilitate more precise surgical planning. In other patients, it is necessary to observe the tumor-induced functional changes and determine the relationship between the tumor and functional brain areas, necessitating the use of more advanced functional MRI (fMRI) techniques. fMRI is a relatively recent imaging technology, which was developed in the 1990s. In a broad sense, fMRI includes diffusion-weighted imaging (DWI), perfusion-weighted imaging (PWI), diffusion tensor imaging (DTI), blood-oxygen-level-dependent (BOLD) imaging, magnetic resonance spectroscopy (MRS), and susceptibility-weighted imaging (SWI). These new MRI techniques have not only enhanced the accuracy of preoperative assessments and promoted the improvement of surgical procedures but have also provided excellent assistance to the formulation of radiotherapy and chemotherapy plans, and have become key tools in the evaluation of treatment prognosis.

11.1.1 Research Applications of DWI in Brain Tumors

DWI reflects the functional characteristics of tumors through the diffusion status of the tumor tissues. The DWI-derived quantitative indicator, the apparent diffusion coefficient (ADC), can describe the rate and range of the free diffusion of water molecules in different directions on the DWI map. It quantifies the diffusion of water molecules in tissues under the action of a diffusion gradient and is related to various factors, including the number, size, and arrangement of cells, extracellular space, nuclear-cytoplasmic ratio, and microcirculatory perfusion. Using ADC values, it is possible to predict the tumor classification and molecular subtype, determine the treatment response and evaluate the prognosis. DWI can also be utilized to quantitatively analyze the diffusion status of brain tumors.

The restricted diffusion characteristic of brain tumors is helpful for the qualitative diagnosis of brain tumors. Compared to normal brain parenchyma, tumorous lesions exhibit varying degrees of restricted diffusion due to increased cell density and reduced extracellular space. DWI can help to determine the tissue of origin for brain metastases as follows: In general, well-differentiated adenocarcinomas present hypointense DWI signals, whereas metastases from small- and large-cell neuroendocrine carcinomas present as hyperintense DWI signals. Furthermore, DWI can discriminate between brain tumors and abscesses, which is immensely helpful for the differential diagnosis of ring-enhancing tumors and abscesses. The ADC value within the cavity of a brain abscess is significantly reduced, whereas restricted diffusion is generally not observed within the intratumoral cavity, but at the tumor wall, of tumors with liquefactive necrosis. High-grade gliomas are characterized by rapid cell proliferation, increased cell density, smaller extracellular spaces, and an increase in the nuclear-cytoplasmic ratio, which can restrict the movement of water molecules, thereby increasing DWI signals and decreasing ADC values (Figs. 11.1 and 11.2). In contrast, low-grade gliomas have relatively high ADC

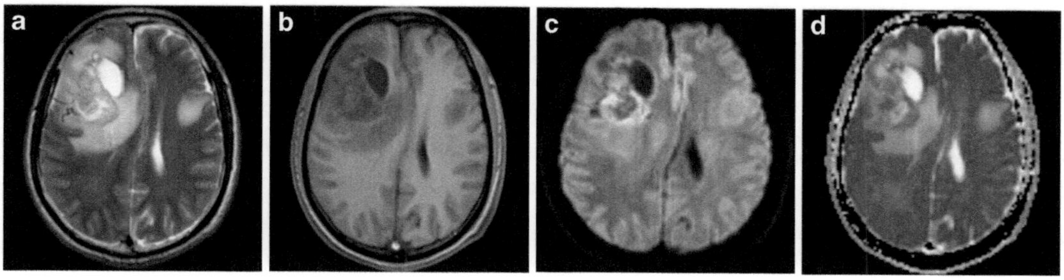

Fig. 11.1 IDH-wildtype glioblastoma, WHO grade IV. A 56-year-old male patient whose MRI shows an irregular, abnormal space-occupying lesion in the right frontal lobe, with significant signal heterogeneity and intralesional cystic changes and necrosis. The solid compartment of the tumor shows isointense and slightly hyperintense T_2WI signals (**a**); slightly hypointense T_1WI signals (**b**); hyperintense DWI signals (**c**); and hypointense ADC signals, signifying the restricted diffusion of the tumor parenchyma (**d**)

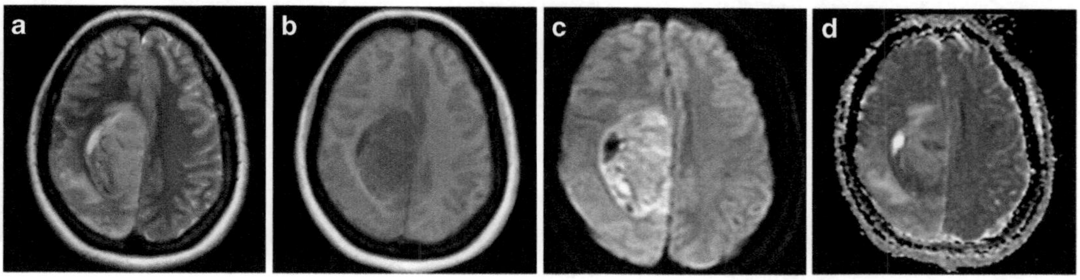

Fig. 11.2 IDH-mutant anaplastic oligodendroglioma, WHO grade III. A 46-year-old female patient whose MRI shows an oval space-occupying lesion in the right parietal lobe, with a lack of intralesional signal homogeneity. Transverse T_2WI shows isointense and slightly hyperintense signals (**a**); transverse T_1WI shows slightly hypointense signals (**b**); transverse DWI shows isointense and hyperintense signals (**c**); and transverse ADC shows hypointense and hyperintense signals, signifying the regional restricted diffusion of the tumor parenchyma (**d**)

values (Fig. 11.3); therefore, an ADC value of 1.185×10^{-3} mm^2/s can be used as a cutoff point to differentiate between low- and high-grade gliomas, with a sensitivity of 97.6% and specificity of 53.1%. A meta-analysis evaluating the use of ADC values to differentiate between the grades of glioma showed that preoperative ADC values had a relatively high accuracy for discriminating between low- and high-grade gliomas. The overall sensitivity and specificity were 0.85 and 0.80, respectively; the positive and negative likelihood ratios were 4 25 and 0.18, respectively, and the area under the receiver operating characteristic curve (AUC) was 0.90. Furthermore, quantitative ADC values showed high discriminatory accuracy for low- and high-grade gliomas.

In 2016, the molecular subtyping of gliomas was incorporated into the WHO classification of CNS tumors, based on histological subtyping. Isocitrate dehydrogenase (IDH) mutations were identified as key biomarkers, and gliomas were divided into IDH-mutant and IDH-wildtype gliomas. Studies have found that IDH-wildtype gliomas have lower ADC values (Fig. 11.1) than IDH-mutant gliomas (Figs. 11.2 and 11.3) and that the minimum ADC value (0.9×10^{-3} mm^2/s) shows the highest sensitivity (91%) and specificity (75%) for predicting IDH-wildtype gliomas. The relative mean ADC could predict IDH mutation status without being affected by the WHO grade of the tumor, and the optimal cut-off value for differentiating between IDH-mutant and wildtype gliomas was 1.2, with a sensitivity of 81.9%, specificity of 74.6%, and AUC of 0.790.

The manifestations of PCNSL in conventional imaging are diverse, which often leads to difficulties in differential diagnosis. DWI is a valuable technique for the diagnosis and differential diagnosis of PCNSL. Due to its high cell density, PCNSL is characterized by restricted diffusion,

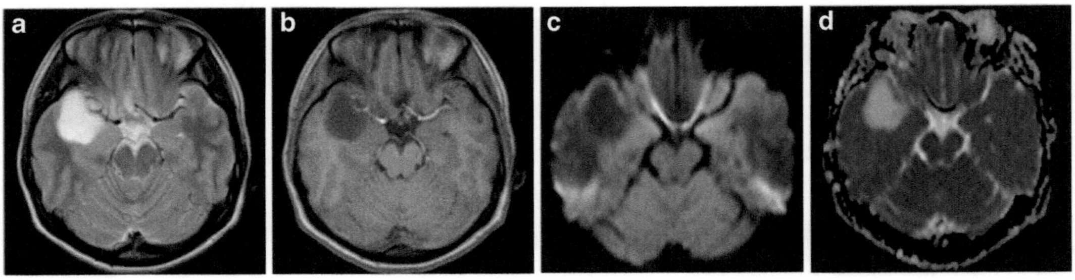

Fig. 11.3 IDH-mutant oligodendroglioma, WHO grade II. A 26-year-old female patient whose MRI shows an abnormal circular lesion in the right temporal lobe with homogenous signal intensity. Transverse T_2WI shows hyperintense signals (**a**); transverse T_1WI shows hypointense signals (**b**); transverse DWI shows hypointense signals (**c**); and transverse ADC shows hyperintense signals, signifying the absence of restricted diffusion (**d**)

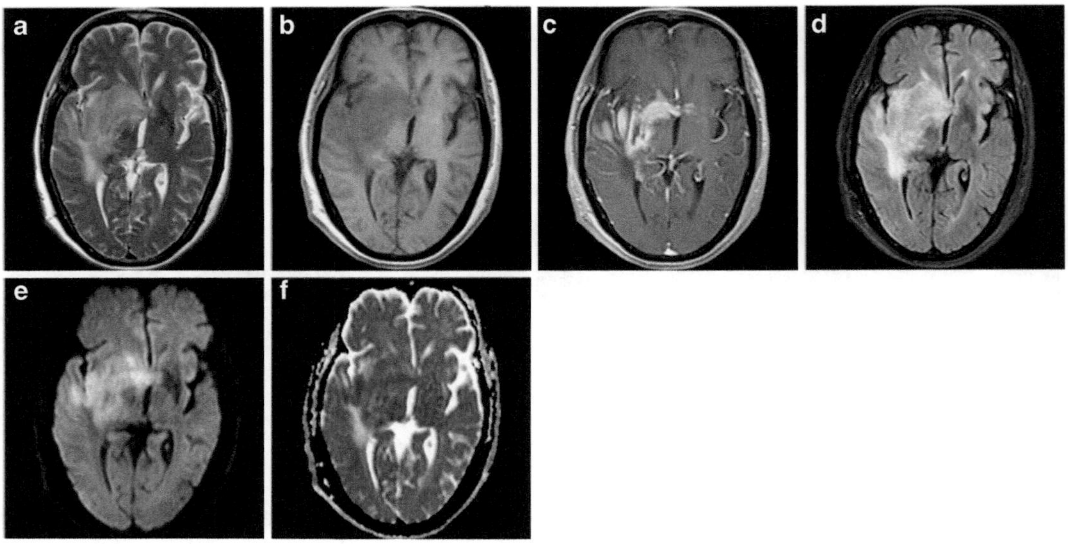

Fig. 11.4 Flaky space-occupying lesion of the right basal ganglia. T_2WI shows heterogeneous hyperintensity (**a**); T_1WI shows hypointensity (**b**); contrast-enhanced T_1WI shows homogenous enhancement (**c**); FLAIR shows heterogenous hyperintensity (**d**); DWI (b-value = 800) shows hyperintensity of the lesion in the right basal ganglia (**e**); and transverse ADC value shows heterogeneous decrease, signifying restricted diffusion (**f**)

which presents as hyperintense signals on DWI maps with decreased ADC values (Fig. 11.4). Although glioblastomas and metastases can also exhibit restricted diffusion, PCNSL tends to have lower ADC values. Additionally, ADC values can aid in the prediction of prognosis, as previous studies have shown that PCNSL patients with lower ADC values in the tumor enhancement area before treatment had shorter survival times. Furthermore, ADC values can also be used to determine treatment response, as repeat testing of ADC values in patients with PCNSL after different chemotherapy regimens allows the monitoring of significant changes in ADC values, which were found to be significantly associated with patient survival. In fact, one study showed that lymphoma patients whose minimum ADC value before treatment was $<384 \times 10^{-6}$ mm^2/s had faster disease progression and poorer prognosis.

11.1.2 Research Applications of DTI in Brain Tumors

DTI, a more recent imaging technique based on DWI, can be used to accurately display the direction and quantification of the diffusion motion exhibited by the water molecules in lesions.

When applied to the diagnosis of brain tumors, physicians can utilize DTI to measure fractional anisotropy (FA) and ADC values, to determine the diffusion direction of the water molecules in brain tissues, while also determining the integrity of the nerve fiber structures and the relationship of white matter fiber bundles with tumors, thereby facilitating more precise surgical planning. Holodny et al. used DTI to determine the positional relationship between corticospinal tracts and adjacent brain tumors, which helped delineate the extent of surgical resection. Three different types of relationship were identified between infiltrative brain tumors and neighboring corticospinal tracts: (1) the corticospinal tract was unaffected by the tumor; (2) the tumor was adjacent to the corticospinal tract, and involvement was suspected; and (3) the tumor had infiltrated the corticospinal tract, leading to the breakage, displacement, and deformation of adjacent white matter tracts. In a randomized prospective study, Wu et al. performed preoperative DTI on patients with gliomas and found that a more involved surgical resection in patients with corticospinal tract involvement ensured an increased preservation of postoperative nerve function, as well as a longer survival time compared to patients who did not undergo a preoperative evaluation. Chen et al. utilized DTI to track the white matter fibers in the peritumoral edema zone of glioma patients and found that the degree of fiber bundle destruction directly reflected the extent of tumor cell infiltration, helping to confirm the boundary of the tumor infiltration zone. In another study, DTI was used to reconstruct white matter fiber bundles dominated by the effective fibers of pyramidal tracts, to ensure the maximum surgical resection of tumors and the preservation of the effective fibers of pyramidal tracts. The results of that study indicated that the disability rate 3 months after surgery was significantly lower in these patients than in those who underwent conventional total tumor resections. Therefore, the DTI-guided resection of gliomas involving crucial nerve fiber bundles not only assists surgeons in ensuring maximum tumor resection but can also reduce the postoperative disability rate, improving the patient's postoperative quality of life.

11.1.3 Research Applications of PWI in Brain Tumors

The methods of perfusion MRI currently utilized to evaluate the hemodynamic changes of brain tumors primarily include dynamic susceptibility contrast (DSC)-PWI, dynamic contrast-enhanced (DCE)-MRI, and arterial spin labeling (ASL). Both DSC-PWI and DCE-MRI require the injection of a contrast agent, and by detecting the signal changes induced by the bolus of contrast agent, these techniques can be used to acquire signal intensity-time curves, which can be converted to tissue contrast agent concentration-time curves, and regional hemodynamic parameters can be calculated by fitting different mathematical models. Commonly used parameters in DSC-PWI include relative cerebral blood volume (rCBV), regional cerebral blood flow (rCBF), mean transit time (MTT), and time to peak (TTP). Of these, rCBV is the most commonly utilized parameter in the assessment of brain tumors. Commonly used parameters in DCE-MRI include the plasma-to-extravascular volume transfer (K^{trans}), fractional volume of the extravascular extracellular space (V_e), fractional plasma volume (V_p), and extravascular-to-plasma volume transfer (K_{ep}), of which, K^{trans} is most commonly utilized. Due to the complexities of quantifying DCE parameters, the clinical applications of this technique are limited. ASL does not require the injection of contrast agents, but instead uses the hydrogen protons of arterial blood as an endogenous tracer to acquire information on the perfusion of brain tissues, and accurately assess tumor angiogenesis in a non-invasive manner.

Early studies have shown that elevated rCBV is associated with more active angiogenesis and aggressiveness of malignant tumors; therefore, rCBV is a potential imaging biomarker for preoperative tumor grading. Furthermore, significant differences have been found between the rCBV values of high- and low-grade brain tumors, with high-grade gliomas (WHO grades III and IV) having higher rCBV values than low-grade gliomas (WHO grades I and II). However, there is currently no unified standard for rCBV cut-off values for the classification of high- and low-grade gliomas. Some studies have defined $rCBV_{max}$ = 1.7 as the cut-off value to differentiate between the two, whereas others have recommended a cut-off value of $rCBV_{max}$ = 2.01. Additionally, brain tumors of different pathological types also present different perfusion manifestations. For example, even though oligodendrogliomas are low-grade tumors, they tend to exhibit relatively high rCBV, which may be due to the abundant blood vessels and dense capillary networks present in the tumors. In addition to exhibiting restricted diffusion, CNS lymphomas are characterized by distinct perfusion imaging features. In conventional contrast-enhanced MRI, lymphomas are significantly enhanced, with findings similar to those of glioblastomas, brain abscesses, and demyelinating lesions, which may cause difficulties in the differential diagnosis. Perfusion imaging shows that lymphomas are hypoperfused compared to glioblastomas and other lesions, which is a helpful imaging feature for differential diagnosis.

Perfusion imaging can also help to determine the molecular characteristics of gliomas. Many studies have found that compared with IDH-wildtype (Fig. 11.5), IDH-mutant gliomas have lower rCBV values (Fig. 11.6), while all IDH-wildtype gliomas, regardless of the histological grade, show significantly elevated perfusion. This may be related to the more active angiogenesis and less heterogenous microenvironment of IDH-wildtype gliomas. rCBV can serve as a robust, non-invasive imaging biomarker for predicting IDH mutation status. Additionally, DSC-PWI can be performed to discriminate the treatment responses of gliomas, especially between tumor pseudo-progression and tumor recurrence, which is an issue of significant clinical concern. More specifically, tumor pseudo-progression exhibits a lower level of perfusion than tumor recurrence, which may be attributed to the decreased cell density and vascularization of pseudo-progressive lesions, as opposed to the neovascularization that frequently occurs in tumor recurrence, resulting in increased intralesional blood supply and elevated rCBV. Furthermore, both the rCBV value of DSC-PWI and the K^{trans} of DCE have good discriminant abilities for radiation necrosis and tumor recurrence. One study using 1.23 as the rCBV cut-off value found that the sensitivity of discriminating between the two was 88% and specificity was 75%; whereas adopting a K^{trans} cut-off value of 28.76 gave a sensitivity of 89% and specificity of 97%.

Owing to its convenience and speed, ASL perfusion imaging also plays a vital role in the preoperative classification, treatment follow-up, and differential diagnosis of gliomas. High-grade gliomas exhibit significantly higher rCBF than low-grade gliomas (Fig. 11.7). However, one study demonstrated that ASL imaging could not differentiate between WHO grade III and IV gliomas, because WHO grade III gliomas are pri-

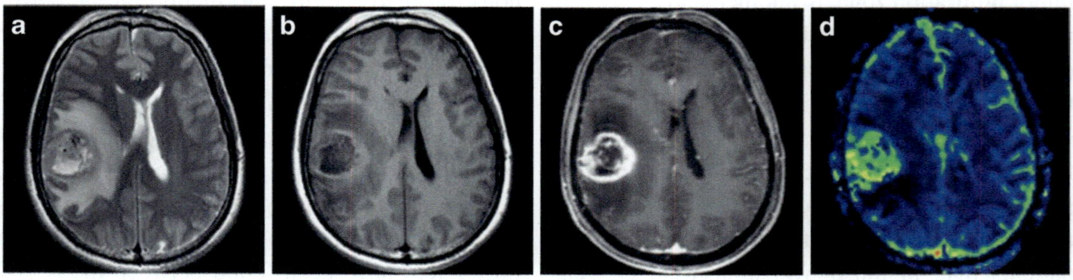

Fig. 11.5 IDH-wildtype glioblastoma, WHO grade IV. A 53-year-old male patient whose MRI shows a circular mass in the right parietal lobe. Transverse T_2WI shows heterogenous mixed hyper- and hypointense signals (**a**); transverse T_1WI shows heterogenous iso- to hypointense signals (**b**), surrounded by finger-like edema; contrast-enhanced scan shows significant heterogenous ring-like enhancement (**c**); and the solid component of the lesion shows significantly elevated CBV, with relative mean CBV and relative maximum CBV of 2.78 and 6.63, respectively (**d**)

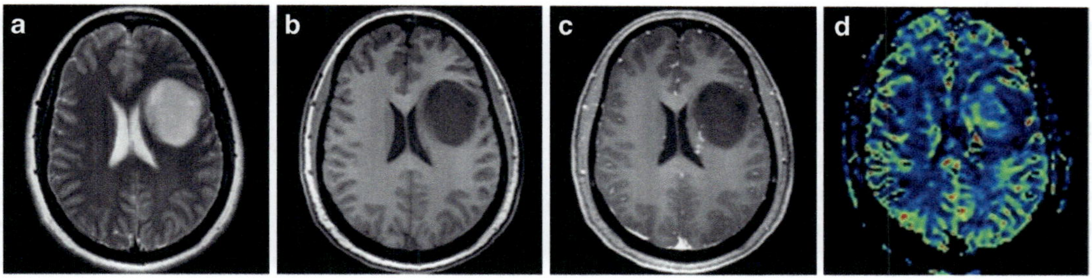

Fig. 11.6 IDH-mutant astrocytoma. A 31-year-old female patient whose MRI shows a circular mass in the left frontoparietal lobe. Transverse T_2WI shows heterogeneous hyperintense signals (**a**); transverse T_1WI shows homogeneous hypointense signals (**b**), without no obvious signs of edema around the lesion; contrast-enhanced scan shows no significant enhancement (**c**); and the lesion shows slightly elevated CBV, with relative mean CBV and relative maximum CBV of 0.83 and 3.24, respectively, which were both lower than those of IDH wild-type glioma (**d**)

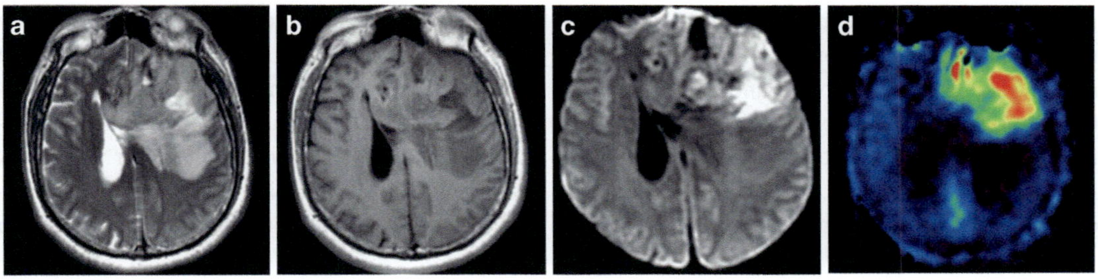

Fig. 11.7 IDH-mutant and 1p/19q co-deleted oligodendroglioma. A 43-year-old male patient whose MRI shows an irregular mass in the left frontotemporal lobe. Transverse T_2WI show heterogeneous hyperintense signals (**a**); transverse T_1WI shows homogeneous iso- to hypointense signals (**b**); transverse DWI shows mixed hyper- and hypointense signals (**c**); and lesion CBF is significantly higher than the contralateral side (**d**)

marily oligodendrogliomas with hyperperfusion, whereas WHO grade IV gliomas are primarily glioblastomas that may exhibit a variety of perfusion changes due to intratumoral cystic necrosis. Additionally, ASL can help differentiate post-treatment responses in high-grade gliomas. One key point in the evaluation of glioblastomas following chemotherapy and radiotherapy is to determine whether the MRI T_1-enhanced region is tumor recurrence or tumor pseudo-progression. Studies have found a significant difference in rCBF between the two, with postoperative brain tumor recurrence showing a significantly higher rCBF than tumor pseudo-progression, clearly differentiating between the two conditions. Another study found that ASL can be used to rapidly and easily differentiate between PCNSL and glioblastoma, as PCNSL shows a significantly lower CBF than glioblastoma, while the AUC value for the differential diagnosis between the two is >0.9.

11.1.4 Research Applications of Proton MRS in Brain Tumors

MRS can provide information on various metabolites in brain tumors, which can facilitate the differential diagnosis while also providing valuable information for the biopsy localization, grading, treatment evaluation, and prognostic determination of brain tumors. MRS is divided into single- and multi-voxel spectroscopy. Single-voxel spectroscopy is easy to operate and suitable for clinical applications, whereas multi-voxel spectroscopy can evaluate the spatial distribution of metabolites within a lesion in one scan session, which is helpful for assessing the extent and malignancy of the lesion, formulating treatment plans, and determining the site of biopsy.

Different types and grades of brain tumors exhibit different MRS findings. For most brain tumors, MRS reveals an increased choline (Cho) peak, decreased N-acetylaspartate (NAA) peak, and increased Cho/creatine (Cr) and Cho/NAA ratios. The increase in Cho peak is associated with increased tumor cell density and accelerated cell membrane Cho metabolism, whereas the decrease in NAA peak is associated with reduced neuronal function and damaged neuronal structure in the tumor area. Generally speaking, the Cr peak remains relatively unchanged in low-grade gliomas, but shows a decrease in high-grade gliomas. Nevertheless, despite the frequent occurrence of increased Cho/Cr and Cho/NAA in high-grade gliomas, there are overlaps in MRS findings among different grades of tumors. The lactate (Lac) and lipid (Lip) peaks cannot be observed in normal brain tissues, and are found only in tumor tissues, especially high-grade tumors. The Lac peak can be seen across all grades of gliomas, whereas the combination of the Lac and Lip peaks allows the discrimination of high-grade (Fig. 11.8) from low-grade gliomas (Fig. 11.9).

The MRS findings of PCNSL also involve elevated Cho/Cr and Cho/NAA ratios, but studies have found that more than 90% of cases exhibited Lac and Lip peaks, which were not proportional to the degree of intralesional necrosis. This feature may help to distinguish PCNSL from glioblastoma. MRS can also be applied to discriminate brain tumors from non-neoplastic lesions; however, relying on MRS alone can often lead to difficulties in differential diagnosis. For example, demyelinating lesions can exhibit increased Cho/Cr and decreased NAA/Cr, which are similar to the MRS findings of tumors. Therefore, the combination of conventional MR findings with clinical presentations is critical for similar lesions. A meta-analysis showed that MRS can also be utilized to differentiate high-grade gliomas that are

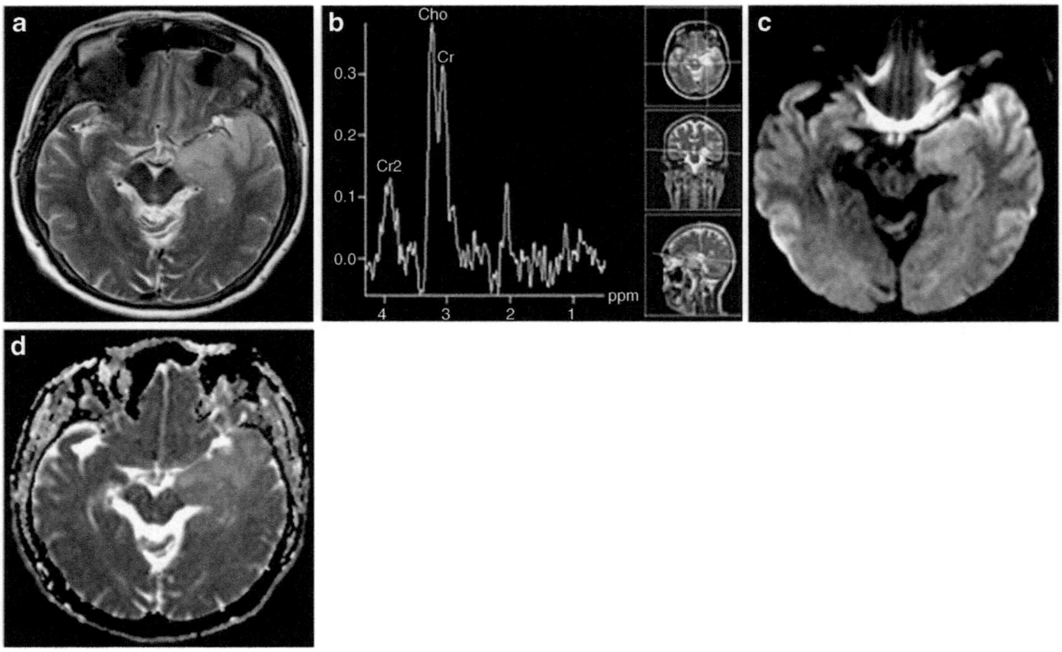

Fig. 11.8 Left temporal lobe glioma, WHO grade II. MRI shows glioma of the left temporal lobe, with hyperintense signals observed in transverse T2WI (**a**). Multivoxel MRS shows elevated Cho/Cr and reduced NAA/Cr (**b**). Transverse DWI (b-value = 800) shows mixed signals in the left temporal lobe mass, dominated by iso- to hyperintense signals (**c**), whereas no significant decrease was observed in ADC value (**d**)

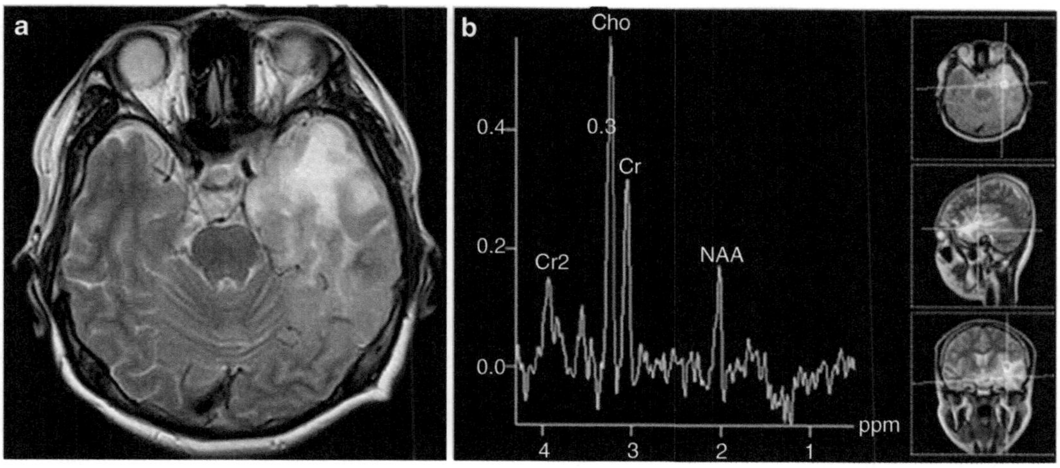

Fig. 11.9 Left temporal lobe glioma, WHO grade III. Transverse T_2WI shows hyperintense signals in the left temporal lobe (**a**); multi-voxel proton MRS shows increased Cho/Cr, decreased NAA/Cr, and an inverted Lac peak at 1.33 ppm (**b**)

treatment-responsive from true tumor progression, attaining a sensitivity of up to 91% and specificity of 95% in the differential diagnosis between the two. Among all indicators, the Cho/Cr ratio showed the greatest significance in differential diagnosis.

11.1.5 Research Applications of SWI in Brain Tumors

At present, SWI is not routinely performed as part of head MRI sequences. Information on the morphology and distribution of hemorrhage and calcification in gliomas is very valuable for the diagnosis and differential diagnosis of such tumors. However, the display of intratumoral calcification and microbleeds is difficult to achieve using conventional spin-echo (SE) sequences (i.e., T_1WI and T_2WI), but this can be easily accomplished using SWI, which can also produce phase images to differentiate between calcification and hemorrhage. Therefore, SWI is a useful tool for the non-invasive evaluation of CNS gliomas. SWI can increase the detection rate of intratumoral hemorrhage in the brain, which has significant implications for the quantitative diagnosis of tumors and guidance of clinical surgery. Furthermore, since SWI mainly relies on the magnetic susceptibility differences among tumor tissues to form image contrast, it can more clearly display tumor boundaries. As for the qualitative aspects of brain tumors, SWI can provide useful information for qualitative diagnosis with respect to vascular proliferation and microbleeds. Early manifestations of basal ganglia germinoma include patchy lesions in the basal ganglia without space-occupying effects, accompanied by atrophy of the ipsilateral sulci and midbrain, which can easily be confused with cerebral infarction. SWI can aid in the identification of neovascularization within germinomas, facilitating early diagnosis. Solitary-enhancing nodules in the brain may be solitary granulomas, demyelinating pseudotumor, lymphomas or glioblastomas. These lesions may sometimes be difficult to differentiate, and SWI can provide valuable information for their differential diagnosis. Studies have shown almost all glioblastomas exhibit hypointense SWI signals representing blood metabolites, calcifications, and veins, whereas these signals are rarely observed in non-neoplastic lesions and lymphomas. Therefore, this sign can be exploited for differential diagnosis, attaining a specificity of nearly 100% for discrimination.

Invasive brain tumors tend to exhibit rapid intratumoral vascular growth and multiple microbleeds. During the course of brain glioma growth, the increased secretion of vascular endothelial growth factor (VEGF) promotes the growth of immature new microvessels and increases microvascular density. Therefore, the detection of such intratumoral alterations facilitates the qualitative diagnosis of brain tumors. Furthermore, microvascular density is positively correlated with the pathological grade of gliomas. Therefore, the presence of SWI hypointensities, the proportion of the entire tumor occupied by hypointensities, and the morphology of hypointensities can also assist with the preoperative classification and evaluation of brain tumors. Researchers have observed that tumor classification based on SWI showed good concordance with T_1 enhancement. Mittal et al. found that brain tumors with higher PWI-derived rCBV values and MRS-derived Cho/Cr ratios showed more hypointensities on SWI. Additionally, the presence of intratumoral calcification, as well as the morphology and level of calcification, are important features in the evaluation of brain tumors, while SWI can display the calcified components of brain tumors. When detecting calcification in brain tumors such as oligodendrogliomas, the addition of SWI sequences led to a statistically significant increase in sensitivity (from 33 to 86%) but did not affect the specificity. SWI was also helpful in discriminating vestibular schwannomas from cerebellopontine angle meningiomas, as microbleeds can be observed in schwannomas but not meningiomas.

11.1.6 Research Applications of fMRI in Brain Tumors

The principle of craniocerebral tumor resection is the safe and maximal removal of tumors, while its challenge lies in grasping the balance between complete tumor resection and the preservation of function. However, functional localization is difficult due to a variety of factors, including individual differences in brain functional areas, the compression and displacement of functional areas by lesions, and the remodeling of functional areas. Therefore, it is extremely unreliable to depend solely on the surgeon's subjective judgment to achieve the localization and protection of functional areas, while the objective and accurate localization of brain functional areas has now become a key technique that can determine the success of brain tumor surgery in functional areas. The most common imaging method currently used in the localization of brain functional areas is fMRI. By performing task-based fMRI research on patients with brain tumors, it is possible to identify and confirm the functional areas of language with a sensitivity and specificity of up to 90%. On top of this, task-based fMRI is also convenient and non-invasive, which has enabled this technique to play a crucial role in the intraoperative localization of cortical language areas in brain tumor surgery. Additionally, fMRI has shown a similar performance to invasive techniques in displaying motor networks or motor areas, and can therefore also serve as a simple and effective method for the preoperative evaluation of motor areas. Preoperative task-based fMRI has shown a relatively good performance in localizing the motor and supplementary motor areas; therefore, it is frequently integrated into neuronavigation systems to assess the spatial positional relationship of brain tumors with adjacent functional areas, in order to guide surgical resection (Fig. 11.10).

During the surgical process, factors such as the opening of the skull, loss of cerebrospinal fluid, and traction often lead to "shifts" in the actual intraoperative position of lesions. In most craniotomies, shifts of up to or even exceeding 1 cm can occur in brain tissues, which substantially reduces the accuracy of surgical procedures. However, since the advent of intraoperative MRI (iMRI), the real-time MRI-based acquisition of brain deformation and shift errors during the surgical process has become a reality, leading to significant improvements in the precision of navigation and localization. Many studies have shown that the application of iMRI can significantly increase the tumor resection rate and postoperative survival rate of patients, while its long-term clinical efficacy has also been verified. Additionally, the application of intraoperative fMRI in brain tumor surgery can also assist neu-

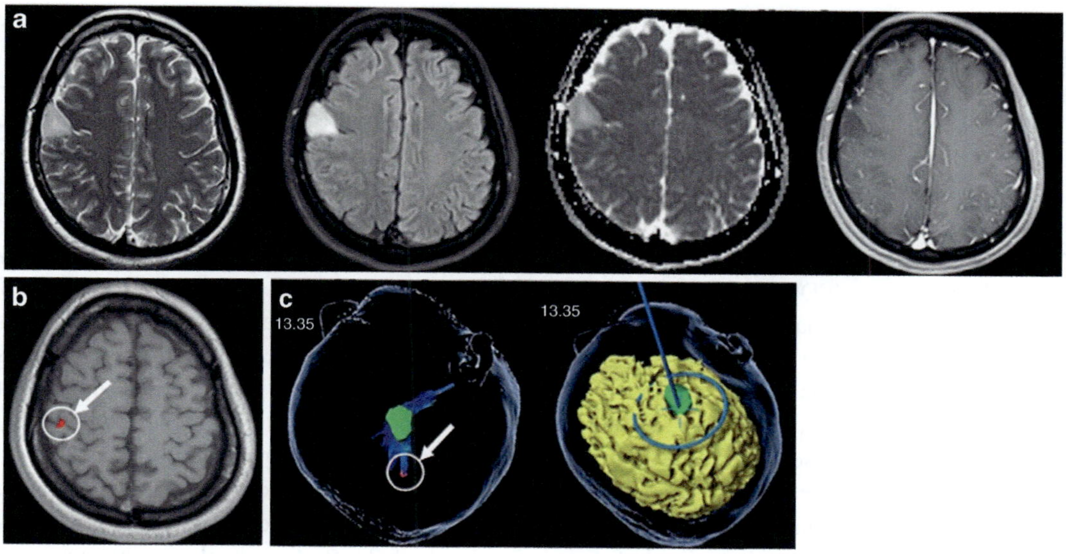

Fig. 11.10 Right frontal lobe oligodendroglioma, WHO grade II. A 27-year-old female patient, in whom a space-occupying lesion was discovered in the right frontal lobe 3 months ago. Patient's preoperative MRI, which revealed that the lesion was adjacent to the motor areas (**a**). Patient's preoperative fMRI motor activation map during hand movements (**b**). The tumor boundary and functional activation map were integrated into 3D navigation to assist in the avoidance of motor activation areas during surgery (**c**). Arrow: motor activation area

rosurgeons with avoiding cortical functional areas, thereby achieving precise resection. Wu et al. implemented intraoperative fMRI in the resection of patients with gliomas in the Broca area. In their study, patients underwent intraoperative awakening to perform language tasks in an awake state under anesthesia, which were combined with the simultaneous acquisition of fMRI information, in order to collect real-time activation information of the patient's cortical language areas during the operation. This approach not only enabled maximal tumor resection but also ensured the preservation of the patient's language function.

With the advancements in modern neurosurgery, the gradual deepening of our understanding on brain tumors is closely related to progress in neuroimaging. An increasing number of neurosurgeons are now implementing advance preoperative neuroimaging methods to facilitate surgical planning. Most fMRI techniques have good reproducibility, do not involve ionizing radiation, and incur relatively low costs; therefore, these techniques have significant implications for brain tumors with respect to surgical planning, prognosis prediction, reduction of surgery-induced functional impairments and postoperative complications, improvement of postoperative quality of life, and promotion of further rehabilitation in postoperative neural function.

11.2 Research Applications of PET Imaging in Brain Tumors

With the rapid development of imaging techniques, the use of PET imaging has gradually become more widespread for the clinical diagnosis and treatment of brain tumors, demonstrating unique advantages in displaying the overall expression of tumor markers. PET imaging is now a new method for analyzing the molecular pathological characteristics of tumors and screening for targeted drugs. This technique allows the direct visualization of tumor biological processes at the molecular and cellular levels and enables the direct measurement of sugar, protein, lipid, and nucleotide metabolism; it is extensively applied in the diagnosis, classification, and efficacy evaluation of brain tumors. Different PET imaging agents can reflect different characteristics in tumor cells.

11.2.1 Common PET Imaging Agents

11.2.1.1 Glucose Metabolism

Fluorodeoxyglucose (FDG) is currently the most frequently used PET imaging agent that reflects glycolysis in tissues and cells. The pathological basis of ^{18}F-FDG PET is that the cells of malignant tumors exhibit a higher uptake and utilization of glucose than those of normal tissues. The majority of brain tumors are characterized by glucose hypermetabolism, while the level of ^{18}F-FDG uptake is associated with the level of tumor malignancy. More specifically, CNS tumors with relatively low malignancy show a similar level of ^{18}F-FDG uptake to that of normal white matter, whereas tumors with relatively high malignancy tend to have elevated ^{18}F-FDG uptake, but which is often similar to that of gray matter.

11.2.1.2 Amino Acids and Choline

PET imaging agents for amino acid transport that are currently in common use include ^{11}C-methionine (^{11}C-MET), O-(2-[^{18}F]fluoroethyl)-L-tyrosine (^{18}F-FET), and ^{11}C-choline (^{11}C-CH). At present, ^{11}C-MET is the most established imaging agent for amino acids in clinical research, and its retention in gliomas mainly reflects the increase in amino acid transport activity, that is, the increase of protein synthesis in tumor cells. Under normal circumstances, brain tissues (except for the pituitary) tend to exhibit very low ^{11}C-MET uptake, implying that this compound can serve as an excellent imaging agent for brain tumors. ^{11}C-MET imaging is superior to ^{18}F-FDG imaging with respect to the diagnosis of gliomas, discrimination between tumor recurrence and necrosis, early evaluation of therapeutic efficacy, and the diagnosis of peritumoral tissues and low-grade gliomas. However, ^{11}C-MET has a relatively short half-life (about 20 min), which has restricted its application in clinical practice. ^{18}F-FET has a longer half-life (110 min) than ^{11}C-MET, and its uptake does not depend on the disruption of the blood-brain barrier; therefore, it is more widely accepted in clinical applications. ^{18}F-FET PET imaging can facilitate the discrimination between brain tumors and non-neoplastic lesions, showing high sensitivity and specificity for the diagnosis of primary intracranial tumors. Furthermore, the time-activity curve acquired using dynamic ^{18}F-FET PET imaging can aid the classification and diagnosis of gliomas. This is because high-grade gliomas reach an early peak of ^{18}F-FET uptake at 10–15 min after injection, which is followed by a decrease, whereas low-grade gliomas tend to exhibit a delayed peak of ^{18}F-FET uptake that continues to rise steadily thereafter. In meta-analysis of 23 studies involving 994 patients, ^{18}F-FET PET showed a significantly higher sensitivity than ^{18}F-FDG PET for the preoperative classification of gliomas (88 vs 63%), as well as a higher specificity (89 vs 57%). In 2016, new content on molecular subtypes was added to the WHO classification of CNS tumors, which stipulated that histological morphology, WHO grade, and biomarkers must be combined in order to form an integrated diagnosis of gliomas. The most important among the molecular features are IDH mutation and chromosomal 1p/19q co-deletion status, which are intimately linked with the molecular subtyping of gliomas, formulation of individualized treatment plans, and efficacy of postoperative chemotherapy and radiotherapy. ^{18}F-FET PET imaging is useful for the prediction of glioma genotype, while also contributing clinically to prognostic prediction and the discrimination of metastasis from recurrence following radiosurgery. ^{11}C-CH is currently the most commonly applied imaging agent for Cho that can reflect its metabolism in tumors. ^{11}C-CH imaging can obtain a higher tumor-to-peripheral tissue uptake ratio than ^{11}C-MET imaging, producing better-quality images. However, ^{11}C-CH is also a non-specific tumor imaging agent, which may give rise to false positives and false negatives in tumor tests. For example, tuberculous meningiomas are positive for ^{11}C-CH, whereas some low-grade gliomas may be negative for ^{11}C-CH.

11.2.1.3 Cell Proliferation

^{18}F-fluorothymidine (^{18}F-FLT) is a PET imaging agent commonly used to reflect the activity level of cell proliferation. ^{18}F-FLT is a thymidine analog that can be acted on by thymidine kinase I to enter cells and participate in metabolism, a process similar to the reaction between ^{18}F-FDG and hexokinase. However, unlike thymidine, ^{18}F-FLT has a low affinity for mitochondrial thymidine kinase II, and can therefore serve as a tracer that specifically targets the cell cycle. Therefore, ^{18}F-FLT PET can be used to quantify mitotic activity and cell division. Furthermore, since ^{18}F-FLT is only taken up by tumor cells in the S phase of the cell cycle, it has some level of specificity for the diagnosis of brain tumors. In terms of evaluating the efficacy of radiotherapy, the decrease in ^{18}F-FLT uptake value occurs earlier than that of ^{18}F-FDG, which implies that the former can be used to differentiate between radiation necrosis and tumor recurrence. Additionally, ^{18}F-FLT PET has shown superior accuracy and higher correlation with prognosis than ^{18}F-FDG PET for the diagnosis of recurrence in high-grade gliomas.

11.2.1.4 Others

Hypoxia is a key factor contributing to the progression and drug resistance of malignant tumors; therefore, the PET imaging of hypoxia occupies a crucial position in metabolic imaging, especially for post-radiotherapy brain tumors, and can serve as a non-invasive evaluation method. ^{18}F-fluoromisonidazole (^{18}F-FMISO) is currently the most commonly applied imaging agent for hypoxia. It can freely cross the blood-brain barrier and diffuse rapidly within tissues to attain equilibrium. This diffusion process is not affected by perfusion, and ^{18}F-FMISO will only be taken up by severely hypoxic cells. ^{18}F-FMISO PET images need to be calibrated using blood samples in order to calculate the tumor-to-blood ratio of ^{18}F-FMISO uptake, while a ratio of >1.2 indicates a higher ^{18}F-FMISO uptake in hypoxic tissues compared to normal tissues. This ratio can be combined with MRI anatomical images to delineate ROIs for the calculation of hypoxic tumor volume, which is an independent factor for determining the poor prognosis of malignant gliomas.

11.2.2 Applications of PET in Brain Tumors

PET imaging is able to reflect the biochemical, metabolic, and functional status of tumor tissues. There is a wide variety of intracranial tumors, about 90% of which can be localized and qualitatively diagnosed using CT and MRI, without the use of PET. In this section, we will focus on describing the application of PET imaging in gliomas, intracranial lymphomas, and brain metastases.

11.2.2.1 Glioma

Gliomas account for 40–50% of all intracranial tumors, while different grades of gliomas exhibit different levels of ^{18}F-FDG uptake. Some studies have shown that 86% of gliomas with decreased ^{18}F-FDG uptake are classified as grades I and II, whereas 94% of those with increased ^{18}F-FDG uptake are classified as grades III and IV (Fig. 11.11). Nevertheless, there are certain drawbacks to using ^{18}F-FDG PET imaging for the clinical classification of tumors. ^{18}F-FDG is a glucose analog that can directly reflect cellular energy metabolism. However, hexokinase II is overexpressed in some brain tumors, and its catalytic effect on ^{18}F-FDG entails that PET imaging may overestimate the glucose metabolic levels of these brain tumors to a certain extent, giving rise to false positive results. Examples of such tumors include pilocytic astrocytomas and gangliogliomas. Moreover, inflammation, active tuberculosis, granulation tissues, and certain benign tumors can also present high ^{18}F-FDG uptake. Additionally, owing to the relatively high glucose metabolism of the cerebral cortex, difficulties may arise in the accurate delineation of tumor boundaries and differentiation from surrounding normal tissues. In such cases, delayed ^{18}F-FDG imaging can be implemented, as it exploits the longer retention time of radioactive tracers in tumors compared to normal gray matter, thereby improving the discriminant ability between tumors and normal tissues. Another valuable contribution of ^{18}F-FDG PET imaging in brain tumors is the ability to discriminate between tumor recurrence and radiation necrosis. More

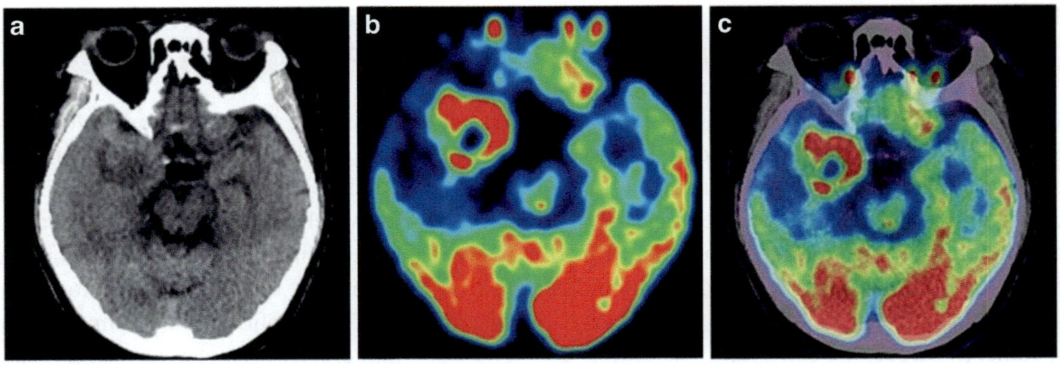

Fig. 11.11 High-grade glioma of the right temporal lobe. A 52-year-old male patient whose transverse brain CT shows a mass in the right temporal lobe, with a hypodense center and slightly hyperdense rim (**a**). Transverse ^{18}F-FDG PET (**b**) and integrated ^{18}F-FDG PET/CT (**c**) show significantly increased glucose metabolism at the rim, with a maximum standardized uptake value (SUV) of 5.75. Impaired glucose metabolism can be seen around the tumor, which signifies peritumoral edema

specifically, increased glucose uptake is observed in recurrent brain tumors, whereas decreased glucose metabolism is found in radiation necrosis. A recent meta-analysis reported that utilizing ^{18}F-FDG PET in the diagnosis of primary glioma recurrence gave an acceptable level of accuracy, with a diagnostic sensitivity of 0.77 [95% confidence interval (CI): 0.66–0.85] and specificity of 0.78 (95% CI: 0.54–0.91). Furthermore, this technique is suitable for gliomas of any histological type. However, occasionally in clinical practice, ^{18}F-FDG PET cannot clearly differentiate between tumor recurrence and radiotherapy-induced injury, regardless of whether gray or white matter is used as the reference standard. The main reason for this may be that normal brain tissue shows a relative increase in glucose uptake following radiotherapy, while the inflammatory changes caused by radiotherapy-induced injury also lead to varying degrees of increased FDG uptake.

^{11}C-MET PET imaging of brain gliomas can produce positive results in more than 90% of cases, and significant ^{11}C-MET retention can be observed even in low-grade primary brain tumors, which are clearly demarcated from normal brain tissues. ^{11}C-MET can also be utilized in the identification and localization of malignant gliomas with a high risk of post-radiotherapy recurrence. A recent meta-analysis on the post-treatment recurrence of gliomas found that ^{11}C-MET PET showed a good accuracy for high-grade gliomas, with a sensitivity of 70% (95% CI: 50–84%) and specificity of 93% (95% CI: 44–100%).

^{18}F-FET is currently the most commonly used PET tracer for gliomas. There are overlaps in the levels of ^{18}F-FET uptake among different grades of gliomas. The tumor-to-brain ratio (TBR) derived from ^{18}F-FET PET can be used to differentiate between high- and low-grade gliomas with a sensitivity of 71–80% and a specificity of 56–85%, while the cutoff values of mean TBR and maximum TBR for the differentiation between high- and low-grade tumors are 1.9–2.9 and 2.5–2.7, respectively. A meta-analysis of 23 studies involving 994 patients showed that ^{18}F-FET PET had a significantly higher sensitivity than ^{18}F-FDG PET for the preoperative classification of gliomas (88 vs 63%), whereas ^{18}F-FDG PET had a higher specificity than ^{18}F-FET PET (89 vs 57%). In addition to providing information for the preoperative classification of gliomas, ^{18}F-FET PET can also supplement the prediction of glioma molecular subtypes (Figs. 11.12 and 11.13). Verger et al. divided 90 newly diagnosed, and untreated patients with gliomas into three groups: IDH-mutant and 1p/19q co-deleted oligodendrogliomas (16 cases), IDH-mutant astrocytomas (27 cases), and IDH-wildtype glioblastomas (47 cases). The results of their

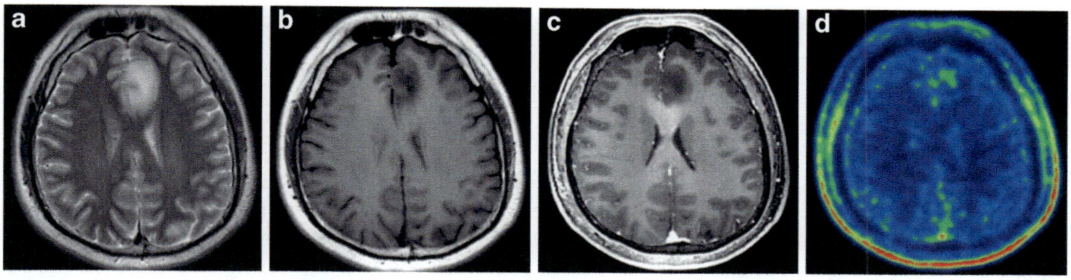

Fig. 11.12 Left frontal lobe oligodendroglioma, WHO grade II. A 19-year-old male patient whose MRI shows an oval mass in the left frontal lobe. Transverse T_2WI shows heterogeneous hyperintense signals (**a**); transverse T_1WI shows hypointense signals without significant edema (**b**); contrast-enhanced scan shows no significant enhancement (**c**); and transverse ^{18}F-FET PET shows slightly increased uptake within the lesion (**d**)

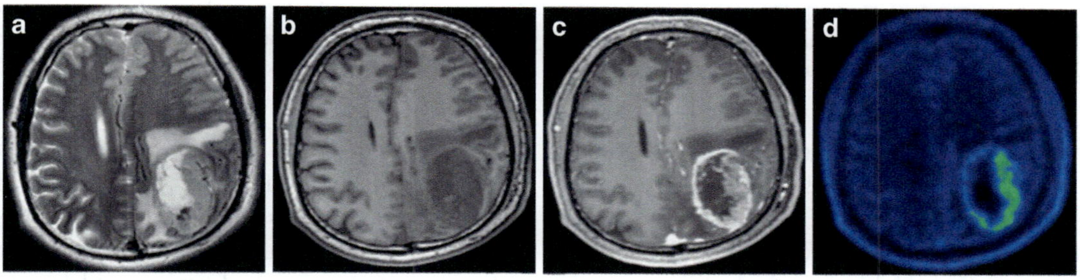

Fig. 11.13 Left parietal lobe glioblastoma, WHO grade IV. A 41-year-old male patient whose MRI shows an oval mass in the left parietal lobe. Transverse T_2WI shows heterogeneous mixed isointense and hyperintense signals (**a**); transverse T_1WI shows hypointense signals surrounded by finger-like edema signals (**b**); contrast-enhanced scan shows significant ring-like enhancement (**c**); and transverse ^{18}F-FET PET shows significantly increased uptake within the lesion (**d**)

study revealed that the mean TBR, maximum TBR, time-to-peak (TTP), and slope of ^{18}F-FET uptake could each discriminate between IDH-mutant astrocytomas and IDH-wildtype glioblastomas. Of these, mean TBR showed the best diagnostic performance, with an optimal cutoff value of 1.95, and a sensitivity, specificity, and accuracy of 89, 67, and 81%, respectively. Mean TBR, maximum TBR, TTP, and slope were all useful for predicting IDH mutation status, with the combined multiparametric prediction reaching an accuracy of up to 73%.

11.2.2.2 Intracranial Lymphoma

PCNSL is a rare malignant tumor of the CNS. It is classified as an invasive extranodal non-Hodgkin's lymphoma, and its pathological type is mostly diffuse large B-cell lymphoma. Despite its low incidence, PCNSL has a very high level of malignancy. Primary intracranial lymphomas generally do not involve the whole body and are mostly found in immunocompromised patients, such as patients with AIDS or patients receiving long-term immunosuppressive therapy after organ transplantation. PCNSL frequently occurs in the frontal lobe, temporal lobe, basal ganglia, corpus callosum, periventricular white matter, and cerebellum, either as single or multiple lesions. At present, the preliminary diagnosis of PCNSL depends primarily on CT and MRI. However, intracranial PCNSL shares many similar CT and MRI findings with other common intracranial space-occupying diseases (e.g., gliomas, and intracranial metastases of malignant tumors), which has led to a high rate of misdiagnosis. ^{18}F-FDG PET/CT is an imaging approach that integrates anatomical with functional information. It combines anatomical structural information with glucose metabolic status, in order to analyze the characteristics of lesions, which can

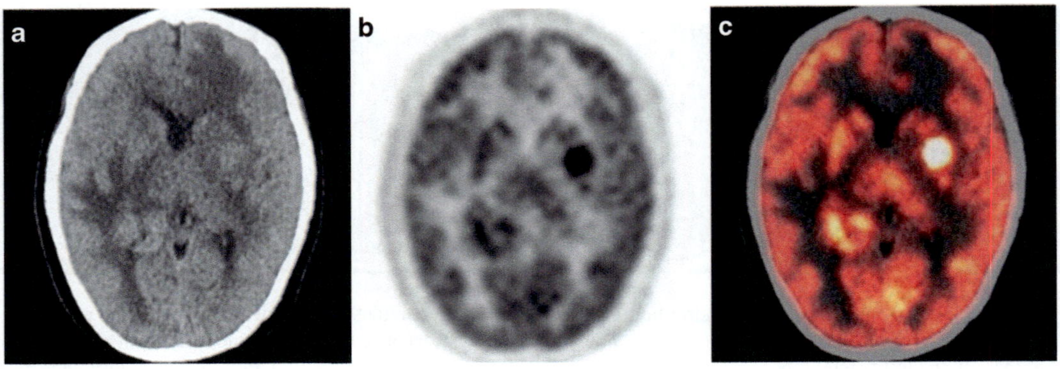

Fig. 11.14 Central nervous system lymphoma (diffuse large B-cell). A 68-year-old female patient whose transverse brain CT shows multiple hyperdense masses in the left basal ganglia, left frontal lobe, and right posterior horn of the lateral ventricle, surrounded by flaky hypodensities (**a**). Transverse ^{18}F-FDG PET (**b**) and integrated ^{18}F-FDG PET/CT (**c**) shows significant glucose hypermetabolism in the lesions above, showing a maximum standardized uptake value (SUV) of 10.49, and large areas of peripheral edema

facilitate the diagnosis of intracranial primary lymphomas. ^{18}F-FDG PET imaging of untreated intracranial lymphomas will reveal a clearly demarcated radioactive foci with a high level of retention (Fig. 11.14), but which still needs to be differentiated from single intracranial metastases. ^{18}F-FDG PET imaging can also be utilized in the evaluation of therapeutic efficacy in primary intracranial lymphomas. Additionally, ^{11}C-MET imaging can display clear radioactive foci, but the extent of these foci tends to be larger than that revealed in CT.

11.2.2.3 Brain Metastasis

MRI can be implemented to obtain a large amount of information related to brain metastases. Additionally, conventional structural imaging, MRI can also acquire functional metabolic information through diffusion, perfusion, and spectroscopic imaging. PET imaging is a useful supplement to MRI and can provide further metabolic information on brain metastases (Fig. 11.15). The principle of ^{18}F-FDG imaging for brain metastases is the same as that for primary intracranial tumors, which also implies it has a number of similar shortcomings in clinical application. For example, the high background noise in the cortex and basal ganglia can significantly reduce the signal-to-noise ratio of PET imaging, and its resolution is also relatively low, which has restricted its wider clinical application. In addition to ^{18}F-FDG, other tracers, such as those reflecting the level of amino acid metabolism, can also be utilized in the diagnosis and efficacy evaluation of brain metastases. The active transport process of amino acid tracers can provide metabolic information without relying on impairments to the blood-brain barrier. Furthermore, the significantly lower background activity of amino acid tracers in the brain than ^{18}F-FDG is also another major advantage. However, neither ^{18}F-FDG nor amino acid PET imaging can accurately discriminate brain metastases from common primary malignant tumors of the brain, such as glioblastomas. Although ^{18}F-FET uptake may be higher in high-grade gliomas than low-grade gliomas, there are overlaps in the uptake values among glioblastomas, metastases, and inflammatory diseases such as multiple sclerosis. Even epileptogenic foci may cause abnormal ^{18}F-FET uptake. A large-scale study using ^{18}F-FET for the diagnosis of brain space-occupying lesions found no difference between the standardized uptake values (SUV) of high-grade gliomas and non-neoplastic lesions. Furthermore, ^{18}F-FET PET imaging showed a low sensitivity for micrometastases. Therefore, there has been an intensification in the research and development of novel PET tracers, with the aim of overcoming the limitations of PET imaging in clinical applications.

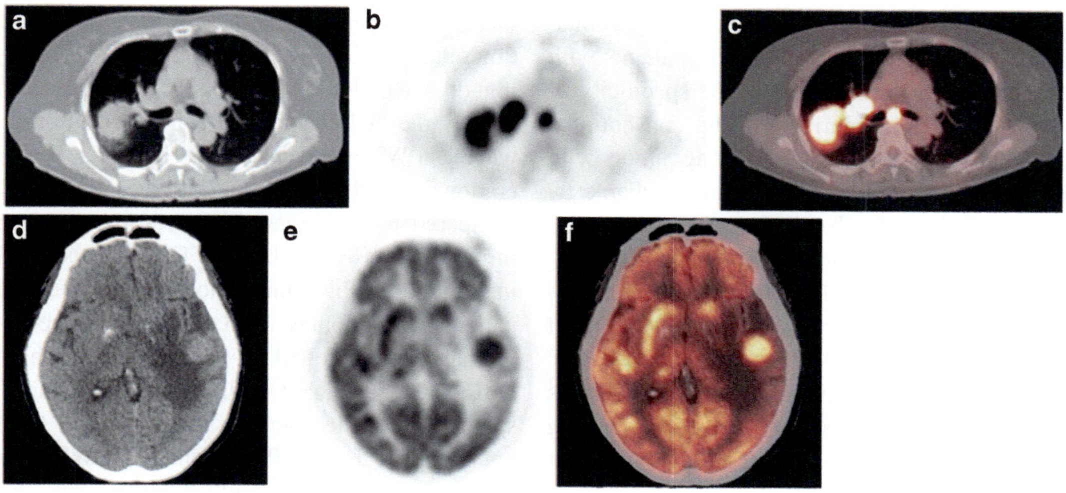

Fig. 11.15 Adenocarcinoma of the right upper lobe of the lung with mediastinal, right hilar, and brain metastases. A 70-year-old male patient. Transverse ^{18}F-FDG PET/CT shows soft tissue masses in the right upper lobe of the lung, with lobular and spiculate edges (**a**). Transverse ^{18}F-FDG PET (**b**) and integrated ^{18}F-FDG PET/CT (**c**) show significant glucose hypermetabolism of the lesion in the right lung, and right hilar and mediastinal metastatic lymph nodes. Transverse ^{18}F-FDG PET/CT shows hyperdense nodules in the left temporal lobe (**d**). Transverse ^{18}F-FDG PET (**e**) and integrated ^{18}F-FDG PET/CT (**f**) show significant glucose hypermetabolism of the lesions, with a large area of peripheral edema, suggestive of metastatic lesions

PET plays an important role in the formulation of treatment plans for brain metastases. A study reported on the use of MRI and ^{11}C-MET PET to evaluate the recurrence of brain metastasis treated with γ-knife radiosurgery. It was found that the irradiation field delineated based on ^{11}C-MET PET was smaller than that formulated under MRI guidance, but led to a longer patient survival time, suggesting that ^{11}C-MET PET can more effectively guide the delineation of the irradiation target. Similar findings were observed for ^{18}F-FET imaging. The increase in brain metastasis volume is not a marker of tumor progression. As with gliomas, radiation-induced changes may be mistaken for tumor progression; therefore, PET imaging can assist with the differentiation from radiation necrosis. In terms of ^{11}C-MET, its uptake in brain metastases is higher than that in radiation necrosis, with a sensitivity of 79% and specificity of 75%, while ^{18}F-FET uptake is significantly correlated with ^{11}C-MET uptake (r = 0.84). Furthermore, the results of dynamic ^{18}F-FET imaging showed that combining TBR (>1.9) with time-activity curves can achieve a diagnostic accuracy of up to 93%.

One of the current research hotspots is the discovery of early imaging-based markers for the evaluation of therapeutic efficacy, to improve the treatment strategies of patients. Therefore, there is a need to fully develop and validate imaging markers, whether they are based on MRI or PET, to fulfill their clinical applications.

11.3 Research Applications of PET/MR in Brain Tumors

Although MRI is a routine scan performed in brain tumors, conventional structural MRI may not be able to reliably predict the malignancy or growth potential of lesions. Furthermore, damage to normal brain structures caused by postoperative injury and chemoradiotherapy-induced necrosis, as well as non-specific treatment-induced signals such as inflammation, edema, demyelination, ischemia, and metal implants, have all increased the challenges faced by the clinical application of MRI. A number of new treatment strategies, such as anti-angiogenesis therapy or immunotherapy, may obscure or cause the enhancement of the affected area, which further affects the diagnostic accuracy in the evaluation of post-treatment response. In patients with glioma receiving radiotherapy, the specificity of detecting glioma recurrence using conventional MRI may be as low as 50%. Among tumors with imaging features of low-grade gliomas characterized by the lack of enhancement, 40% of the final pathological confirmation may consist of high-grade components. fMRI, PET, and other functional imaging techniques can also reflect tissue-specific biological characteristics. Therefore, the combination of PET with MRI has potential implications for further improving overall diagnostic accuracy and patient management.

11.3.1 Advantages of Integrated PET/MR over Conventional Equipment

In recent years, a large number of studies have stressed on the potential application value of multiparametric integrated PET/MR in brain tumors. Preliminary studies have mainly focused on the practicality and consistency of multimodal imaging based on integrated PET/MR, and few have examined diagnostic accuracy. The earliest study on the accuracy of integrated PET/MR involved the comparison between PET/CT and PET/MR in evaluating the relationship of primary CNS tumors. The results revealed that the imaging quality of PET/MR and PET/CT both satisfied the diagnostic criteria, and the resulting TBR showed excellent concordance, with a Pearson's correlation coefficient of 0.98. Furthermore, compared to PET/CT, PET/MR had higher sensitivity and showed no artifacts or distortions in all images produced. Integrated PET/MR enables the simultaneous acquisition of PET and MRI, which allows the comparison of direction correlations among different imaging parameters obtained during a single scan session. This, in turn, helps us to explore the complementarity of metabolic or anatomical information provided by different modalities.

The preliminary investigations on PET/MR were mostly bimodal studies, mainly comparing the concordance and variability in the information obtained using either amino acid PET imaging or MRI alone. ^{18}F-FET PET imaging can display the malignancy and activity of gliomas, whereas PWI can reveal the microvascular proliferation and perfusion of tumor tissues. Filss et al. compared the differences between the imaging information provided by ^{18}F-FET PET and PWI in patients with brain tumors. A total of 56 patients with gliomas and 8 patients with meningiomas were enrolled in the study, for whom TBRs were calculated, while the tumor volumes, spatial congruence, and distance between local hot spots in ^{18}F-FET PET scans and PWI maps were assessed. Their results revealed that ^{18}F-FET PET could clearly discriminate between tumor tissues and normal regions, which was more difficult to accomplish using rCBV maps. Furthermore, in patients with gliomas, the TBR and tumor volumes based on ^{18}F-FET PET were significantly larger than in rCBV maps [TBR: 2.28 ± 0.99 vs. 1.62 ± 1.13, $P < 0.001$; tumor volume: (24.3 ± 26.5) cm^3 vs. (8.9 ± 13.9) cm^3; $P < 0.001$], while the spatial congruence between the two was poor, and the mean distance between local hot spots was (25.4 ± 16.1) mm. In patients with meningiomas, the TBR in ^{18}F-FET PET was significantly larger than in rCBV maps [TBR: $(5.33 \pm 2.63$ vs. 2.37 ± 0.32, $P < 0.001)$], but the spatial distribution of tumors was similar between the two. These findings imply that performing tumor imaging with ^{18}F-FET PET and rCBV in patients with gliomas can yield different information. Compared to rCBV maps, ^{18}F-FET PET showed significantly higher TBRs and tumor volumes, with a poor spatial congruence between the two parameters and a large variability in local hot spots. Taken together, the results indicate that rCBV as measured by PWI does not reflect the metabolically active tumor tissues of gliomas as depicted by amino acid PET. Apart from PWI, there is also an ongoing debate as to whether DWI indicators, such as minimum ADC, can be applied clinically in preoperative tumor classification and treatment planning. In order to establish the pathological correlate of minimum ADC, Rose et al. examined the relationship between minimum ADC and maximum ^{18}F-fluorodopa

(^{18}F-FDOPA) PET uptake in patients with newly diagnosed glioblastoma multiforme. In this study, MRI and ^{18}F-FDOPA PET data were acquired preoperatively from 15 patients with high-grade brain tumors (WHO grade III or IV), and regions of minimum ADC value within the tumor volume defined by ^{18}F-FDOPA PET was correlated with regions of maximum ^{18}F-FDOPA uptake. The results showed limited anatomical overlap between regions with minimum ADC and maximum TBR. Compared to the region with maximum ^{18}F-FDOPA TBR (2.45 ± 0.88) within the tumor tissues, the region with minimum ADC had a significantly lower ^{18}F-FDOPA TBR (1.36 ± 0.22, $P = 0.0001$). This implies that there is a poor correlation between minimum ADC and the most aggressive component of high-grade gliomas. Therefore, other factors, such as tissue compression or local ischemia, may have contributed to the restricted diffusion of glioblastomas. Therefore, caution should be exercised when utilizing minimum ADC as a marker of tumor grade and as a preoperative guidance for tumor biopsies in clinical practice.

11.3.2 Clinical Applications of Integrated PET/MR

11.3.2.1 Guidance for Preoperative Needle Biopsy

As the clinical application of PET/MR in brain tumors continues to advance, studies have found that this technique can provide useful guidance for the preoperative needle biopsy of brain tumors. Masada et al. reported the case of a 53-year-old male patient with malignant lymphoma who complained of walking and gait disturbances. MRI revealed multiple lesions of the bilateral frontal lobe, with significant enhancements in contrast-enhanced scan, while ^{18}F-FDG PET showed significant heterogeneous increases in lesion ^{18}F-FDG uptake. Needle biopsy was performed under the guidance of PET and MRI co-registration, and histological examination confirmed the lesion as malignant lymphoma, indicating that PET/MR co-registration can help to determine the most active component of brain tumors. MRS and PET are both non-invasive imaging methods of proliferation-related cell metabolism and are therefore more likely to detect highly active tumor regions. Some researchers have attempted to incorporate preoperative MRS and PET into the intraoperative navigation system to guide the surgical biopsy and tumor sampling of gliomas, thereby improving the intraoperative characterization of tumor tissues and verification of imaging biomarkers. Their results demonstrated that this approach enabled neurosurgeons to sample the tumor region based on physiological and molecular imaging markers. In a case of needle biopsy performed within a pathologically confirmed astrocytoma (WHO grade II), a region without marked enhancement but with elevated local Cho peak and increased ^{11}C-MET uptake was confirmed through needle biopsy as an early malignant transformation zone. MRI is the most common method utilized to determine the location and extent of gliomas. In a prospective study, Pauleit et al. explored whether diagnostic accuracy could be improved by combining MRI with ^{18}F-FET PET. Co-registration was performed between the ^{18}F-FET PET and MRI images of 31 patients with suspected gliomas, followed by needle biopsies at regions with both abnormal MRI signals and increased ^{18}F-FET uptake (match), as well as regions with abnormal MRI signals but normal ^{18}F-FET uptake or vice versa (mismatch), which gave a total of 52 biopsy samples. The results showed that the diagnostic performance (as measured using AUC) of needle biopsies based on MRI alone was 0.80, with a sensitivity of 96% for detecting tumor tissues, and a specificity of only 53%; whereas the diagnostic performance of MRI combined with ^{18}F-FET PET increased to 0.98, with a sensitivity of 93% and specificity of 94%. These findings indicate that the combined use of MRI and ^{18}F-FET PET in patients with gliomas significantly improves the identification of glioma tissues, which has significant implications for target selection in the diagnostic biopsies and treatment planning of gliomas.

Several studies have demonstrated that amino acid PET imaging shows a different glioma extent from conventional plain and contrast-enhanced MRI (Fig. 11.16), while the combination of the two can help to guide the extent of surgical resection and determine the target area of radiotherapy. In a study on 50 patients with newly diagnosed, untreated glioblastoma, Lohmann et al. performed a retrospective analysis on the tumor volumes delineated by ^{18}F-FET PET (V_{PET}) and by contrast-enhanced and FLAIR MRI (V_{MRI}). They found that 43 patients (86%) showed significantly larger V_{PET} than V_{MRI} [(21.5 ± 14.3) mL vs. (9.4 ± 11.3) mL; $P < 0.001$], while 40 patients (80%) showed both increased FET uptake and significant contrast enhancement, but with low spatial similarity in tumor volume between the two, and 10% of patients showing increased ^{18}F-FET uptake beyond the areas of abnormal FLAIR signals. Taken together, this study has shown that the tumor volume delineated by ^{18}F-FET PET is significantly larger than that by MRI contrast enhancement, which strongly suggests that the information derived from the two modalities should be combined to guide the treatment and diagnosis of patients with newly diagnosed glioblastomas. Some researchers argue that contrast-enhanced MRI cannot reflect the entire infiltration extent of gliomas, whereas the amino acid tracer, ^{18}F-DOPA, shows a higher TBR and sensitivity for gliomas. Therefore, they compared between the tumor extents delineated by PET and conventional MRI in 10 patients with glioma and obtained 23 biopsy samples from matched or mismatched areas between metabolism and contrast enhancement. Their findings revealed that among the 16 samples histopathologically confirmed as high-grade gliomas, 13 were obtained from areas with increased metabolism, whereas only 6 were obtained from areas with contrast enhancement in contrast-enhanced images. Given these results, they concluded that ^{18}F-DOPA PET metabolism

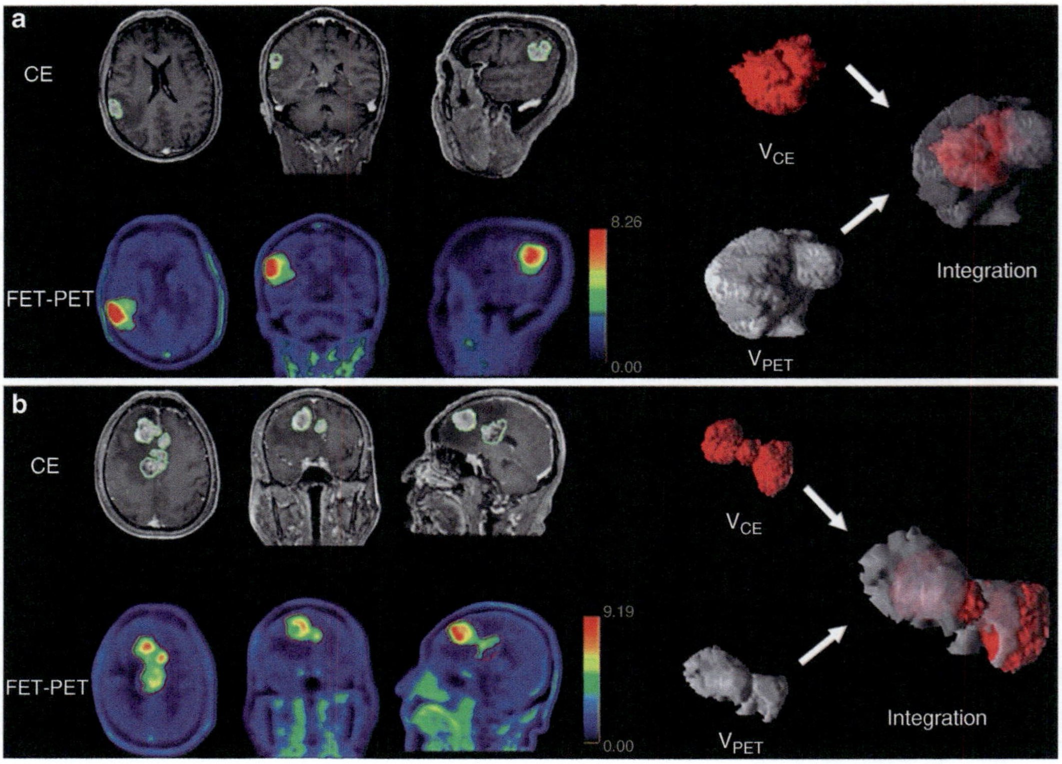

Fig. 11.16 Integrated ^{18}F-FET PET/MR improves the presentation of glioma spatial distribution. ^{18}F-FET-PET and contrast-enhanced (CE) MRI show low spatial similarity but large overlaps. V_{PET} is significantly larger than V_{CE}, and most of V_{CE} is contained within V_{PET} (**a**). There is high spatial dissimilarity between V_{PET} and V_{CE} (**b**), and the two are mutually complementary in the delineation of the entire tumor. Arrows: integration

can more accurately identify higher-grade regions within gliomas, and is therefore valuable in guiding the target selection of stereotactic biopsies.

11.3.2.2 Assistance for Preoperative Diagnosis of Brain Tumors

PET/MR is also valuable for the preoperative diagnosis of brain tumors. Findings on the use of MRI features alone to discriminate between high- and low-grade gliomas have remained controversial. In view of this, a retrospective analysis was performed on 127 patients with MRI-suspected low-grade gliomas, who were enrolled based on the following inclusion criteria: lesions with no significant contrast enhancement, showing hyperintense T_2WI signals, hypointense T_1WI signals, and no intralesional hemorrhage or necrosis. The final pathological confirmation revealed that 47 patients had high-grade glioma, and 7 had non-neoplastic lesions; 97 patients exhibited ^{18}F-FET hypermetabolism, of whom 93 patients with neoplastic lesions, 69% with low-grade gliomas, and 89% with high-grade gliomas showed increased ^{18}F-FET uptake; the kinetic analysis of ^{18}F-FET showed that the sensitivity for high-grade gliomas was 95%; specificity, 72%; positive predictive value, 74%; and negative predictive value, 95%. Based on these findings, it can be seen that among MRI-suspected low-grade gliomas, the kinetic analysis of ^{18}F-FET showed an extremely high sensitivity for the detection of high-grade gliomas. Given that PWI and ^{18}F-FET PET can both provide grading information for gliomas, researchers have compared the diagnostic value of ^{18}F-FET PET and PWI for the tumor grading of patients with newly diagnosed, untreated gliomas using an integrated PET/MR scanner. They found that both techniques showed high accuracy in the discrimination of high- and low-grade gliomas. In order to further elucidate the value of molecular imaging for exploring intratumoral heterogeneity in low-grade gliomas. Kunz et al. designed a prospective study involving 55 patients with MRI-suspected WHO grade II gliomas. By analyzing the kinetic curve characteristics of ^{18}F-FET, the patients were divided into three subgroups: (1) a homogeneous WHO grade II glioma group (30 patients), (2) a homogeneous malignant glioma group (10 patients), and (3) a heterogeneous group exhibiting both low- and high-grade characteristics at different sites (15 cases). The assessment of 373 biopsy samples obtained from these patients revealed a strong correlation between tumor grade and uptake kinetics ($P < 0.0001$). Homogeneous patterns of uptake kinetics were associated with homogeneous histopathological findings, while heterogeneous patterns were associated with histopathological heterogeneity. Furthermore, local hot spots exhibiting characteristics of malignant glioma accounted for 4–44% of the entire tumor volume; therefore, the researchers concluded that in MRI-suspected WHO grade II gliomas, ^{18}F-FET uptake kinetics were closely linked with intratumoral histopathology, which can facilitate the accurate identification of local anaplastic foci and has significant implications for prognostic evaluation and treatment planning. Haubold et al. utilized radiomics to analyze the value of multiparametric ^{18}F-FET PET/MR in guiding the preoperative grading and genotype prediction of 42 patients with gliomas. They found that the combination of contrast-enhanced MRI, ^{18}F-FET PET, and SWI showed the best performance in discriminating between high- and low-grade gliomas, with an AUC, sensitivity, and specificity of 0.85, 83.1%, and 79.6%, respectively; the AUC and sensitivity were lower than those of this study. Moreover, the AUCs of this combination in predicting glioma IDH1 mutation, 1p/19q co-deletion, and MGMT promoter methylation status were 0.887, 0.978, and 0.757, respectively. Another study found that multimodal imaging using integrated ^{18}F-FET PET/MR allows the non-invasive prediction of glioma IDH mutation status, and the discrimination of IDH-wildtype glioblastomas (Fig. 11.17) from IDH-mutant astrocytomas without 1p/19q co-deletion (Fig. 11.18), providing imaging evidence for the accurate preoperative diagnosis of gliomas, guidance of clinical treatment decisions, and evaluation of patient prognosis. However, this technique had limited value in discriminating between IDH-mutant, 1p/19q co-deleted oligodendrogliomas and IDH-mutant astrocytomas without 1p/19q co-deletion (Fig. 11.19), and therefore requires further investigation.

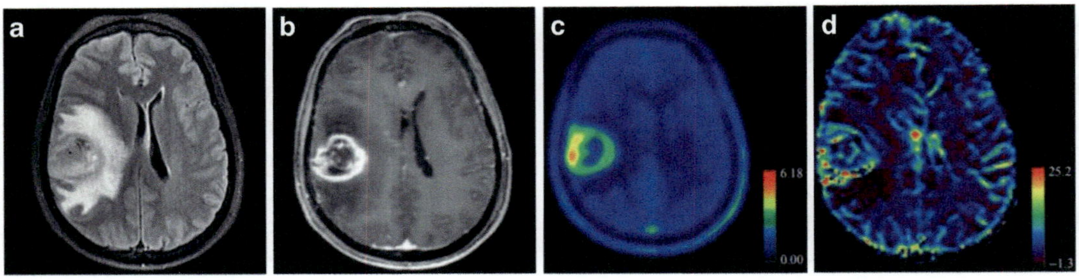

Fig. 11.17 IDH-wildtype glioblastoma, WHO grade IV. A 53-year-old male patient, whose integrated PET/MR shows a round mass in the right parietal lobe. Transverse FLAIR shows heterogeneous mixed hyper- and hypointense signals with finger-like perilesional edema (**a**); contrast-enhanced scan shows a heterogeneous ring-enhancing lesion (**b**); transverse ^{18}F-FET PET shows significantly enhanced uptake within the lesion, with TBR_{mean} and TBR_{max} values of 2.48 and 4.83, respectively (**c**); and the solid component of the lesion shows significantly elevated CBV, with relative mean and maximum CBV values of 2.78 and 6.63, respectively (**d**)

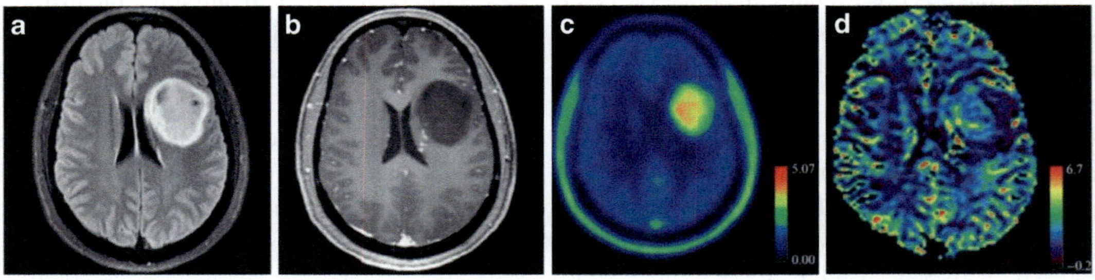

Fig. 11.18 IDH-mutant astrocytoma without 1p/19q co-deletion. A 31-year-old female patient, whose integrated PE/MRI shows a round mass in the left frontoparietal lobe. Transverse FLAIR shows heterogeneous hyperintense signals without significant perilesional edema (**a**); contrast-enhanced scan shows no significant contrast enhancement (**b**); transverse ^{18}F-FET PET shows significantly enhanced uptake within the lesion, with TBR_{mean} and TBR_{max} values of 2.35 and 3.74, respectively, which are both lower than those of IDH-wildtype glioblastoma and IDH-mutant, 1p/19q co-deleted oligodendroglioma (**c**); and lesion CBV is slightly elevated compared to the contralateral side, with relative mean and maximum CBV values of 0.83 and 3.24, respectively, which are both lower than those of IDH-wildtype glioblastoma and IDH-mutant, 1p/19q co-deleted oligodendroglioma (**d**)

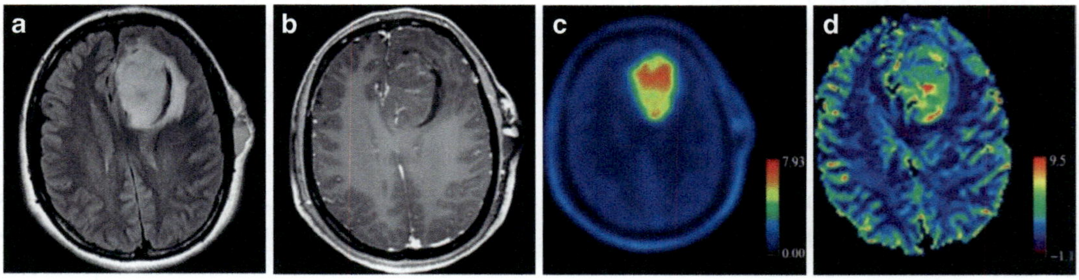

Fig. 11.19 IDH-mutant, 1p/19q co-deleted oligodendroglioma, WHO grade III. A 34-year-old female patient, whose integrated PET/MR shows a round mass in the left frontal lobe. Transverse FLAIR shows heterogeneous hyperintense signals with patchy perilesional edema (**a**); contrast-enhanced scan shows mild punctate enhancement within the lesion (**b**); transverse ^{18}F-FET PET shows significantly enhanced uptake within the lesion, with TBR_{mean} and TBR_{max} values of 3.98 and 7.35, respectively (**c**); and lesion CBV is significantly elevated, with relative mean and maximum CBV values of 1.08 and 3.33, respectively (**d**)

11.3.2.3 Evaluation of Therapeutic Efficacy and Prognosis in Brain Tumors

PET/MR is an important approach in the follow-up and evaluation of therapeutic efficacy in the treatment of brain tumors (Fig. 11.20), discrimination between true recurrence and pseudoprogression, and prognostic prediction. In a study involving 16 patients with glioma undergoing standard radiotherapy, preoperative ^{18}F-FET PET/CT, and ^{18}F-FET PET/MR (including DWI, PWI, etc.) were performed, and the correlation between multimodal imaging parameters and tumor recurrence was analyzed. The results of the study indicated that performing multiparametric imaging before radiotherapy was feasible, and significant parametric differences were observed between the recurring and non-recurring groups at the voxel level. Furthermore, combining the imaging parameters is a logistic regression model allowed the prediction of recurrence probability in glioma patients, in which ^{18}F-FET was found to be the most important predictor. Quantitative volumetric (3D-VOI) lesion analysis has also been utilized to examine the diagnostic potential of integrated ^{18}F-FET PET/MR for the differentiation between recurrent gliomas and post-treatment-related effects (PTRE). In this retrospective study, recurrence was evaluated in 42 patients, including 32 patients with histologically confirmed glioma recurrence and 10 patients with PTRE, for whom, the mean (relative) ADC (ADC_{mean}, $rADC_{mean}$) and TBR were calculated. The results indicated that the glioma recurrence group showed higher ADC_{mean} and TBR_{max} than the PTRE group ($P < 0.05$). Both ADC_{mean} and TBR_{max} demonstrated reliable diagnostic performance in differentiating between glioma recurrence and PTRE. Furthermore, the bivariate analysis based on ADC_{mean} and TBR_{max} showed the highest diagnostic accuracy of up to 90% and is therefore useful for providing clinical guidance.

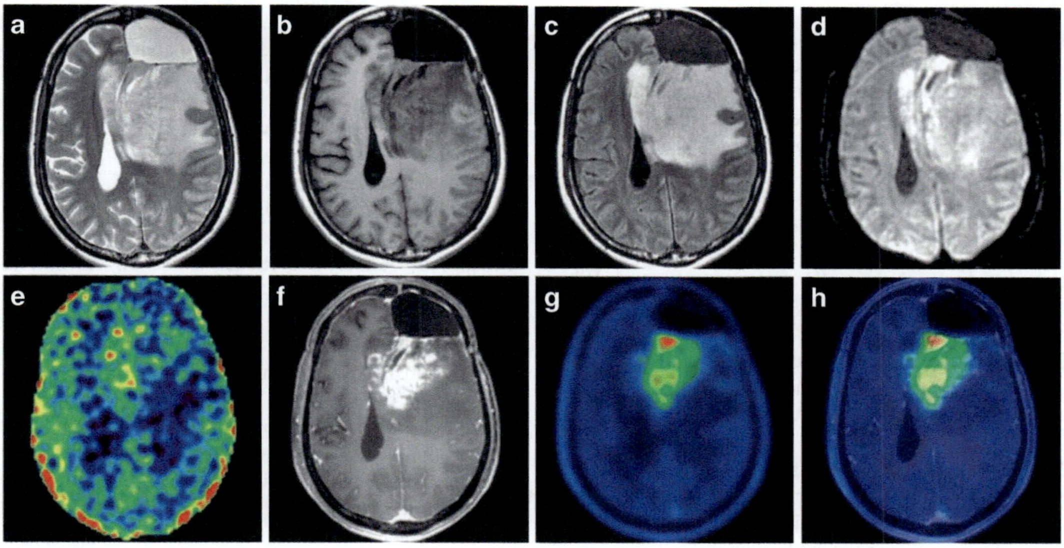

Fig. 11.20 Diagnosis of postoperative glioma recurrence using integrated ^{18}F-FET PET/MR. Integrated PET/MR shows an irregular mass in the left frontoparietal lobe, as well as a residual postoperative cavity situated anterior to the lesion. Transverse T_2WI shows heterogeneous hyperintense signals (**a**); transverse T_1WI shows heterogeneous hypointense signals (**b**); transverse FLAIR shows heterogeneous hyperintense signals with a small amount of perilesional edema (**c**); transverse DWI shows heterogeneous hyperintense signals (**d**); transverse ASL shows heterogeneous increases in lesion CBF (**e**); contrast-enhanced scan shows significant contrast enhancement (**f**); transverse ^{18}F-FET PET shows significant heterogeneous increased uptake within the lesion (**g**, **h**)

In summary, the clinical applications of combining PET and MRI are extremely valuable in neuro-oncology. Regardless of using separate scans that are subsequently merged, or one-stop scanning using integrated PET/MR, the use of such techniques will increase over the next few years. Although exciting results have been achieved through the combination of amino acid PET and advanced MRI techniques, more research is needed to determine its best applications. Integrated PET/MR scanners are expected to improve patient comfort and their potential as a one-stop imaging technique in neuro-oncology will be fully realized in the future.

Suggested Reading

Wang LL, Leach JL, Breneman JC, et al. Critical role of imaging in the neurosurgical and radiotherapeutic management of brain tumors. Radiographics. 2014;34(3):702–21.

Leu K, Ott GA, Lai A, et al. Perfusion and diffusion MRI signatures in histologic and genetic subtypes of WHO grade II-III diffuse gliomas. J Neurooncol. 2017;134(1):177–88.

Barajas RFJR, Rubenstein JL, Chang JS, et al. Diffusion-weighted MR imaging derived apparent diffusion coefficient is predictive of clinical outcome in primary central nervous system lymphoma. AJNR Am J Neuroradiol. 2010;31(1):60–6.

Huang WY, Wen JB, Wu G, et al. Diffusion-Weighted Imaging for Predicting and Monitoring Primary Central Nervous System Lymphoma Treatment Response. AJNR Am J Neuroradiol. 2016;37(11):2010–8.

Farquharson S, Tournier JD, Calamante F, et al. White matter fiber tractography: why we need to move beyond DTI. J Neurosurg. 2013;118(6):1367–77.

Delgado AF, Delgado AF. Discrimination between Glioma Grades II and III Using Dynamic Susceptibility Perfusion MRI: A Meta-Analysis. Am J Neuroradiol. 2017;38(7):1348–55.

Morabito R, Alafaci C, Pergolizzi S, et al. DCE and DSC perfusion MRI diagnostic accuracy in the follow-up of primary and metastatic intra-axial brain tumors treated by radiosurgery with cyberknife. Radiat Oncol. 2019;14(1):65.

Nakamura H, Doi M, Suzuki T, et al. The Significance of Lactate and Lipid Peaks for Predicting Primary Neuroepithelial Tumor Grade with Proton MR Spectroscopy. Magn Reson Med Sci. 2018;17(3):238–43.

Dimou S, Battisti RA, Hermens DF, et al. A systematic review of functional magnetic resonance imaging and diffusion tensor imaging modalities used in presurgical planning of brain tumour resection. Neurosurg Rev. 2013;36(2):205–14.

Zulfiqar M, Dumrongpisutikul N, Intrapiromkul J, et al. Detection of intratumoral calcification in oligodendrogliomas by susceptibility-weighted MR imaging. Am J Neuroradiol. 2012;33(5):858–64.

Zhang L, Min Z, Tang M, et al. The utility of diffusion MRI with quantitative ADC measurements for differentiating high-grade from low-grade cerebral gliomas: evidence from a meta-analysis. J Neurol Sci. 2017;373:9–15.

Chen Z, Tie Y, Olubiyi O, et al. Reconstruction of the arcuate fasciculus for surgical planning in the setting of peritumoral edema using two-tensor unscented Kalman filter tractography. Neuroimage Clin. 2015;7:815–22.

Chen W, Cloughesy T, Kamdar N, et al. Imaging proliferation in brain tumors with 18F-FLT PET: comparison with ^{18}F-FDG. J Nucl Med. 2005;46(6):945–52.

Spence AM, Muzi M, Mankoff DA, et al. ^{18}F-FDG PET of gliomas at delayed intervals: improved distinction between tumor and normal gray matter. J Nucl Med. 2004;45(10):1653–9.

Nihashi T, Dahabreh IJ, Terasawa T. Diagnostic accuracy of PET for recurrent glioma diagnosis, a meta-analysis. Am J Neuroradiol. 2013;34(5):944–50.

Hutterer M, Nowosielski M, Putzer D, et al. [^{18}F]-fluoro-ethyl-L-tyrosine PET: a valuable diagnostic tool in neuro-oncology, but not all that glitters is glioma. Neuro Oncol. 2013;15(5):341–51.

Unterrainer M, Galldiks N, Suchorska B, et al. ^{18}F-FET PET uptake characteristics in patients with newly diagnosed and untreated brain metastasis. J Nucl Med. 2017;58(4):584–9.

Momose T, Nariai T, Kawabe T, et al. Clinical benefit of ^{11}C-methionine PET imaging as a planning modality for radiosurgery of previously irradiated recurrent brain metastases. Clin Nucl Med. 2014;39(11):939–43.

Grosu AL, Astner ST, Riedel E, et al. An interindividual comparison of O-(2[18F]fluoroethyl)-L-tyrosine(FET)-and L-[methyl-11C] methionine(MET)-PET in patients with brain gliomas and metastases. Int J Radiat Oncol Biol Phys. 2011;81(4):1049–58.

Ceccon G, Lohmann P, Stoffels G, et al. Dynamic O-(2-18F-fluoroethyl)-L-tyrosine positron emission tomography differentiates brain metastasis recurrence from radiation injury after radiotherapy. Neuro Oncol. 2016;19(2):281–8.

Jansen N, Graute V, Armbruster L, et al. MRI-suspected low-grade glioma: is there a need to perform dynamic FET PET? Eur J Nucl Med Mol Imaging. 2012;39(6):1021–9.

Kunz M, Thon N, Eigenbrod S, et al. Hot spots in dynamic(FET)-F-18-PET delineate malignant tumor parts within suspected WHO grade II gliomas. Neuro Oncol. 2011;13(3):307–16.

Galldiks N, Langen K, Pope WB. From the clinician's point of view-What is the status quo of positron emission tomography in patients with brain tumors? Neuro Oncol. 2015;17(11):1434–44.

Albert NL, Weller M, Suchorska B, et al. Response Assessment in Neuro-Oncology working group and European Association for Neuro-Oncology recommendations for the clinical use of PET imaging in gliomas. Neuro Oncol. 2016;18(9):1199–208.

Fink JR, Muzi M, Peck M, et al. Multimodality brain tumor imaging: MR imaging, PET, and PET/MR imaging. J Nucl Med. 2015;56(10):1554–61.

Catana C, Drzezga A, Heiss W, et al. PET/MRI for neurologic applications. J Nucl Med. 2012;53(12):1916–25.

Werner P, Barthel H, Drzezga A, et al. Current status and future role of brain PET/ MRI in clinical and research settings. Eur J Nucl Med Mol Imaging. 2015;42(3):512–26.

Filss CP, Galldiks N, Stoffels G, et al. Comparison of ^{18}F-FET PET and perfusion-weighted MR imaging: a PET/MR imaging hybrid study in patients with brain tumors. J Nucl Med. 2014;55(4):540–5.

Rose S, Fay M, Thomas P, et al. Correlation of MRI-derived apparent diffusion coefficients in newly diagnosed gliomas with [18F]-Fluoro-L-Dopa PET: what are we really measuring with minimum ADC? Am J Neuroradiol. 2013;34(4):758–64.

Pauleit D, Floeth F, Hamacher K, et al. O-(2-[18F] fluoroethyl)-L-tyrosine PET combined with MRI improves the diagnostic assessment of cerebral gliomas. Brain. 2005;128(3):678–87.

Song S, Cheng Y, Ma J, et al. Simultaneous FET-PET and contrast-enhanced MRI based on hybrid PET/MR improves delineation of tumor spatial biodistribution in gliomas: a biopsy validation study. Eur J Nucl Med Mol Imaging. 2020;47(6):1458–67.

Lohmann P, Stavrinou P, Lipke K, et al. FET PET reveals considerable spatial differences in tumour burden compared to conventional MRI in newly diagnosed glioblastoma. Eur J Nucl Med Mol Imaging. 2019;46(3):591–602.

Pafundi DH, Laack NN, Youland RS, et al. Biopsy validation of F-18DOPA PET and biodistribution in gliomas for neurosurgical planning and radiotherapy target delineation: results of a prospective pilot study. Neuro Oncol. 2013;15(8):1058–67.

Verger A, Filss CP, Lohmann P, et al. Comparison of ^{18}F-FET PET and perfusion-weighted MRI for glioma grading: a hybrid PET/MR study. Eur J Nucl Med Mol Imaging. 2017;44(13):2257–65.

Jena A, Taneja S, Gambhir A, et al. Glioma Recurrence Versus Radiation Necrosis: Single-Session Multiparametric Approach Using Simultaneous O-(2-18F-Fluoroethyl)L-Tyrosine PET/MRI. Clin Nucl Med. 2016;41(5):e228–36.

Jena A, Taneja S, Jha A, et al. Multiparametric evaluation in differentiating glioma recurrence from treatment-induced necrosis using simultaneous ^{18}F-FDG-PET/ MRI: a single-institution retrospective study. Am J Neuroradiol. 2017;38(5):899–907.

Tomura N, Kokubun M, Saginoya T, et al. Differentiation between treatment-induced necrosis and recurrent tumors in patients with metastatic brain tumors: comparison among ^{11}C-Methionine-PET, FDG-PET, MR permeability imaging, and MRI-ADC–preliminary results. Am J Neuroradiol. 2017;38(8):1520–7.

Lundemann M, Munck AF, Rosenschöld P, et al. Feasibility of multi-parametric PET and MRI for prediction of tumour recurrence in patients with glioblastoma. Eur J Nucl Med Mol Imaging. 2019;46(3):603–13.

12 Research Applications of Positron Emission Tomography/Magnetic Resonance (PET/MR) Imaging in Cerebrovascular Diseases

Yaqin Hou, Yue Zhang, Fan Fu, Miao Zhang, Xiang Li, and Jie Lu

Cerebrovascular disease is currently one of the foremost diseases in the world with respect to incidence, disability, and fatality rates. As China gradually transitions to an aging society, the incidence rate of cerebrovascular disease has increased each year, accompanied by a trend toward a younger age at onset. The most common type of cerebrovascular disease is ischemic, accounting for 75–90% of all cases. Ischemic cerebrovascular disease has a complicated etiology and complex pathological mechanisms. It generally results from ischemic and hypoxic brain tissue caused by intracranial vessel wall lesions, alterations in blood components, or changes in hemodynamics, leading to brain dysfunction, or even the necrosis and softening of brain tissue. Clinically, this manifests as transient ischemic attacks, reversible ischemic neurological deficits, or cerebral infarctions, subsequently leading to corresponding neurological signs and symptoms. Although most cases of ischemic cerebrovascular disease are non-fatal, the resulting disability rate is very high; therefore, this disease has remained a major research topic in the field of medicine worldwide. The rapid development of neuroimaging, in particular, the ability of functional imaging techniques to not only display morphological changes but also provide information on cerebral blood flow, metabolism, and other aspects, has played a crucial and even decisive role in the early diagnosis and appropriate treatment of ischemic cerebrovascular disease. In this chapter, we will focus on the research advances of MRI, PET, and PET/MR as they relate to the etiology, pathophysiology, treatment decision-making, and efficacy evaluation of ischemic cerebrovascular disease.

Y. Hou · Y. Zhang · F. Fu · M. Zhang · J. Lu (✉)
Department of Radiology and Nuclear Medicine, Xuanwu Hospital, Capital Medical University, Beijing, China

X. Li
Department of Biomedical Imaging and Image-Guided Therapy, Medical University of Vienna, Vienna, Austria

12.1 Research Applications of MRI in Cerebrovascular Diseases

During the pathophysiological process of cerebrovascular disease, cellular and histological damage is preceded by changes in cerebral hemodynamics, which is constantly in a state of dynamic flux. Therefore, these changes in cerebral hemodynamics and the associated changes in brain function are of critical importance to research on the early signs, diagnosis, and pathogenic mechanisms of cerebrovascular disease. Functional MRI (fMRI) techniques include diffusion-weighted imaging (DWI), diffusion kurtosis imaging (DKI), diffusion tensor imaging (DTI), perfusion-weighted imaging (PWI), arterial spin labeling (ASL), magnetic resonance

J. Lu, G. Zhao (eds.), *PET/MR: Functional and Molecular Imaging of Neurological Diseases and Neurosciences*, https://doi.org/10.1007/978-981-19-9902-4_12

spectroscopy (MRS), and blood-oxygen-level-dependent (BOLD) imaging. These techniques can display focal cerebral ischemia at a very early stage, track the course of white matter fibers, reflect the perfusion status of brain tissues, display tissue metabolic and biochemical changes, determine the location of brain functional areas, and reveal whole-brain functional connectivity and functional networks.

12.1.1 Research Applications of DWI in Cerebrovascular Diseases

DWI involves the detection of the diffusion movement of water molecules in human tissues. By measuring the signal intensities before and after the application of diffusion-sensitivity gradient magnetic fields, we can calculate the tissue diffusion coefficient, known as the apparent diffusion coefficient (ADC), and therefore quantify the diffusion rate of water molecules in tissues.

DWI is primarily utilized in the diagnosis of acute and hyperacute cerebral infarction. Due to the occurrence of cytotoxic edema in the early stages of cerebral ischemia, the intracellular water content increases, causing increased cellular swelling and decreased extracellular space, in turn decreasing the diffusion rate of water molecules in the area of infarction. Therefore, at 30 min after the onset of cerebral ischemia, abnormal hyperintensities can be observed in DWI, appearing as hypointensities on the ADC map (Fig. 12.1). ADC values can be used to monitor lesion growth and progression, with areas of cerebral infarction showing a significant reduction in ADC values during the acute stage, followed by the pseudo-normalization or even elevation of ADC values in the late subacute and chronic stages. DWI enables the accurate delineation of the extent and degree of cerebral infarction, the prediction of disease severity, and the dynamic evaluation of therapeutic efficacy. In conventional T_2-weighted imaging (T_2WI), cerebral infarcts appear as homogeneous hyperintensities, which does not allow for the distinction between old and new lesions; whereas in DWI, acute lesions appear as hyperintensities and chronic lesions as hypointensities, which are easily differentiated. Furthermore, DWI can also improve the detection rate of small ischemic lesions, especially small subtentorial lesions that

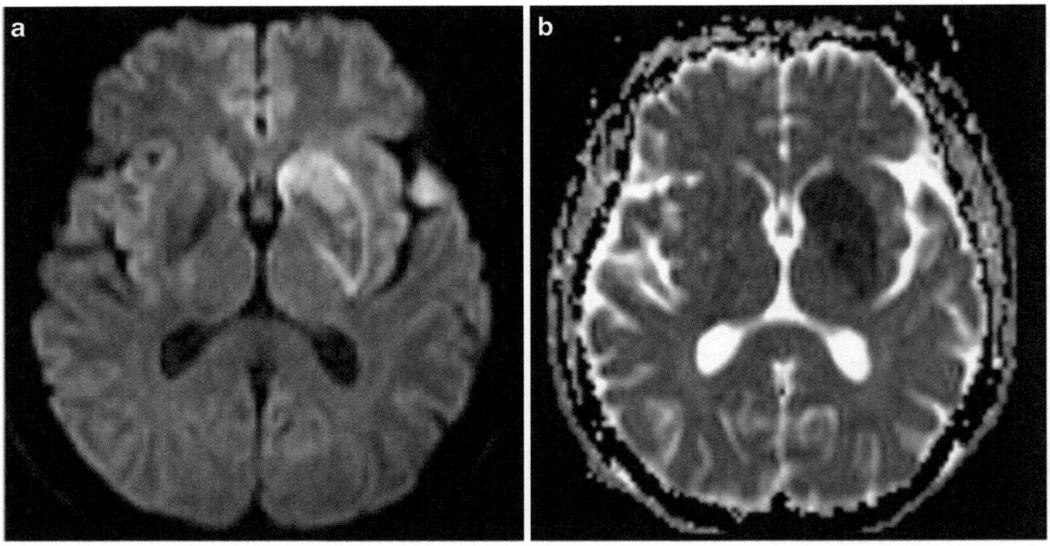

Fig. 12.1 Hyperacute cerebral infarction. A 48-year-old male patient with sudden weakness and numbness in his right limbs. Transverse DWI shows hyperintense signals in the left basal ganglia (**a**). Transverse ADC mapping shows hypointense signals in the left basal ganglia (**b**)

are easily missed in conventional computed tomography (CT) and MRI sequences (Fig. 12.2).

DKI is an extension of DWI. Traditional DWI is based on the normal distribution of diffusion in water molecules, whereas DKI shows the non-normally distributed diffusion of water molecules in tissues. Therefore, DKI is able to provide a more accurate delineation of changes in tissue microstructures and allows for the early evaluation of the extent of any cerebral infarct. Additionally, DKI can simultaneously obtain both DKI and DWI parameters, which primarily include mean kurtosis (MK), mean diffusivity (MD), and ADC values. The size of the MK depends on the complexity of the tissue structures rather than their spatial direction, and can therefore more accurately display the extent of cerebral infarcts and their associated internal microstructural changes. MD is the mean ADC value of the three orthogonal directions and is primarily used to measure the diffusion rate of water molecules, in turn reflecting cellular size and integrity. Compared to ADC, MD provides a more comprehensive reflection of the rate of diffusion movement. In acute cerebral ischemia, MD reflects the extent of cytotoxic edema in tissues, while MK is more sensitive to the disintegration of cytoskeletal structures and mitochondrial swelling. Therefore, regions with mismatched MK and MD abnormalities represent the ischemic penumbra, whereas matched regions represent the area of infarction and severe cell damage (Fig. 12.3). DKI is more accurate than DWI in the diagnosis of early cerebral infarction, and the comparative analysis between the two may have significant implications in both determining the ischemic penumbra and improving patient prognosis. Furthermore, DKI can also

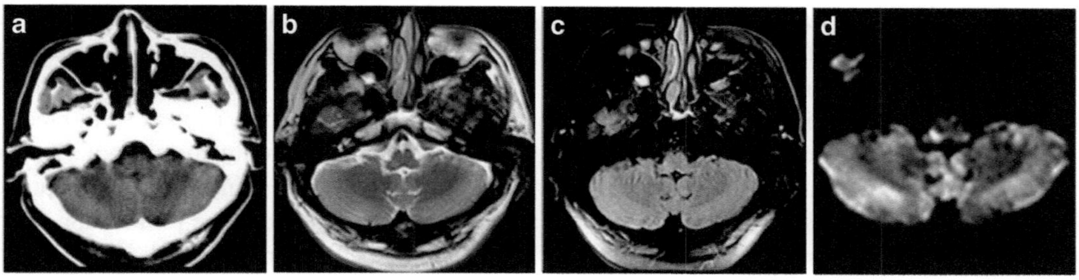

Fig. 12.2 Acute medullary infarction. A 46-year-old female patient who presented with numbness and weakness in her left limbs for 4 h. Transverse plain CT scan shows no abnormalities (**a**). Transverse T_2WI shows slight hyperintensity in the right dorsolateral medulla oblongata (**b**). Transverse FLAIR shows suspicious slight hyperintensity in the right dorsolateral medulla oblongata (**c**). Transverse DWI shows hyperintensity in the right dorsolateral medulla oblongata (**d**)

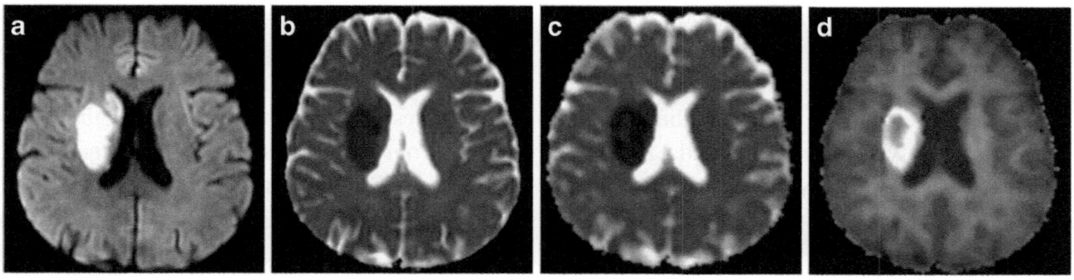

Fig. 12.3 Acute right periventricular cerebral infarction. A 55-year-old male patient who presented with left-sided sensory disturbances for 8 h. Transverse DWI shows homogeneous hyperintense signals in the right periventricular area (**a**). Transverse ADC mapping (**b**) and MD (**c**) show homogeneous hypointense signals. Transverse MK shows heterogeneous hyperintense signals in the right periventricular area, mismatched with the extent of the lesion as determined by DWI, ADC, and MD (**d**)

facilitate the more in-depth analysis of pathological mechanisms at the microscopic level, which can provide useful information for more targeted clinical treatments. Although research on the utilization of DKI in ischemic stroke is currently in its infancy, DKI is ideal for widespread clinical use due to its minimal hardware requirements and short scan time; relevant research will provide new ideas for the diagnosis and treatment of cerebral infarctions.

12.1.2 Research Applications of DTI in Cerebrovascular Diseases

DTI parameters can reflect the integrity of neuronal membrane and nerve fiber myelination. These indicators do not exhibit significant changes during the acute phase of ischemic stroke but are altered significantly in the subacute and chronic phases, due to the loss of fractional anisotropy (FA) caused by the destruction of cellular and/or myelin structures. Despite the extensive utilization of DWI in the evaluation of acute ischemic stroke, its use in chronic ischemic injuries is still limited. In contrast, DTI can provide information on evolving stroke that cannot be acquired using DWI, and is therefore useful for predicting the severity of ischemic injury and patient prognosis in the early stages of ischemic stroke. Studies have found that after the onset of cerebral infarction, dynamic and predictable changes in FA and MD values can be observed over the course of the disease. More specifically, there is a continuous decrease in FA values after cerebral infarction, primarily due to the myelinolysis and axonal disintegration of white matter fibers superior and inferior to the infarct, as well as glial proliferation in the peri-infarct area, leading to the impaired integrity of nerve fibers and a reduction in structural directionality. The trend and timing of changes in FA values concur with Wallerian degeneration. MD values, on the other hand, show an initial decrease followed by a gradual increase and can be attributed to the cytotoxic edema found in acute cerebral infarction, which causes continuous restricted diffusion, significantly reducing the MD values, in turn reflecting the degree of diffusion. When cytotoxic edema progresses to vasogenic edema, there is an increase in extracellular water, elevation of total tissue water content, further exacerbation of cellular damage, and collapse of cellular membrane structure, which produces a large amount of cell debris. This increases intracellular viscosity and causes an elevated level of free diffusion, leading to a gradual rise in MD values. The subsequent necrosis and liquefaction in the area of infarction further enhances the free diffusion of water molecules, resulting in abnormally high MD values. Monitoring the post-infarction changes in DTI parameters can deepen our understanding on the pathophysiological evolution of cerebral infarction and enable a more accurate staging of this disease. The severity of early-stage Wallerian degeneration is related to the recovery of the patient's neurological function. That is, patients with more significant early-stage pyramidal tract degeneration experience more severe neurological impairment, especially with respect to the patient's motor functions. Based on the extent of Wallerian degeneration in the patient's pyramidal tract distal to the lesion, it is possible to predict the long-term recovery of motor function. This is useful for the early determination of patient prognosis, which in turn allows the formulation of an appropriate treatment plan in order to promote functional recovery.

Diffusion tensor tractography (DTT) is an imaging method that involves the use of diffusion tensor data to determine the seed region on the basic images, which are then subjected to fiber tracking or tractography. DTT can accurately determine the anatomical structure of white matter fiber bundles and describe the spatial relationship between the lesion and specific fiber bundles. DTT represents an expansion of imaging techniques from the basics of early diagnosis and evaluation of lesion characteristics to the more involved direct evaluation of relationships between the lesion and key white matter fiber bundles, to predict patient prognosis and functional recovery. The rehabilitation of patients after cerebral infarction depends, to a large extent, on the recovery of limb motor function. Therefore, understanding the degree of damage to the motor tracts after a cerebral infarction is useful for accurately assessing the recovery of motor function. The corticospinal tracts are the largest of the descending pyramidal tracts primarily responsible for controlling voluntary limb movements, and they play a pivotal role in the recovery process of motor functions in stroke patients. DTT can be used to display the spatial relationships between the cerebral infarct and the corticospinal tracts and serve as a reference for predicting motor outcome in several situations.

1. Patients with corticospinal tracts which run adjacent to the infarct area exhibit virtually unaffected motor function, although some patients experience mild limb numbness and weakness, which can be explained by the space-occupying effects of transient peri-infarct edema (Fig. 12.4).
2. Among patients whose corticospinal tracts are compressed or contorted, some of whom experienced significant improvements in motor dysfunction within a short period of time, and essentially recovered during the chronic phase. This may be due to the space-occupying effects caused by the hyperemia and edema of the infarct itself and surrounding brain tissues in the early stages, which led to the contortion and compression of white matter fiber bundles. However, after the hyperemia and edema have subsided and the lesion has decreased in size, the compression of the white matter fiber bundles resolved, leading to significant improvements in the patient's motor dysfunction (Fig. 12.5).
3. Patients in whom a small number of lesions have led to the partial interruption of the corticospinal tracts may still experience a good recovery in motor function, which may be related to the compensation of unaffected motor fibers.
4. In cases where most or all of the corticospinal tracts are involved, causing the majority of fiber bundles to be interrupted or damaged, patients present with severe motor impairments in the acute phase, although some patients may gain some degree of motor function recovery through mechanisms such as the remodeling of white matter fiber bundles and functional compensation. However, such patients experience a slower recovery in motor function compared to patients without corticospinal tract involvement (Fig. 12.6).

Although most patients with cerebral infarction involving the complete corticospinal tract have a poorer prognosis than those with partial involvement, long-term follow-up observations have found that further recovery in motor function is still possible. It is generally believed that motor function recovery in the early post-infarction stages is primarily associated with improvements in lesion ischemia and edema, whereas in the later stages of recovery, it is

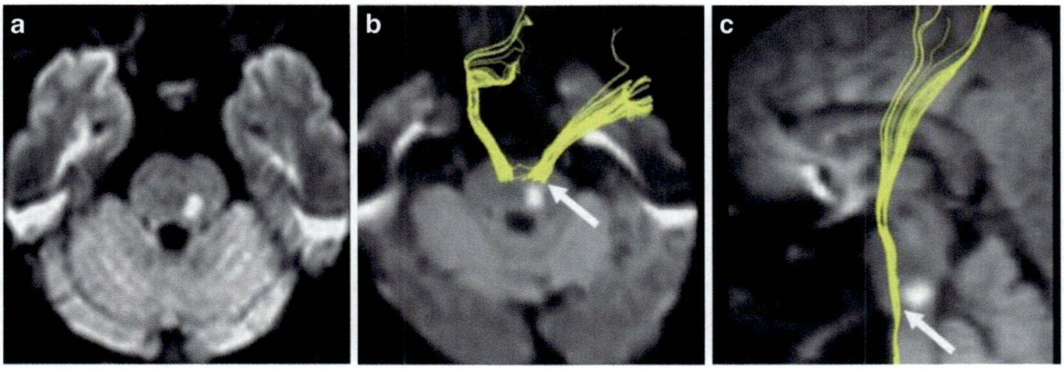

Fig. 12.4 Left pontine infarction. A 57-year-old male patient who presented with numbness and weakness of the right limbs for 1 d. The patient's limb motor dysfunction recovered significantly after 2 weeks. Transverse DWI shows left pontine infarction (**a**). Transverse (**b**) and sagittal (**c**) MRI show that the left corticospinal tracts are located anterior to the infarct, exhibiting good continuity, without compression or interruption (arrows)

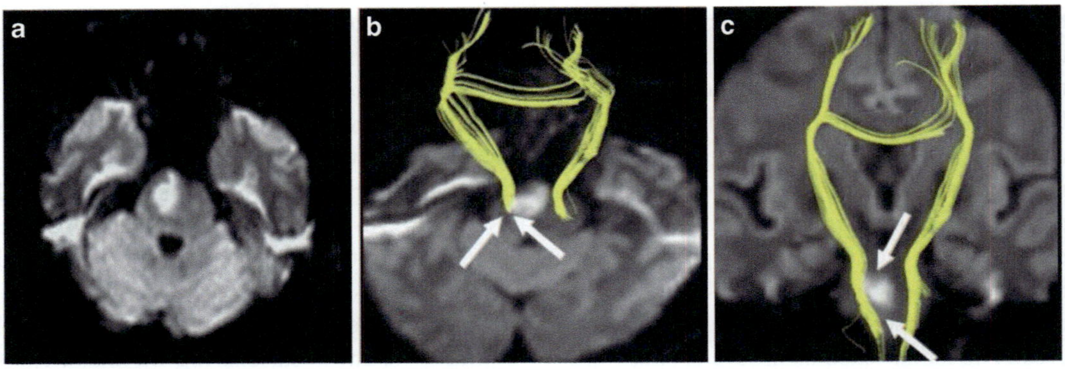

Fig. 12.5 Right pontine infarction. A 59-year-old male patient who presented with left limb weakness and slurred speech for 2 d. The patient recovered after 3 months of routine medical treatment and rehabilitation training. Transverse DWI shows right pontine infarction (**a**). Transverse (**b**) and coronal (**c**) MRI show that the right corticospinal tracts are immediately adjacent to the infarct, exhibiting compression and contortion but without significant interruption (arrows)

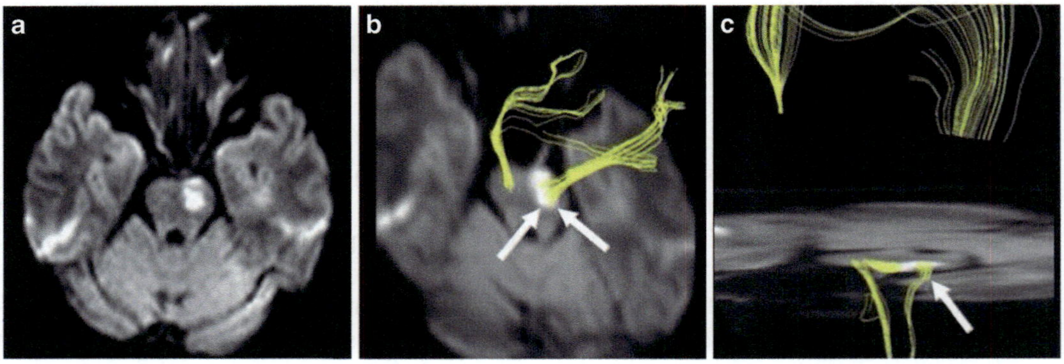

Fig. 12.6 Left pontine infarction. A 62-year-old female patient who presented with right limb weakness and slurred speech for 2 d. Motor dysfunction remained after 3 months of routine medical treatment and rehabilitation training. Transverse DWI shows left pontine infarction (**a**). Transverse (**b**) and sagittal (**c**) MRI show that the left corticospinal tracts pass through the infarct, and the majority of fiber bundles have been interrupted, with only a few fiber bundles remaining inferior to the level of the infarct (arrows)

closely related to functional brain reorganization. Research has shown that multiple cortical areas and conduction pathways are involved in the reorganization of motor function. In addition to the primary motor cortex, the premotor area of the frontal lobe, the supplementary motor area of the insula, and the medial surfaces of the cerebral hemispheres are all associated with motor functional recovery and have nerve fiber connections with the spinal cord. Under normal circumstances, these areas of the brain and their associated descending pathways are in an inhibited state. When the primary motor cortex and its descending pathways are damaged, this inhibition is removed, and the resulting compensatory effects enable patients to restore their motor functions.

The corpus callosum is the largest bundle of commissural fibers connecting the two cerebral hemispheres. In healthy individuals, the callosal fibers are generally in an inhibited state to maintain the functional balance of the cerebral motor cortex between the two hemispheres. After a unilateral ischemic stroke occurs in the cerebral hemisphere, the inhibition on the callosal fibers is removed, allowing the nerve fibers from the contralateral corticospinal tract to traverse to the affected side via the corpus callosum, and then

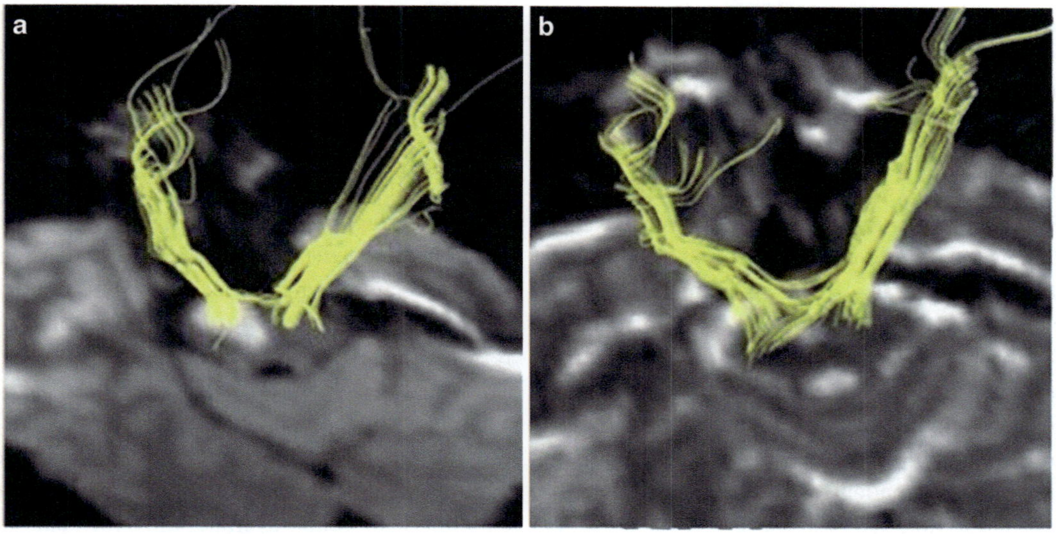

Fig. 12.7 Right pontine infarction. A 60-year-old male patient who presented with left hemiplegia and dizziness. Transverse DWI shows right pontine infarction, and transverse DTT shows that nearly the entire right corticospinal tract has passed through the infarct (**a**). At 180 d after disease onset, DTT shows part of the contralesional fiber bundles crossing over to the ipsilesional side and descending laterally along the infarct (**b**)

descend along the infarct to compensate the function of the damaged corticospinal tract (Fig. 12.7). The contralateral corticospinal tract can also project multiple pontine association fibers to the affected side, even extending up to the motor cortex of the affected hemisphere to compensate for impaired motor functions. Jang et al. performed a DTT study on 40 patients with an infarction of the corona radiata, who were classified according to DTT findings into three types: (1) Type A patients did not have transcallosal fibers originating from contralesional corticospinal tracts; (2) Type B patients had transcallosal fibers originating from contralesional corticospinal tracts that terminated at the corpus callosum or ascended to the cortex of the affected cerebral hemisphere; and (3) Type C patients had transcallosal fibers that projected to the ipsilesional side and descended along the infarct. Patients with severe motor impairment were predominantly type C, implying that severe damage to the motor pathway can remove the inhibited state of dormant fibers, in an effort to compensate for the damaged nerve fibers and restore the patient's motor functions. Damaged corticospinal tracts can also undergo reorganization in the peri-infarct area to restore the patient's motor function. The mechanism underlying this functional recovery is thought to involve the axonal regeneration, dendritic collateral branch formation, and altered synaptic thresholds of unaffected cells around the infarct, mobilizing reserved neural function, rebuilding neural networks, and achieving functional plasticity, subsequently compensating for the brain functions of the affected regions.

12.1.3 Research Applications of Brain Perfusion MRI in Cerebrovascular Diseases

Brain perfusion MRI includes dynamic susceptibility contrast (DSC)-PWI and arterial spin labeling (ASL). DSC-PWI involves the use of rapid scanning and the intravenous bolus injection of contrast agents, so that the changes in tissue magnetic susceptibility caused by the contrast agent lead to changes in MRI signals, which in turn can be used to evaluate the hemodynamics of the brain tissue. Using this imaging technique, parameters such as regional cerebral blood flow (rCBF), relative cerebral blood volume (rCBV), mean transit time (MTT), and time-to-peak (TTP) can be calculated. PWI is highly sensitive to early cerebral ischemia, detecting abnormalities even earlier than DWI. Therefore, performing PWI and DWI at the same time is useful for determining the presence of an ischemic penumbra. During hyperacute cerebral infarction, a larger region of abnormal perfusion is delineated PWI compared to the region of abnormal DWI signals (i.e., the cerebral infarct area), suggesting the presence of an ischemic penumbra. This sign can be used to assist in the selection of patients for thrombolytic therapy, so as to minimize the infarct area, implement individualized therapy for cerebral infarction, and evaluate the efficacy of thrombolytic therapy (Fig. 12.8). The utilization of PWI in patients with chronic middle cerebral artery/internal carotid artery stenosis or occlusion can facilitate the discovery of cerebral ischemic lesions that cannot be detected using conventional MRI. These lesions manifest as delayed TTP and MTT, without significant changes in CBF and CBV, or as normal CBF with slightly elevated CBV. These findings imply that cerebral ischemia induces compensatory cerebrovascular dilation, which decreases circulatory resistance and reduces blood flow velocity and also establishes collateral circulation. Together, these compensatory mechanisms maintain CBF within the normal range (Fig. 12.9). However, compared to healthy individuals, these patients take a longer time for blood supply to reach the ischemic area, decreasing the effective uptake rate of CBF, and diminishing the compensatory and stress response abilities of the cerebral vessels. Therefore, these ischemic areas are at high risk for cerebral infarction and are useful for screening high-risk groups for stroke and performing preventative treatment.

Compared to conventional DSC-PWI, ASL is a brain perfusion imaging technique that does not require the injection of gadolinium-based contrast agents, and as such can be used in patients with renal dysfunction. ASL can be divided based on the labeling method into the following four types: continuous ASL, pulsed ASL, pseudo-continuous ASL, and velocity-selective ASL. Other techniques include territorial ASL and ASL-angiography. ASL can only produce a single parameter, CBF; therefore, it is less effective at evaluating the infarct core during acute cerebral infarction compared to DWI and PWI but is equally sensitive at displaying changes in early cerebral ischemia

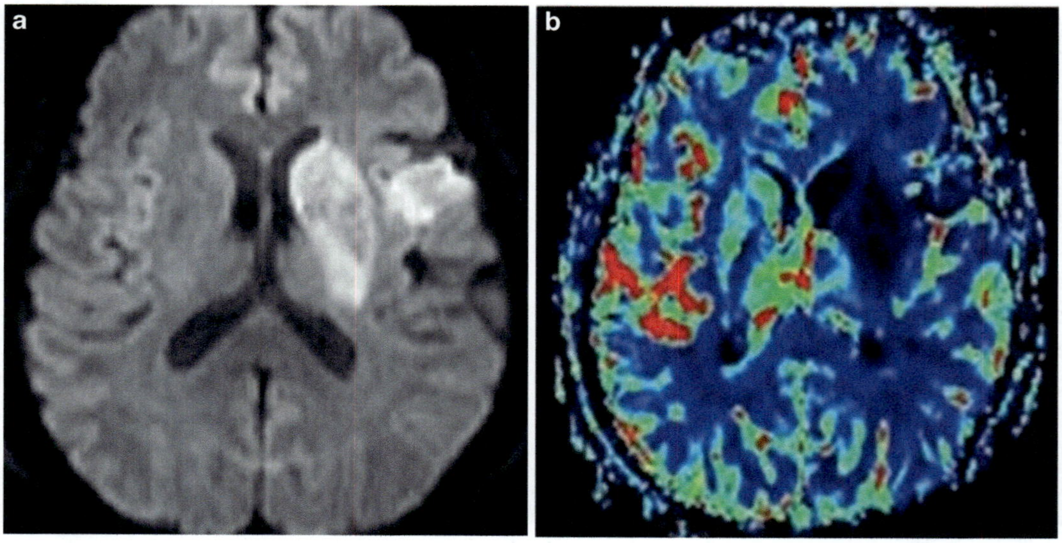

Fig. 12.8 Acute cerebral infarction of the left basal ganglia and left temporal lobe. A 62-year-old male patient who presented with weakness in his right limbs for 3 h. Transverse DWI shows acute cerebral infarction of the left basal ganglia and left temporal lobe (**a**). Transverse PWI CBF shows hypoperfusion of the middle cerebral artery territory, covering a larger area than the extent of DWI hyperintensity (**b**). Therefore, there is a mismatch between CBF and DWI, which implies the presence of an ischemic penumbra

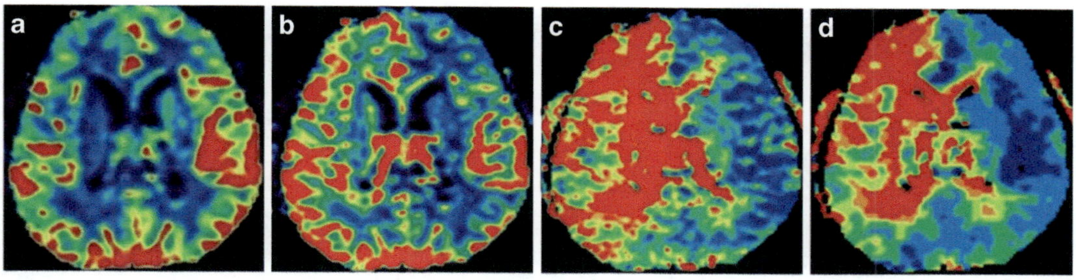

Fig. 12.9 Right internal carotid artery occlusion. A 63-year-old male patient whose MRI shows bilateral periventricular lacunar infarction. Transverse PWI shows roughly symmetric CBF between the bilateral cerebral hemispheres (**a**), as well as slight CBV elevation (**b**), delayed MTT (**c**), and delayed TTP (**d**) in the right cerebral hemisphere

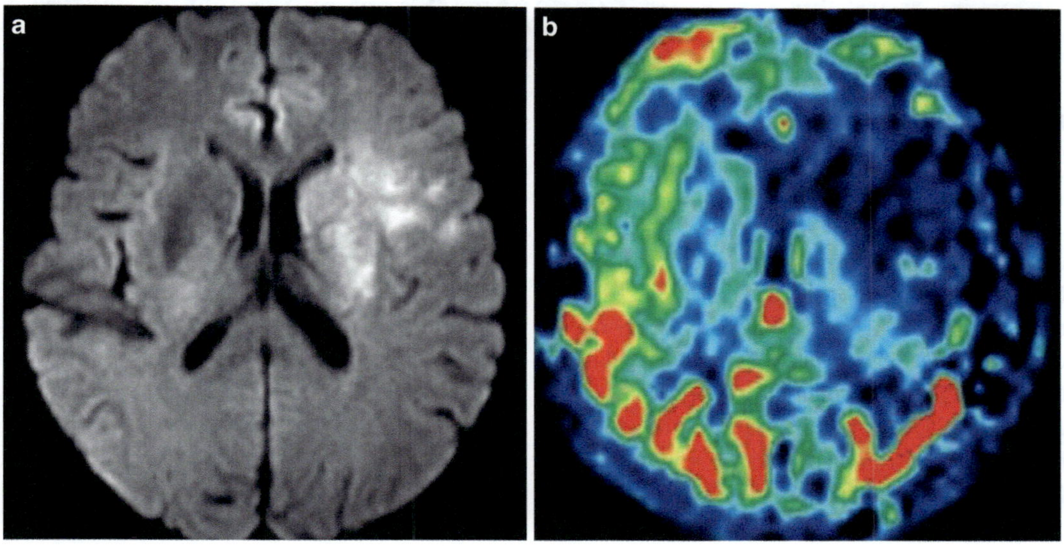

Fig. 12.10 Acute cerebral infarction of the left frontal lobe and left basal ganglia. A 72-year-old female patient who presented with weakness in her right limbs and aphasia for 1 h. Transverse DWI shows acute cerebral infarction of the left frontal lobe and left basal ganglia (**a**). Transverse ASL shows reduced CBF in the left middle cerebral artery territory (**b**)

(Fig. 12.10). Mirasol et al. found that in the assessment of acute ischemic stroke, the regions with decreased CBF as delineated by ASL showed good concordance with the hypoperfused regions determined by DWI-PWI and CT perfusion imaging. As for patients with chronic middle cerebral artery/internal carotid artery occlusion or stenosis whose ischemic lesions cannot be detected using conventional MRI, ASL can be utilized to display abnormal cerebral perfusion in the areas ipsilateral to the affected blood vessels (Fig. 12.11).

During ASL scans, blood labeled by magnetic inversion reaches the capillaries after a period of time, at which point image acquisition can be performed. The interval between labeling and acquisition is known as the post-labeling delay (PLD) and is a key parameter of ASL. The selection of the PLD can affect the determination of CBF and the assessment of perfusion. By adopting two different PLDs when studying chronic ischemic cerebrovascular disease, we can achieve a better evaluation of actual cerebral perfusion levels. More specifically, a shorter PLD can more

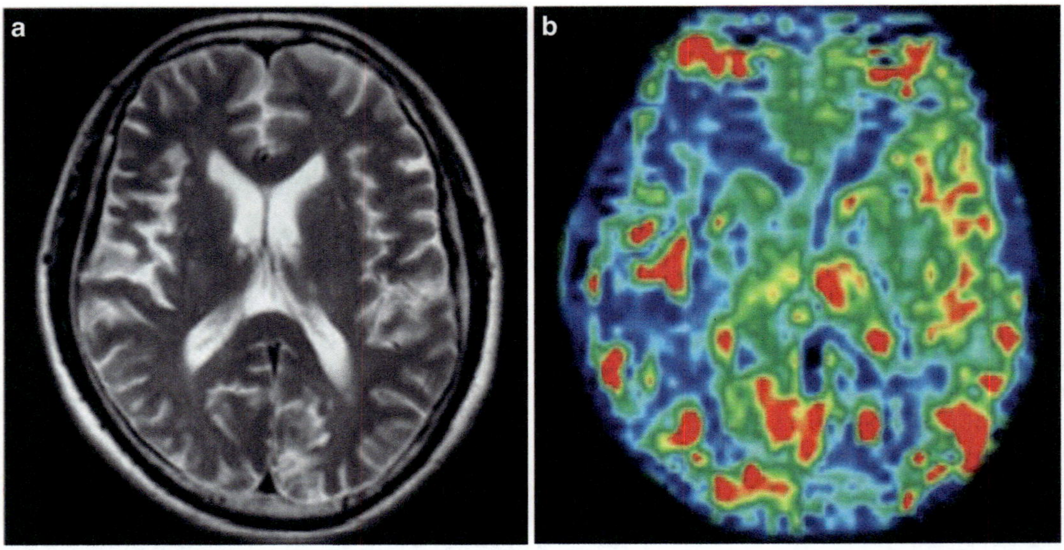

Fig. 12.11 Severe stenosis of the right middle cerebral artery. A 62-year-old male patient, in whom severe stenosis of the right middle cerebral artery had been discovered for 1 year. Transverse T_2WI shows no clear abnormalities (**a**). Transverse ASL shows reduced CBF of the right middle cerebral artery territory (**b**)

easily detect perfusion abnormalities caused by large-vessel stenosis, whereas a longer PLD can more accurately assess actual perfusion levels, owing to the longer time required by collateral circulation pathways than the direct blood supply from normal arteries. Therefore, the contrast between the CBF images derived from these two PLDs can reflect the status of cerebral perfusion compensation or the level of cerebrovascular reserve, which is of practical significance in clinical settings for the accurate assessment of ischemic levels and determination of prognosis. Using ischemic moyamoya disease in children as an example, performing scans with two different PLDs enables the level of perfusion compensation to be assessed more accurately, which can then be applied to the formulation of individualized treatment plans (Fig. 12.12). Lyu et al. performed ASL using two different PLDs to differentiate between antegrade and collateral blood flow in patients with middle cerebral artery stenosis and proposed the possibility of quantifying collateral blood flow using ASL.

Territorial ASL, also known as vessel-selective ASL, involves labeling the blood in specific blood vessels to observe the compensatory effects of collateral vessels on the territory of occluded vessels following a proximal large-vessel occlusion. This technique is now widely used in the determination of collateral blood flow in patients with carotid artery stenosis and moyamoya disease (Fig. 12.13).

12.1.4 Research Applications of MRS in Cerebrovascular Diseases

MRS is an effective technique for the noninvasive in vivo evaluation of tissue metabolism. The progressive decline, or even disappearance, of intralesional N-acetylaspartate (NAA) can be observed in acute cerebral infarction, while patients with a more significant decrease in NAA levels have poorer prognosis. In contrast, the decline in the choline (Cho) and creatinine (Cr) peaks tend to be less significant than that of NAA. Lactate (Lac) is a product of anaerobic glycolysis that cannot be detected in normal brain tissues. Therefore, elevated Lac concentrations imply that tissue ischemia and hypoxia have resulted in impairments in normal aerobic metabolism. In fact, Lac can be detected using ^{1}H-MRS a few minutes after the onset of cerebral ischemia, following which Lac increases rapidly,

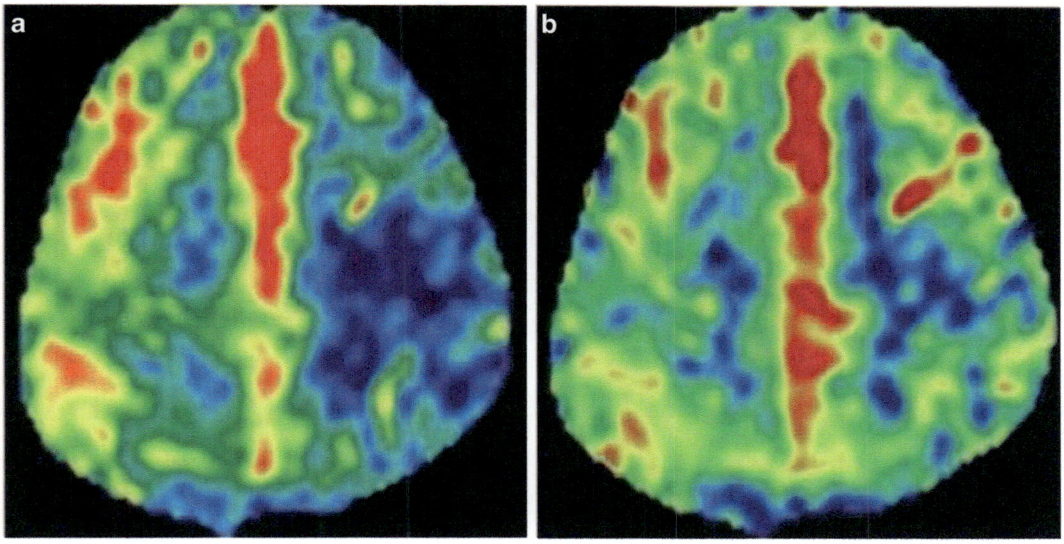

Fig. 12.12 Moyamoya disease. A 9-year-old male patient. Transverse ASL with PLD = 1.5 s shows reduced CBF in the left frontoparietal lobe (**a**). Transverse ASL with PLD = 2.5 s shows a smaller extent of CBF reduction in the left frontoparietal lobe (**b**)

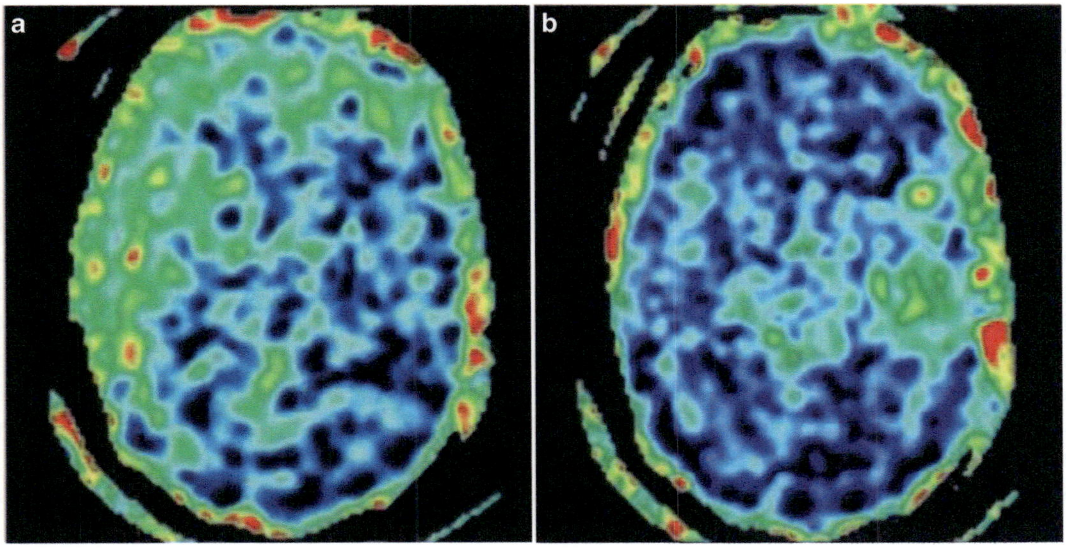

Fig. 12.13 Severe stenosis of the right internal carotid artery. A 64-year-old male patient. MRI performed with selective labeling of the right internal carotid artery. Transverse territorial ASL shows perfusion defects in the right frontoparietal lobe (**a**). Selective labeling of the left internal carotid artery. Transverse territorial ASL shows normal perfusion in the left hemisphere, while perfusion can be observed in the right prefrontal lobe, suggesting compensatory blood supply by the left internal carotid artery to the right frontal lobe (**b**)

reaching its peak during the hyperacute phase. Therefore, Lac is considered a sensitive marker in the early stages of cerebral infarction (Fig. 12.14). ^{1}H-MRS is a valuable technique for differentiating between the area of cerebral infarction and the ischemic penumbra. In acute cerebral infarction, the extent of Lac presence is often larger than the infarct area as delineated by conventional MRI. Therefore, a region with normal MRI findings and normal or slightly reduced

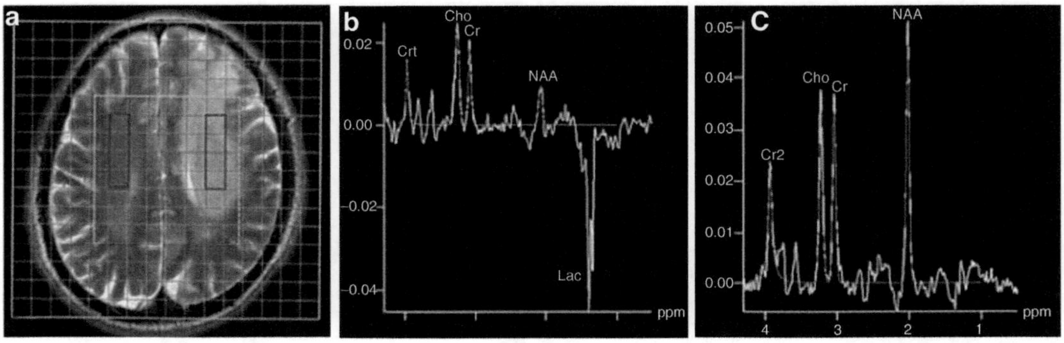

Fig. 12.14 ^{1}H-MRS localization. Transverse T_2WI shows a large area of infarct in the left centrum semiovale. MRI-based ^{1}H-MRS localization map: four symmetric voxels were selected at the lesion center and corresponding contralateral site (**a**). The infarct ^{1}H-MRS curve shows a significant decrease in NAA, varying extents of decreases in Cho and Cr, and a deep inverted Lac peak at 1.33 ppm (**b**). ^{1}H-MRS of normal contralateral brain tissues shows the NAA, Cho, and Cr peaks, and the absence of a Lac peak (**c**)

NAA, but with the presence of a Lac peak, can be regarded as an ischemic penumbra. Additionally, the Lac/NAA ratio can also be used to determine the infarct area, where a ratio > 1.0 denotes the infarct area, and < 1.0 indicates the non-infarct area. However, further investigations are needed to determine whether the degree of NAA and Lac changes can be used to discriminate among the infarct core, ischemic penumbra and benign hypoperfusion.

For patients with chronic cerebral ischemia accompanied by intra- and extracranial large-vessel stenosis or occlusion, but are in the compensatory phase, the level of cerebral ischemia is often not completely consistent with the degree of vascular stenosis, due to factors such as compensatory blood supply via collateral circulation. Therefore, conventional imaging techniques often reveal no abnormalities, or only small lacunar infarcts, in most patients. At this point, patients may appear to have an essentially normal regional blood flow but may experience a decrease in cerebrovascular reserve capacity, and their brain tissue may have a reduced capacity for effective blood uptake, leaving the neurons in a functionally inhibited and hypometabolic state. The occurrence of acute decompensation at this point can easily cause a stroke, which can then lead to severe neurological impairments. A ^{1}H-MRS study on patients with chronic internal carotid artery/middle cerebral artery stenosis or occlusion found that white matter which appeared without abnormal findings on conventional MRI exhibited metabolic abnormalities, manifesting as decreased NAA and increased Cho concentrations, with a Lac peak observed in some patients (Fig. 12.15). Although there is no fundamental difference in the cerebral metabolic changes detected by ^{1}H-MRS between chronic cerebral ischemia and infarction, their respective underlying mechanisms are not completely the same.

During cerebral infarction, neurons are subjected to irreversible damage, the number of cells is reduced, and NAA undergoes a progressive and irreparable decline. In chronic cerebral ischemia, however, the functional changes indicated by the decrease in NAA are relatively mild, while the neuronal structure of ischemic tissues remain intact, and may return to normal once blood circulation is restored. The mechanisms underlying ipsilesional Cho elevation are the same as those involved in the early stages of cerebral infarction. Both are the result of the degradation of cell membrane components in ischemic tissues and the release of large amounts of phosphatidylcholine, suggesting that metabolic abnormalities of the cell membrane may occur in the early stages of ischemia prior to the onset of cerebral infarction. This implies that such patients have sustained an ischemic brain injury, but the metabolic state of their brain tissue is still in the transitional stage toward cerebral infarc-

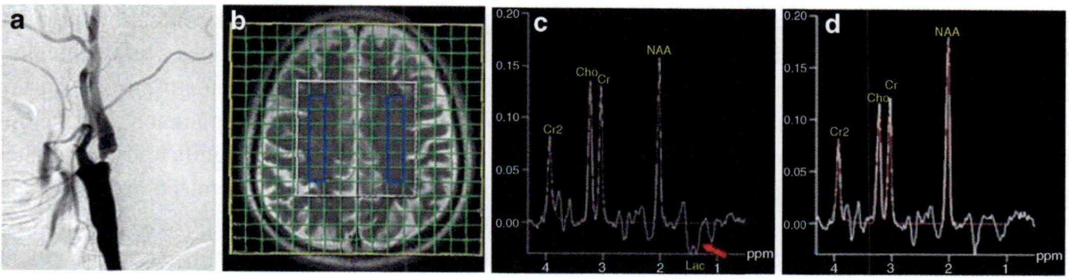

Fig. 12.15 Severe stenosis in the initial segment of the right internal carotid artery. A 45-year-old male patient who presented with recurrent left limb weakness for 3 years. Digital subtraction angiography shows severe stenosis in the initial segment of the right internal carotid artery (**a**). ^{1}H-MRS localization map: six symmetrical voxels were selected each in the bilateral centrum semiovale (**b**). Right ^{1}H-MRS curve shows decreased NAA, increased Cho, and inverted Lac peak at 1.33 ppm (**c**) (arrow). Left ^{1}H-MRS curve at a symmetrical site shows the NAA, Cho and Cr peaks, and the absence of a Lac peak (**d**)

tion. The appearance of Lac is related to anaerobic glycolysis and the cellular infiltration of the infarcted area, and the presence of a Lac peak in patients with chronic cerebral ischemia can be attributed to the anaerobic glycolysis induced by the continuous hypoxic state of the brain tissue. Although such patients experience significantly lower levels of ischemia and hypoxia than those with cerebral infarction, the appearance of a Lac peak within a given region indicates that there is greater decrease in the cerebral perfusion of this particular area, which is more likely to develop cerebral infarction. Therefore, ^{1}H-MRS enables the early detection of high-risk areas for cerebral infarction, which can facilitate the accurate determination of the level of cerebral ischemia and patient's prognosis, while also providing a new evaluation method for patients in the compensatory phase of chronic cerebral ischemia.

12.1.5 Research Applications of BOLD Imaging in Cerebrovascular Diseases

BOLD imaging is primarily utilized in chronic cerebrovascular disease, especially in research of the mechanisms underlying post-infarction recovery. BOLD-fMRI studies on the recovery of motor function following cerebral ischemia revealed that hand movements performed by patients in the early stages after the onset of ischemia elicited extensive activation of the contralesional cerebral hemisphere. Furthermore, during the slow process of functional recovery, the extent of contralesional activation gradually decreased, whereas the ipsilesional hemisphere showed a tendency toward re-activation. The expansion of activated areas in the contralesional hemisphere was more common among patients with poor recovery, suggesting that activation in the contralesional hemisphere during the early stages of ischemia is not a key factor contributing to the recovery of motor function. This phenomenon is most likely due to the disinhibition of non-crossing corticospinal tracts in the contralesional hemisphere by the ipsilesional hemisphere. Following cerebral infarction, the non-injured, peri-infarct area in the ipsilesional cerebral hemisphere exhibits some degree of plasticity. Both human and animal studies have found that the peri-infarct area in the ipsilesional cerebral hemisphere can play a role in motor recovery. Additionally, one study found that the activation volume of the contralesional cerebellar hemisphere showed a positive linear association with the patient's recovery of motor function, implying that the cerebellum plays a mediating role in functional recovery from cerebral infarction. As with motor function, the recovery of language, sensory, cognitive, and other functions in patients with cerebral infarction is also closely related to the plasticity of brain tissues and the dynamic reorganization of neural networks. In BOLD-fMRI studies on patients with aphasia in the recovery phase of cerebral infarction, it was found that language-related activation areas shifted from the left to the right cerebral hemisphere. This redistribution and reorganization indicate that the location of functional language areas of the cerebral cortex can be altered through sensory input, learning, and experience. The utilization of BOLD imaging in conjunction with simple language tasks is an effective method for evaluating the functional language status of aphasic patients with cerebral infarction. By monitoring the dynamic changes of the corresponding functional areas, as well as their relationship with the patient's functional recovery, we are able to gain a deeper understanding of the neural mechanisms of brain functional recovery.

However, patients with cerebral infarction often find it difficult to perform tasks and maintain task consistency. The general linear model (GLM) of BOLD imaging assumes that the patient's hemodynamic responses are normal, although the reduction in cerebral perfusion can lead to decreased BOLD signals. Additionally, the interconnectivity between brain areas is overlooked in task-based BOLD imaging. As research in functional brain imaging is carried out in greater depth, researchers have begun paying more attention to the information obtained by BOLD-fMRI in the resting state. Resting-state fMRI is beneficial to patients with cerebral infarction who are unable to perform tasks and is especially suitable for large-sample, long-term, longitudinal studies on patients with cerebral infarction. Extensive abnormalities can be observed in the functional networks of the brain after cerebral infarction. Current research has demonstrated that the functional motor network has been damaged in patients with cerebral infarction and that the improvement of motor function is closely linked with the remodeling of brain functions. Therefore, the analysis and evaluation of the whole-brain functional network are of crucial significance to studying the dynamic mechanisms underlying the process of motor function reorganization after cerebral infarction.

Carter et al. performed a cross-sectional study on patients with subacute stroke and found reduced interhemispheric functional connectivity in the somatomotor network, including the bilateral primary motor cortices, supplementary motor area, secondary somatosensory cortex, cerebellum, thalamus, and putamen. Upper limb motor dysfunction was significantly correlated with the decreased interhemispheric functional connectivity of the bilateral primary motor cortices, but not with intrahemispheric functional connectivity. Furthermore, a follow-up study demonstrated that the decrease in the interhemispheric functional connectivity of the bilateral primary motor cortices can be detected within a few hours after the onset of cerebral infarction, and this functional connectivity was gradually strengthened with the recovery of motor function. Another study found that in the early stages of cerebral infarction, the interhemispheric functional connectivity between the bilateral primary motor cortices was more lateralized to the ipsilesional side. This asymmetry was greatest at 1 month after onset, and then gradually returned to normal levels, which was consistent with the redistribution of brain activation between the bilateral hemispheres as seen in task-based fMRI.

Longitudinal studies of patients with subcortical infarction revealed a decrease in functional connectivity between the ipsilesional primary motor cortex and relevant brain areas during the initial stages of recovery, whereas the functional connectivity of the ipsilesional thalamus and cerebellum with the main contralesional motor areas gradually decreased over the course of recovery. These findings indicate that the enhancement of the connectivity of the ipsilesional primary motor cortex is beneficial to motor function recovery. The dynamic changes in the functional connectivity between the ipsilesional primary sensorimotor cortex and the bilateral motor areas after cerebral infarction are significantly correlated with clinical motor function scores, suggesting that enhanced interhemispheric functional connectivity of the motor cortex may be the underlying brain mechanism of motor function recovery. By performing resting-state fMRI on patients with unilateral pontine infarction, Lu et al. showed that pontine infarction led to reduced functional connectivity in ipsilesional cerebro-cerebellar motor pathways (decreased connectivity between ipsilesional motor cortex and contralesional cerebellum), as well as reduced functional connectivity in ipsilesional cerebro-cerebellar non-motor pathways (ipsilesional prefrontal cortex and contralesional cerebellum). Such cerebrocerebellar functional disconnectivity demonstrates that anatomical neurocircuits are the biological basis of functional connectivity (Fig. 12.16). Additionally, resting-state fMRI can also be used to observe the impairments in the white matter functional connectivity of patients with cerebral infarction. Using white matter fMRI data, Wang et al. explored the changes in the white matter functional tensors of the sensorimotor system in patients with acute pontine infarction. They found that using fMRI and DTI for white matter tractography produced essentially the same results with respect to the morphology of patients' pontine-thalamic bundles. Furthermore, compared to healthy controls, patients with pontine infarction showed reduced functional tensor values of ipsilesional fiber bundles related to the thalamus-motor cortex, which were also significantly positively associated with the patients' upper limb motor scores at the six-month follow-up. These findings indicate that resting-state fMRI can uncover the dynamic patterns of repair in the white matter remodeling of patients with cerebral infarction, and may serve as a biomarker to predict the prognosis of motor patients' motor function.

Nevertheless, the vast majority of existing resting-state fMRI studies have utilized group analysis at the cohort level in the post-processing step, due to the low signal-to-noise ratio of BOLD data, which can be improved by implementing group analysis. Therefore, their findings can only reflect overall trends in functional brain networks, whereas inter-individual variability is discarded as noise, and as such does not meet the requirements for the individualized diagnosis and treatment of patients with clinical neurological diseases. Lu et al. challenged the post-processing models of traditional analysis methods and performed an in-depth analysis of the individual differences of functional connectivity in healthy adults. Their results revealed that inter-individual variability in functional connectivity is dependent on brain networks and \evolution. Specifically, brain networks involved in higher-order cognition (language, control, and attention networks) exhibited significant inter-individual variability, whereas the primary visual, sensory, and motor cortices showed smaller inter-individual variability. Furthermore, the degree of variability in functional connectivity was positively correlated with the variability in sulcal depth, but not cortical thickness. The degree of variability in connectivity was also significantly negatively correlated with short-range connectivity but was significantly positively correlated with long-range connectivity (Fig. 12.17).

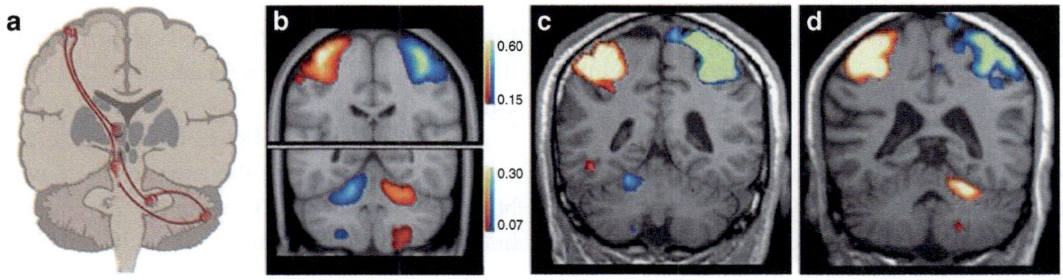

Fig. 12.16 Schematic diagram of a coronal section of the cerebro-ponto-cerebellar circuit. Main components of the cerebrocerebellar circuit. The polysynaptic efferent pathway between the cerebral cortex and the pons is mainly projected to the contralateral cerebellum. The afferent pathway is first projected to the deep cerebellar nuclei, then to the thalamus, and finally to the cerebrum (**a**). Resting-state fMRI of healthy adults shows the intrinsic functional connectivity between the bilateral cerebrum and cerebellum (**b**). Cerebrocerebellar functional connectivity is present in patients with left (**c**) and right (**d**) pontine infarction. Functional connectivity is impaired in the affected circuit, but remains unchanged in the unaffected circuit

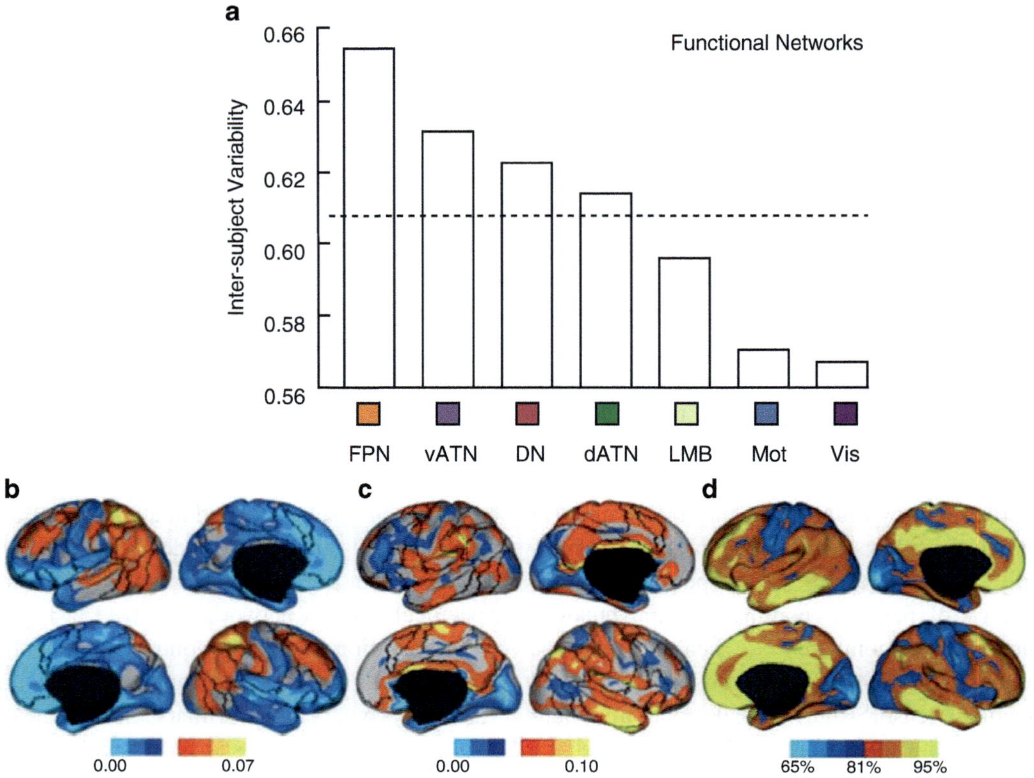

Fig. 12.17 Inter-individual variability in the functional connectivity of brain networks. Brain networks involved in higher-order cognition (control and attention network) showed greater variability, whereas the sensory, motor, and visual networks showed smaller variability (**a**). Brain regions that are phylogenetically the youngest (frontal lobe, temporal lobe and parietal lobe) showed the highest variability. Inter-individual variability was correlated with sulcal depth (**b**), not significantly correlated with cortical thickness (**c**), and positively correlated with long-range connectivity (**d**)

Additionally, the inter-individual variability of functional connectivity was also significantly associated with behavioral differences, in that brain regions with high connectivity variability were consistent with regions of high variability in cognitive or behavioral domains as determined by behavioral studies. Taken together, these findings demonstrate that inter-individual variability in functional connectivity can characterize the different manifestations of human behavior, and therefore serve as a theoretical basis for the formulation of individualized treatment plans for patients with cerebral infarction.

With the gradual advances of resting-state fMRI technology and the continuous improvements in its data analysis methods, the multi-perspective, longitudinal evaluation of whole-brain functional connectivity and functional networks will undoubtedly further elucidate the brain mechanisms underlying the functional reorganization after cerebral infarction, which will provide valuable information for clinical rehabilitation.

The wide range of MRI techniques have provided more options for the assessment of cerebrovascular diseases. The ability to combine histomorphological changes with data such as cerebral hemodynamics, brain metabolism, biochemical changes, white matter integrity, and functional connectivity has significant implications for attaining an in-depth understanding on the pathophysiological mechanisms underlying the pathogenesis of cerebral ischemia, and accurately evaluating the functional state of ischemic brain tissues. Therefore, MRI continues to play a crucial role in the early diagnosis, differential diagnosis, treatment selection, dynamic lesion monitoring, efficacy evaluation, and prognostic determination of ischemic cerebrovascular disease.

12.2 Research Applications of PET Imaging in Cerebrovascular Diseases

Several ischemic cerebrovascular diseases are the result of the transient or permanent occlusion or stenosis of cerebral blood vessels, which leads to metabolic and molecular changes in brain cells, thereby causing brain dysfunction and morphological damage. The blood flow and metabolic changes of brain tissues in the ischemic core and its adjacent regions can be assessed using radionuclide imaging, especially PET, for which there are currently a variety of different tracers, such as $^{15}O\text{-}H_2O$, $^{13}N\text{-}NH_3{\cdot}H_2O$, and ^{18}F-fluorodeoxyglucose (^{18}F-FDG), imaging agents for neuroinflammatory factors, imaging agents for benzodiazepine receptors, and imaging agents for hypoxia, among others. In this chapter, we have focused on the applications of PET in ischemic cerebrovascular disease and atherosclerotic plaque.

12.2.1 Applications of PET in Ischemic Cerebrovascular Diseases

12.2.1.1 Applications of PET in Acute Ischemic Cerebrovascular Diseases

CBF refers to the volume of blood passing through 100 g of brain tissue per unit of time and plays a decisive role in the maintenance of brain tissue function and metabolic levels. $^{15}O\text{-}H_2O$ PET is currently recognized as the gold standard for the quantitative measurement of CBF and is able to accurately quantify CBF values and clarify the extent of the ischemic penumbra, which is critical to facilitating early diagnosis and thrombolytic therapy in clinical settings. In healthy brains, the average whole-brain CBF is about 50 mL/(100 g·min), the average CBF of gray matter is higher, at 80 mL/(100 g·min), and the average CBF of white matter is about 20 mL/(100 g·min). In addition to obtaining CBF values, $^{15}O\text{-}H_2O$ PET can also be used to obtain oxygen extraction fraction (OEF) and cerebral blood metabolic rate of oxygen ($CMRO_2$). OEF is the percentage of oxygen taken up by a tissue after blood passes through the capillary bed, while $CMRO_2$ reflects the metabolic activity of brain tissues, and is a comprehensive indicator of the oxygen metabolism and utilization of the brain. Under normal physiological conditions, resting-state CBF is proportional to $CMRO_2$ and OEF, i.e., $CMRO_2 = CBF \times OEF$.

The conversion of cerebral ischemia to cerebral infarction is a process of dynamic change, with irreversible damage spreading from the ischemic core to the periphery. For patients with acute cerebral ischemia, the early treatment of reversible brain tissue damage is an important goal. Studies have shown that the cerebral infarct core has a CBF of <12 mL/(100 g·min) or a $CMRO_2$ of <65 μmol/(100 g·min). When CBF drops to 12–22 mL/(100 g·min), the ischemic region has the potential of either progressing to infarction or achieving recovery. This region is also known as the region of "misery perfusion". Its pathophysiological mechanism involves the decrease in rCBF caused by an increased capacity for compensatory vasodilation, which implies that in order to meet their metabolic needs, neurons must extract more oxygen from inflowing blood, causing OEF to increase to as high as 80% (normal value, 40%). At this point, CBF is still higher than 22 mL/ (100 g·min), however, the normal range of CBF cannot be attained due to the inadequacy of the blood supply, and this area is therefore defined as the hypoperfused region. The recovery potential of functional impairments in post-ischemic cells does not depend solely on the residual blood flow in the ischemic phase, but also on the duration of the blood flow disturbance. Preliminary PET imaging studies conducted on the duration of local ischemia in animal and human stroke models have found that PET can be used to observe four stages of focal cerebral ischemia. The first stage is when the decrease in regional cerebral perfusion pressure (CPP) matches the decrease in the regional blood flow of cerebrovascular tissues, while the decrease in CBF induces the increase in CBV via vasodilation in order to maintain CBF stability. The second stage involves the increase in OEF as CBF decreases in order to maintain $CMRO_2$. In the third stage, the CBF and $CMRO_2$ of the infarcted brain area decrease, while OEF increases to maintain tissue metabolism as far as possible. Brain tissues in this stage are defined as the ischemic penumbra. In the fourth stage, CBF, $CMRO_2$, and OEF are all at very low levels, and brain tissues in this stage have undergone irreversible ischemic injury or infarction. A number of studies have demonstrated that determining the ischemic penumbra after stroke is the key to successful treatment and that some patients may have very a long window for effective treatment.

Brain weight accounts for only 2% of total body weight, but its oxygen consumption at rest accounts for 20% of the total basal oxygen consumption in humans, most of which is used for the oxidative metabolism of glucose. Under normal physiological conditions, glucose is the only substrate consumed in the energy metabolism of the brain. ^{18}F-FDG is the most widely used imaging agent for glucose metabolism in clinical settings. As with glucose, ^{18}F-FDG is transported into cells via glucose transporters and phosphorylated by hexokinase to form ^{18}F-FDG-6-phosphate (^{18}F-FDG-6P). However, the absence of a hydroxyl group in ^{18}F-FDG-6P prevents its further metabolism, resulting in the retention of this reaction product within the cell. Therefore, ^{18}F-FDG-6P can be used to display the distribution of glucose uptake by cells in the body. Under normal physiological conditions, neurons in cortical gray matter, basal ganglia, cerebellum, and brainstem have the greatest demand for glucose, leading to a significant elevation in ^{18}F-FDG uptake. The cerebral metabolic rate of glucose (CMRGlc) is an objective indicator that can reflect human glucose metabolism, and in a healthy human brain is approximately 25 μmol/(100 g·min). CMRGlc is significantly correlated with CBF, and studies have shown that when rCBF >40 mL/(100 g·min), CMRGlc will remain within the normal range, but when rCBF decreases from 35 mL/(100 g·min) to 20 mL/(100 g·min), CMRGlc will undergo a sharp increase, followed by a decrease, and finally cease almost completely when rCBF <20 mL/(100 g·min). Therefore, in regions with reduced CBF, this sharp increase in glucose metabolism may be of critical clinical significance and may serve as an imaging feature of the ischemic penumbra.

Although experimental stroke studies involving ^{18}F-FDG have been performed for more than 20 years, these have primarily been restricted to animal experiments, whereas clinical studies have been relatively scarce, with the majority limited to patients in the subacute phase. This may be linked, to some extent, with the long preparation process of ^{18}F-FDG and the need to wait for at least 40 min after injection before imaging can be performed. Experimental studies on ischemic stroke models in small animals and primates have demonstrated consistent trends in the reduction of ^{18}F-FDG uptake in the infarct core but found substantial spatiotemporal variations in ^{18}F-FDG uptake in the peri-infarct area. The research team led by Walberer found in a rat model of stroke that elevated ^{18}F-FDG uptake could not be observed in the peri-infarct area during the acute ischemic phase and appeared only at 1 d after onset, which was more consistent with the timing of the neuroinflammatory response. In another study, Heiss and his research team examined the PET findings of 16 patients with acute ischemic stroke at onset and during follow-up, in which the changes in the CBF, CBV, $CMRO_2$, OEF, and CMRGlc of ipsilesional and contralesional brain tissues were compared between the two time points. Their results revealed that in the infarct core, blood flow, and metabolism were significantly lower than the corresponding contralesional regions, and did not change significantly at follow-up. When the peri-infarct area was defined based on decreased $CMRO_2$, no significant changes in CBF were observed at follow-up, but there were significant reductions in $CMRO_2$, OEF, and CMRGlc, and this region was

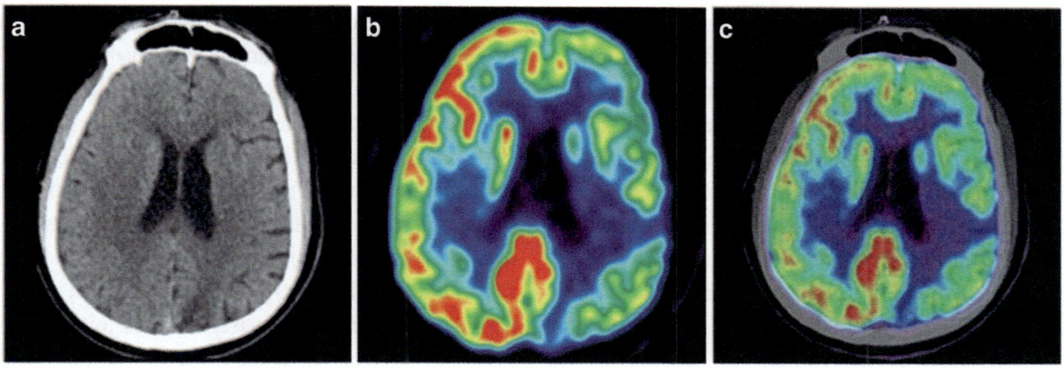

Fig. 12.18 Left intracranial artery stenosis. A 60-year-old male patient. Transverse head CT plain scan shows foliate hypodense shadows in the left parietal lobe (**a**). Transverse ^{18}F-FDG PET (**b**) and integrated ^{18}F-FDG PET/CT (**c**) show impaired ^{18}F-FDG uptake of the left parietal lobe, which was 59% lower than the corresponding contralateral region; as well as reduced ^{18}F-FDG uptake in the left frontal and parietal lobes, which was 18% lower than the corresponding contralateral region

later confirmed as an infarcted area using CT. When the peri-infarct area was defined based on increased OEF, only regions with elevated OEF and slightly impaired $CMRO_2$ showed metabolism levels that were close to normal values (Fig. 12.18).

Hypoxia markers play an important role in the identification of ischemic tissues. Increased uptake of radiolabeled nitroimidazole derivates can be observed in the histologically damaged ischemic core, as well as adjacent intact tissues at follow-up. ^{18}F-fluoromisonidazole (^{18}F-FMISO) is a common hypoxia marker utilized in clinical settings. Yeh et al. were the first to use ^{18}F-FMISO to examine patients with ischemic stroke and found increased ^{18}F-FMISO uptake in the peri-infarct area during the acute phase, while the decrease in this elevated uptake during the chronic stage indicated that tissues that were initially positive for ^{18}F-FMISO uptake had either been infarcted or had recovered.

12.2.1.2 Applications of PET in Chronic Cerebrovascular Diseases

Chronic ischemic cerebrovascular disease, which accounts for about 70% of all cerebrovascular disease, is largely the result of the stenosis or occlusion of the internal carotid or middle cerebral artery. In the chronic phase, CBF remains an important metric for evaluation, but measuring CBF alone is insufficient. When CPP decreases, normal blood flow can still be maintained via the autoregulatory vasodilation of distal resistance vessels, and this autoregulatory function is known as the cerebrovascular reserve (CVR). CVR refers to the ability of distal cerebral arteries to perform compensatory dilation or constriction to maintain normal CBF under the effects of normal physiological or pathological stimuli. Clinically, resting-state, acetazolamide-challenged $^{15}O\text{-}H_2O$ PET is a key technique for measuring CVR. Based on the known physiological responses of CBF, CBV, and OEF to CPP reduction, researchers have proposed three stages that describe the regional cerebral hemodynamics resulting from chronic carotid occlusion. In stage 0, CPP is normal, due to the complete compensation of the occluded artery by collateral circulation; CBF and $CMRO_2$ are closely matched; OEF is normal; CBV is not elevated; CBF responds normally to vasodilatory stimuli; and CVR is normal. In stage I, CPP reduction is reflected in the hemodynamic impairment, and CBF is maintained via the autoregulatory vasodilation of small arteries. At this point, CBV is increased, CVR is decreased, and CBF shows a weaker response to vasodilatory stimuli, although OEF remains normal. In stage II hemodynamic failure, CPP drops below the lower limit of autoregulation, CBF decrease is more prominent than $CMRO_2$ decrease, and CVR is reduced. At this point, OEF increases to maintain brain oxygen metabolism and tissue function, while ischemic injury may cause $CMRO_2$ to drop below the normal range. This stage is also known as "misery perfusion." Kuroda et al. performed long-term follow-up on 77 patients with ischemic cerebrovascular disease and found that the degree of CVR impairment was better at predicting stroke risk than the degree of vascular stenosis. Therefore, the evaluation of CVR is useful for the early clinical detection of high-risk groups for stroke, enabling the implementation of early interventions.

The ^{13}N-labeled PET tracer, ^{13}N-ammonia (^{13}N-NH_3), is a small-molecule, neutral aqueous solution that can freely pass through the blood-brain barrier and into brain tissues with blood flow, where it is converted into glutamine and retained. Stress tests conducted using ^{13}N-$NH_3{\cdot}H_2O$ PET/CT have demonstrated that ^{13}N-$NH_3{\cdot}H_2O$ PET can reflect CVR capacity and improve the diagnostic rate of ischemic cerebrovascular disease. Researchers have combined ^{13}N-$NH_3{\cdot}H_2O$ with ^{18}F-FDG to study CBF and cerebral metabolism in ischemic cerebrovascular disease. One-day integrated CBF-cerebral metabolism imaging techniques have been developed for the assessment of cerebral ischemia patients with varying extents of cerebrovascular stenosis, in order to examine the characteristics of impaired brain function. Based on qualitative and semi-quantitative analysis, CBF and metabolism were shown to match in a number of different ways, and it was therefore proposed that the joint evaluation of the two is of great value for patients with chronic ischemic cerebrovascular disease. Additionally, ^{13}N-$NH_3{\cdot}H_2O$ PET/CT was combined with methazolamide challenge to reflect the CVR status of patients with chronic ischemic cerebrovascular disease and evaluate their condition (Fig. 12.19).

Ischemia can cause microglial cells to switch from a quiescent to an activated state, subsequently acting as phagocytes. In this activation process, these cells may undergo morphological changes, undertake proliferation, release pro-inflammatory compounds, and increase immunomodulatory surface antigens, so as to alter their effector program. During the course of this, the

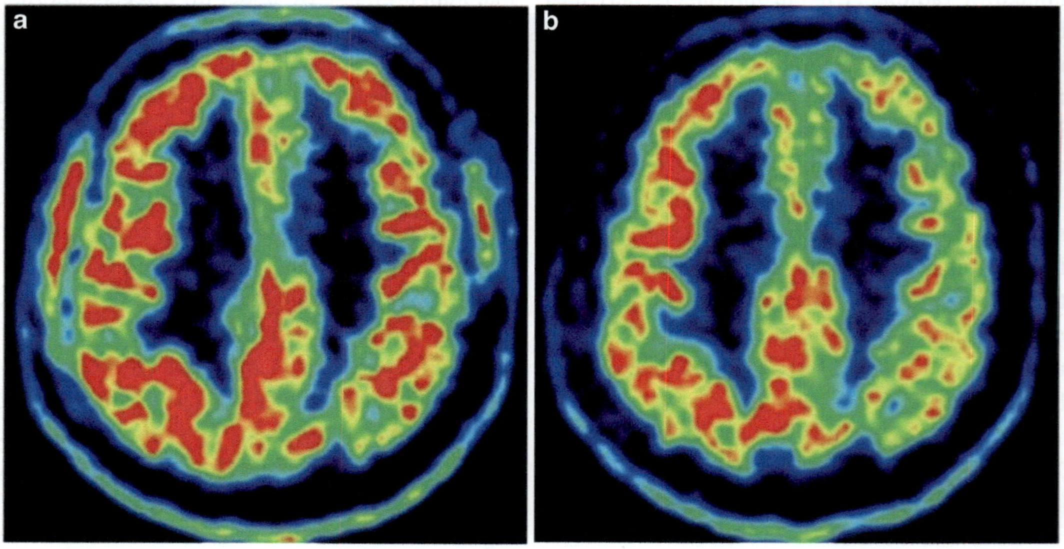

Fig. 12.19 Patient with left intracranial artery occlusion who underwent ^{13}N-$NH_3{\cdot}H_2O$ PET/CT with methazolamide challenge. A 50-year-old male patient. Transverse resting-state ^{13}N- $NH_3{\cdot}H_2O$ PET shows hypoperfusion in the left parietal lobe (**a**). Transverse ^{13}N- $NH_3{\cdot}H_2O$ PET after methazolamide challenge shows new hypoperfused regions in the left frontal lobe in addition to the left parietal lobe (**b**)

translocator protein 18 kDA (TSPO), also known as benzodiazepine receptor, is upregulated on the mitochondria of activated microglial cells, and can therefore serve as an inflammatory biomarker. ^{11}C-PK11195 is a commonly used inflammatory tracer in clinical practice. Studies have observed that ^{11}C-PK11195 uptake is elevated in the ischemic core and its peripheral areas within a few days after ischemia onset.

12.2.1.3 Applications of PET in the Efficacy Evaluation of Treatments for Ischemic Cerebrovascular Disease

The prevention and treatment of ischemic cerebrovascular disease consist of medical and surgical treatments. PET imaging plays a crucial role in the preoperative assessment and prognostic determination of surgical treatment. ^{15}O-H_2O PET can accurately determine the CBF, $CMRO_2$, and OEF values of brain tissues in patients with acute ischemic cerebrovascular disease. According to experimental results, CBF values less than 60% of the normal range, and $CMRO_2$ values greater than 40% of the normal range can be used to accurately identify the ischemic penumbra of stroke patients for intervention, thereby effectively reversing the ischemic penumbra. However, the short half-life of ^{15}O-H_2O, and therefore its need for an on-site cyclotron for production, have substantially restricted the clinical application of this technique in acute ischemic cerebrovascular disease. Surgical treatments for chronic ischemic cerebrovascular disease include endarterectomy and arterial bypass, among others, of which extracranial artery-middle cerebral artery bypass surgery is one of the most commonly utilized methods. Indications for surgery primarily include recurrent transient ischemic attacks and mild neurological impairment induced by cerebral artery stenosis or occlusion, but without symptoms such as severe hemiplegia and aphasia, perfusion imaging showing reduced CBF of the affected brain areas, and nonresponsiveness to medical treatment, among others. Bypass surgery attempts to improve the patient's CBF by adding or completely replacing the blood supply from a cerebral artery to the brain, with the goal of preventing stroke recurrence. In a prospective evaluation of 40 patients with symptomatic unilateral vascular occlusion, it was found that patients with elevated OEF had a higher risk for stroke, while the risk of recurrent stroke increased markedly with increasing OEF. Therefore, ^{15}O-H_2O PET is an important imaging technique for evaluating the therapeutic efficacy of bypass surgery. Powers et al. performed a multi-center, randomized trial involving 195 patients with symptomatic atherosclerotic internal carotid artery occlusion to investigate the therapeutic efficacy of medical and surgical treatments. Their results demonstrated that OEF values as measured by ^{15}O-H_2O PET were crucial in identifying patients at high risk for recurrent stroke due to poor collateral circulation. They also found that compared with medical treatment alone, bypass surgery plus medical treatment did not reduce the risk of recurrent ipsilateral ischemic stroke within 2 years. However, this study has been criticized for its poor design and implementation, and therefore, further investigations are currently ongoing concerning the evaluation of specific indications for bypass surgery.

^{18}F-FDG PET has also been utilized to evaluate the efficacy of surgical and interventional treatments for chronic ischemic cerebrovascular disease. An ^{18}F-FDG PET study on 19 patients with chronic carotid artery stenosis or occlusion found that carotid artery stent placement led to improvements in postoperative cerebral glucose metabolism and neurocognitive function. The research team led by Yu performed pre- and postoperative imaging assessments on patients with chronic cerebral ischemia undergoing bypass surgery. Their results indicated that ipsilesional CBF and ^{18}F-FDG uptake were both higher than preoperative levels, and patients experienced improvements in all symptoms within 1 month after surgery. Furthermore, surgery can help to increase the CBF and ^{18}F-FDG uptake of regions with hypoperfusion and reduced ^{18}F-FDG uptake. However, in-depth studies have not been conducted on the long-term changes in cerebral metabolic levels.

12.2.2 Applications of PET in Atherosclerotic Plaque

Carotid atherosclerosis is currently the primary cause of ischemic stroke in China, with about 70% of ischemic strokes resulting from the rupture of carotid atherosclerotic plaques. Therefore, the early identification of vulnerable plaques and the evaluation of plaque stability are of utmost importance in preventing and controlling the onset of ischemic stroke events. Atherosclerosis is a systemic, chronic, inflammatory disease of the vessel walls caused by vascular risk factors that can gradually progress into vulnerable plaques, and eventually result in the occurrence of cerebrovascular events. Studies have shown that vulnerable plaques can rupture to form emboli that enter the bloodstream and cause thromboembolisms, which in turn can lead to ischemic stroke. Intraplaque neovascularization and macrophage inflammation are key factors contributing to the vulnerability of carotid plaques. Plaque vulnerability is determined by plaque composition, while the different stages in plaque progression are characterized by different inflammatory responses. Common characteristics of vulnerable plaques include a large lipid-rich necrotic core with a thin overlying fibrous cap, containing abundant macrophages, T lymphocytes, and some smooth muscle cells.

Morphological imaging has certain drawbacks in the diagnosis of vulnerable carotid plaques. Therefore, molecular imaging techniques, especially molecular probes for nuclear imaging, have now become a hotspot of research in this field. Every step in the pathophysiological mechanism underlying the onset of carotid plaques and their development into vulnerable plaques is an important target for molecular imaging. The primary processes include inflammatory cell aggregation, endothelial cell activation, macrophage apoptosis, intraplaque hypoxia, neovascularization and subsequent microcalcification, fibrous cap degradation, and thrombosis, which ultimately lead to ischemic stroke onset. PET is a common molecular imaging technique that involves the specific radiolabeling of molecular tracers to achieve the visual, non-invasive analysis of in vivo cellular metabolic activity. At present, a wide range of molecular imaging methods have been established for tumor imaging, and have been utilized to clarify the molecular mechanisms of tumorigenesis. Owing to the similarities in molecular imaging targets, these techniques can also be applied to carotid atherosclerotic plaques. However, due to the poor resolution of PET imaging, it is essentially unable to discriminate among the various anatomical features. Therefore, many multimodal imaging techniques have emerged recently, and the application of PET/CT and PET/MR techniques has gradually enhanced the specificity and sensitivity of PET scans. The combination of PET with CT or MRI can be used to identify the components of atherosclerotic plaques and the degree of inflammatory response, which allows us to accurately assess the vulnerability of carotid plaques.

12.2.2.1 Applications of ^{18}F-FDG PET in Carotid Atherosclerotic Plaque

^{18}F-FDG is currently the most widely used molecular imaging tracer for the evaluation of plaque inflammation. ^{18}F-FDG is phosphorylated by hexokinase to form ^{18}F-FDG-6P, which cannot undergo further glycolysis due to its lack of a hydroxyl group, and is therefore retained intracellularly, while its retention is especially prominent in metabolically active inflammatory cells, such as intraplaque activated macrophages. This, therefore, is the basis for the ^{18}F-FDG PET molecular imaging of inflammatory vulnerable carotid plaques. In animal models and clinical studies, ^{18}F-FDG uptake was found to be closely associated with macrophage aggregation. Hyafil et al. showed that the lipid-rich necrotic core of non-stenotic carotid plaques as detected by MRI was significantly associated with high ^{18}F-FDG uptake. Tawakol et al. demonstrated that ^{18}F-FDG PET can be used to evaluate the inflammatory activity of plaques after drug therapy. Therefore, ^{18}F-FDG PET can monitor the degree of inflammatory response in vulnerable plaques, and hence predict the risk of ischemic stroke onset, which facilitates the clinical risk stratification of stroke onset among patients with carotid atherosclerosis, and the formulation of individualized treatment plans.

A study involving patients with recently symptomatic carotid stenosis found that ^{18}F-FDG uptake related to intraplaque inflammation was associated with the risk of early stroke recurrence. Furthermore, ^{18}F-FDG PET studies have revealed significant differences in the target-to-background ratio (TBR) between symptomatic and asymptomatic plaques, as well as between plaques positive and negative for microembolic signals. Therefore, ^{18}F-FDG PET can accurately detect high-risk carotid plaques, and predict the risk of atherosclerosis progression and thrombotic complications.

12.2.2.2 Applications of Other PET Tracers in Vulnerable Carotid Plaques

In addition to ^{18}F-FDG, a number of other tracers can also be utilized in the imaging of carotid plaques, so as to determine their level of vulnerability. These include tracers specific to the occurrence of hypoxia, neovascularization, and microcalcification in the pathological process of plaque formation, as well as novel PET tracers for atherosclerosis.

1. Other PET tracers based on the plaque formation process:
   (a) ^{18}F-FMISO: The lack of normal blood vessels in carotid atherosclerotic plaques often gives rise to hypoxia, while hypoxia is closely related to plaque volume and plaque inflammation. ^{18}F-FMISO PET has been extensively utilized in the imaging of hypoxic atherosclerosis. Researchers have demonstrated using a rabbit model of hyperlipidemia that ^{18}F-FMISO uptake is significantly elevated in atherosclerotic areas. Studies have also shown that ^{18}F-FMISO PET allows the visual analysis of hypoxic regions in atherosclerosis.
   (b) ^{68}Ga-NOTA-RGD: Neovascularization frequently occurs within vulnerable carotid plaques. Over the course of plaque progression, new blood vessels are prone to rupture and hemorrhage, which causes thromboembolism, and eventually leads to the occurrence of ischemic stroke. ^{68}Ga-NOTA-RGD targets integrin $\alpha v\beta 3$ which is specifically expressed on the surface of vascular endothelial cells and macrophages. Therefore, PET/CT imaging performed on mouse models of atherosclerosis and patients' blood vessels enables the visual assessment of atherosclerosis.
   (c) ^{18}F-sodium fluoride (^{18}F-NaF): Calcification is the final outcome of inflammation, and one of the key features of atherosclerosis. Microcalcification primarily occurs in the fibrous cap overlying the plaque surface, and contributes significantly to plaque vulnerability. ^{18}F-NaF is a specific tracer commonly used to detect bone metastases. Studies have shown that ^{18}F-NaF can be taken up by atherosclerotic vessel walls, and is associated with the risk factors of atherosclerosis. Other studies have found that ^{18}F-NaF uptake is significantly higher in vulnerable carotid plaques than in contralateral asymptomatic plaques and the control group. The study by Li et al. demonstrated that ^{18}F-NaF PET/CT was useful in the detection of microcalcification activity in carotid atherosclerosis, and can assess the stability of carotid plaques, while low-dose CT can help to determine the degree of plaque calcification and plaque localization (Fig. 12.20).
2. Novel PET tracers:
   (a) ^{99m}Tc-HYNIC-IL-2: Interleukin 2 (IL-2) and scavenger receptors are expressed on the surface of macrophages. ^{99m}Tc-HYNIC-IL-2 is a biological probe targeting IL-2 and has been widely utilized in the imaging of carotid plaques.
   (b) ^{64}Cu-DOTA-DAPTA: As an effective molecular probe for carotid atherosclerosis, this compound has a strong affinity for various chemokine receptors.
   (c) ^{68}Ga-DOTA-TATE: This compound has a specific affinity for type II somatostatin (SST) receptor, which is overexpressed in activated macrophages and injured endothelial cells. Studies have shown that atherosclerotic vessels exhibited a significant

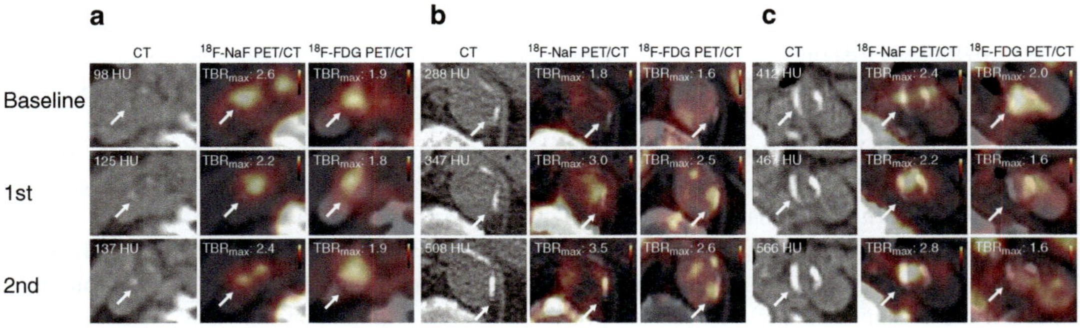

Fig. 12.20 Comparative study of ^{18}F-FDG PET/CT and ^{18}F-NaF PET/CT in carotid atherosclerosis progression. Transverse ^{18}F-NaF-PET/CT scan of myeloma patients with varying degrees of carotid artery calcification. In non-calcified lesions, the location of ^{18}F-NaF uptake in the carotid plaque was consistent with that of ^{18}F-FDG, and both showing increased calcium uptake (**a**). In mildly calcified lesions, after progressive arterial calcium accumulation, ^{18}F-NaF uptake showed significant increases from baseline to follow-up (**b**). In severely calcified lesions, dense calcium components can be observed (**c**). Arrows indicate calcified lesions

correlation between ^{68}Ga-DOTA-TATE and ^{18}F-FDG uptake.

(d) ^{18}F-FMCH: Cho plays an important role in the process of cell membrane formation. Studies on atherosclerotic plaques in mice found that tracing with ^{18}F-FMCH (targeting macrophage cell membrane receptors) and ^{11}C-Cho enhanced the detection of macrophages in the inflammatory response.

(e) ^{11}C-PK11195: TSPO is widely found in the outer mitochondrial membrane and expressed in some macrophages. Gaemperli et al. performed ^{11}C-PK11195 (targeting TSPO) PET/CT imaging in carotid plaques and found that this technique significantly increased the detection of vulnerable carotid plaques.

(f) ^{99m}Tc-RP805: During proteolysis, macrophages produce a variety of proteases, of which matrix metalloproteinase (MMP) is the most common and can be specifically tagged using the ^{99m}Tc-RP805 tracer. Studies have demonstrated that this tracer can be used for plaque imaging in animal models.

(g) ^{99m}Tc-cAbVCAM1–5: Endothelial cells are activated during the inflammatory response of atherosclerosis, while the vascular cell adhesion molecule 1 (VCAM-1) found on their cell surface can serve as a target for tracers. Studies have shown that PET imaging of vulnerable plaques in mouse models could be carried out effectively using ^{64}Cu-P-selectin monoclonal antibody ($T_{1/2}$ = 12.7 h) and ^{99m}Tc-cAbVCAM1–5.

(h) ^{68}Ga-pentixafor: This compound can trace the type 4 chemokine receptor (CXCR4) found on macrophages involved in atherosclerosis progression. Kircher et al. performed a retrospective analysis on 92 patients with atherosclerosis who underwent ^{68}Ga-pentixafor PET/CT and ^{18}F-FDG PET/CT imaging. They found that ^{68}Ga-pentixafor PET/CT identified more atherosclerotic plaques than ^{18}F-FDG PET/CT, and the two showed a weak correlation. Therefore, their findings demonstrate that ^{68}Ga-pentixafor could serve as a useful tracer for the evaluation of vulnerable atherosclerotic plaques.

PET is a valuable molecular imaging technique for the quantification of CBF and metabolism, which allows the accurate evaluation of CVR function through its intrinsic connections and dynamic evolution. Therefore, this technique can provide objective imaging evidence for the risk stratification of patients with cerebral ischemia, thereby achieving the early warning of cerebral infarction as well as the individualized and precise diagnosis and treatment of patients, which effectively reduces the incidence rate of cerebral infarction.

12.3 Research Applications of PET/MR in Cerebrovascular Diseases

MRI is commonly utilized for the examination of cerebrovascular diseases, as it provides detailed anatomical images as well as information on brain function, perfusion, tissue biochemical changes, and other characteristics. PET is also an important tool in the study of neurological diseases, while the development and application of a wide variety of specific tracers have played a crucial role in studying the pathogenic mechanisms of cerebrovascular diseases, as well as guiding its early diagnosis and treatment. Integrated PET/MR combines PET molecular imaging techniques with multiparametric MRI techniques for the acquisition of comprehensive imaging information in a single scan session. This approach not only allows the visualization of metabolic levels in brain tissue lesions, but also the precise anatomical location, hemodynamic changes, diffusion characteristics, and biochemical information of these lesions. Therefore, PET/MR can provide a strong support for further investigating the pathophysiological mechanisms of ischemic cerebrovascular disease, elucidating the trends in its pathogenesis, and guiding individualized clinical treatment.

12.3.1 Applications of Integrated PET/MR in Cerebrovascular Diseases

12.3.1.1 Applications of Non-invasive Quantitative Methods with Integrated PET/MR

Integrated PET/MR not only enables the precise co-registration of PET and MRI data, but also allows the simultaneous acquisition of information on CBF, cerebral metabolism, brain functional network connectivity, and white matter fiber bundles. There is currently an urgent clinical need to further understand the pathophysiological mechanisms of ischemic cerebrovascular disease. CBF is one of the key quantitative indicators of ischemic cerebrovascular disease. As mentioned previously, the gold standard for the quantification of CBF is ^{15}O-H_2O PET, the traditional method of which involves administering a bolus of ^{15}O-H_2O, and tracking the dynamic processes as the tracer reaches the brain, while also sampling arterial blood from the radial artery at different time points during the acquisition process. Then, using arterial blood as the input function, image processing is performed to obtain a time-radioactivity curve of specified brain areas, in order to calculate the CBF values. However, this method requires the sampling of arterial blood, which has restricted its widespread application in clinical settings. Su et al. proposed an image-derived arterial input function (IDAIF) method of CBF quantification involving the co-registration of PET and MRA images acquired using separate scanners. In their study, 8 healthy volunteers underwent either the conventional arterial sampling method or the IDAIF method for the calculation of whole-brain CBF, and the correlation between the two methods was examined. Their results revealed that the CBF calculated using these two methods were highly correlated ($r = 0.93$), implying that the IDAIF method could replace the conventional arterial sampling method for the calculation of CBF. Integrated PET/MR offers the unique advantage of simultaneous scanning, allowing both PET and MRI data to be acquired at the same time in a single scan session. Therefore, the precise co-registration between the two sets of images enables the easy and accurate acquisition of IDAIF information, and as such is more suitable for the non-invasive and absolute quantitative research on CBF.

In 2017, the same research team built upon their previous study involving separate scanners and performed integrated PET/MR on 7 healthy volunteers to compare the calculation results between the arterial sampling and IDAIF methods. The CBF calculated using the two methods showed strong agreement ($r = 0.88$), and the difference between them was not statistically significant. In current clinical settings, ASL and PWI are often used to replace ^{15}O-H_2O PET for the quantitative measurement of CBF. Zaro et al. used the ischemic regions delineated by ^{15}O-H_2O PET to guide the selection of PWI maps. Their results indicated that PWI achieved the highest accuracy at predicting the CBF critical flow threshold when time-to-maximum (T_{max}) > 6.1 s and TTP > 4.8 s. Therefore, the integration of ^{15}O-H_2O PET and PWI to evaluate the differences in perfusion as displayed by PWI and PET can help to address the current bottleneck in the development of perfusion imaging in acute ischemic stroke and has significant implications for further elucidating the pathophysiological changes in this disease. ASL is a non-invasive MRI technique that can also provide quantitative rCBF images. Using integrated PET/MR, Okazawa et al. performed a quantitative comparison of ^{15}O-H_2O PET and ASL in 11 healthy volunteers, which revealed that the quantitative results from ASL were slightly higher than those of ^{15}O-H_2O PET, and compared the differences between the two techniques can help to guide the clinical application of ASL. Additionally, Puig et al. performed integrated PET/MR on 14 healthy volunteers, in order to perform a quantitative comparison of ASL and ^{15}O-H_2O PET perfusion parameters in the resting state, during hyperventilation, and after acetazolamide use. No significant differences in CBF values were found between the two techniques in any state.

12.3.1.2 Evaluation of Chronic Ischemic Cerebrovascular Disease with Integrated PET/ MR

PET studies have found that some patients with ischemic cerebrovascular disease exhibit crossed cerebellar diaschisis (CCD), in which supratentorial brain lesions result in reduced blood flow and metabolism of the contralateral cerebellum. This phenomenon was first reported by Baron et al. in 1980. They utilized non-invasive ^{15}O-H_2O PET imaging to reveal the decreases in blood flow and oxygen metabolic rates of the contralesional cerebellar hemisphere in patients with supratentorial brain infarction. Researchers have subsequently utilized other techniques, such as $CMRO_2$ and CMRGlc, to further investigate this phenomenon, and confirmed the existence of CCD. The occurrence of CCD may be the result of pathologies in the cortico-ponto-cerebellar pathway and can appear immediately after the onset of ischemic stroke. This phenomenon, however, can be reversed with successful reperfusion therapy. The occurrence of CCD is closely related to the inadequate perfusion of the frontal lobe and thalamus. fMRI studies have demonstrated the presence of CCD in patients with acute, subacute, and chronic ischemic cerebrovascular disease, while the severity of CCD in subacute patients was associated with their neurological severity and clinical outcomes. Researchers at the University of Zurich found that among patients with ischemic cerebrovascular disease, the detection of CCD using BOLD fMRI with a carbon dioxide challenge demonstrated a similar sensitivity compared to acetazolamide-challenged ^{15}O-H_2O PET. In the study by Kim et al. on patients with CCD after cerebral infarction, PET imaging showed reduced metabolism in the contralateral cerebellum, while DTI also revealed significantly lower FA values in the contralesional middle cerebellar peduncle, signifying the presence of damage to the cortico-ponto-cerebellar pathway. Nevertheless, the specific mechanisms underlying the onset of CCD are poorly understood, while findings on the impairments and dynamic changes of functional connectivity and fiber bundles in CCD, as well as their relationship with CBF and metabolic changes, remain inconclusive. Furthermore, this phenomenon can occur in both acute and chronic ischemia, while similar effects have also been observed in non-ischemic lesions such as brain tumors.

Brain perfusion and metabolism are both inextricably linked with neural activity and are therefore crucial physiological indicators of the state of brain function. Due to the extremely high energy demand of nervous tissues, the oxidative metabolism of glucose is virtually the only substrate for brain energy metabolism under normal physiological conditions. The glucose metabolized within neurons is primarily used to support cellular nutrition and maintain cellular functions. Generally speaking, the energy consumed by signal conduction, such as the propagation of action potentials and postsynaptic ion channels, accounts for 87% of total energy consumption, while the remaining 13% is used to maintain the resting membrane potential of neurons. Research has shown that blood flow is highly correlated with metabolism and that this correlation decreases with increasing age. Among patients with chronic ischemic cerebrovascular disease, the early, comprehensive, and meticulous assessment of brain function, as well as the timely intervention in high-risk groups, can facilitate the prevention of stroke recurrence. In a study previously conducted by the authors, we found that performing simultaneous ^{18}F-FDG PET and ASL on patients with chronic ischemic cerebrovascular disease who required bypass surgery reflected the patient's preoperative hemodynamic and metabolic status in the non-infarcted area. After surgery, significant increases were observed in the blood flow and metabolism of ipsilesional brain areas, and patients experience marked improvement in symptoms. Therefore, this technique is essential for the prevention of stroke recurrence and the evaluation of surgical efficacy (Fig. 12.21). Additionally, we have also analyzed the combination of ^{18}F-FDG PET and DWI when utilized in the evaluation of chronic ischemic cerebrovascular disease, which revealed reduced ^{18}F-FDG uptake in the infarct core, whereas peri-infarct tissue that appeared normal in structural MRI showed reduced ^{18}F-FDG uptake and elevated ADC values. These findings may have been due to ischemia-induced microcirculatory dys-

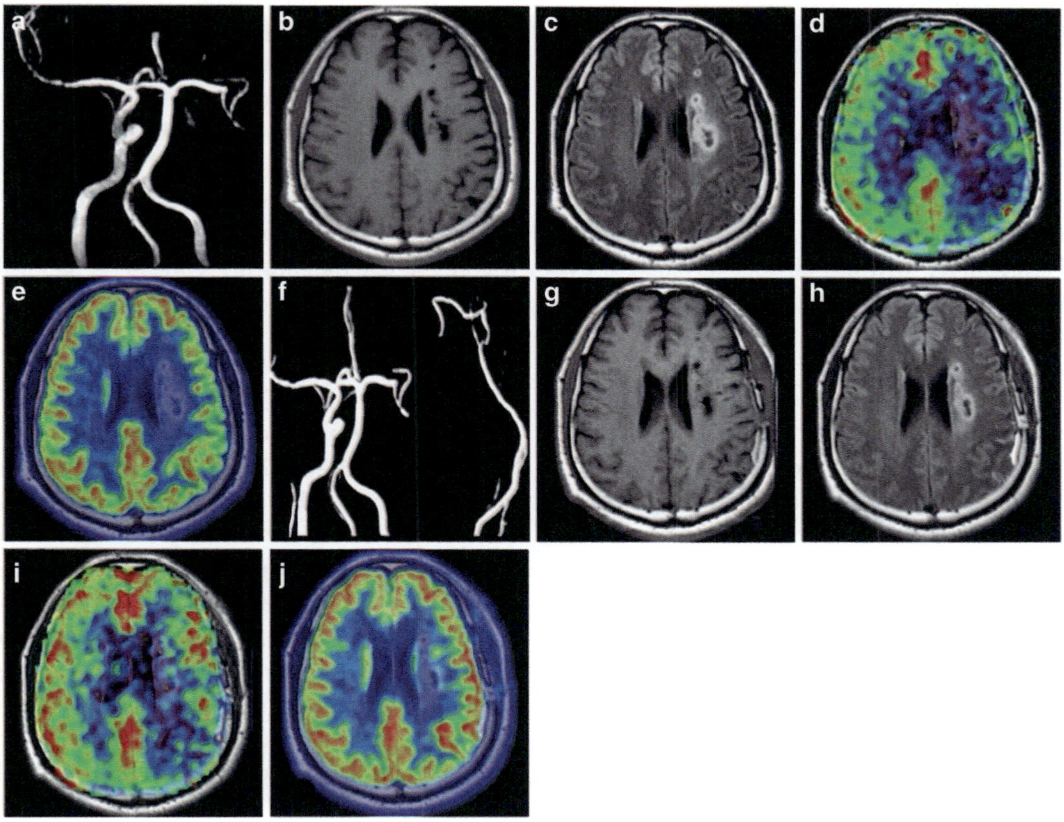

Fig. 12.21 Left internal carotid artery occlusion treated with bypass surgery. A 45-year-old male patient who presented with restricted movement of the right limbs for 7 months. Preoperative images of bypass surgery. MRA shows left carotid artery occlusion (**a**). MRI shows infarcts in the left corona radiata, manifesting as T_1WI hypointensities (**b**), and FLAIR hyperintensities (**c**). Integrated ASL-MRI shows decreased CBF (**d**), which was approximately 30 mL/(100 g·min). ^{18}F-FDG PET/MR shows reduced ^{18}F-FDG uptake (**e**), and a mean standardized uptake value (SUVmean) of about 7.51. Postoperative images of bypass surgery. MRA shows the left bypass graft (**f**). MRI with T_1WI (**g**) and FLAIR (**h**) reveals the same left corona radiata infarcts as in preoperative imaging. Increases can be observed in the CBF measured by ASL-MRI (**i**) and cerebral metabolism measured by ^{18}F-FDG PET/MR (**j**), showing a CBF of about 50 mL/(100 g·min) and SUVmean of about 8.0

function, which led to increased cellular permeability, increased extracellular water, and other factors. However, further investigation is needed to elucidate the exact mechanisms involved in this process.

12.3.2 Applications of Integrated PET/MR in Carotid Atherosclerotic Plaque

PET/MR is currently the most advanced imaging technique available that can implement the simultaneous acquisition of MRI and ^{18}F-FDG PET data in a single session, and can therefore achieve the precision co-registration of the two sets of images. Additionally, this technique can also provide information on the inflammatory response of carotid atherosclerotic plaques at the morphological and molecular levels, which permits the real-time fusion of anatomical, functional, and metabolic information, thereby more accurately evaluating the stability of carotid plaques. Furthermore, MRI has obvious advantages over PET/CT, including its lack of radiation and ability to achieve high-resolution imaging of soft tissues, allowing carotid atherosclerotic plaques to be displayed more clearly.

12.3.2.1 Research Applications of ^{18}F-FDG in Carotid Atherosclerotic Plaque

^{18}F-FDG is the most common PET tracer used in clinical settings, and studies have demonstrated the benefit of performing ^{18}F-FDG PET/MR to evaluate the stability of atherosclerotic plaques. Li et al. compared the value of ^{18}F-FDG PET/MR and ^{18}F-FDG PET/CT in the evaluation of carotid plaques, and found no significant differences in PET findings between the two hybrid systems in the case of vein bypass surgery, whereas the errors resulting from different attenuation correction algorithms used could be ignored. Therefore, these findings are a direct reflection of the reliability of the PET/MR system, while the higher soft tissue contrast and multiple sequences of high-resolution MRI could better display the structure of the carotid artery wall than CT (Fig. 12.22). Ripa et al. performed ^{18}F-FDG PET/MR and ^{18}F-FDG/CT on the carotid arteries of six male patients positive for the human immunodeficiency virus (HIV), and found significant correlations in the mean standardized uptake value (SUV_{mean}) and maximum SUV (SUV_{max}) between the two imaging techniques (SUV_{mean}: $r = 0.98$; SUV_{max}: $r = 1.00$; both: $P < 0.001$). Therefore, they concluded that ^{18}F-FDG PET/MR can effectively be used to evaluate the stability of carotid atherosclerotic plaques. Mootaz et al. performed ^{18}F-FDG PET/MR on seven patients with carotid plaques, who were divided according to scan times into standard and low dose groups. They found that the standard ^{18}F-FDG dose in ^{18}F-FDG PET/MR scans could be reduced by 75% while still ensuring high image quality and precise quantification. The results of the study by Rischpler et al. demonstrated that after the administration of drug therapy in patients with carotid atherosclerotic plaques, ^{18}F-FDG PET/MR could detect the metabolic changes of inflammatory cells in carotid plaques, and was therefore useful for determining the efficacy of clinical drug therapies.

12.3.2.2 Research Applications of Other Tracers in Carotid Atherosclerotic Plaque

In addition to ^{18}F-FDG, the utilization of other novel tracers can enhance the accuracy and specificity of PET/MR in evaluating the stability of carotid plaques. ^{68}Ga-pentixafor can trace CXCR4 in macrophages over the course of atherosclerosis progression, which has significant implications in the quantitative evaluation of the stability of carotid atherosclerotic plaques. Li et al. performed ^{68}Ga-pentixafor PET/MR on the atherosclerotic lesions of 38 tumor patients, and their TBR values were calculated. Their results indicated that the TBR value of the descending aorta wall was significantly higher in men than in women [(1.9 ± 0.3) vs. (1.7 ± 0.2), respectively; $P < 0.05$], and that compared with patients with a mean TBR ≤ 1.70, those with a mean TBR > 1.70 had significantly higher incidence rates of diabetes, hypertension, hypercholesterolemia, and cardiovascular disease. Furthermore,

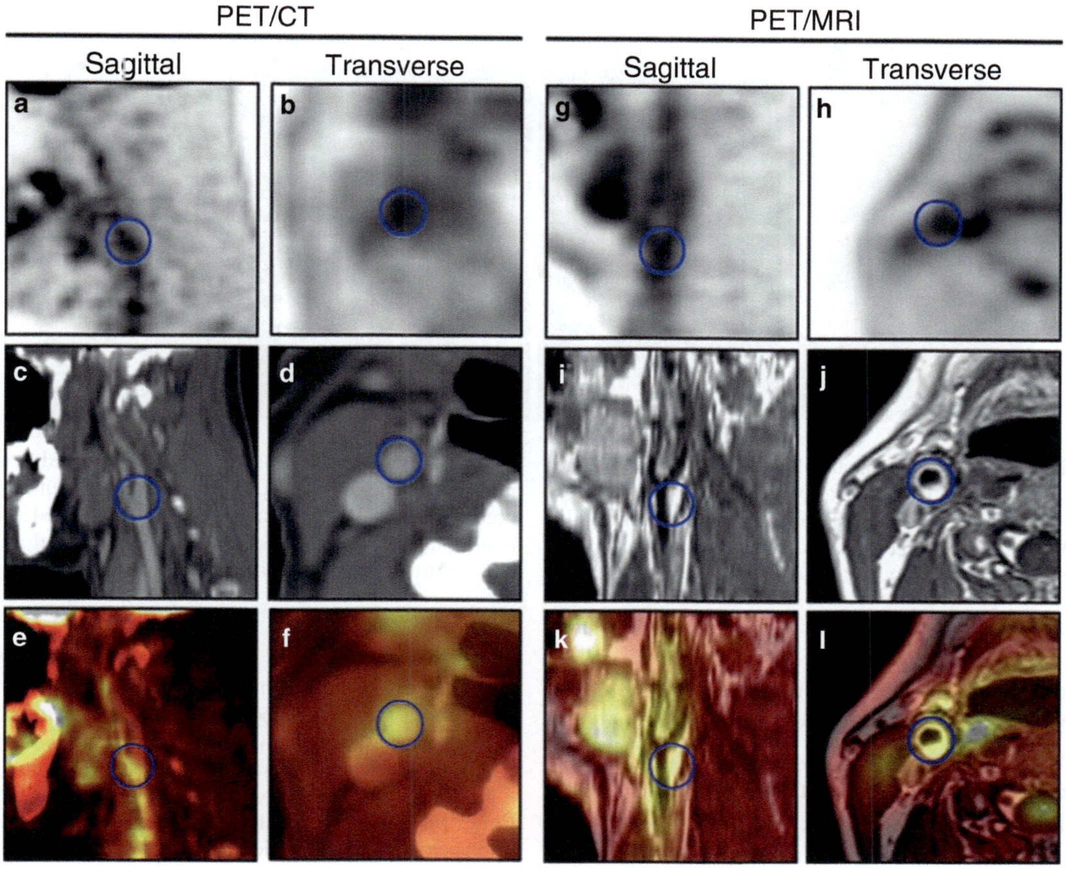

Fig. 12.22 Integrated PET/CT and MR images of the right carotid artery in a patient with head and neck cancer. A 52-year-old male patient whose right carotid plaque shows focal ^{18}F-FDG uptake (the blue circle indicates the plaque at the carotid bifurcation)

^{68}Ga-pentixafor uptake has good reproducibility (r = 0.60, $P < 0.01$), and studies have shown that patients with high ^{68}Ga-pentixafor uptake have an elevated incidence of cardiovascular risk factors. Therefore, ^{68}Ga-pentixafor PET/MR is a powerful imaging technique that can be utilized to evaluate the stability of atherosclerotic plaques.

Subsequently, Li et al. performed ^{68}Ga-pentixafor PET/MR on 72 patients with lymphoma to examine carotid plaques with various lesions and confirmed through histopathology and immunohistochemistry analyses that the CXCR4 expression of atherosclerotic plaques can serve as a surrogate marker for inflammatory atherosclerosis. They concluded, therefore, that ^{68}Ga-pentixafor PET/MR can quantify the CXCR4 expression of atherosclerotic plaques to assess plaque stability (Fig. 12.23).

The rupture of carotid atherosclerotic plaques is a major cause of ischemic stroke and represents a serious threat to human health. Therefore, the early identification of vulnerable plaques, along with the evaluation of plaque stability, is critical for achieving early clinical intervention. High-resolution MRI can accurately provide morphological information on plaque composition but cannot accurately assess intraplaque inflammation. In contrast, PET can quantify intraplaque macrophage-mediated inflammation but has a relatively poor spatial and tissue resolution. Therefore, combining PET with high-resolution MRI allows us to accurately assess the vulnerability

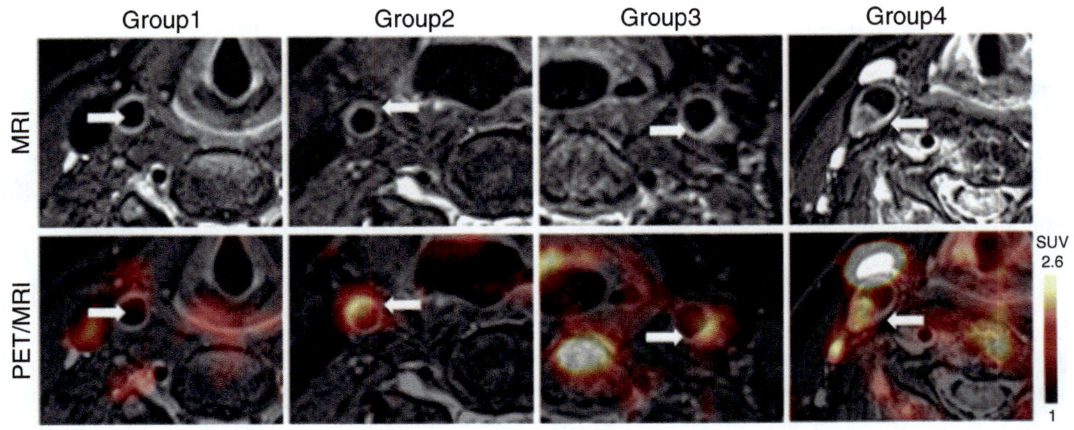

Fig. 12.23 ^{68}Ga-pentixafor PET/MR of carotid plaques with different lesions. Transverse MRI of carotid artery (**a**). Transverse integrated PET/MR of carotid artery (**b**). Focal ^{68}Ga-pentixafor uptake can be observed in a mildly atherosclerotic carotid artery with slightly eccentric thickening. Significant ^{68}Ga-pentixafor can be observed in a moderately atherosclerotic carotid artery with significant eccentric thickening. No increased uptake is observed in a non-significantly eccentric control carotid artery (arrows indicate arterial regions of interest)

of carotid plaques. Integrated PET/MR allows the simultaneous acquisition of MRI and PET within a single scan session, ensuring the precise co-registration between the two sets of images. Therefore, it can be utilized for the qualitative and quantitative analysis of carotid intraplaque inflammation, while also providing information on plaque morphological structure and inflammatory cell metabolism, thereby achieving a more accurate assessment of plaque stability. This technique, therefore, holds great value for the early warning and effective prevention of ischemic stroke in clinical practice.

Suggested Reading

Baskin A, Buchegger F, Seimbille Y, et al. PET molecular imaging of hypoxia in ischemic stroke: an update. Curr Vasc Pharmacol. 2015;13(2):209–17.

Calcagno C, Ramachandran S, Izquierdo-Garcia D, et al. The complementary roles of dynamic contrast-enhanced MRI and ^{18}F-fluorodeoxyglucose PET/ CT for imaging of carotid atherosclerosis. Eur J Nucl Med Mol Imaging. 2013;40(12):1884–93.

Carter AR, Astafiev SV, Lang CE, et al. Resting interhemispheric functional magnetic resonance imaging connectivity predicts performance after stroke. Ann Neurol. 2010;67(3):365–75.

Cui C, Cui C, Ma Y, et al. Characteristics of cerebral blood flow and glucose metabolism in patients with different severities of cerebrovascular stenosis evaluated by one-day PET cerebral blood flow and metabolism combined imaging. J Clin Exp Med. 2020;19(4):427–30.

Cui C, Ma Y, Wang M, et al. Preliminary research on the impairment characteristics of cerebral metabolism and blood flow in patients with severe cerebrovascular stenosis. Int J Radiat Med Nucl Med. 2014;3:141–7.

Cui B, Zhang T, Ma Y, et al. Simultaneous PET-MRI imaging of cerebral blood flow and glucose metabolism in the symptomatic unilateral internal carotid artery/middle cerebral artery steno-occlusive disease. Eur J Nucl Med Mol Imaging. 2019a;47(7):1668–77.

Cui B, Zhang M, Ma J, et al. Integrated ^{18}F-FDG PET/ MRI evaluation of ischemic cerebrovascular disease. Chin J Med Imaging Tech. 2019b;35(12):1817–22.

Evans NR, Tarkin JM, Buscombe JR, et al. PET imaging of the neurovascular interface in cerebrovascular disease. Nat Rev. Neurol. 2017;13(11):676–88.

Golestani AM, Tymchuk S, Demchuk A, et al. Longitudinal evaluation of resting-state fMRI after acute stroke with hemiparesis. Neurorehabil Neural Repair. 2013;27(2):153–63.

Heiss WD. Radionuclide imaging in ischemic stroke. J Nucl Med. 2014;55(11):1831–41.

Heiss W, Zaro WO. Validation of MRI determination of the penumbra by PET measurements in ischemic stroke. J Nucl Med. 2017;58(2):187–93.

Hyafil F, Schindler A, Sepp D, et al. High-risk plaque features can be detected in non-stenotic carotid plaques of patients with ischaemic stroke classified as cryptogenic using combined ^{18}F-FDG PET/MR imaging. Eur J Nucl Med Mol I. 2016;43(2):270–9.

Kao H, Lin M, Wu W, et al. Improvement of cerebral glucose metabolism in symptomatic patients with carotid artery stenosis after stenting. Clin Nucl Med. 2015;40(9):701–7.

Kircher M, Tran-Gia J, Kemmer L, et al. Imaging inflammation in atherosclerosis with CXCR4-directed ^{68}Ga-pentixafor PET/CT: correlation with ^{18}F-FDG PET/CT. J Nucl Med. 2020;61(5):751–6.

Li X, Heber D, Gonzalez JC, et al. Association between osteogenesis and inflammation during the progression of calcified plaque evaluated by ^{18}F-Fluoride and ^{18}F-FDG. J Nucl Med. 2017;58(6):968–74.

Li X, Heber D, Rausch I, et al. Quantitative assessment of atherosclerotic plaques on ^{18}F-FDG PET/MRI: comparison with a PET/CT hybrid system. Eur J Nucl Med Mol Imaging. 2016;43(8):1503–12.

Li X, Yu W, Wollenweber T, et al. ^{68}Ga-pentixafor PET/MR imaging of chemokine receptor 4 expression in the human carotid artery. Eur J Nucl Med Mol Imaging. 2019;46(8):1616–25.

Lu J, Liu H, Zhang M, et al. Focal pontine lesions provide evidence that intrinsic functional connectivity reflects polysynaptic anatomical pathways. J Neurosci. 2011;31(42):15065–71.

Lyu JH, Ma N, Liebeskind D, et al. Arterial spin labeling MRI estimation of antegrade and collateral flow in unilateral middle cerebral artery stenosis. Stroke. 2016;47(2):428–33.

Mateo J, Izquierdo-Garcia D, Badimon J, et al. Noninvasive assessment of hypoxia in rabbit advanced atherosclerosis using ^{18}F-fluoromisonidazole positron emission tomographic imaging. Circ Cardiovasc Imaging. 2014;7(2):312–20.

Mirasol RV, Bokkers RP, Hernandez DA, et al. Assessing reperfusion with whole-brain arterial spin labeling:a noninvasive alternative to gadolinium. Stroke. 2014;45(2):456–61.

Mueller S, Wang D, Fox MD, et al. Individual variability in functional connectivity architecture of the human brain. Neuron. 2013;77(3):586–95.

Okazawa H, Higashino Y, Tsujikawa T, et al. Noninvasive method for measurement of cerebral blood flow using O-15 water PET/MRI with ASL correlation. Eur J Radiol. 2018;105:102–9.

Park CH, Chang WH, Ohn SH, et al. Longitudinal changes of resting-state functional connectivity during motor recovery after stroke. Stroke. 2011;42(5):1357–62.

Powers WJ, Clarke WR, Grubb RL, et al. Extracranial-intracranial bypass surgery for stroke prevention in hemodynamic cerebral ischemia. JAMA. 2011;306(18):1983–92.

Puig O, Henriksen OM, Vestergaard MB, et al. Comparison of simultaneous arterial spin labeling MRI and ^{15}O-H_2O PET measurements of regional cerebral blood flow in rest and altered perfusion states. J Cereb Blood Flow Metab. 2020;40(8):1621–33.

Quality Management and Safety Management Group of the Chinese Society of Radiology, Magnetic Resonance Group of the Chinese Society of Radiology. Expert consensus on the standardized application of arterial spin labelling cerebral perfusion MRI. Chin J Radiol. 2016;50(11):817–24.

Reynolds MR, Derdeyn CP, Grubb RL, et al. Extracranial-intracranial bypass for ischemic cerebrovascular disease: what have we learned from the Carotid Occlusion Surgery Study? Neurosurg Focus. 2014;36(1):E9.

Rudd JH, Warburton EA, Fryer TD, et al. Imaging atherosclerotic plaque inflammation with [18F]-Fluorodeoxyglucose positron emission tomography. Circulation. 2002;105(23):2708–11.

Saba L, Anzidei M, Marincola BC, et al. Imaging of the carotid artery vulnerable plaque. Cardiovasc Inter Rad. 2014;37(3):572–85.

Sebok M, Van Niftrik CHB, Piccirelli M, et al. BOLD cerebrovascular reactivity as a novel marker for crossed cerebellar diaschisis. Neurology. 2018;91(14):e1328–37.

Shen K, Hutchison RM, Bezgin G, et al. Network structure shapes spontaneous functional connectivity dynamics. J Neurosci. 2015;35(14):5579–88.

Small SL, Hlustik P, Noll DC, et al. Cerebellar hemispheric activation ipsilateral to the paretic hand correlates with functional recovery after stroke. Brain. 2002;125(7):1544–57.

Su Y, Arbelaez AM, Benzinger TL, et al. Noninvasive estimation of the arterial input function in positron emission tomography imaging of cerebral blood flow. J Cereb Blood Flow Metab. 2012;33(1):115–21.

Su Y, Vlassenko AG, Couture LE, et al. Quantitative hemodynamic PET imaging using image-derived arterial input function and a PET/MR hybrid scanner. J Cereb Blood Flow Metab. 2017;37(4):1435–46.

Su Y, Wang H, Liang Z, et al. Evaluation of cerebrovascular reserve in patients with unilateral internal carotid artery or middle cerebral artery stenosis: A study on ^{13}N-Ammonia PET/CT cerebral perfusion imaging combined with methazolamide challenge. Chin J Rehabil Theory Pract. 2016;22(11):1304–9.

Van Golen LW, Kuijer JPA, Huisman MC, et al. Quantification of cerebral blood flow in healthy volunteers and type 1 diabetic patients: comparison of MRI arterial spin labeling and [^{15}O]H_2O positron emission tomography(PET). J Magn Reson Imaging. 2014;40(6):1300–9.

Vesey AT, Jenkins W, Forsythe R, et al. 18F-Fluoride and 18F-Fluorodeoxy- glucose positron emission tomography after transient ischemic attack or minor ischemic stroke: case-control study. J Am Coll Cardiol. 2016;67(13):1616.

Walberer M, Backes H, Rueger MA, et al. Potential of early [^{18}F]-2-Fluoro2-Deoxy-D-Glucose positron emission tomography for identifying hypoperfusion and predicting fate of tissue in a rat embolic stroke model. Stroke. 2012;43(1):193–8.

Wang M, Ma Y, Ji X, et al. Imaging characteristics and patterns of simultaneous cerebral metabolism and cerebral blood flow imaging in ischemic cerebrovascular disease. J Capital Med Univ. 2013;34(1):43–8.

Wang J, Yang Z, Zhang M, et al. Disrupted functional connectivity and activity in the white matter of the sen-

sorimotor system in patients with pontine strokes. J Magn Reson Imaging. 2019;49(2):478–86.
Wang L, Yu C, Chen H, et al. Dynamic functional reorganization of the motor execution network after stroke. Brain. 2010;133(Pt 4):1224–38.
Xu HJ, Qin W, Chen H, et al. Contribution of the resting-state functional connectivity of the contralesional primary sensorimotor cortex to motor recovery after subcortical stroke. PLoS One. 2014;9(1): e84729.
Yin L, Cheng S, Xiao J, et al. 3D pseudocontinuous arterial spin-labeling perfusion imaging detected crossed cerebellar diaschisis in acute, subacute and chronic intracerebral hemorrhage. Clin Imaging. 2018;50:37–42.
Yu Z, Shi X, Zhou Z, et al. Cerebral glucose metabolism changes in chronic ischemia patients following subcranial-intracranial bypass. Neurosurg Rev. 2020;43(5):1383–9.
Zaro-Weber O, Moeller-Hartmann W, Siegmund D, et al. MRI-based mismatch detection in acute ischemic stroke: optimal PWI maps and thresholds validated with PET. J Cereb Blood Flow Metab. 2017;37(9):3176–83.
Zhang M, Lu J, Jiao L, et al. Proton magnetic resonance spectroscopy in patients with symptomatic unilateral internal carotid artery/middle cerebral artery stenosis or occlusion. J Magn Reson Imaging. 2011;34(4):910–6.

Research Applications of Positron Emission Tomography/Magnetic Resonance (PET/MR) Imaging in Traumatic Brain Injury (TBI)

13

Feng Xiong, Yizhen Pan, Chuxin Huang, Lijun Bai, and Jun Liu

Traumatic brain injury (TBI) refers to changes in the local anatomical and pathological structures of the head caused by trauma, often from an external physical force such as impact or an external blow to the head and exposure to shock waves in war, subsequently leading to further impairments in brain function. The changes in brain function can present as the loss or decrease of consciousness, alterations in mental state, incomplete memory of events after the injury, and neurological impairments. Under normal circumstances, patients with TBI are generally classified as mild, moderate, or severe, based on the initial Glasgow Coma Scale (GCS) score documented in the emergency department, the duration of the loss of consciousness, and the duration of post-traumatic amnesia (i.e., memory loss after the injury). Age groups at high risk for TBI mainly include children aged 4 years or younger, adolescents aged 15–19 years, and older adults aged over 65 years. Approximately 30% of patients with TBI suffer from persistent post-traumatic neurological and psychiatric disorders and are unable to revert to normal levels, severely affecting their quality of life. Falls account for about 38% of TBIs and occur primarily in children and older adults. It is estimated that mild TBIs (mTBIs) account for 80–90% of all TBI cases, the high incidence and prevalence of which have resulted in an immense economic and social burden.

TBIs can further be classified as primary or secondary, and the neuropathological and microvascular changes related to primary TBI include white matter hemorrhage, neuronal degeneration, epidural/subdural hematoma, venous hyperemia, and enlarged perivascular spaces. One of the most common injuries is traumatic axonal injury (TAI), also known as diffuse axonal injury (DAI), which is caused by the stretching of axons. TAIs frequently occur at gray-white matter interfaces, the cerebral cortex, the corpus callosum (CC), and the brainstem, all of which have been verified through postmortem studies as common sites for injury. Patients with TAI/DAI typically undergo anterograde/retrograde axonal degeneration and fragmentation within a few months after the initial injury, which in some cases last for several years. The axonal degeneration and fragmentation can subsequently give rise to neurocognitive and behavioral impairments. Secondary injury is due to the cellular destruction induced by the ini-

F. Xiong · Y. Pan · L. Bai (✉)
The Key Laboratory of Biomedical Information Engineering, Ministry of Education, Department of Biomedical Engineering, School of Life Science and Technology, Xi'an Jiaotong University, Xi'an, Shaanxi, China
e-mail: bailijun@xjtu.edu.cn

C. Huang · J. Liu
Department of Radiology, The Second Xiangya Hospital of Central South University, Changsha, Hunan, China
e-mail: junliu123@csu.edu.cn

J. Lu, G. Zhao (eds.), *PET/MR: Functional and Molecular Imaging of Neurological Diseases and Neurosciences*, https://doi.org/10.1007/978-981-19-9902-4_13

tial trauma and is related to the overlapping effects of post-traumatic stress disorder (PTSD) on cerebral metabolism, cerebral blood flow (CBF) changes, ion homeostasis, and other factors.

With the advances in imaging technology over the last few decades, we have gained a deeper understanding on the pathophysiology of TBI. Structural and functional imaging made possible by various modalities and techniques is suitable for visualizing the hemodynamic and metabolic changes in the brain, while also aiding in the evaluation of primary injuries and prevention of further deterioration, thereby providing more treatment options for TBI patients. Conventional imaging techniques are relatively poor predictors of the prognostic symptoms of TBI (especially mTBI). Therefore, basic research on the development of MRI-based techniques for the accurate diagnosis and prognostic identification of TBI has gradually garnered the interest of the international medical community. In fact, a review article entitled "CT scan does not predict outcome of mild traumatic brain injury" published in *Nature Reviews Neurology* in 2012 stated that "of the 1,292 patients with mTBI, 97% did not show relevant or suspected pathological findings according to CT scan…CT scans are poor predictors of clinical outcome following mild TBI." The review also highlighted the fact that the local injury status detected by conventional computed tomography (CT) and MRI in patients with TBI has a relatively poor predictive ability for clinical symptoms, while the techniques for analyzing the covariation of structural and functional characteristics in TBI are particularly underdeveloped. At present, MRI-based TBI research is focused on brain structural and functional studies involving the mechanisms of brain damage and related neuropsychological symptoms, primarily utilizing techniques such as functional MRI (fMRI), three-dimensional T_1 weighted imaging (3D-T_1WI), diffusion tensor imaging (DTI), and susceptibility weighted imaging (SWI).

13.1 Research Applications of MRI in TBI

MRI is the preferred imaging modality for visualizing the subacute and chronic phases of TBI. However, its limitations in evaluating skull fractures and allowing patient monitoring, relatively long scan times, and sensitivity to head motion have hindered the utilization of MRI in the acute phase of TBI. Nevertheless, MRI is more sensitive than CT in detecting DAIs and non-hemorrhagic contusions, particularly in the frontal and temporal lobes, as well as small subdural hematomas and brain stem injuries. In approximately $^1/_3$ of patients with mild-to-moderate TBI, MRI reveals focal atrophy of the frontal and temporal regions during the chronic phase, which can predict the patient's prognosis. In addition to whole-brain atrophy, the number, size, and depth of the lesions are also associated with the level of consciousness and prognosis. MRI scans have shown that lesion resolution was accompanied by improved neuropsychological test results. However, approximately 15% of patients with normal MRI findings still had a poor prognosis and were unable to return to work. Therefore, given the inconsistency between lesion manifestation and patient prognosis, it is of crucial significance that appropriate MRI sequences are obtained. The advantages of multiparametric MRI have provided new possibilities for the detection of different injury sites and methods. For many years, T_1- and T_2-weighted spin-echo and fluid-attenuated inversion recovery (FLAIR) sequences have been the most commonly used MRI sequences in the evaluation of head injuries. Compared to the T_1-weighted spin-echo sequence, the T_2-weighted spin-echo sequence is more sensitive for detecting contusions. In terms of the evaluation of traumatic lesions, FLAIR has comparable or better sensitivity than the T_2-weighted spin-echo sequence. During the acute phase of TBI, FLAIR can be used to detect DAI and edema; during the subacute and chronic phases, FLAIR is primarily utilized in the detection of gliosis. The T_2*-

weighted gradient-echo sequence can display the hemosiderin deposits caused by hemorrhage and is superior to T_1- and T_2-weighted imaging in the detection of TBI. A study on patients with varying severities of TBI found that the clinical outcome was correlated with the number of lesions detected by the T_2*-weighted gradient-echo sequence, but not with T_2-weighted imaging. In patients with mTBIs, MRI abnormalities detected within 72 h were associated with neuropsychological impairments but not with the time taken to return to work or the occurrence of post-concussion sequelae. SWI is a recently developed MRI technique with a high sensitivity to hemosiderin and may, in fact, be more sensitive than conventional MRI sequences at detecting hemorrhagic lesions. In general, MRI is the preferred method for detecting abnormalities during the subacute and chronic phases of TBI, provided that the appropriate MRI sequence has been selected.

13.1.1 DTI Findings in TBI

DTI is a relatively new MRI technique that allows the visualization of the white matter tracts of the central nervous system (CNS). By measuring the degree and direction of diffusion in the water molecules, DTI can be used to observe the major pathological changes in TBI-related axonal injuries. The diffusion of water molecules within bodily tissues is influenced by their structural environment, and the greatest diffusion in white matter tracts can be observed along the direction parallel to the myelin sheaths. The two parameters measured using DTI, mean diffusivity (MD) and fractional anisotropy (FA), are both indicators of axonal integrity. Therefore, DTI can be utilized to reconstruct color maps reflecting the direction of diffusion, which show the location and direction of major white matter tracts in the CNS. In patients with mTBI, DTI performed during the acute phase of TBI revealed reduced white matter FA, primarily in the CC and internal capsule, which is likely the result of axonal injury. In fact, this injury pattern can still be observed a few days to a few years after the initial injury (Fig. 13.1). Furthermore, the extent of abnormal diffusion is also associated with the GCS score, while a decrease in FA is related to the presence of cognitive dysfunction more than one year after the initial injury. The results regarding changes in TBIs as visualized on DTI have, thus far, remained inconsistent, which may be due to the different pathophysiological processes involved. In patients with chronic TBIs, however, the increased diffusion in extensive cortical regions was found to be positively associated with learning and memory. In general, structural techniques, such as conventional CT and structural MRI (sMRI), can be used to describe primary TBIs. The information acquired through CT scans is most suitable for detecting lesions in the early stages of the injury, whereas MRI techniques are more useful during the recovery stage. Nevertheless, the negative predictive value of conventional CT and MRI is limited,

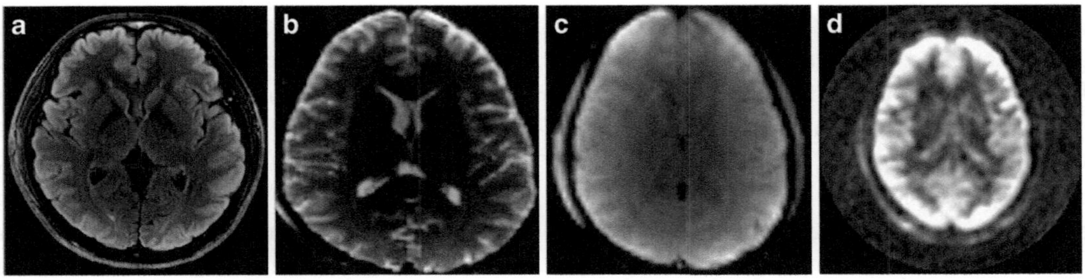

Fig. 13.1 MRI findings in patients with mTBIs. Transverse T_2-weighted FLAIR MRI (**a**); DTI (**b**); BOLD imaging (**c**); ASL imaging (**d**)

indicating that the absence of abnormalities does not guarantee the most ideal outcome. Newer MRI techniques, such as DTI, have promising prospects for utilization in TBI. Since diffusion-based imaging methods are indirectly dependent on the energy state of the imaged cells, these techniques can also provide information on secondary injury. Furthermore, given that conventional structural CT and MRI are unable to show the functional changes of the brain, fMRI techniques may be more valuable in predicting the cognitive changes and prognosis of patients with mTBIs, which can facilitate the implementation of clinical treatment plans.

13.1.2 fMRI Findings in TBI

fMRI is a functional neuroimaging technique based on MRI, which involves the detection of changes in blood flow in order to measure the relevant brain activity. fMRI is a non-invasive MRI technique, and the majority of existing fMRI studies are based on the utilization of the blood-oxygen-level-dependent (BOLD) method to T_2*-weighted imaging. Deoxyhemoglobin and oxyhemoglobin have different magnetic properties, that is, deoxyhemoglobin is paramagnetic whereas oxyhemoglobin in diamagnetic. Therefore, changes in the relative proportions of the two will cause temporary changes in the MR signals of the target area relative to surrounding tissues. During specific tasks or in the resting state, changes in the regional blood flow of the corresponding cortical areas will give rise to changes in cerebral microcirculatory blood flow, which affects the amount of oxygen consumption, leading therefore to regional changes in the ratio of deoxyhemoglobin to oxyhemoglobin. fMRI has excellent value in clinical practice, as it combines the anatomical precision of MRI with functional information, in turn enabling the mapping of brain areas activated by specific language or cognitive tasks, improving our understanding of neuropsychological dysfunction. At present, the primary aim of standardized fMRI is to evaluate and visualize the areas of the brain involved in cognition and behaviors.

Studies on the different levels of TBI have demonstrated the presence of changes in brain activity, suggesting that post-TBI in neural network alterations may mediate cognitive control and may be an indirect consequence of DAI. Compared to healthy controls, patients with DAI alone showed the compensatory activation of brain function in the prefrontal cortex (PFC). A research team led by McAllister performed fMRI to study the working memory of patients with mild-to-moderate TBI and found significant differences in the activation patterns of working memory circuits between TBI patients and healthy controls within one month, and even more than one year, after the original injury. Under a moderate working memory load, patients showed significantly higher activations in the parietal and prefrontal lobes than healthy controls. Task-based fMRI showed no significant difference between TBI patients and healthy controls, suggesting that following TBI, impairment-related changes in the regulation of working memory may be the basis for the cognitive impairment symptoms related to working memory. A study on athletes with mTBIs found that mTBI patients had lower task-related activation in the right PFC. However, another study involving football players demonstrated that in the absence of impaired neurobehavioral performance, concussed players had significant increases in the amplitude and extent of brain activation during a finger sequencing task performed under fMRI, and these increases were primarily observed in the parietal, lateral frontal, and cerebellar regions. In summary, fMRI is an effective imaging technique for the evaluation of cognitive function during the subacute and chronic phases of TBI. The advantage of fMRI is that the same patient can undergo multiple scans within a short period of time without exposure to ionizing radiation. Therefore, this technique has the potential for broad research and clinical applications, while its unique features have facilitated baseline measurements of neurological function in prospective research.

13.1.3 Research Applications of Multimodal MRI on the Mechanisms of mTBI

Based on the current epidemiological status of and imaging studies involving mTBIs, we can see that mTBI has garnered growing interest in the international medical community, but there remain numerous challenges in its clinical diagnosis and treatment. First, the majority of mTBI patients "appear" to be fully recovered, but early clinical examinations have revealed that patients with persistent symptoms or neuropsychological impairments still experience certain difficulties. Second, the traditional methods for evaluating TBIs are primarily aimed at patients with more serious TBIs (i.e., moderate-to-severe TBIs) and are therefore not sufficiently sensitive to evaluate the subtle cognitive changes and behavioral sequelae that are most commonly caused by mTBIs. Third, the long-term consequences of many brain injuries resulting from mTBIs may only manifest several months to several years after the initial injury. For example, mTBIs in the preschool years may alter the developmental potential of the brain, eventually leading to drug abuse, emotional disorders, and behavioral disorders during adolescence. In short, there is a major clinical need for the early detection and diagnosis of mTBIs, as well as the evaluation of individual differences among mTBI patients, so as to implement an effective treatment regimen.

According to current research, using multimodal imaging techniques to investigate the mechanisms underlying the structural and functional covariation of mTBIs are more useful for exploring the post-traumatic changes of cognitive function in patients with mTBI, thereby providing more effective detection methods for clinical treatment. Unlike patients with moderate-to-severe TBIs, mTBI patients may exhibit clear hematoma, edema, or contusion in CT images, and their pathological characteristics are often manifested as DAI. DAIs are caused by the sudden acceleration, deceleration, or rotational distortion of the brain, resulting in large shearing forces that give rise to the diffuse injury of white matter tracts. Studies have found that white matter tracts connecting the different functional areas of the brain are relatively long and curved, which makes them more susceptible to the impact of blunt forces. Compared to the clear presence of intracranial edema and contusion on imaging findings, DAIs may be more closely related to post-TBI sequelae and neuropsychological symptoms, leading to impairments in higher-order cognitive functions. Therefore, the accurate determination of the severity and extent of DAIs is of crucial significance for the timely implementation of interventional measures, prediction of the patient's prognosis, and evaluation of therapeutic efficacy in mTBIs.

Given the complex pathogenic mechanisms of mTBI and the diversity of its clinical symptoms, it is difficult to diagnose mTBI-specific neurological dysfunctions using a single imaging technique. Therefore, some researchers have proposed that the combination of two or more imaging modalities can serve as effective markers for studying the mechanisms and achieving the accurate diagnosis of mTBIs. To that end, most of the systematic studies on mTBIs thus far have utilized multimodal imaging techniques.

13.1.3.1 Modulatory Effects of the Catechol-O-Methyltransferase (*COMT*) Gene on the Functional Brain Networks of mTBI Patients

Sharp et al. discovered that among the subdivisions of the striatum (i.e., the caudate nucleus, putamen, and nucleus accumbens), patients with TBIs only showed a significant reduction in the functional connectivity between the caudate nucleus and the rest of the brain, accompanied by varying degrees of damage to the white matter tracts connecting the caudate nucleus and the PFC. These findings indicate that the caudate nucleus is a key area targeted by the TBI-related disruptions in the functional networks of the brain. Furthermore, the neural projections from the striatum to the frontal lobe form one of the main dopaminergic pathways in the brain, and the effect of dopamine on cognitive function is widely acknowledged. COMT is an enzyme that degrades dopamine and is widely distributed in the frontal lobe. The rs4680 single-nucleotide polymorphism of the *COMT* gene causes the *Val* allele to be replaced by the *Met* allele. The resulting *Met/Met* genotype causes poor thermal stability and lower enzymatic activity (only $^1/_3$ that of the *Val/Val* genotype), leading individuals with the *Met/Met* genotype to exhibit a higher content of dopamine in the frontal lobe. These observations have led to speculations of a non-linear relationship between dopamine content and cognitive function in patients with mTBIs.

One study reported the use of BOLD-fMRI data to calculate the whole-brain voxel-wise functional connectivity with the caudate nucleus, in order to explore the impact of mTBIs on the functional networks, using the caudate nucleus as the seed region (Fig. 13.2). The same study also compared whether functional network changes caused by mTBIs were modulated by the *COMT* genes and/or accompanied by corresponding changes in cognitive function. The results of the aforementioned study demonstrated that the modulatory effects of the *COMT* gene on the mTBI-related functional networks were primarily concentrated in the frontal regions of the brain, including the middle frontal gyrus and orbitofrontal cortex, and that they evolved over time. The structural and functional connections between the caudate nucleus and frontal cortex constitute an important conduction pathway for dopamine, while the frontal cortex plays an important role in regulating the cognitive functions of patients with mTBIs. Based on non-parametric permutation testing, the differences in resting-state functional networks of the brain were compared between healthy controls and patients with mTBIs and revealed that mTBI patients had significantly less functional connectivity of the four subdivisions of the caudate nucleus than healthy controls. Furthermore, these differential brain areas were primarily located in the frontal lobe and included the orbitofrontal cortex (BA11), superior frontal gyrus (BA8), inferior frontal gyrus (BA44), and middle frontal gyrus (BA9), while differential brain areas of the right ventral caudate nucleus also included the anterior cingulate cortex (BA32) (Fig. 13.3). The modulatory effects of the *COMT* gene on the functional connectivity between the caudate nucleus and the frontal lobe had a direct impact on the recovery of cognitive dysfunction in mTBI patients. Research has shown that mTBI patients carrying the *Met* gene experienced persistent cognitive impairments (i.e., slower information processing speed), whereas patients with the *Val/Val* genotype showed some recovery in cognitive function. These findings further demonstrate the heterogeneity of the presentation of injuries in mTBI patients, while also providing support for the in-depth exploration of the pathogenic mechanisms of mTBI and its interventional treatments.

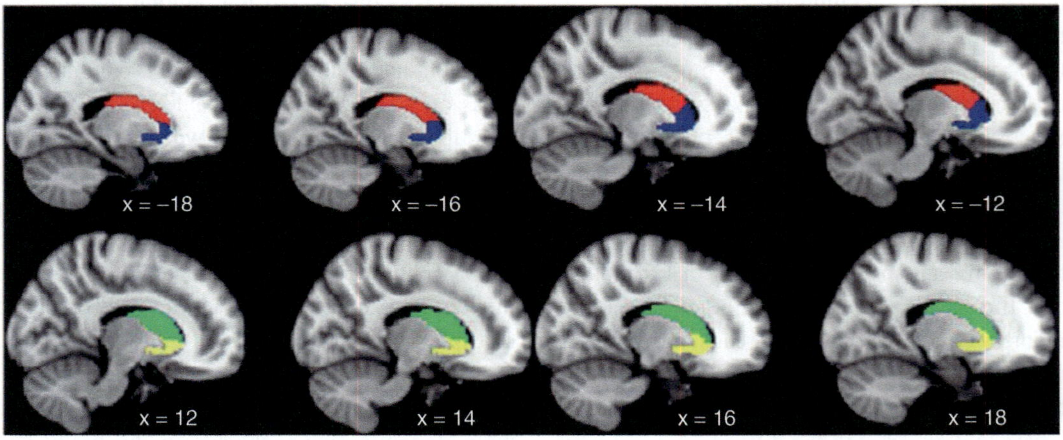

Fig. 13.2 Four subregions of the caudate nucleus

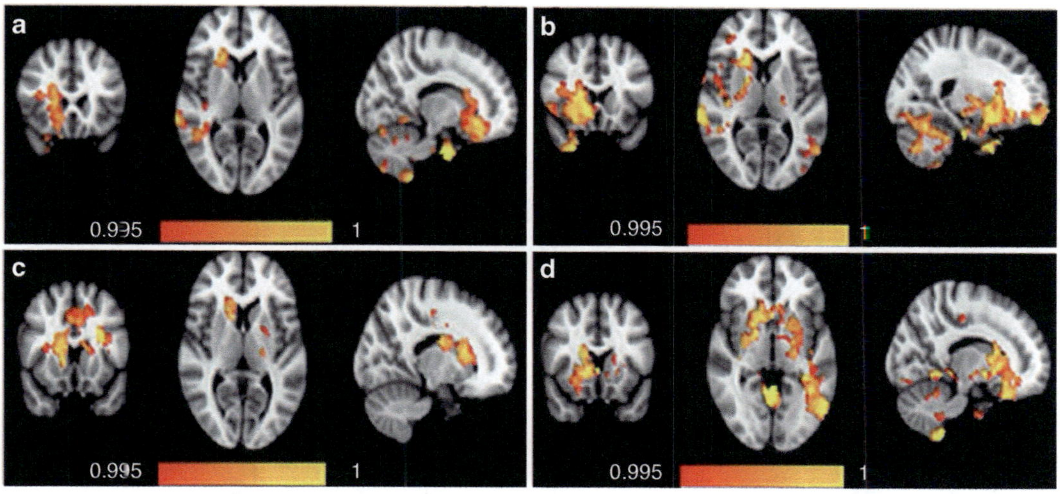

Fig. 13.3 Reduced functional connectivity in patients with mTBIs. Reduced mTBI functional network activated by the left ventral caudate nucleus (**a**); reduced mTBI functional network activated by the left dorsal caudate nucleus (**b**); reduced mTBI functional network activated by the right ventral caudate nucleus (**c**); and reduced mTBI functional network activated by the right dorsal caudate nucleus (**d**)

13.1.3.2 Modulatory Effects of the Bone-Derived Neurotrophic Factor (*BDNF*) Gene on Cortical Thickness in mTBI Patients

BDNF is a neurotrophic factor that can promote the growth, proliferation, and differentiation of neurons. It exerts a regulatory effect on the morphological structure of the cerebral cortex, including the hypothalamus and other brain nuclei, and plays an important role in learning, memory, and emotional regulation. Mutations of the *BDNF* gene can lead to reductions in activity-dependent BDNF levels, causing a susceptibility to neurodegenerative diseases. Liguori et al. discovered, in a study on multiple sclerosis, that patients carrying the *Met* allele showed a significantly lower volume of cerebral gray matter and a higher risk of developing global gray matter atrophy. Moreover, when performing an episodic memory task, *Met* carriers showed significantly stronger functional connectivity between the hippocampus and the posterior cingulate cortex (PCC). BDNF is abundantly expressed in the frontal and temporal lobes, including the hippocampus, where it functions to regulate cortical plasticity. These regions, in turn, play a crucial role in fear extinction and, as such, are key targets for treating PTSD and other emotional disorders. Studies have found that patients with PTSD symptoms have significantly lower levels of serum BDNF, while the formation and extinction of fear memories in PTSD patients are associated with BDNF levels. Therefore, researchers have combined sMRI data with *BDNF* polymorphisms to examine the structural damage of the brain caused by mTBIs and further explore the modulatory effects of the *BDNF* gene on the structural damage of the brain and the PTSD severity of mTBI patients. The aforementioned study confirmed that mTBI is a potential factor for triggering PTSD and that the PTSD symptoms of mTBI patients changed over time (Fig. 13.4). By utilizing linear mixed models and other methods of analysis, that study also showed that the modulatory effects of *BDNF* on regional cortical thickness in mTBI patients were primarily found in the frontal lobe cingulate gyrus and occipital lobe (Fig. 13.5). In addition to the above, extensive connections can also be found between the frontal cortex and the limbic system (e.g., amygdala, hippocampus, etc.), which are key targets in the process of fear extinction learning. The PCC serves to integrate visual cognition and emotional process and exerts regulatory effects on negative emotions. Given that the core symptoms of PTSD

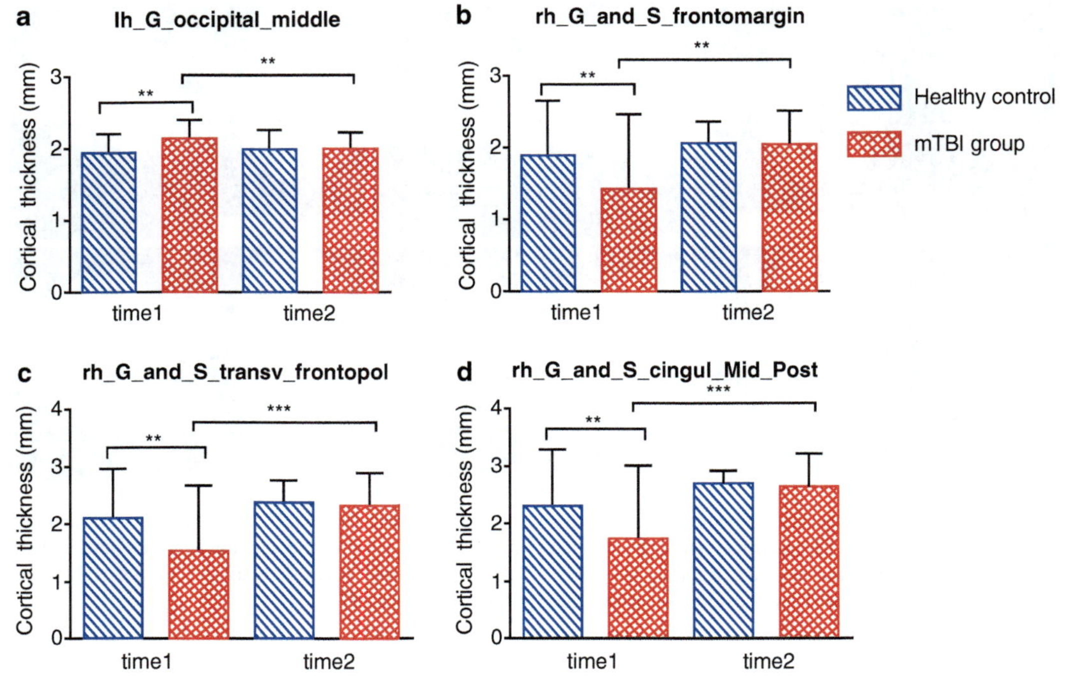

Fig. 13.4 Changes in the cortical thickness of *Met* allele carriers. Effect of the *Met* allele on the thickness of the middle occipital gyrus (**a**); effect of the *Met* allele on the thickness of the fronto-limbic cortex (**b**); effect of the *Met* allele on the thickness of the frontal pole cortex (**c**); and effect of the *Met* allele on the thickness of the middle and posterior cingulate cortex (**d**)

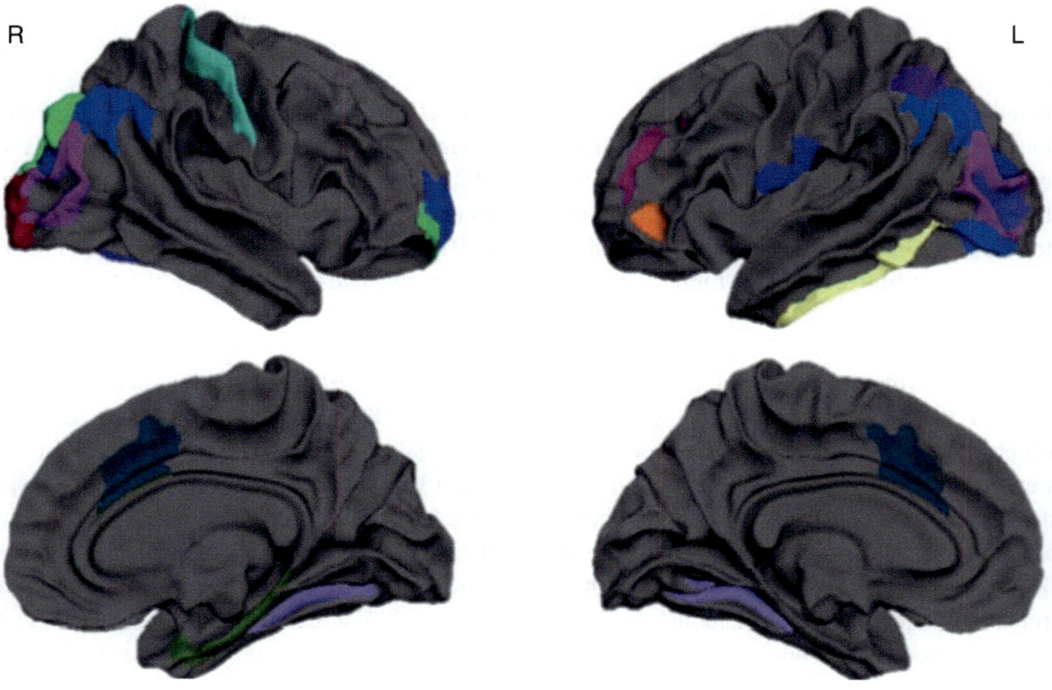

Fig. 13.5 Changes in the cortical thickness of mTBI patients

are all directly related to fear, changes in the morphological structure of the frontal lobe and cingulate gyrus lead to disruptions in intrinsic functional connectivity, which in turn lead to an imbalance in emotional control strategies, therefore resulting in an inability to cope with the fear stimuli produced by PTSD. Furthermore, a study on mTBI patients carrying the *Met* allele found that PTSD symptoms continued to persist 3 to 6 months after the initial injury, and patients with a thinner PCC thickness at the initial stages of the injury showed more severe PTSD symptoms. These findings demonstrate that the *BDNF* gene exerts regulatory effects on the changes in the PTSD symptoms of mTBI patients. Therefore, it can serve as a biomarker and be combined with imaging techniques to identify effective treatment plans for mTBI patients with PTSD symptoms.

13.1.3.3 Automatic Diagnosis of mTBI Subtypes Based on Machine Learning

mTBIs can lead to persistent cognitive impairments and significant PTSD symptoms in TBI patients. However, the early diagnosis of mTBI patients with persistent cognitive impairments or those who may later develop chronic PTSD is extremely difficult to achieve using traditional imaging techniques. Furthermore, the heterogeneity and variability of mTBI presents a challenge to the management and interventional treatment of patients. The combination of machine learning and MRI techniques for diagnosis and classification has been applied to research on a variety of neurodegenerative diseases, such as attention deficit hyperactivity disorder, Alzheimer's disease (AD), and Parkinson's disease (PD). At present, research involving the application of machine learning to TBI classification has been limited to feature extraction to discriminate between TBI patients and healthy subjects, and few studies have examined the classification of patients with different pathological subtypes of TBI.

One study combined DTI with machine learning algorithms to develop an objective and accurate automatic diagnosis and classification method for mTBI subtypes, so as to provide technological support for the early clinical diagnosis of patients with different mTBI subtypes. In the aforementioned study, the FA value (which can characterize the microstructural damage of white matter tracts) was utilized as a classification feature, leave-one-subject-out validation was performed to train the support vector machine (SVM) classification model, and permutation testing was implemented 5000 times to test the performance of this classifier. The SVM-based diagnosis and classification was divided into four steps: feature extraction, feature selection, classification training and testing, and classifier performance evaluation. The results of this study indicated that this diagnosis and classification model could objectively and effectively discriminate mTBI patients with different prognoses (Fig. 13.6), with an accuracy of up to 84%. The results of permutation testing were $P < 0.001$, which indicate that this model is markedly superior to random empirical distribution and was statistically significant. Therefore, this study has provided the scientific basis for a clinical classification and diagnosis method for mTBI patients and demonstrated to some extent that FA and other imaging parameters can serve as imaging biomarkers for mTBIs.

13.1.4 Structural-Functional Coupling of the Brain in TBI-Induced Cognitive Aging Impairments

TBIs often result in damage to long-range white matter connections, generally appearing as white matter hyperintensities (WMHs) in early conventional MRI scans. Studies have shown that WHMs may be caused by damage to white matter tracts and the rupture of microvessels. In addition, TBIs can lead to deficits in interhemispheric integrity, especially in the CC. According to DTI studies, the decrease in FA reflects the damage to the CC microstructure post-TBI. The special role of the CC in the structural connectivity between the cerebral hemispheres, as well as the correspondence of anatomical structures between the

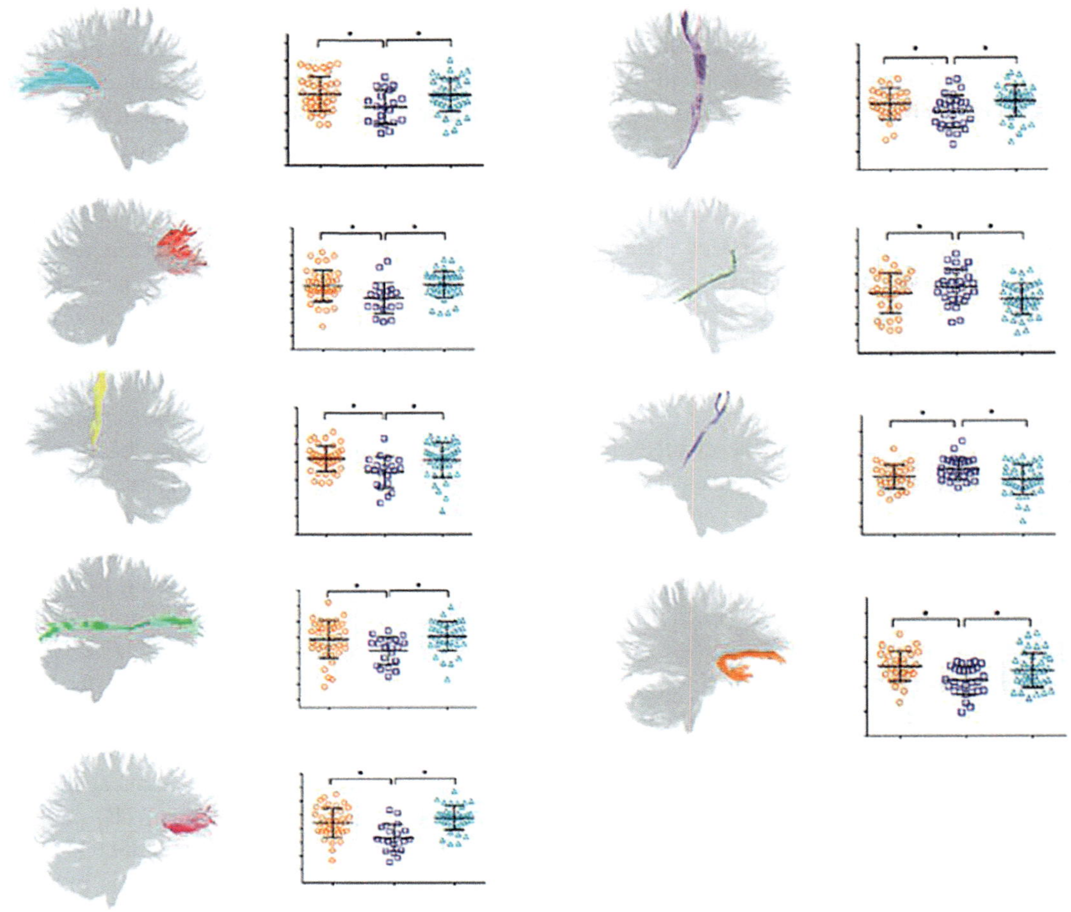

Fig. 13.6 Combination of early DTI with SVM classifiers for the identification of deficits in information processing speed among mTBI patients 6–12 months post-injury (Reproduced with permission from BAI LJ, BAI GH, WANG S, et al. Strategic white matter injury associated with long-term information processing speed deficits in mild traumatic brain injury. *Human Brain Mapping*, 2020, 41(15):4431–4441). Diffusion values of the thalamus-superior frontal gyrus tract, anterior thalamic radiation, cingulum bundle, uncinate fasciculus, and genu of the corpus callosum can be used to implement the effective, early determination of whether a specific cognitive impairment, i.e., deficits in information processing speed, will occur in patients 6–12 months post-injury, and therefore serve as a feasible method for the identification of high-risk groups

fiber bundles projecting from different CC subregions to different functional regions of the cerebral cortex, has made it feasible to more precisely examine the impact of mTBI-induced CC injuries on cognitive function. This approach can be used to analyze the covariation characteristics of structural damage in different CC subregions and the functional connectivity of the corresponding areas of the brain.

According to reports, CC structural connectivity may play a decisive role in the stability of interhemispheric voxel-mirrored homotopic connectivity (VMHC). However, there is a certain level of heterogeneity in the results produced by different models, which may be due to limitations of research on the covariation mechanisms of structure and function after mTBI, thereby preventing a convergent conclusion at the systems level from a pathological perspective. Furthermore, as the largest bundle of commissural fibers between the two hemispheres, the CC plays a critical role in cognitive function, and the loss of its structural integrity contributes directly to the decline in executive function.

The specificity of CC abnormalities to mTBIs, as well as the impact of such abnormalities on interhemispheric functional connectivity and cognitive function, implies that the CC plays an important coordinating role in these processes. Moreover, extensive and persistent changes are observed following WMH regression, which suggests that the core area of damage in white matter tracts caused by white matter injuries may be located in the CC.

One year after the initial injury, the loss of integrity in different CC regions showed significant persistence and time-dependent regional specificity. The extent of the injury began from CC zone II within 14 days of the injury (T-1), then spread to CC zones I, II, VI, and V at 3 months (T-2), and finally to all CC subregions (zones I–V) at 6–12 months (T-3) (Fig. 13.7). Furthermore, the regions with changes in interhemispheric structural connectivity caused by damage to the CC corresponded to the regions with changes in interhemispheric functional connectivity. The decrease in the interhemispheric functional connectivity of the dorsolateral PFC (DLPFC) also led to impaired executive function in mTBI patients. The CC promotes the interhemispheric transmission of information, and as such, the multiple areas of the bilateral cerebral hemispheres connected via the five different subregions of the CC can affect recovery from mTBIs (Fig. 13.8). Therefore, as demonstrated by previous studies, mTBI is a concept involving widespread brain network disturbances.

The extensive and persistent differences exhibited by CC fiber bundles before and after WMH regression suggest that the damage to the microstructure of CC white matter fibers might be caused by the WMHs. Therefore, the CC may be core area of microstructural damage affected by WMHs in mTBIs. One study found that as the FA values decreased, CC zone II was the first to sustain damage. This area is generally located in the anterior part of the CC trunk and differs with respect to the locations of CC injury reported by

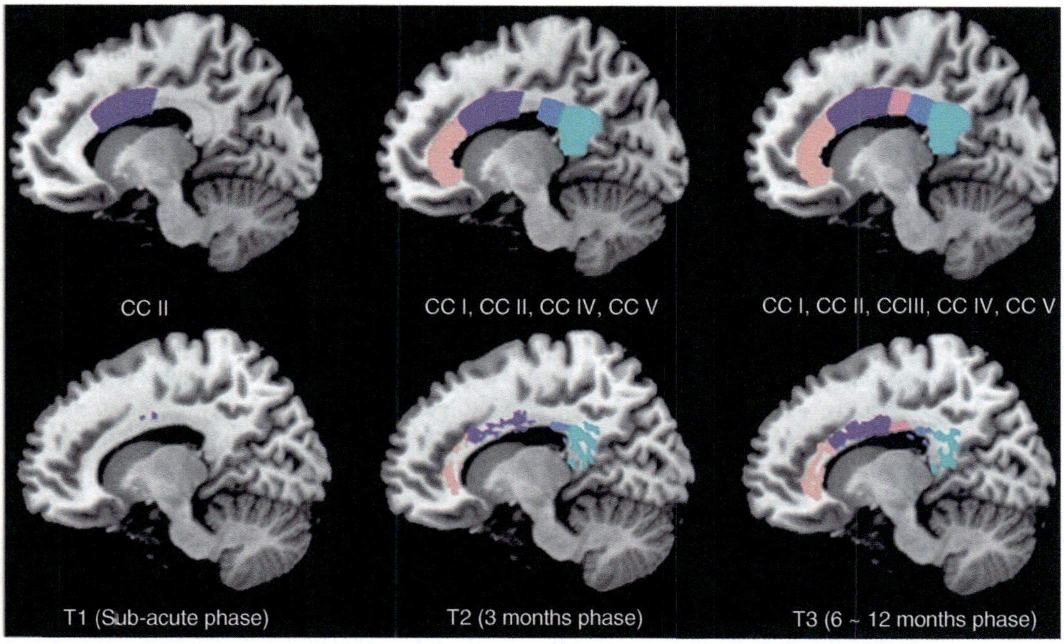

Fig. 13.7 Loss of integrity at different CC subregions within one year after TBI. A general linear model and Bonferroni correction were performed to compare the damage in the subregions of the corpus callosum (CC) between different mTBI phases and healthy controls. The adjusted *P*-value is <0.01. The sites of injury in the CC subregions during the subacute and follow-up phases (first row) show a spatial correspondence with the statistical maps of FA reductions based on between-group comparisons (second row). Injury first occurred in CC zone II (T-1); then in CC zones I, II, IV, and V (T-2); and finally, in all five subregions (zones I-V) (T-3)

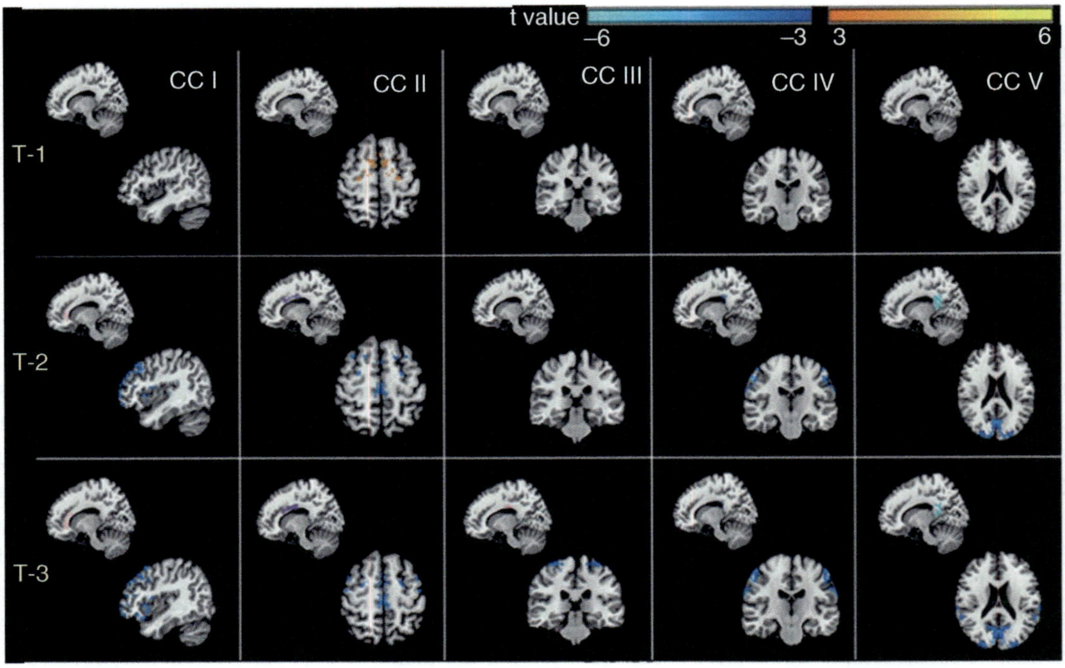

Fig. 13.8 Spatial correspondence between diffusion index (FA value) reductions and changes in voxel-mirrored homotopic connectivity (VMHC). The color bar represents the statistical map of significant t-values for the comparison of voxel-mirrored homotopic connectivity (VMHC) between mTBI patients and healthy controls. Multiple comparisons correction was performed with a cluster size >160 mm^3, and the significance level was $P < 0.05$. The subregions of the corpus callosum corresponding to FA reductions are shown in the coronal and axial images in the different columns (from subacute to follow-up phases). The image in the upper left is the left cerebral hemisphere. Subacute phase (T-1); 3 months post-injury (T-2); and 6–12 months post-injury (T-3)

previous studies in the subacute phase, which were in the body and genu of the CC. Other studies have also found a significant increase in the FA values of the CC genu during the subacute phase (within 21 days). Possible reasons contributing to this controversy may include the following: (1) differences in sample sizes; (2) differences in injury time, mainly with respect to the time between the injury and first MRI scan; (3) differences in injury type, as some studies included sports-related concussions and did not exclude mTBI patients based on whether abnormalities were present in conventional imaging scans; and (4) differences in techniques of DTI analysis, as among these studies, the measurement area of the CC was typically located in the mid-sagittal plane, and the CC is generally divided into three or five subregions. In sum, these differences may partially explain the variability of the research findings.

The clinical symptoms of mTBIs can continue to appear for a few months after injury and may even persist for a year or longer, with some neuropsychological tests showing no signs of improvement. These findings suggest that recovery from mTBIs is a non-linear process, and some patients may require a longer time to attain complete recovery, which is different from other reports indicating that cognitive symptoms can be alleviated within three months. One possible explanation for this discrepancy is that among the subgroups of mTBI patients, there may be some patients whose clinical symptoms may never fully recover. In view of the central role played by the CC, a major transhemispheric white matter tract, in the coordination of cognitive functions, a recent study explored the relationship between CC atrophy and cognitive impairment in PD. They found that the volume loss in multiple segments of the CC was different between most cognitively impaired subjects (dementia patients) and cognitively intact subjects. Therefore, an expansion in the extent of post-mTBI CC damage may be a risk factor for neurodegenerative diseases such as PD and AD.

Interhemispheric communication is an important organizing principle of the human brain and reflects the individual differences in the process of brain development. Given the role of the CC in coordinating interhemispheric functional connectivity, and the effects of CC morphology on interhemispheric functional connectivity, special attention should be paid to CC damage induced by mTBI. A recent study on the interhemispheric structural and functional connectivity of patients with amyotrophic lateral sclerosis showed that impairments to CC-mediated interhemispheric neuronal communication may promote changes in interhemispheric functional connectivity.

Research has shown that athletes with sports-related concussions showed a stronger regional homogeneity (ReHo) in the supplementary motor area (SMA) during the subacute phase of the injury than healthy athletes. Another study was the first to demonstrate that even in injuries with rapid neuropsychological changes, performing VMHC within 14 days of the initial injury to analyze interhemispheric functional connectivity also revealed enhanced functional connectivity. A recent study found that acute stress can cause the brain to enter a state that promotes rapid defense mechanisms, which in turn can induce the enhancement of intra-network functional connectivity, including relevant areas of the temporal lobe. This enhanced functional connectivity is only attained seven days post-injury but did not persist beyond four weeks post-injury. Some researchers believe that this "pruning" may signify the initial physiological response of reorganization, triggering synaptic strengthening through co-activation inputs, thereby giving rise to extensive enhancements in functional connectivity. The expansion of CC structural damage in mTBIs may alter the connectivity of the corresponding functional projection areas, thereby affecting cognitive function.

Studies have shown that at 7 or 28 months (mean value) after injury, impairments can be observed in the functional connectivity of the PFC, premotor area/SMA, and temporo-parieto-occipital association area. Furthermore, a decline in the VMHC of the primary motor cortex was observed after 6–12 months (T-3). Patients with mTBIs generally exhibit impairments in memory, information processing speed, and attention. Therefore, the decrease in VMHC of motor-related cortical areas may further signify multi-system damage 6 months or more after the initial injury. One study has provided strong evidence that the early diagnosis of motor-related dysfunctions in PD can mitigate the burden of injury in mTBIs. In addition to this, among the large-scale functional networks corresponding to the functional projection areas of the CC, persistent impairments have been observed in the functional connectivity of the PFC (the core region of the brain's default mode network) in mTBIs.

There are several limitations to currently available research. First, the human brain is not completely symmetrical, whereas the assumptions of VMHC analysis are based on a symmetrical standard template. Second, although some studies have found that impairments in interhemispheric transcallosal structural connectivity corresponded well with regions exhibiting alterations in interhemispheric functional connectivity, there was no significant correlation between interhemispheric functional connectivity (VMHC) and structural connectivity (FA values of different CC subregions). This discrepancy may have stemmed from the different spatial resolutions of the fMRI (voxel-based) and DTI (region of interest-based) analyses.

13.2 Research Applications of PET Imaging in TBI

TBI is a major cause of death and disability, encompassing penetrative (when objects breach the skull and dura mater, directly damaging the brain parenchyma) and closed injuries (when the skull and dura mater remain intact), and can be clinically classified according to severity as mild, moderate, or severe. mTBI, which is more common, is generally caused by blunt, nonpenetrative head trauma. Patients often present with mild symptoms, which generally need to be correlated with their medical history to reach a clinical diagnosis. There are currently no fully validated imaging or humoral biomarkers to determine the presence of nerve damage in patients with mTBIs. Moderate-to-severe TBIs can cause axonal stretching and shearing or DAI. Therefore, non-invasive imaging techniques are of crucial significance to the evaluation of severity and prognosis. Current imaging studies are focused on the different severities of TBIs, some of which are based on structural and functional MRI, whereas others have adopted PET imaging to target the metabolic changes involved.

PET is a powerful molecular imaging modality that can help us to understand normal and abnormal brain functions at the molecular level. It involves the use of radiopharmaceuticals to measure the various metabolic processes of the brain. These radiotracers emit positrons, which undergo radioactive decay and subsequently collide with electrons in the surrounding tissue to produce two photons. The PET scanner can detect these photons, or gamma (γ)-rays, in order to reconstruct images of the spatial density of the functional activities and metabolic processes within the brain. As targeted radiotracers display similar biological behaviors to the corresponding natural elements of their compounds in the body, they can participate in normal or abnormal metabolic processes in vivo, thereby reflecting the biological processes of the relevant metabolic substrates. Therefore, different radiotracers can be utilized to explore the pathophysiological manifestations of different diseases. At present, a number of studies have been conducted on PET findings in TBI. Different metabolic changes over the course of different diseases have been uncovered through medical imaging, which can improve our judgment concerning the clinical significance of different imaging findings, while also providing guidance for clinical diagnosis, treatment, and prognosis. In this section, we will describe PET studies on TBI involving various radiotracers.

13.2.1 ^{18}F-FDG Pet

Glucose metabolism is the primary source of energy in cells. Through the use of ^{18}F-labelled fluorodeoxyglucose (FDG) PET, it is possible to measure the glucose uptake and metabolism of different areas of the brain. ^{18}F-FDG is currently the most widely-used PET imaging agent, with extensive clinical applications in diseases of the brain, cardiovascular system, and malignant tumors, among others. For example, PET imaging has revealed abnormal ^{18}F-FDG uptake in the brain in neurodegenerative diseases (including AD) and mental disorders (including schizophrenia and bipolar disorder), as well as a reduced cerebral metabolic rate of glucose (CMRGlc) during the loss of consciousness.

According to PET studies on TBIs, a largely consistent trend of metabolic changes in the brain can be observed across different studies in moderate-to-severe TBIs. During the acute phase, a general increase in glucose metabolism can be detected across all brain regions, which is followed by a long-term decrease in metabolism from the subacute-to-chronic phases. In contrast, the ^{18}F-FDG PET evaluation of metabolism in mTBIs is fraught with inconsistencies (Fig. 13.9). A few studies have found decreased glucose metabolism in the frontal and temporal lobes during task execution, whereas other studies have revealed both increases and decreases in symptom-related metabolic activity. Similarly, there are controversies regarding the evaluation of glucose uptake during the resting state, with some studies detecting alterations in the frontal and temporal lobes, and others detecting no significant differences. These inconsistencies could be attributed to the inherent heterogeneity of the mTBI patient population, as well as discrepancies in analysis methods. Therefore, further investigations are needed to determine the role of ^{18}F-FDG PET in TBIs more clearly, particularly mTBIs.

The neurological manifestations of chronic severe TBIs include severe motor dysfunction, sensory disturbances, and disorders of consciousness. Therefore, assessing the longitudinal

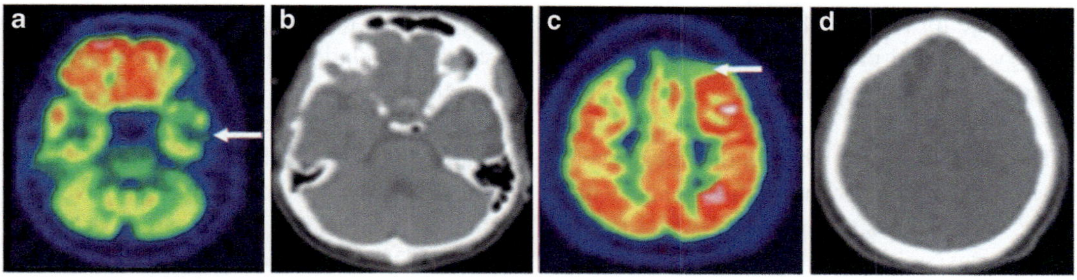

Fig. 13.9 ^{18}F-FDG PET/CT images of patients with TBIs. A 25-year-old male patient with a moderate TBI who underwent an ^{18}F-FDG PET/CT scan 5 months after his initial injury: transverse ^{18}F-FDG PET shows decreased metabolism of the left temporal lobe (**a**, arrow), accompanied by mild brain volume reduction and cerebral softening (**b**). A 28-year-old male patient with a severe TBI who underwent an ^{18}F-FDG PET/CT scan 12.5 months after his initial injury: transverse ^{18}F-FDG PET shows significantly decreased metabolism of the left frontal lobe (**c**, arrow), accompanied by significant cerebral softening (**d**)

changes of brain metabolism is critical to guiding and supporting rehabilitation and prognosis. ^{18}F-FDG PET/CT can facilitate the evaluation of brain metabolism and its changes over time in patients with severe TBIs. In an ^{18}F-FDG PET/CT study involving 45 patients with chronic severe TBIs, changes in cerebral glucose metabolism were observed, while the increase in ^{18}F-FDG uptake over time was associated with higher levels of arousal and increased heart volumes. During the course of long-term follow-up, the increase in ^{18}F-FDG uptake was found to be related to the discontinuation of anticonvulsants, as well as improvements in verbal expression, postural changes, and communication abilities. Improvements in verbal expression, in particular, could significantly increase brain glucose metabolism, which is the result of neurorehabilitation in the chronic phase. Some studies recommend that patients with a TBI or lowered level of consciousness should undergo additional resting-state ^{18}F-FDG PET scans and single venous sample testing, in order to combine radioactive uptake in the brain with plasma tracer concentrations for analysis, followed by a comprehensive analysis and quantification of CMRGlc.

Based on the data discussed above, we can see that ^{18}F-FDG PET imaging is not only useful for the evaluation of brain metabolic activity and pathophysiological mechanisms in TBI patients but can also provide guidance for their longitudinal recovery and prognostic evaluation.

13.2.2 Tau and Beta-Amyloid (Aβ) PET

The aggravation of TBI severity can lead to higher incidences of dementia and disability, and some patients may develop chronic traumatic encephalopathy (CTE), which is often closely related to clinical symptoms such as cognitive impairment. Current research shows that TBI is linked to an increased risk of and is considered a major risk factor for dementia. mTBIs result in a higher risk of dementia among older adults, whereas moderate-to-severe TBIs are associated with an elevated risk of dementia across all age groups. A meta-analysis of 15 case–control studies revealed that head injuries can increase the risk of AD. Furthermore, some studies have suggested that the occurrence of TBI can directly trigger the aggregation of tau protein and Aβ, which are involved in the pathophysiological processes of AD, while diffuse Aβ plaques have been observed in some young patients with severe TBIs. Similar results have also been obtained in animal experiments. Therefore, tau and Aβ are considered biomarkers of TBIs.

Tau protein is ubiquitous in the brains of healthy adults and is an abundant microtubule-associated protein that is harmless when bound normally with microtubules. Under normal conditions, tau is a fundamental substance for maintaining neuronal integrity and axoplasmic transport. It can promote the assembly and maintenance of microtubules, which in turn are responsible for intracellular transport, axon morphology, and cell physiology. The normal functioning of tau depends on the balance, phosphorylation state, and structural integrity of different tau isoforms, whereas the imbalance of these states may lead to tau dysfunction, in which tau no longer binds to microtubules, but instead accumulates as insoluble neurofibrillary tangles within the CNS. These tangles ultimately lead to neurodegeneration, including the appearance of CTE following TBIs.

Post-TBI TAI is one potential mechanism for the production of Aβ. A large number of Aβ plaques are formed in damaged axons, while the enzymes necessary for the cleavage of amyloid precursor protein to form Aβ can accumulate at the site of TAI. One study found that Aβ aggregates can be observed in the brains of patients with both moderate-to-severe TBI and AD. Furthermore, Aβ aggregation was found in approximately $^1/_3$ of patients who died acutely post-TBI, while the same proportion of patients who survived at least a year post-TBI also showed Aβ aggregation.

In recent years, the development of novel PET tracers, such as tau and Aβ ligands, have received attention in the research of TBIs. As TBIs are closely associated with tau and Aβ, PET bioligand tracers that can bind with increased aggregations of tau and Aβ have been developed, thereby quantitatively detecting the amount of tau and Aβ deposition in different regions of the brain. AD patients generally exhibit a 50–70% higher Aβ detection rate in cortical regions than elderly controls. At the one-year follow-up of young and middle-aged patients with moderate-to-severe TBI, higher Aβ deposition was observed in the cortical gray matter and striatum than that in controls. Another study found that at 11 months to 17 years post-TBI, patients with severe TBI showed increased accumulations of ^{11}C-Pittsburgh compound B (^{11}C-PiB, an Aβ ligand tracer) in the precuneus, PCC, and cerebellum. In order to explore the possible link between TBI and AD, some studies have performed Aβ PET imaging on patients with moderate-to-severe TBI, AD patients, and healthy controls, in order to compare the deposition status of Aβ in different brain regions. Taken together, these studies have demonstrated the relationship between TBI and AD to a certain extent.

At present, a wide range of PET tracers with binding affinity and selectivity for intracerebral tau and Aβ deposition have been developed, including ^{11}C-PiB, ^{18}F-Florbetapir, ^{11}C-PBB3, and ^{18}F-FDDNP. However, only some studies have utilized these tracers in the investigation of TBIs or CTE, and further validation is needed with respect to their basic and clinical mechanisms. Therefore, PET imaging studies on the detection of tau and Aβ deposition in patients with TBIs or suspected CTE, as well as the analysis of the relationship between tau and Aβ deposition with clinical symptoms, stages, and prognosis, will remain important research directions in the future.

13.2.3 $CuCl_2$ PET

Copper (Cu) is a trace element necessary for cell proliferation and wound repair, and some studies have found that increased Cu uptake may serve as a biomarker for TBIs. A wide range of positron-emitting Cu isotopes can be used for PET imaging of Cu metabolism, including ^{60}Cu, ^{61}Cu, ^{62}Cu, and ^{64}Cu. Of these, the physical half-life of the ^{64}Cu radionuclide is 12.7 h, which can facilitate the transport of ^{64}Cu radiopharmaceuticals from the production site to remote imaging equipment. Currently, a number of PET studies involving the evaluation of Cu metabolism have utilized $^{64}CuCl_2$ as a radiotracer for non-invasive evaluation based on PET/CT imaging. The physiological transport of ^{64}Cu through the blood-brain barrier is mediated by human copper transporter 1 or other copper transporters. Its radiation dose in humans is similar to that of ^{18}F-FDG, and its cytotoxicity is minimal. Therefore, it has previously been used in studies on Cu metabolism in both healthy subjects and patients with Wilson's disease.

In an animal experiment involving the use of C57BL/6 mice to establish mouse models of TBI through controlled cortical impact, PET/CT imaging was performed 24 h after intravenous injection of the $^{64}CuCl_2$ tracer. Higher regional ^{64}Cu uptake was observed in the injured cortical tissues than in the contralateral cortical tissues of TBI mice and the corresponding cortical regions of non-TBI mice. Therefore, it is believed that $CuCl_2$ can be used as a tracer to detect increased ^{64}Cu uptake in injured brain tissues, which may serve as a novel PET/CT biomarker for the non-invasive evaluation of TBIs. The increased uptake of ^{64}Cu in injured brain tissue may have resulted from the joint effects of increased Cu uptake by activated microglial cells, Cu/Zn superoxide dismutase, and other Cu transporters or concomitants. Given the potential differences in the injury response to Cu between rodents and humans, further clinical studies are still needed, whereas the current data from preclinical studies can serve as a reference for future clinical studies on the use of $^{64}CuCl_2$ as a PET/CT tracer for the non-invasive evaluation of TBIs in humans.

13.3 Research Applications of PET/MR in TBI

Several patients with TBI develop brain dysfunction, and continuous improvements have been achieved in the imaging methods for detecting and assessing brain damage. There is a heterogeneity between MRI and PET findings, and TBI patients may exhibit concordant or discordant findings between the two modalities. For example, TBI patients may have concordant MRI and ^{18}F-FDG PET findings in the frontal and temporal regions but not in other areas of the brain. Furthermore, some patients may suffer from severe brain dysfunction but may not exhibit abnormalities on MRI. Therefore, the combination of PET and MRI enables the integrated analysis of the results from the two imaging modalities, maximizing the mutual complementarity of their respective advantages.

An increasing number of recent studies are combining functional PET imaging with structural and functional MRI. With respect to TBI research, the combination of these two imaging modalities can be used to determine the effects of post-TBI inflammation and glial changes. Furthermore, multimodal imaging is playing an increasingly important role in guiding the diagnosis, treatment, and prognosis of diseases. In the previous section, we primarily focused on the different types and principles of PET tracers. In this section, we will continue the discussion along with examples of studies that have combined PET and MRI in different situations.

13.3.1 Combination of ^{18}F-FDG PET and MR-DWI in the Evaluation of TBI

^{18}F-FDG PET, MRI, and histological evaluation were performed on adult male Sprague–Dawley rat models of TBI established through controlled cortical impact. T_2-weighted imaging (T_2WI) of the rat TBI model showed increased signal intensities in the CC, hippocampus, and amygdala at different time points post-injury; the decrease in apparent diffusion coefficient (ADC) signals of the hippocampus and amygdala during the subacute phase indicates cytotoxic edema, whereas the increase in ADC signals of the CC indicates vasogenic edema. Unlike the MRI findings, the relative uptake curve of ^{18}F-FDG showed different results in these three regions of the brain: in the subacute phase, the CC showed a significant increase in ^{18}F-FDG uptake, the amygdala showed a significant decrease, and the hippocampus did not show any significant change. The hippocampus, however, was the only region with significant changes during the acute and chronic phases. These results imply that a relatively "focal" injury from a controlled cortical impact can also cause global changes in the brain. The combination of ^{18}F-FDG PET with T_2WI and DWI can be used to assess glial changes after inflammation and injury. By labelling astrocytes and microglial cells through histological methods, it was found that their ^{18}F-FDG uptake peaked or increased significantly at the same time, showing good agreement. Neuronal dysfunction can lead to a decrease in ^{18}F-FDG uptake, whereas the activation of astrocytes and microglial cells can cause an increase. Therefore, if responses are present in both cell types (neurons and glial cells), their effects will "cancel" each other out, causing ^{18}F-FDG uptake to approach baseline levels. In general, glial activation and cell damage during ^{18}F-FDG PET imaging affect the uptake of ^{18}F-FDG. Therefore, the combined application of ^{18}F-FDG and MRI can help improve our understanding of the complex changes that occur following TBIs.

In the assessment of brain injury among patients with TBIs, it is also possible to combine ^{18}F-FDG PET with MRI to analyze the changes in brain dysfunctions. In a study on patients with severe TBI, ^{18}F-FDG PET imaging was combined with DWI to explore the relationship between functional changes and structural damage of the brain. The results revealed the presence of a functional-structural relationship between the functional metabolism of the inferior parietal lobe, precuneus, and frontal lobe with the structural integrity of the frontal-inferior parietal, precuneus-inferior parietal, thalamic-hypothalamic, and thalamic-prefrontal tracts.

13.3.2 Combination of ^{11}C-PiB PET and DTI in the Evaluation of TBI

As mentioned in the previous section, PET can be used to achieve the in vivo localization of Aβ. ^{11}C-PiB is an Aβ ligand tracer, and images of its binding potential can reflect the density of Aβ plaques. Research has shown that the distribution of ^{11}C-PiB in the brains of AD patients is consistent with the distribution of Aβ plaques found in neuropathological studies, showing an initial increase in the precuneus/PCC, frontal cortex, and caudate nucleus, followed by increases in the lateral temporal and parietal cortices.

In TBI patients, the resulting axonal injury may trigger the production and pathological aggregation of Aβ. The biomechanical effects of torsion and shear stress on white matter tracts can cause axonal injury, which leads to an increase in Aβ production and its aggregation in the acute phase of the injury. The pathological effects of damage to axons and their encapsulating myelin sheaths can still be observed several years after the injury, especially in long-range white matter tracts. ^{11}C-PiB PET can be utilized to reveal the white matter integrity and anisotropy of TBI patients. Post-TBI ^{11}C-PiB binding is related to white matter damage and time after injury, while the degree of white matter damage is also associated with ^{11}C-PiB binding in the PCC of TBI patients. The white matter may act as both the source of Aβ production and the channel of Aβ spreading. In the PCC, the correlation between axonal injury and the pathological elevation of Aβ may reflect the role of this region as a highly-connected cortical center that has integrated the spreading of damage from injured white matter tracts. The time after injury is also correlated with ^{11}C-PiB binding, suggesting the presence of a neurodegenerative process.

By combining ^{11}C-PiB PET with DTI, researchers have attempted to verify the Aβ pathology of long-term TBI survivors without dementia, as well as the relationship of Aβ pathology after moderate-to-severe TBI with the number and distribution of axonal injuries. Patients with moderate-to-severe TBIs at 11 months to 7 years post-injury were enrolled in one study. The patients underwent ^{11}C-PiB PET, sMRI, and DTI (which can be used to evaluate the degree of post-TBI axonal injury), as well as relevant neuropsychological assessments. Age-matched healthy controls and AD patients were also enrolled for PET and sMRI. Comparisons between TBI patients and healthy elderly controls revealed increases in the ^{11}C-PiB binding potential post-TBI, which were most prominent in the precuneus/PCC and cerebellum, while the increase in the ^{11}C-PiB binding of regional gray matter was found to be correlated with the FA decrease in the cingulum bundle, which is directly connected to the PCC. These findings indicate that Aβ pathology of the PCC is associated with the degree of axonal injury in patients with TBI (Fig. 13.10).

TBIs may increase the incidence rates of various types of dementia, and these patients usually experience a gradual exacerbation in clinical degenerative symptoms post-TBI. Regarding whether this clinical presentation is related to the TBI, researchers have observed through in vivo

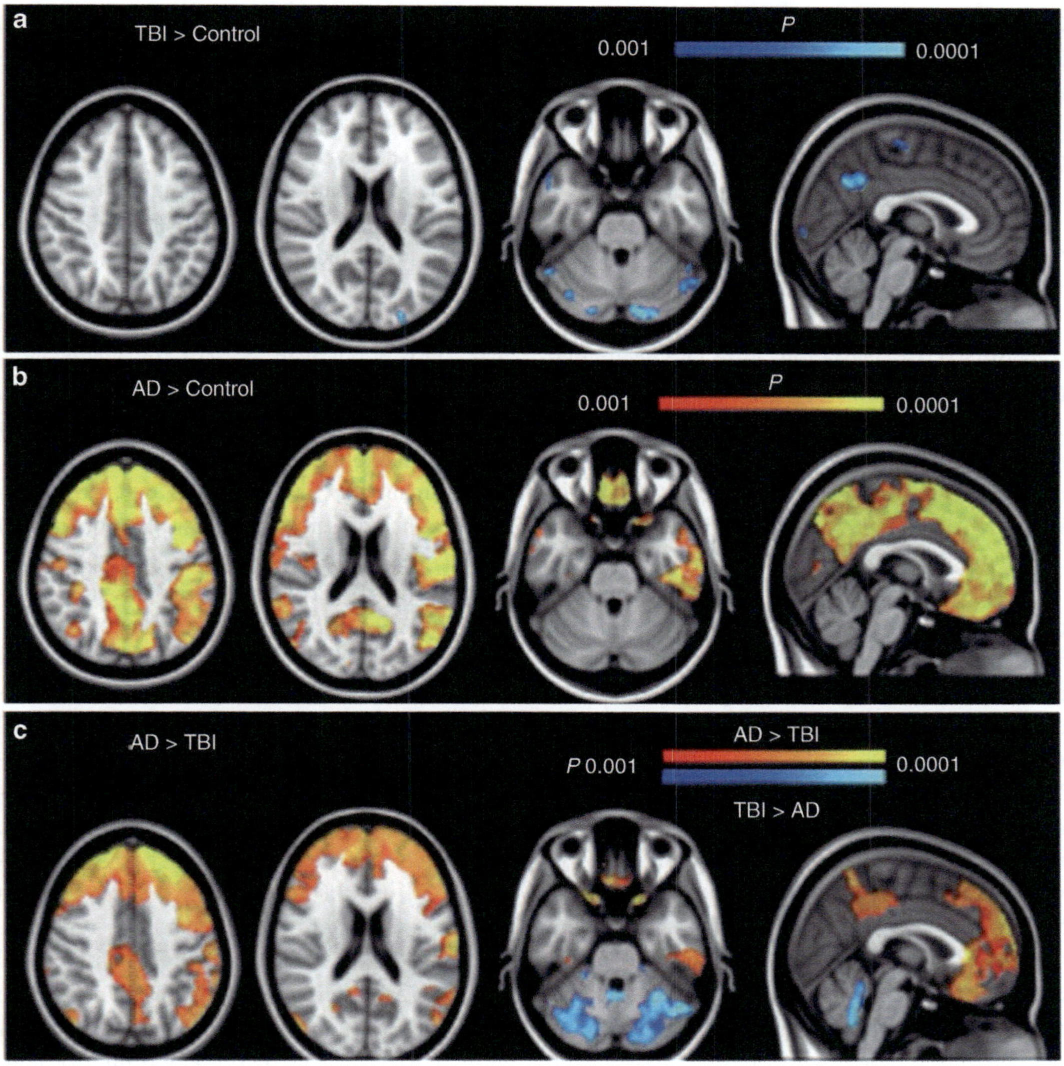

Fig. 13.10 Differences in ^{11}C-PiB binding potential among TBI patients, AD patients, and healthy elderly controls. Compared to healthy elderly controls, TBI patients showed significantly elevated ^{11}C-PiB binding potential in the blue-light blue regions (**a**). Compared to healthy controls, AD patients showed significantly elevated ^{11}C-PiB binding potential in the red-yellow regions (**b**). Compared to AD patients, TBI patients showed significantly elevated ^{11}C-PiB binding in the light blue regions, and compared to TBI patients, AD patients showed significantly elevated ^{11}C-PiB binding potential in the red-yellow regions (**c**). Control: control group

studies that long-term TBI survivors had increased ^{11}C-PiB binding, which showed an overlapping distribution with AD patients, but also involved the cerebellum. These findings indicate that performing Aβ imaging of chronic TBIs may help us understand the development of neurodegenerative diseases in long-term TBI survivors. Furthermore, elucidating the relationship between cortical ^{11}C-PiB and white matter damage in connective tracts also signifies the presence of a link between axonal injury and Aβ pathology.

Studies based on ^{11}C-PiB PET imaging have found that unlike AD, post-TBI Aβ pathology is triggered by a different set of mechanisms, which may be related to the pathology of Aβ plaques in

CTE. Overall, the results of these studies suggest that ^{11}C-PiB binding, white matter structure, age, and injury time are interrelated, but more longitudinal studies are needed to verify their causal relationships.

13.3.3 Evaluation of TBI under Discordant PET and sMRI Data

Repetitive TBIs, caused by mild and accumulative brain damage, is a type of degenerative disease that occurs in patients with a history of multiple concussions or head injuries. Boxers have consistently been the most frequently studied patient group, as they may undergo thousands of concussions over the course of their careers.

DTI and magnetic resonance spectroscopy (MRS) are commonly used to detect axonal injury or potential chemical changes in TBI patients. However, these imaging methods cannot clearly elucidate the mechanisms underlying repetitive TBIs. ^{18}F-FMZ PET can be used to reflect brain metabolic function and neuronal integrity. ^{18}F-FMZ is a neutral antagonist showing selective, reversible binding and high affinity with the central benzodiazepine receptor (BZR) binding site of the gamma-aminobutyric acid type A ($GABA_A$) receptor. The $GABA_A$ receptor is abundantly distributed in the cortex and reflects neuronal density and integrity. The benzodiazepine binding site on $GABA_A$ has previously been used as a marker of neuronal viability. The binding potential of ^{18}F-FMZ can serve as a sensitive marker of neuronal viability, receptor density, and binding affinity. Previous imaging studies on the binding potential of ^{18}F-FMZ have shown that the selective loss of injured neurons could still be detected, even in the presence of normal MRI findings. TBI patients with metabolic abnormalities exhibit certain symptoms following brain injury. Despite the absence of MRI abnormalities, they show a lower binding potential on ^{18}F-FMZ PET imaging, which reflects the destruction of neuronal integrity and the loss of neurons. It is currently believed that ^{18}F-FMZ PET imaging can discriminate hypometabolism caused by neuronal loss from that caused by other factors.

In one study, researchers performed structural and biomolecular imaging of the brain to examine the imaging findings in repetitive TBIs. All subjects underwent neuropsychological assessments and behavioral tasks, as well as structural and functional molecular imaging, in order to explore whether their neuropsychological characteristics and cognitive-motor-related functional impairments were associated with their imaging findings. In the neuropsychological tests, boxers showed deficits in visuospatial memory and motor coordination, which showed significant correlations with the biomolecular imaging results of neuronal injury. In contrast, sMRI did not reveal any morphometric abnormalities in professional boxers. PET imaging of boxers revealed that the impaired glucose metabolism of the frontal areas of the brain was associated with cognitive dysfunction, similar to findings in AD. ^{18}F-FMZ showed a relatively low binding potential in the angular gyrus and temporal cortex, which is indicative of neuronal deficits. These results reflect the chronic neuronal damage inflicted by repetitive TBI in professional boxers, which in turn led to cognitive impairment and motor dysfunction. The ^{18}F-FMZ PET results of this study are consistent with the neuronal loss induced by repetitive TBI. In the intergroup comparison, boxers showed significantly lower ^{18}F-FMZ uptake than the healthy control group in the left angular gyrus, left orbitofrontal cortex, left inferior temporal cortex, left superior temporal cortex, right precuneus, and right cerebellum. These regions of low uptake indicate the presence of neuronal damage.

Suggested Reading

Annen J, Heine L, Ziegler E, et al. Function-structure connectivity in patients with severe brain injury as measured by MRI-DWI and FDG-PET. Hum Brain Mapp. 2016;37(11):3707–20.

Bang SA, Song YS, Moon BS, et al. Neuropsychological, metabolic, and GABAA receptor studies in subjects with repetitive traumatic brain injury. J Neurotrauma. 2016;33(11):1005–14.

Blennow K, Brody DL, Kochanek PM, et al. Traumatic brain injuries. Nat Rev Dis Primers. 2016;2:16084.

Brabazon F, Wilson CM, Shukla DK, et al. ^{18}F FDG-PET combined with MRI elucidates the pathophysiology of traumatic brain injury in rats. J Neurotrauma. 2017;34(5):1074–85.

Byrnes KR, Wilson CM, Brabazon F, et al. FDG-PET imaging in mild traumatic brain injury: a critical review. Front Neuroenergetics. 2014;5:13.

Chen JK, Johnston KM, Frey S, et al. Functional abnormalities in symptomatic concussed athletes: an fMRI study. Neuroimage. 2004;22(1):68–82.

Chen SH, Kareken DA, Fastenau PS, et al. A study of persistent post-concussion symptoms in mild head trauma using positron emission tomography. J Neurol Neurosurg Psychiatry. 2003;74(3):326–32.

Frank MJ, Doll B, Oas-Terpstra J, et al. Prefrontal and striatal dopaminergic genes predict individual differences in exploration and exploitation. Nat Neurosci. 2009;12(8):1062–8.

Heiss WD, Kracht L, Grond M, et al. Early [(11)C] Flumazenil/H(2)O positron emission tomography predicts irreversible ischemic cortical damage in stroke patients receiving acute thrombolytic therapy. Stroke. 2000;31(2):366–9.

Hong YT, Veenith T, Dewar D, et al. Amyloid imaging with carbon 11-labeled pittsburgh compound B for traumatic brain injury. JAMA Neurol. 2014;71(1):23–31.

Jantzen KJ, Anderson B, Steinberg FL, et al. A prospective functional MR imaging study of mild traumatic brain injury in college football players. AJNR Am J Neuroradiol. 2004;25(5):738–45.

Johnson VE, Stewart JE, Begbie FD, et al. Inflammation and white matter degeneration persist for years after a single traumatic brain injury. Brain. 2013;136(Pt 1):28–42.

Johnson VE, Stewart W, Smith DH. Traumatic brain injury and amyloid-beta pathology: a link to Alzheimer's disease? Nat Rev. Neurosci. 2010;11(5):361–70.

Johnson VE, Stewart W, Smith DH. Widespread tau and amyloid-beta pathology many years after a single traumatic brain injury in humans. Brain Pathol. 2012;22(2):142–9.

Johnson VE, Stewart W, Smith DH. Axonal pathology in traumatic brain injury. Exp Neurol. 2013;246:35–43.

Klunk WE. Amyloid imaging as a biomarker for cerebral beta-amyloidosis and risk prediction for Alzheimer dementia. Neurobiol Aging. 2011;32(Suppl 1):S20–36.

Levin HS, Diaz-Arrastia R. Diagnosis, prognosis, and clinical management of mild traumatic brain injury. Lancet Neurol. 2015;14(5):506–17.

Liguori M, Fera F, Gioia MC, et al. Investigating the role of brain-derived neurotrophic factor in relapsing-remitting multiple sclerosis. Genes Brain Behav. 2007;6(2):177–83.

Madsen K, Hesby S, Poulsen I, et al. Comparison of analytical methods of brain ^{18}F FDG-PET after severe traumatic brain injury. J Neurosci Methods. 2017;291:176–81.

Odano I, Halldin C, Karlsson P, et al. [18F]flumazenil binding to central benzodiazepine receptor studies by PET-quantitative analysis and comparisons with [11C] flumazenil. Neuroimage. 2009;45(3):891–902.

Peng F, Muzik O, Gatson J, et al. Assessment of traumatic brain injury by increased ^{64}Cu uptake on $^{64}CuCl_2$ PET/CT. J Nucl Med. 2015;56(8):1252–7.

Rathore S, Habes M, Iftikhar MA, et al. A review on neuroimaging-based classification studies and associated feature extraction methods for Alzheimer's disease and its prodromal stages. Neuroimage. 2017;155:530–48.

Salat DH, Robinson ME, Miller DR, et al. Neuroimaging of deployment-associated traumatic brain injury (TBI) with a focus on mild TBI (mTBI) since 2009. Brain Inj. 2017;31(9):1204–19.

Scholl M, Damian A, Engler H. Fluorodeoxyglucose PET in neurology and psychiatry. PET Clin. 2014;9(4):371–90.

Scott G, Ramlackhansingh AF, Edison P, et al. Amyloid pathology and axonal injury after brain trauma. Neurology. 2016;86(9):821–8.

Smith DH, Johnson VE, Stewart W. Chronic neuropathologies of single and repetitive TBI: substrates of dementia? Nat Rev. Neurol. 2013;9(4):211–21.

Stein TD, Montenigro PH, Alvarez VE, et al. Beta-amyloid deposition in chronic traumatic encephalopathy. Acta Neuropathol. 2015;130(1):21–34.

Sundman M, Doraiswamy PM, Morey RA. Neuroimaging assessment of early and late neurobiological sequelae of traumatic brain injury: implications for CTE. Front Neurosci. 2015;9:334.

Umile EM, Sandel ME, Alavi A, et al. Dynamic imaging in mild traumatic brain injury: support for the theory of medial temporal vulnerability. Arch Phys Med Rehabil. 2002;83(11):1506–13.

Whiteneck G, Cuthbert JP, Corrigan JD, et al. Risk of negative outcomes after traumatic brain injury: a statewide population-based survey. J Head Trauma Rehabil. 2016;31(1):E43–54.

Wu X, Kirov I, Gonen O, et al. MR imaging applications in mild traumatic brain injury: an imaging update. Radiology. 2016;279(3):693–707.

Yamaki T, Uchino Y, Henmi H, et al. Increased brain glucose metabolism in chronic severe traumatic brain injury as determined by longitudinal ^{18}F-FDG PET/CT. J Clin Neurosci. 2018;57:20–5.

Research Applications of Positron Emission Tomography/Magnetic Resonance (PET/MR) Imaging in Depression

14

Mingrui Xia, Jiakai He, Junling Xu, Jiliang Fang, and Yong He

Depression is a mood and affective disorder, primarily characterized by a marked and persistent depressed mood. A 2017 epidemiological survey by the World Health Organization (WHO) revealed that the incidence of depression in China was 4.2%, and it has been increasing every year. Current treatment options for depression primarily include pharmacotherapy, psychotherapy, and physical therapy.

14.1 Research Applications of MRI in Depression

Ongoing advancements in multimodal MRI techniques have enabled researchers to conduct noninvasive, in vivo observations on the structural and functional characteristics of the human brain, abnormalities of which can serve as sensitive features for the diagnosis and treatment of neurological diseases. Of these newer techniques, functional MRI (fMRI) primarily involves the use of blood-oxygen-level-dependent (BOLD) imaging to acquire information on brain activity. In task-based fMRI, different experimental paradigms are performed to observe the responses elicited in the brain by different stimuli, whereas resting-state fMRI is used to examine regional brain activity and network connectivity patterns while at rest. These techniques have now been widely implemented in the evaluation of abnormal brain mechanisms involved in depression, and in the exploration of imaging markers that can be used for the diagnosis and treatment evaluation of this mood disorder.

14.1.1 Task-Based and Resting-State fMRI

14.1.1.1 Primary Principles and Methods

BOLD-fMRI, in which the images are generated based on the changes in the oxygen level of different brain areas induced by changes in blood flow, is currently the most widely used fMRI technique. Ogawa et al. demonstrated that hemoglobin exhibits different magnetic properties in its oxidized and reduced forms, which can be visualized using MRI. Therefore, BOLD-fMRI is a functional brain imaging technique that indirectly measures neuronal activity based on blood

M. Xia · Y. He (✉)
National Key Laboratory of Cognitive Neuroscience and Learning, Beijing Normal University, Beijing, China
e-mail: yong.he@bnu.edu.cn

J. He · J. Fang (✉)
Department of Radiology, Guang An Men Hospital, China Academy of Chinese Medical Science, Beijing, China

J. Xu
Department of Radiology and Nuclear Medicine, Henan Provincial People's Hospital, Zhengzhou, Henan, China

J. Lu, G. Zhao (eds.), *PET/MR: Functional and Molecular Imaging of Neurological Diseases and Neurosciences*, https://doi.org/10.1007/978-981-19-9902-4_14

oxygen levels and utilizes T_2*-weighted imaging to detect paramagnetic deoxyhemoglobin and diamagnetic oxyhemoglobin. BOLD-fMRI is also a dynamic imaging technique that can indirectly measure the metabolic levels of the brain, reflecting the correlation of time-dependent cerebral cortical signals during neurophysiological processes. As such, BOLD-fMRI can provide strong technological support for investigating changes in the functional networks of the brain.

Facial expressions are the most intuitive means to convey human emotions. Based on the theory that "patients with depression have negative cognitive schemas for facial expressions" fMRI studies on depression using facial expression paradigms have found abnormal activity in the "prefrontal-striatal-thalamic circuit" of patients. However, these findings have been inconsistent due to the presence of numerous influencing factors. In recent years, this theory has been extensively studied using a number of imaging methods, including electroencephalography (EEG), PET, and single-photon emission computed tomography (SPECT). BOLD-fMRI has been widely utilized in task-based fMRI studies since its inception. One common approach in task-based fMRI is to present subjects with emotional stimuli consisting of different facial expressions and to then calculate the responses evoked by these stimuli in various brain areas; the findings can be used for lesion localization, disease monitoring, efficacy evaluation, and prognosis determination in patients with depression. Common emotional stimuli for facial expressions can be classified as positive or negative, which can represent acceptance or rejection, respectively, in social interactions, whereas neutral facial expressions rarely contain immediate social information. Therefore, the facial expressions used in fMRI studies on depression primarily include the following: acceptance-type stimuli (positive), i.e., happy and surprised; rejection-type stimuli (negative), i.e., sad, angry, fearful, and disgusted; and neutral stimuli. Of these stimuli, happy and sad facial expressions are the most commonly used, whereas surprised expressions may be mistaken for fear and are therefore less commonly used in studies.

As with task-based fMRI, resting-state fMRI is also based on the BOLD theory. There are two categories of calculation methods for resting-state fMRI: (1) detection of regional activity characteristics, activity intensity, or regional similarity in brain activity, which primarily includes amplitude of low-frequency fluctuation (ALFF) and regional homogeneity (ReHo); or (2) observation of synchronous activity signals between regions of interest (ROIs), which primarily includes seed-based functional connectivity (FC). However, since the selection of seed regions is subjective, differences in selection methods can lead to substantial variability in the final calculation results.

14.1.1.2 fMRI Studies on Brain Functional Abnormalities in Depression

According to the results of task-based fMRI studies on patients with depression, areas of the brain with abnormal activation elicited by emotional facial expression paradigms are primarily found in the amygdala, hippocampus, cingulate cortex, prefrontal cortex (PFC), fusiform gyrus, thalamus, insula, and basal ganglia. The amygdala and hippocampus are located in the medial temporal lobe, and when presented with facial expression stimuli, patients with depression exhibit activation of the amygdala and inhibition of hippocampal and PFC activity. These abnormal changes in brain function showed a trend of improvement after treatment with antidepressants. Dysfunction of the amygdala can give rise to affective disorders, while the degree of activation can serve as an indicator of the severity of depression. Patients with depression showed hyperactivation of the amygdala when presented with sad (negative) facial stimuli, which was reduced after short-term antidepressant treatment. Furthermore, studies have shown that negative stimuli can induce the hyperactivation of the PFC, hippocampus, and parahippocampal gyrus in patients with depression. The cingulate cortex is an important component of the reward and emotional cognition systems. After viewing facial stimuli with negative emotions, patients with depression were found to exhibit enhanced activation of the anterior cingulate cortex (ACC). The frontal lobe is closely associated with cognition, emotion, and execution. Studies have found that when presented with sad facial stimuli, patients with depression exhibited a lower extent of activation in the left inferior frontal, middle frontal, and postcentral gyri than healthy controls, but a higher extent of activation in the ipsilateral amygdala, ventral striatum, insula, caudate nucleus, thalamus, dorsal ACC, and inferior parietal lobule. Another study demonstrated that when processing negative facial emotions, first-episode patients with mild to moderate depression showed significantly increased activation of the right middle frontal gyrus compared to healthy controls. These findings indicate that the right PFC is involved in the processing of negative facial emotions, which can explain the clinical presentations of cognitive impairments in the emotion recognition, reward processing, and other functions of patients with depression. The temporal lobe is intimately associated with mental activity and plays a crucial role in the processing of emotions, memory, and mental activity. The amygdala is a key center of human emotional regulation and plays a critical role in the onset of depression. The abnormal increase of activity in the amygdala is a specific indicator of primary depression, which can promote the onset or recurrence of depression. Dannlowski et al. performed a task-based fMRI study on patients with chronic depression, the results of which revealed that when presented with negative emotional stimuli, patients showed reduced functional connectivity of the amygdala and PFC with the occipital lobe, further confirming that the occipital lobe is one of the pathogenic mechanisms of depression. During the discrimination of negative facial stimuli, patients with depression showed significantly enhanced activation of the fusiform gyrus, which is located at the occipitotemporal junction.

Another study found that in contrast to healthy controls, patients with depression exhibited a relative decrease in the level of activation of the bilateral fusiform gyrus and right putamen when presented with increasingly happy facial expressions; as task difficulty increased, patients with depression showed increases in the level of activation of the right fusiform gyrus, left putamen, and left hippocampus–amygdala complex. The parietal lobe is closely related to the frontal lobe and has extensive functional connectivity with multiple regions of the brain, including the temporal and occipital lobes. The anterior parietal lobe is predominantly connected with the frontal lobe and is responsible for sensation and proprioception; the middle parietal lobe is primarily connected with the temporal lobe and is related to cognitive language processing; and the posterior parietal lobe is primarily connected with the occipital lobe and is involved in logical thinking. The postcentral gyrus is involved with the cognitive processing of various sensations, while the supramarginal and angular gyri are closely related to sensory and language impairments. Therefore, patients with depression who exhibit abnormal parietal function may present with somatization disorder, memory impairments, and impaired logical reasoning. Functional abnormalities of the inferior parietal lobule may be associated with the repetitive confirmation of negative self-referent information in patients with depression. Studies have also found that during depressive episodes, patients showed stronger activation of the left fusiform gyrus and left amygdala when processing facial expressions of disgust compared to healthy controls.

Resting-state fMRI studies on patients with depression primarily involve the observation of changes in local brain activity and those in synchronicity among various areas of the brain. Observational studies on regional brain activity in patients with depression showed abnormal ALFF in the PCC, orbitofrontal cortex (OFC), PFC, fusiform gyrus, and subcortical nuclei. Another study found that ALFF changes in the left perigenual ACC and left hippocampus were correlated with scores on depression clinical rating scales. Patients with recurrent depressive disorder (RDD) exhibit extensive, whole-brain ALFF abnormalities, which are primarily located in the visual recognition circuit and default mode network (DMN). A meta-analysis revealed that patients with depression had increased ReHo values in the left superior frontal and fusiform gyri, as well as decreased ReHo values in the left cerebellum, postcentral and superior temporal gyri, right cuneus, and inferior parietal gyrus. Patients with recurrent depression also showed specific increases in the ReHo values of the medial PFC, as the ReHo values of the right insula and left inferior frontal gyrus were correlated with disease duration, while the ReHo values of the left middle occipital gyrus, calcarine fissure, inferior parietal gyrus, putamen, right middle frontal gyrus, and precentral gyrus were correlated with symptom severity.

There are currently a host of urgent problems that need to be addressed in the studies described above, such as the standardization of facial expression stimuli and the impact of environmental factors, necessitating the exploration of new ideas, techniques, and methods based on these existing studies. In summary, the abnormally functioning areas of the brain in patients with depression are primarily located in the frontal, temporal, and parietal lobes, the cingulate gyrus, and the amygdala, and as such, the abnormal connectivity of the cortico-limbic system may also be involved in the pathogenesis of depression.

14.1.1.3 Hypotheses on Abnormal Mechanisms of Functional Networks of the Brain Proposed by fMRI Studies

FC is defined as the temporal correlation of the activity signals between different areas of the brain, which can be used to evaluate the functional interactions between these various areas. The primary methods for studying FC include model-driven FC analysis and data-driven FC analysis. Model-driven FC analysis first requires the selection of a seed region based on prior knowledge (e.g., based on the results of previous task-based fMRI studies), and the extraction of the associated time series. This is followed by the calculation of the correlation between the seed region and other voxels of the whole brain or other ROIs, and subsequent statistical analysis to determine the FC of the seed region and other brain areas. Data-driven methods were later introduced to study whole-brain FC patterns. Since these methods do not require the subjective definition of seed regions, they can avoid the problem of subjectivity in seed selection. The primary methods of data-driven analysis include principal component analysis (PCA), cluster analysis, and independent component analysis (ICA), of which ICA has produced relatively consistent research findings. By utilizing FC methods, we can reveal functional networks composed of brain areas that have close functional relationships, known as functional brain networks. There is a strong concordance between resting-state and task-based studies on the functional networks of the brain. Based on current research, it is believed that there are two mutually antagonistic systems in the brain, one of which is the DMN, and the other is a task-related system that encompasses the frontoparietal and attention networks. Smith et al. performed an ICA study on resting-state and task-related brain networks and were able to reliably identify a number of resting-state networks in the human brain, including the DMN, visual network, central executive network (CEN), sensorimotor network, attention network (salience network, SN), cerebellar network, and auditory network. Of these networks, the DMN, CEN, and SN have garnered the most attention in current research on patients with depression. The DMN, which is divided into the anterior DMN, found in the medial PFC, and the posterior DMN, located in the PCC and precuneus, is functionally active in the resting state and deactivated when performing tasks. The CEN is functionally antagonistic to the DMN, as the former is most active when completing cognitive tasks, and is involved in the formation of attention, memory, and other cognitive functions. The SN is significantly activated during stress and is closely connected with the emotional processing circuit of the limbic system. It is involved in the transition between DMN and SN.

Greicius et al. found that the FC of the ACC, OFC, precuneus, and thalamus was significantly enhanced in patients with depression. Other studies have also observed increased FC within the anterior DMN and decreased FC within the posterior DMN in patients with depression. This regional inconsistency within the DMN suggests the presence of a functional dissociation between the anterior and posterior DMN in patients with depression. The current consensus is that the FC is enhanced between the anterior DMN and medial PFC, although this is related to the patient's drug therapy status. The anterior insula is a key node in the SN, as patients with depression exhibit increased FC between the bilateral ACC and decreased FC between the bilateral anterior insula, while the intraregional FC of the right insula is negatively correlated with the severity of depression. The insula and amygdala are major seed regions in studies on the SN, and patients with depression show reductions in the FC between the insula and amygdala which vary with affective changes. Furthermore, the results of ICA and FC analysis revealed increased FC of the SN with the ACC, insula, medial OFC, and anterior DMN. As an important component of the SN, the amygdala showed decreased FC with multiple areas of the brain, including the ACC and left ventrolateral PFC. Conversely, the amygdala showed increased FC with the temporal pole. Manoliu et al. were the first to propose the CEN and divided it into three sub-networks. They found that patients with depression showed increased FC between the left ventromedial angular and dorsal postcentral gyri within the CEN; significantly elevated FC of the dorsolateral PFC with the lateral ACC, left parahippocampal gyrus, thalamus, and precentral gyrus; and reduced intra-network FC among other areas of the brain within the CEN, and between the precuneus and the insula of the SN (Figs. 14.1 and 14.2).

A meta-analysis on patients with depression revealed an increased FC between the frontoparietal network and posterior parietal cortex, the DMN and medial PFC, and the hippocampus and dorsolateral PFC, as well as a decreased FC between the frontoparietal network and the inferior parietal lobule in the dorsal attention network, the affective network and medial PFC, the ventral attention network and precuneus, and the occipital lobe and PCC. These FC abnormalities can partially explain the clinical symptoms of patients with depression. For example, a reduced FC within the frontoparietal network can affect patient's cognitive control; enhanced FC between the frontoparietal network and DMN and reduced FC between the frontoparietal network and dorsal attention network can explain patient's indecisiveness toward external stimuli. Patients with RDD display similar FC abnormalities as those with depression, but with a greater magnitude of decrease and involving more extensive brain areas. These abnormalities mainly appear in the ACC, amygdala, hippocampus, and insula, even exhibiting impaired FC in multiple functional brain networks. When different emotional experiences were induced in patients during depressive episodes, not only was differential activation detected in the PFC, limbic system, and cingulate gyrus, but changes in activation intensity were also detected in other areas of the brain, including the hypothalamus, hippocampus, amygdala, globus pallidus, and cerebellar vermis.

In recent years, there has been a rapid development in neuroimaging-based human connectomics, which strives to achieve the mapping and topological description of network connectivity patterns in the human brain at a macroscopic level. Using this approach, the human brain is regarded as a complex network composed of a large number of anatomical units linked together through structural connections (white matter tracts, gray matter morphological associations) or functional connections (temporal correlations), such that mathematical graph theory and other computational methods can be utilized to quantitatively, comprehensively, and meticulously describe the rules of connectivity governing human brain networks. Based on this, we can gain a deeper understanding of the abnormal mechanisms of depression from the perspective of neural circuits. Zhang et al. were the first to introduce large-scale, complex network analysis (i.e., brain connectomics) to the imaging-based evaluation of depression. They discovered small-world properties in the functional brain networks of both first-episode, treatment-naïve patients with depression and healthy controls. However, the brain networks of patients with depression had a smaller shortest path length and higher global efficiencies, therefore exhibiting a shift toward a random network. Additionally, the abnormal nodes in the brain networks of patients

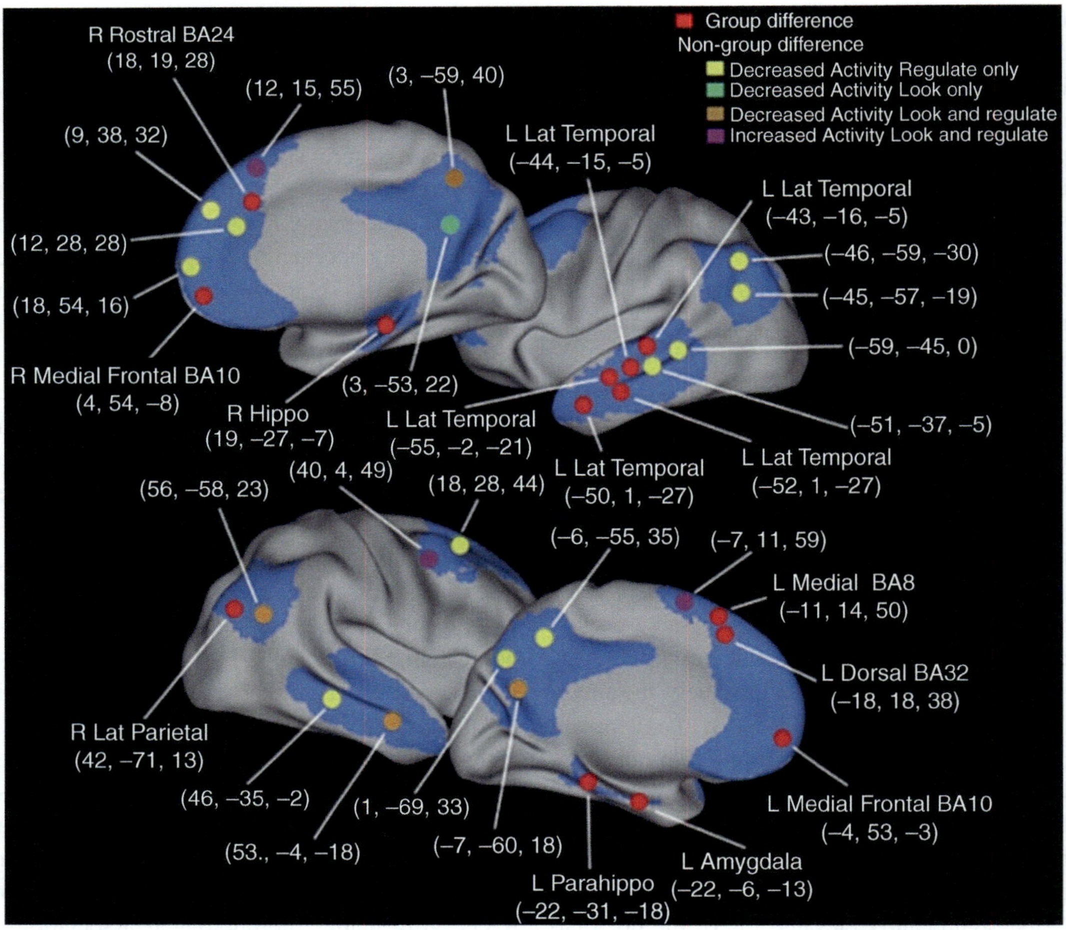

Fig. 14.1 Abnormal areas of the brain in the DMN of patients with depression (Reproduced with permission from SHELINE Y I, BARCH D M, PRICE J L, et al. The default mode network and self-referential processes in depression. Proc Natl Acad Sci USA, 2009, 106(6):1942–1947). Areas of the brain in the DMN with increased or decreased functional connectivity based on different studies and task-induced activity. The DMN is shown in light blue. The top left figure shows the medial surface of the right hemisphere, and the top right figure shows the lateral surface of the left hemisphere. The bottom left figure shows the lateral surface of the right hemisphere, and the bottom right figure shows the medial surface of the left hemisphere. The red overlapping areas represent regions with task-induced differences within the DMN, which can be used to distinguish between patients with depression and healthy controls. The remaining regions do not have between-group differences, but showed decreased activity in the regulate (i.e., emotional regulation) condition only (yellow) and look (i.e., passive viewing) condition only (green), both regulate and look conditions (orange), or increased activity in both the regulate and look conditions (fuchsia)

were primarily located in the hippocampus, DMN, OFC, and occipital lobe. By utilizing a high-precision brain connectomics analytical framework, Xia et al. also revealed disrupted brain FC patterns in patients with depression who exhibited a tendency toward randomization. Furthermore, they identified increased long-range connectivity within the higher-order medial/lateral frontoparietal system, and decreased short-range connectivity within the primary cortices, as well as significant associations between brain network abnormalities and the clinical symptoms of depression. Xia et al. further performed an fMRI-based multi-center

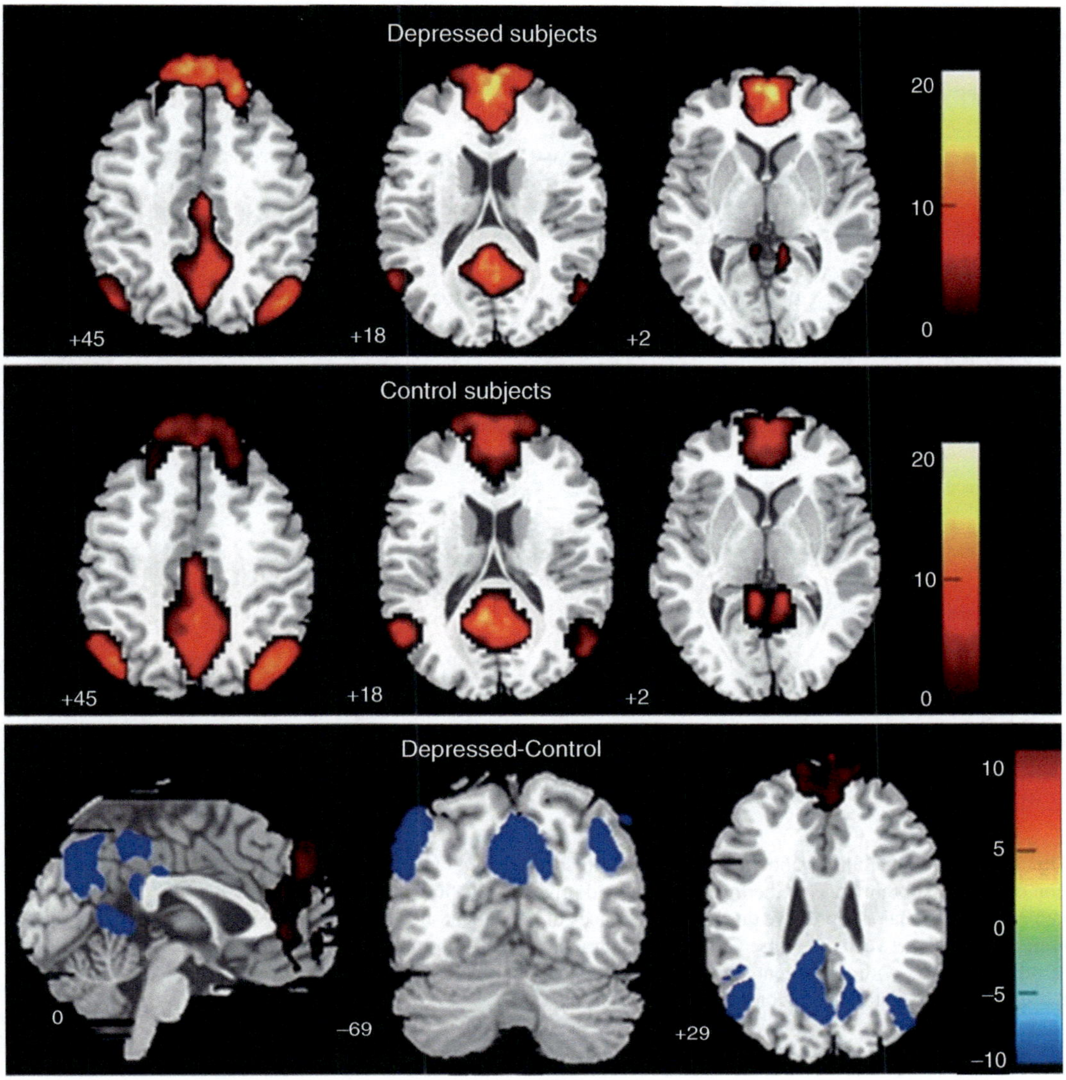

Fig. 14.2 Abnormal functional connectivity patterns within the DMN of patients with depression (Reproduced with permission from ZHU X, WANG X, XIAO J, et al. Evidence of a dissociation pattern in resting-state default mode network connectivity in first-episode, treatment-naive major depression patients. Biol Psychiatry, 2012, 71(7):611–617). Patients with depression showed significant increases in FC between the medial PFC and ACC (dark red) compared to control subjects, and significant decreases in FC between the PCC and precuneus (blue). Depressed subjects: patients with depression; Control subjects: healthy controls; Depressed-Control: Depressed group—control group

big data (1434 subjects) analysis to systematically evaluate the impact of key analytical strategies for brain connectomics on identifying the core nodes of abnormal brain function in patients with depression. Their results confirmed the reproducibility of abnormal functional activities and connectivity in the higher-order medial/lateral frontoparietal system and primary cortices, thereby providing a reproducibility validation framework and methodological guidance for studying brain imaging connectomic markers for depression (Fig. 14.3).

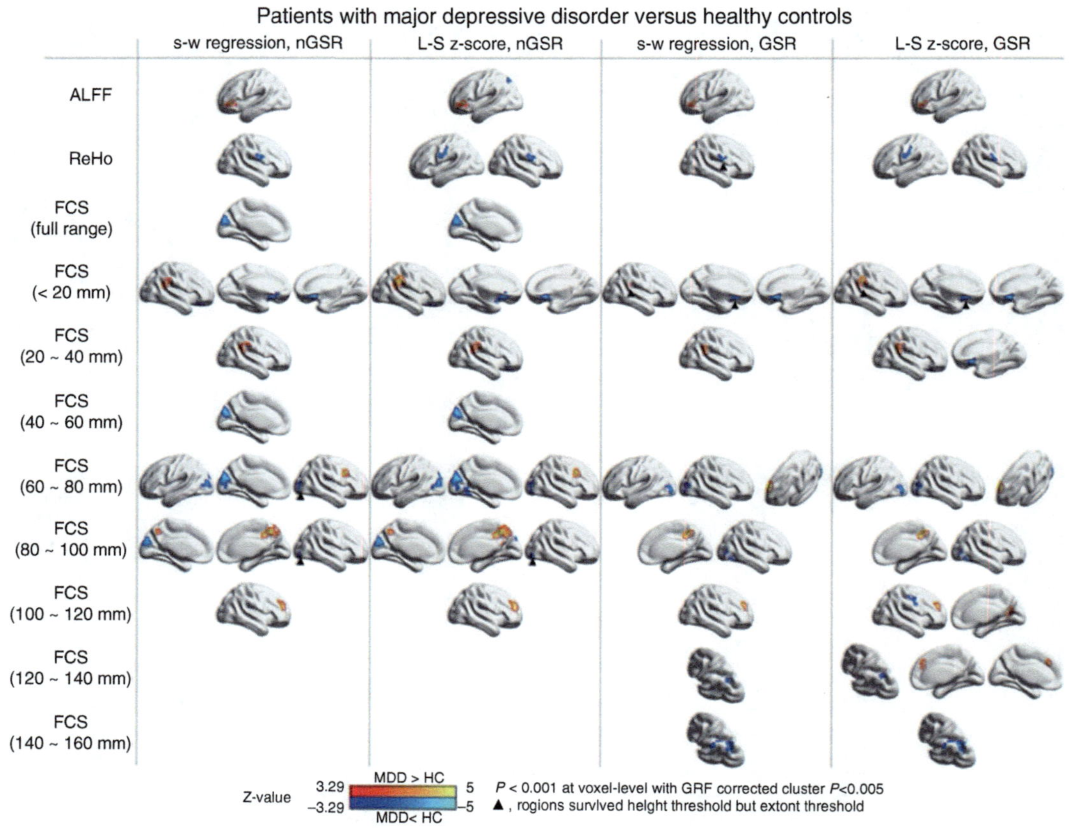

Fig. 14.3 Reproducibility validation for the identification of abnormal brain areas in the frontoparietal and primary cortices of major depressive disorder. Differences in brain function between patients with depression and healthy controls, with consistent conclusions obtained through multiple data calculation methods (i.e., ALFF, ReHo, FCS). Patients with major depressive disorder versus healthy controls: Comparison of patients with depression and healthy controls; $P < 0.001$ at voxel level with GRF corrected cluster $P < 0.005$: voxel-level GRF correction

14.1.2 Research Applications of Structural MRI in Depression

Past research described depression as a typical functional disease, but subsequent studies gradually uncovered the presence of micro- and macroscopic anatomical abnormalities in patients with depression. At present, gray matter density and volume analyses based on structural MRIs have been extensively utilized in research on depression. A meta-analysis of major depressive disorder (MDD) found that affected patients had significantly reduced gray matter volume in the rostral ACC and dorsal PFC, and that these alterations were more prominent in patients with multiple depressive episodes. Further subgroup analysis also revealed that patients with comorbid anxiety and first-episode, treatment-naïve patients also had significant atrophy of the hippocampus and amygdala. Another meta-analysis on voxel-based morphometry (VBM) studies, which covered a variety of mental illnesses including depression, found extensive atrophy of the dorsal ACC and bilateral insula in all patient groups, of which patients with depression showed more significant gray matter atrophy of the anterior hippocampus and amygdala compared to other mental illnesses. Surface-based morphometry (SBM) studies involve the reconstruction of gray matter surfaces and gray–white matter junction surfaces to calculate a series of surface-based metrics (cortical thickness, surface area, curvature, etc.). The ENIGMA project is currently the most representative SBM study on depression, involving the analysis of cortical thickness and surface area based on a large multi-center sample (20 centers, 2148 MDD patients, 7957 healthy controls). The findings of this project revealed that the OFC, ACC, insula, and temporal cortex of adult MDD patients were significantly thinned, whereas adolescent MDD patients had significantly smaller surface areas in the frontal, visual, and sensorimotor cortices.

In summary, patients with depression exhibited reduced gray matter volume in the PFC, ACC, hippocampus, and amygdala, and other areas of the brain, as well as a significantly thinner OFC, ACC, insula, and temporal cortex. These alterations can explain the clinical presentations related to the executive function and emotional control of patients with depression. Interventional treatments for depression can increase regional gray matter volume, while improvements in clinical presentations are associated with gray matter alterations in different brain areas.

14.1.3 Research Applications of Diffusion MRI in Depression

Unlike VBM-based structural imaging studies, diffusion MRI can be used to examine tissue microstructure, such as the neurocytoskeleton and axons. Diffusion MRI exploits the different characteristics exhibited by the Brownian motion of water molecules restricted by various cellular structures and is primarily utilized to examine the structural changes in white matter (predominantly axons). This technique can be utilized to calculate structural, morphological, intensity, and other information related to the connective pathways of white matter fibers. Current research concerning this topic is relatively scarce. White matter abnormalities in patients with depression are chiefly manifested as microstructural alterations of white matter fibers in the frontal lobe, parietal lobe, thalamus, and other areas of the brain, such as the connective circuits of the frontal lobe with the limbic system and reward system, and the frontal lobe with the executive network and emotion network.

14.1.4 Research Applications of Arterial Spin Labelling (ASL) Imaging in Depression

ASL imaging utilizes the subject's own water molecules as a tracer to quantify their cerebral blood flow (CBF), obtaining results similar to BOLD imaging findings. Patients with depression exhibit abnormal perfusion in the DMN (PFC and ACC), which reflects the hemodynamic basis of abnormal brain functions in depression.

14.1.5 Research Applications of Magnetic Resonance Spectroscopy (MRS) in Depression

MRS is currently the only technique available for in vivo metabolite detection. This technique can be used to determine neurotransmitter concentrations [i.e., N-acetylaspartate (NAA), glutamate, glutamine, γ-aminobutyric acid (GABA), and choline (Cho)] in target brain areas. Patients with depression exhibit a wide range of neurotransmitter changes in the PFC and ACC, including: (1) decreased concentrations of glutamate, glutamine–glutamate complex, and GABA; (2) increased concentrations of Cho and creatine (Cr); and (3) decreased ratios of NAA/Cr and Cho/Cr. These findings can reflect the pathogenic and therapeutic mechanisms of depression at the molecular level.

14.1.6 Research on the Mechanisms of Therapeutic Efficacy

According to imaging studies on the use of pharmacotherapy in patients with depression, antidepressants can mitigate the hyperactivation of patients' ACC and amygdala to negative facial stimuli. A meta-analysis found that pharmacotherapy can significantly reduce the ReHo values of patients' left dorsomedial PFC, right insula, and bilateral thalamus, while also significantly elevating the ReHo values of their right superior frontal gyrus. Furthermore, pharmacotherapy can enhance the ability of the ACC to regulate the subcortical circuit involving the amygdala, striatum, thalamus, and hippocampus, and improvements in this regulation were correlated with symptom remission. Some forms of pharmacotherapy can mitigate damage to white matter fibers in the frontal lobe, parietal lobe, thalamus, and other regions of the brain. Antidepressants have also been shown to exert significant regulatory effects on functional brain networks. By adopting a longitudinal study design, Wang et al. examined the brain network mechanisms underlying the treatment of depression with escitalopram, which revealed that the drug exerted different regulatory effects on key connective pathways of the dorsomedial/lateral PFC and hippocampus. Moreover, changes in connectivity strength were significantly correlated with improvements in clinical symptom scores (Fig. 14.4).

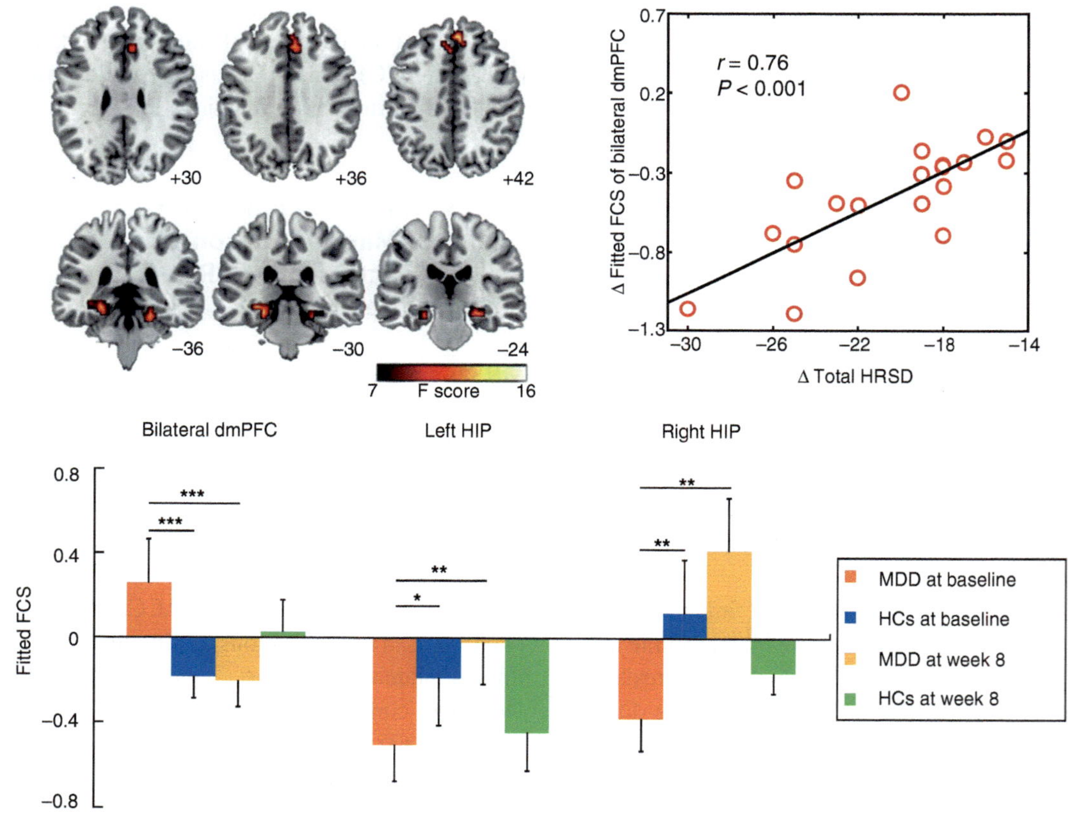

Fig. 14.4 Research on the brain network mechanisms of antidepressants in depression. In patients with depression, antidepressants exerted inhibitory effects on the functional connectivity strength of the dorsomedial prefrontal cortex and enhanced the regulatory effects on the connectivity between the bilateral hippocampus and cerebellum. Changes in the functional connectivity strength of the dorsomedial prefrontal cortex were significantly correlated with the changes in the clinical symptom scores of patients. Bilateral dmPFC: bilateral dorsomedial prefrontal cortex; Score: clinical rating scale scores; Left HIP: left hippocampus; △ Fitted FCS of bilateral dmPFC: Changes in fitted functional connectivity strength of bilateral dorsomedial prefrontal cortex; △ Total HRSD: Changes in total Hamilton Depression Rating Scale; Right HIP: right hippocampus; Fitted FC: standardized functional connectivity; MDD at baseline: patients with major depressive disorder at baseline; HCs at baseline: healthy controls at baseline; MDD at week 8: patients with major depressive disorder at week 8; HCs at week 8: healthy controls at week 8

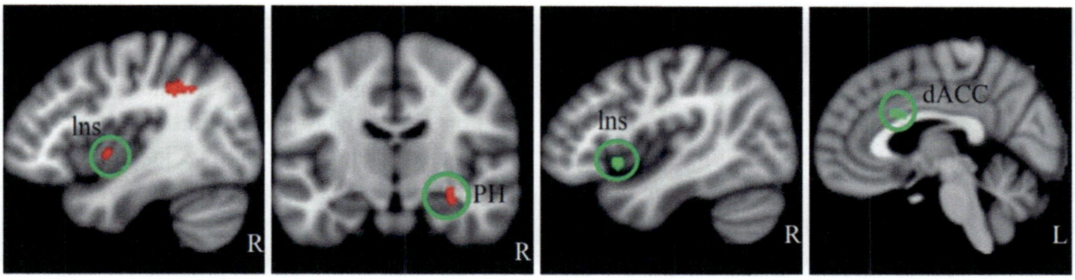

Fig. 14.5 Modulation of DMN function by transcutaneous auricular vagus nerve stimulation (taVNS). *Ins* Insula, *PH* parahippocampus, *dACC* dorsal anterior cingulate cortex

Electroconvulsive therapy can increase the gray matter volume of the caudate nucleus, hippocampus, amygdala, insula, and posterior superior temporal gyrus in the right cerebral hemisphere among patients with depression. Perrin et al found significant reductions in the whole-brain FC strength of the left dorsolateral PFC after electroconvulsive therapy, as well as a significant correlation between the extent of the decrease in connectivity strength and improvements in clinical symptoms. Repetitive transcranial magnetic stimulation (rTMS) has been shown to improve abnormal intra- and inter-network FC in the DMN, frontoparietal control network, and SN of patients with depression. Transcranial direct current stimulation (tDCS) is similar to rTMS, both of which can affect the functional states of the amygdala and hippocampus. tDCS can improve the abnormal FC of depression-related brain networks, while pharmacotherapy has also been shown to be effective in improving the DMN. Additionally, Fang et al. demonstrated that transcutaneous vagus nerve stimulation at auricular acupoints could modulate the functional status of the DMN and dorsolateral PFC-amygdala circuit, and these changes were significantly associated with improvements in patients' clinical symptoms (Fig. 14.5). Taken together, these findings suggest that the regulatory effects of various treatments for depression on the brain networks of patients are primarily concentrated in the frontal lobe and limbic system, which can serve as potential therapeutic targets.

14.2 Research Applications of PET in Depression

Depression is currently one of the most common mental disorders seen in clinical settings, and its pathogenic mechanism remains a hot spot for research and a challenge in the medical field. Research involving medical imaging is an important means by which to explore the pathogenesis of depression, and the continuous advancement of functional imaging techniques has further highlighted their advantages in exploring treatment responses and therapeutic efficacy in depression. PET involves the real-time in vivo observation of functional activity of the brain, thereby objectively displaying regional CBF (rCBF), regional cerebral metabolic rate of glucose (GMRglc), and the binding of neurotransmitters with their corresponding receptors under normal physiological or pathological states. Therefore, PET has gradually evolved into an effective tool for research on depression and will play an increasingly important role in the etiological investigation, early diagnosis, and treatment evaluation of depression.

14.2.1 Research on Brain Perfusion Imaging

Commonly used PET imaging agents for brain perfusion include $^{13}N\text{-}NH_3{\cdot}H_2O$ and $^{15}O\text{-}H_2O$. The majority of brain perfusion imaging studies have discovered varying degrees of brain perfusion changes in patients with depression, but with inconsistent findings reported in the literature. These changes are primarily found in the frontal, temporal, occipital, and parietal lobes, in addition to the cingulate gyrus. Some researchers who conducted perfusion PET studies on patients with depression have concluded that patients in the resting state had increased rCBF in the right thalamus and caudate nucleus, as well as decreased cerebral perfusion in the left PFC and right ACC.

Savitz et al. performed PET imaging of the brain on treatment-naïve patients with bipolar depression, the results of which revealed the hyperperfusion of the left ventral frontal lobe and left amygdala. Furthermore, Hamilton Depression Rating Scale (HAM-D) scores were found to be positively correlated with perfusion in the left amygdala, and negatively correlated with perfusion in the left frontal lobe. The study by Videbech et al. on patients with moderate-to-severe depression revealed increased perfusion in the right hippocampus and left cerebellum. Ji et al. showed that patients with bipolar depression had increased perfusion in the bilateral basal ganglia, which they speculated may be physiological basis for manic episodes in bipolar depression. Monkul et al. showed that patients with depression had increased perfusion in the right ACC, bilateral PCC, left parahippocampal gyrus, and right caudate nucleus. Furthermore, they found that the severity of depression was negatively correlated with CBF in the left middle and frontal gyri, right medial frontal gyrus, and right ACC, but positively correlated with CBF in the right thalamus. As such, their results support the presence of abnormalities in the resting-state CBF in the cortical pathways of the limbic system. Their study also found that anxiety in patients with depression was positively correlated with CBF in the bilateral PCC and inferior parietal lobule, whereas depressed mood was negatively correlated with CBF in the left dorsolateral PFC and left angular gyrus. Fu et al. performed ASL and ^{18}F-fluorodeoxyglucose (^{18}F-FDG) PET/CT on patients with MDD to examine the functional changes of CBF and glucose metabolism in the PFC. Their results revealed reductions in the CBF and standardized uptake value (SUV) of the PFC (Figs. 14.6 and 14.7), which were closely associated with patients' depressive symptoms. Therefore, the PFC may be a key functional region in severe depression, and ^{18}F-FDG PET/CT was found to be more sensitive than ASL at identifying functional abnormalities in the PFC. Additionally, other PET imaging studies have shown hypoperfusion in the cerebellum and thalamus of patients with depression. Therefore, it has been speculated that the cerebellum is involved in the recognition and expression of negative emotions, whereas long-term severe depression may affect the cerebellum by damaging the functional connections between the cerebellum and frontal lobe. Nevertheless, there is currently no data to verify whether cerebellar hypoperfusion is a risk factor for depression or a consequence resulting from the progression of depression.

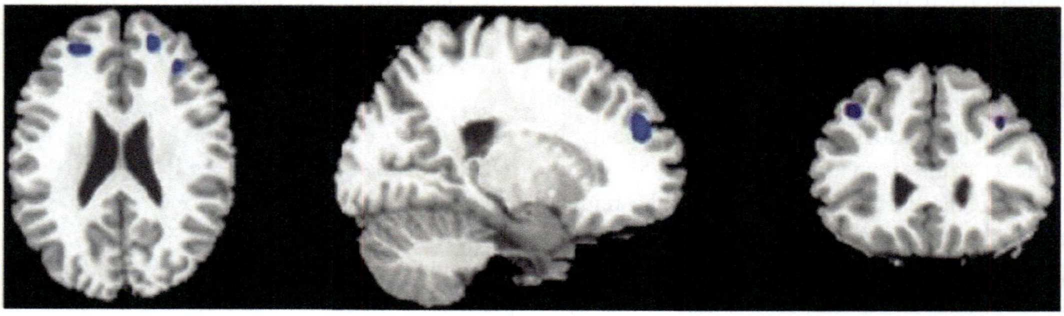

Fig. 14.6 Schematic diagram of areas of the brain with abnormal rCBF in patients with first-episode depression. Decreased rCBF (blue regions) in the left middle frontal gyrus, and right superior and middle frontal gyri of the experimental group (18 patients with first-episode depression) compared to the control group (17 subjects)

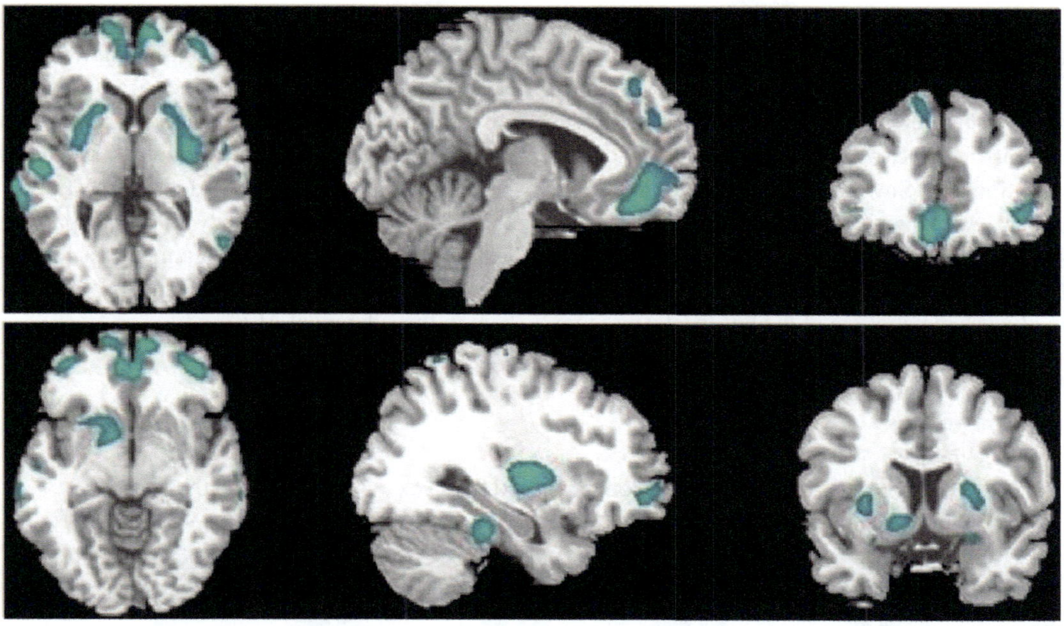

Fig. 14.7 Schematic diagram of areas of the brain with abnormal regional glucose metabolism in patients with first-episode depression. Decreased ^{18}F-FDG metabolism (green regions) in the bilateral superior, middle, and inferior frontal gyri, bilateral superior and middle temporal gyri, bilateral lentiform nuclei, caudate nucleus, left globus pallidus, and bilateral ACC of the experimental group (18 patients with first-episode depression) compared to the control group (17 subjects)

14.2.2 Research on Brain Metabolic Imaging

14.2.2.1 Research on Brain Glucose Metabolic Imaging

Glucose is virtually the only source of energy for brain tissues, and extensive abnormalities in brain glucose metabolism can be detected in patients with depression. ^{18}F-FDG is a classic imaging agent for carbohydrate metabolism which can enter the cell via glucose transporters on the cell membrane. Me-4^{18}FDG is a novel imaging agent for glucose metabolism which can enter the cell via sodium–glucose cotransporters (SLGTs) on tumor cell membrane. Drevets et al. found that treatment-naïve patients with depression exhibited increased glucose metabolism in the bilateral OFC, bilateral ventral frontal lobe, left amygdala, and PCC; decreased glucose metabolism in the subgenual PFC, and anterior and middle dorsolateral PFC; as well as a negative correlation between glucose metabolism in the left dorsolateral PFC and HAM-D scores.

In recent years, some researchers have performed PET imaging to study the changes in brain glucose metabolism before and after treatment with antidepressants. Smith et al. found that patients with MDD treated with citalopram showed decreased glucose metabolism in the anterior cortical regions and increased glucose metabolism in the posterior cortical regions, while these changes were associated with clinical improvements after oral drug administration. By combining PET with HAM-D scores, Kreuzer et al. assessed the relationship between the pre-to post-treatment changes in regional brain glucose metabolism and therapeutic efficacy in RDD patients treated with rTMS. They found that increased regional glucose metabolism of the left dorsal PFC and ACC generally indicated better clinical efficacy. Wu et al. utilized PET imaging to observe the CMRGlc of patients with depression before and after treatment with sertraline for one week. Their results revealed that improvements in depressive symptoms were related to regional CMRGlc decrease in the inferior frontal gyrus and OFC, as well as regional CMRGlc increase in the dorsolateral PFC (Fig. 14.8). Additionally, Suwa et al. reported that RDD patients who received electroconvulsive therapy showed increased glucose metabolism in the left frontal and temporal lobes, whereas the decrease in glucose metabolism of the left frontal and temporal lobes was associated with the increase in glucose metabolism of the right medial temporal lobe. In the study by McGrath et al., insula glucose metabolism was identified as a potential biomarker for treatment evaluation that can guide initial treatment decisions in depression. Baeken et al. applied high-frequency rTMS in patients with RDD and found that treatment responders showed significantly decreased glucose metabolism in the subgenual ACC.

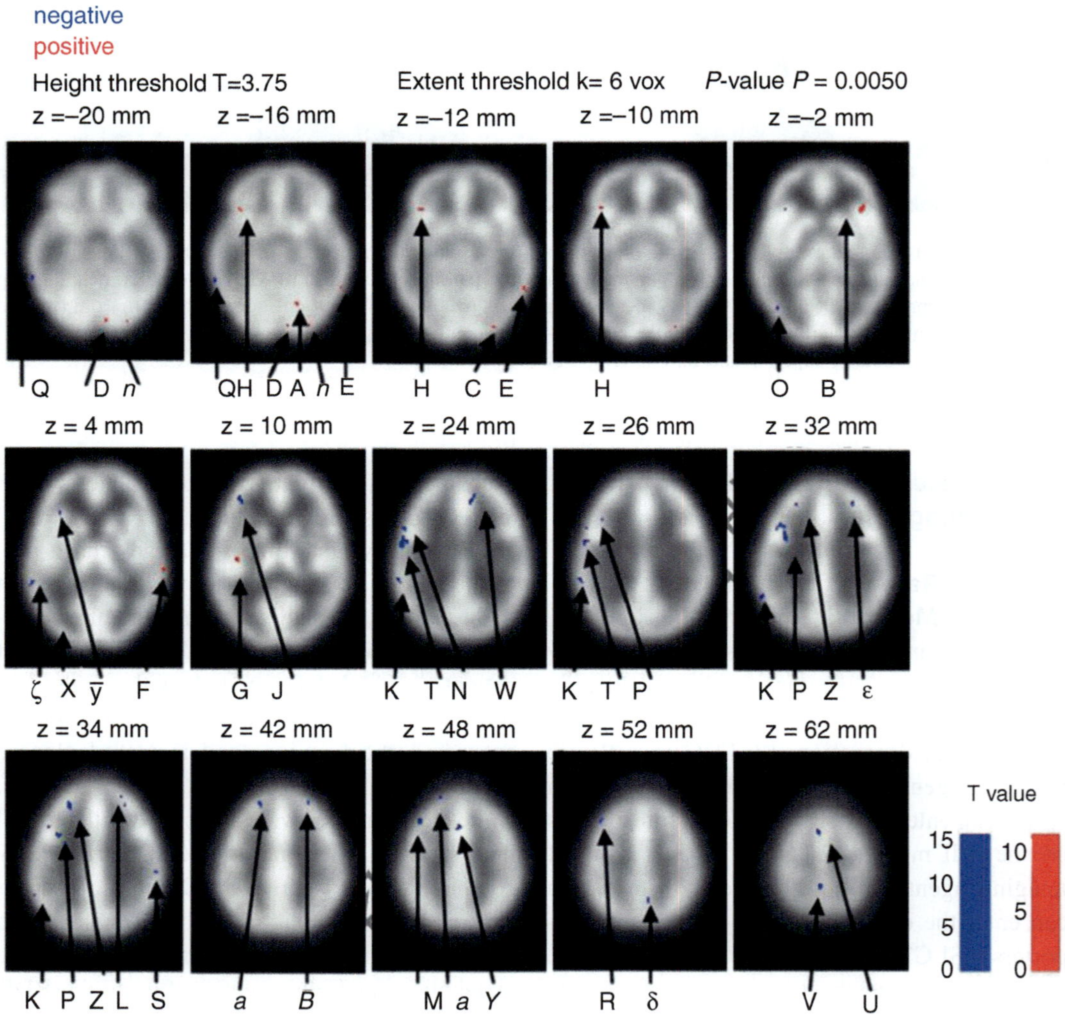

Fig. 14.8 Distribution of brain areas with changes in glucose metabolism after total sleep deprivation (TSD) (Reproduced with permission from WU J C, GILLIN J C, BUCHSBAUM M S, et al. Sleep deprivation PET correlations of Hamilton symptom improvement ratings with changes in relative glucose metabolism in patients with depression. J Affect Disord, 2008, 107(1–3):181–186). Hypometabolic brain regions are located in the inferior frontal gyrus and inferior frontal/orbitofrontal cortex; hypermetabolic regions are located in the dorsolateral prefrontal cortex

14.2.2.2 Research on Brain Oxygen Metabolic Imaging

Ottowitz et al. utilized PET imaging to study the memory processing of patients with depression. Their results indicated that during verbal learning, patients showed elevated oxygen metabolism in the right cingulate gyrus, left ventral PFC, bilateral hippocampus, and left OFC. Moreover, oxygen metabolism of the right ACC was associated with semantic organization, whereas that of the left PFC was related to semantic processing.

14.2.3 Research on Neurotransmitter Receptor Imaging

The pathogenesis of depression is currently still poorly understood. At present, the more widely accepted hypotheses of depression include the monoamine hypothesis and receptor hypothesis of depression. The rapid advancement of neuroreceptor imaging in recent years has permitted the application of 5-hydroxytryptamine (5-HT) transporter (5-HTT), dopamine transporter (DAT), and dopamine receptor imaging techniques in research on the etiological diagnosis and treatment of depression.

14.2.3.1 Research on 5-HT Receptor Imaging

5-HT receptors are associated with a wide range of psychiatric diseases and are key targets of relevant drugs. 5-HT receptors are distributed in the amygdala, central thalamus, caudate nucleus, frontal cortex, occipital cortex, and spinal cord, where they are involved in the regulation of learning, cognition, memory, and motor functions.

5-HT_1A receptors are predominantly expressed at the presynaptic membrane of the raphe nucleus in the brainstem and play a crucial role in treatments for depression. Kaufman et al. performed PET brain imaging using ^{11}C-WAY-100635 (a selective 5-HT_1A receptor antagonist) as an imaging agent for the quantification of 5-HT_1A receptor binding. They found that the ^{11}C-WAY-100635 binding potential of male MDD patients was 67% higher across 13 brain regions than male controls, with the greatest difference appearing in the raphe nucleus. Savitz et al. concluded that patients with depression had decreased 5-HT_1A receptor activity in the medial temporal lobe and limbic regions, which was affected by the level of glucocorticoids; whereas different subregions of the raphe nucleus may exhibit differences in 5-HT_1A receptor binding activity. Furthermore, Boldrini et al. demonstrated enhanced 5-HT_1A receptor activity in the rostral, ventrolateral, and dorsal raphe nucleus, whereas the caudal raphe nucleus showed diminished 5-HT_1A receptor activity.

Pillai et al. further observed the subregional differences of 5-HT_1A receptor binding in the raphe nucleus, which revealed that patients with depression had elevated 5-HT_1A receptor binding in the dorsal raphe nucleus, while 5-HT_1A receptor binding in the dorsal and median raphe nuclei produced a better diagnostic performance than the raphe nucleus as a whole. 5-HT_2A receptors are distributed in human brain tissues, with the highest density in the frontal and temporal lobes, followed by the basal ganglia, parietal lobe, precentral gyrus, and thalamus. Common PET imaging agents for 5-HT_2A receptors include ^{18}F-altanserin, ^{11}C-MDL, ^{18}F-FESP, and ^{18}F-setoperone. ^{18}F-FESP and ^{18}F-setoperone can bind simultaneously with dopamine (DA) receptors. Although current 5-HT_2A receptor PET imaging has shown reduced 5-HT_2A receptor activity in patients with depression, these findings are inconsistent with some prospective clinical studies suggesting that receptor activity may be upregulated. Savitz et al. believe that such contradictory conclusions may have resulted from the interference of antidepressant treatments. Furthermore, the variability of behavioral impairments among patients with depression may also have led to differences in PET imaging.

5-HT_1B receptors are mainly distributed in the basal ganglia. Murrough et al. found reduced 5-HT_1B receptor activity in the ventral striatum of treatment-naïve patients with depression (Fig. 14.9). Additionally, Anisman et al. revealed reduced expression of 5-HT_1B receptors in the PFC, lateral OFC, and hippocampus in suicide survivors with depression. 5-HTT is a mono-

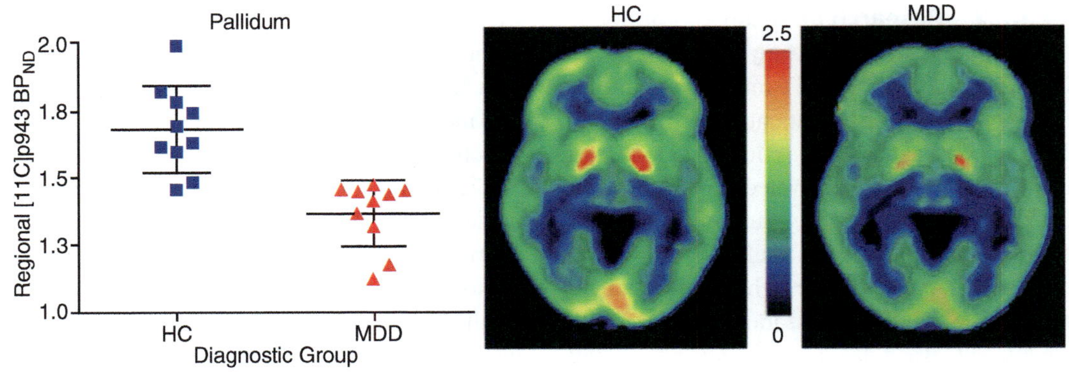

Fig. 14.9 Abnormal reduction of ventral striatum 5-HT_1B function in MDD patients compared to healthy controls (Reproduced with permission from). Regional [^{11}C]p943 BP_{ND}: regional non-displaceable binding potential of ^{11}C-labelled p943

amine transporter that regulates neurotransmission via the removal of 5-HT in the extracellular fluid. It is mainly expressed by serotonergic neurons and plays a critical role in the pathophysiological processes of depression. Research has shown that 5-HTT receptor activity is affected by factors such as the type of imaging agent, season, and body weight. Common 5-HTT imaging agents include ^{11}C-(+)McN5652 and ^{11}C-DASB. Lanzenberger et al. observed that the 5-HTT binding of the median raphe nucleus was more effective at predicting therapeutic efficacy than 5-HTT binding of the amygdala–hippocampus complex, habenula, and subgenual cingulate cortex, which indicates that 5-HTT binding in the median raphe nucleus can be used to predict treatment response. Furthermore, Miller et al. found that patients with severe depression had lower 5-HTT activity than patients with mild depression and healthy controls, suggesting that 5-HTT activity can predict the severity of depression.

14.2.3.2 Research on DA Receptor Imaging

DA receptors are mainly distributed on the dopaminergic pathways of the central nervous system and are involved in the regulation of movement, learning, and memory. By utilizing a PET image database acquired using a highly selective radiotracer, ^{11}C-PE2I, Dubol et al. assessed the striatal and extra-striatal DAT availability of 8 patients treated for depression (compared to 24 healthy controls) and found that reduced presynaptic dopamine function plays a role in the pathophysiology of depression, indicating that extra-striatal dopamine function should be further investigated.

DA1 receptors are primarily distributed in the striatum, nucleus accumbens, optic tract, PFC, precentral gyrus, cingulate gyrus, hippocampus, and amygdala. Common PET imaging agents that are currently used for DA1 receptors include ^{11}C-SCH23390 and ^{11}C-NNC-112. A PET imaging study by Cannon et al. revealed a 14% reduction in DA1 receptor activity in the body of the left caudate nucleus among patients with depression. Additionally, Dougherty et al. found that striatal DA1 receptor activity decreased by 13% when patients with depression experienced anger.

DA2 receptors are predominantly distributed in the striatum. Common PET imaging agents for DA2 receptors include ^{11}C-raclopride (^{11}C-RAC), ^{18}F-fallypride, and ^{11}C-FLB-457 (targeting DA2/DA3 receptors), and ^{11}C-NMSP (targeting DA2/DA4 receptors). By combining PET/CT with HAM-D scores, Sun et al. demonstrated that the decrease in striatal DA2 non-displaceable binding potential (BPND) in patients with first-episode depression was correlated with their depressive symptoms (Fig. 14.10). Their findings, therefore, suggested that abnormalities in

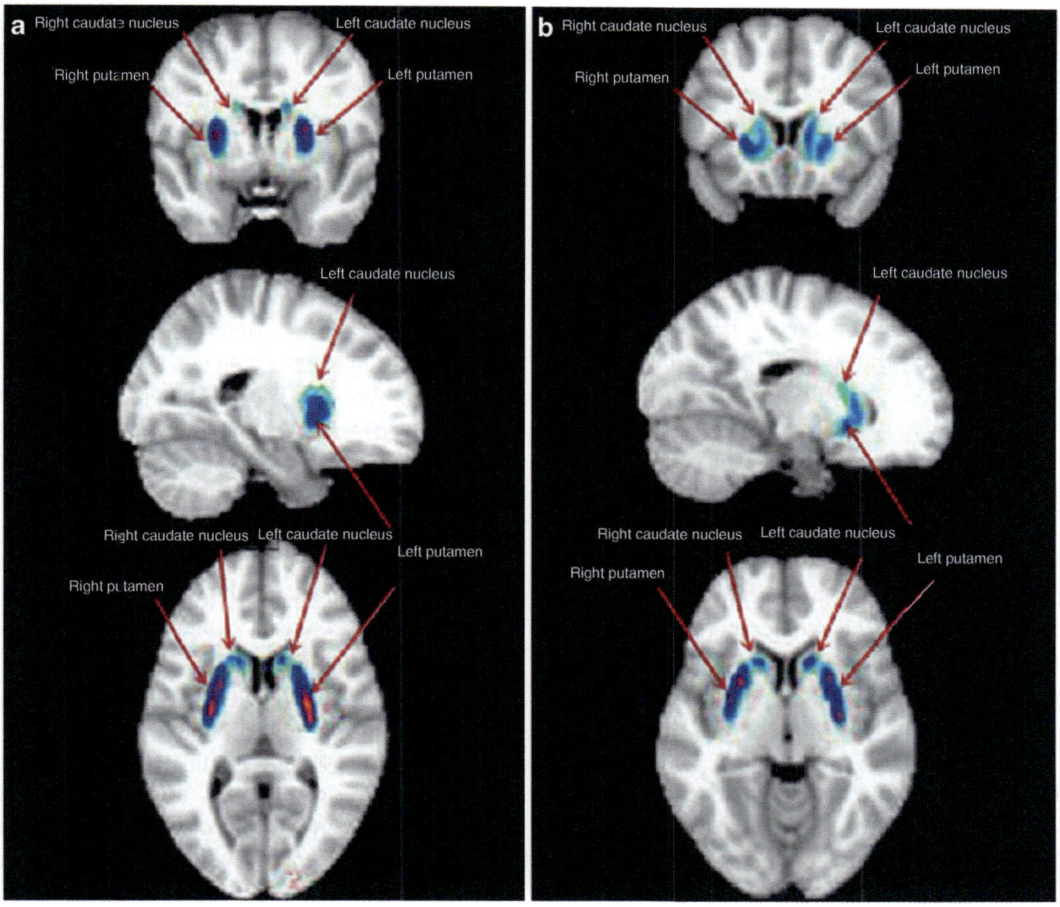

Fig. 14.10 Striatal distribution of ^{11}C-raclopride in the experimental (patients with first-episode depression) and control groups (Reproduced with permission from). Decreased D_2 binding potential in the caudate nucleus and putamen of the experimental group. Coronal, sagittal, and transverse images of average striatal ^{11}C-raclopride binding potential in 20 healthy controls (**a**) and 20 patients with depression (**b**)

the striatal dopamine receptors of patients with depression may be one of the key molecular mechanisms underlying the midbrain dopamine reward circuitry. The PET study by Meyer et al. revealed elevated DA2/DA3 receptor activity in the bilateral insula of patients with depression. Pecina et al. showed that the abnormal elevation of DA2/DA3 receptors in the ventral striatum of MDD patients may be related to the comorbidity of anxiety and depression, or the lack of antidepressant treatment. Saijo et al. observed the efficacy of electroconvulsive therapy in patients with drug-resistant MDD and found no statistically significant difference in D2 receptor binding between MDD patients and healthy controls. Following electroconvulsive therapy, however, MDD patients showed a 25.2% reduction in D2 receptor binding of the right ACC, which suggests that the biological mechanism of electroconvulsive therapy may be related to the dopaminergic system.

DAT PET studies have revealed that alterations in patients with depression occur predominantly in the striatum. Common PET imaging agents for DAT include ^{11}C-CFT and ^{11}C-RTI-32. Meyer et al. demonstrated a 14% decrease in DAT activity among treatment-naïve patients with depression. Furthermore, the PET study by Conway et al. also found reduced DAT activity in the striatum of patients with depression.

14.2.3.3 Research on Norepinephrine Transporter Imaging

Norepinephrine transporters have now become common therapeutic targets in depression. For example, in clinical settings, dual-target drugs, such as venlafaxine, and milnacipran, that target norepinephrine transporters can relieve symptoms more effectively. Moriguchi et al. conducted a PET study on MDD patients and healthy controls, which revealed higher BPND values for norepinephrine transporters in the thalamus of MDD patients, especially in the thalamic subregion anatomically connected to the PFC. These findings suggest antidepressants with a high binding affinity to norepinephrine transporters have an immense potential for the treatment of MDD patients. Remy et al. showed decreased norepinephrine transporter activity in the limbic system of PD patients with comorbid depression, which implies that the occurrence of depression in PD patients is related to impairments in the norepinephrinergic system.

14.2.3.4 Research on Metabotropic Glutamate Receptor (mGluR) Imaging

Glutamate signaling plays a crucial role in the process of emotional regulation, and patients with depression exhibit lower levels of glutamate and glutamine in the brain. Type 5 mGluR (mGluR5) is a targeted glutamate receptor present on the surfaces of and intracellularly in neurons. Ketamine has a rapid antidepressant effect, and its mechanisms include promoting glutamatergic neurotransmission in the PFC. By performing PET imaging, Li et al. found that increased SUV in the PFC was related to treatment with low-dose ketamine, and to the rapid antidepressant effect on the first day of low-dose ketamine. Using PET imaging, Esterlis et al. observed that ketamine could induce a glutamate surge, which led to a decrease in mGluR5 availability in the process, in turn relieving symptoms of anxiety.

14.2.3.5 Other Imaging Research

By utilizing PET imaging, Meyer et al. found a general increase in the activity monoamine oxidase A (MAO-A) across all brain regions in patients with depression, while patients who later underwent recurrence had significantly higher MAO-A activity in the PFC and ACC. These findings indicate that elevated MAO-A activity could serve as one of the characteristic indicators of depression.

14.2.4 Summary

PET imaging has provided some clues for exploring depression response and therapeutic efficacy among patients with depression. Not only does this technique enable the observation of brain perfusion and metabolism at different stages of depression, but also permits the detection of neurotransmitters. Therefore, it can provide objective evidence for the etiological investigation, pathological mechanism, clinical diagnosis, individualized treatment decisions, and prevention of depression, as well as facilitate the research and development of novel antidepressants. At present, one of the more consistent conclusions drawn from current research is the hypothesis on the dysfunction of cortico-limbic circuitry, while the efficacy of antidepressant therapies may be related to whether the abnormal functional activities of the cortico-limbic circuitry can be altered. The basal metabolic activity of the brain in patients with depression may be useful for predicting and evaluating treatment response in depression. However, it is difficult to draw reliable conclusions due to the limitations of factors such as sample size and sample selection. At present, there is a lack of consensus among PET imaging studies on depression owing to a number of factors, including experimental conditions, research methods, and imaging agents, among others. Furthermore, these studies are relatively limited in scope, with the majority focusing on the cortico-limbic system, and fewer on other brain structures. Therefore, future studies on depression will need to expand their sample sizes and conduct more detailed investigations on the biological mechanisms of antidepressant treatments and brain functions, so as to provide guidance for the targeted treatment of depression in clinical practice.

14.3 Research Applications of PET/MR in Depression

Depression is one of the most common mental illnesses in the world. It is chiefly characterized by persistent low mood and anhedonia, sometimes even giving rise to extreme thoughts of self-harm, suicide, or hurting others. Due to the high suicide and disability rates of depression, it places an enormous economic and mental burden on patients, their families, and society as a whole. Our current understanding on depression is still relatively incomplete, and clinicians mainly rely on scales and experience to reach a diagnosis, which is somewhat subjective. In the first two sections, we introduced current research on MRI and PET in depression, which is of significant value to investigating the pathogenic mechanisms and early clinical diagnosis of depression. MRI and PET are both key techniques for understanding and exploring the pathogenic mechanisms of depression. Integrated PET/MR involves performing simultaneous scanning, so as to synchronously acquire anatomical, functional, blood flow, metabolic, and other imaging information from patients with depression under the same physiological state within a single session. This integration of multiparametric imaging data plays an important role in the further, in-depth investigation on the pathogenic mechanisms and pathophysiological changes of depression.

14.3.1 Research Advances of Integrated PET/MR in Depression

There are as yet no published studies related to depression based on integrated PET/MR techniques, and most PET/MR studies on depression involve combining MRI with PET/CT data acquired using different scanners. ^{18}F-FDG is currently the most commonly used radiotracer in clinical practice. ^{18}F-FDG PET imaging reflects the neuronal activity of different brain areas through the uptake of ^{18}F-FDG, whereas fMRI involves the analysis of BOLD signals to reveal the neuronal synchrony among different brain areas. Through the combined application of resting-state ^{18}F-FDG PET/CT and fMRI, researchers have examined the characteristics of changes in glucose metabolism and brain networks in patients with first-episode depression. They found that hypometabolic regions were mainly located in the frontal lobe, while brain areas with reduced functional network connectivity were also found in the frontal lobe. Moreover, the metabolic reductions of the bilateral superior, middle, and inferior frontal gyrus were significantly correlated with resting-state brain network abnormalities. Their findings, therefore, have confirmed that reduced frontal lobe function may be the basis for the onset of depression. On the basis of these results, researchers have further examined the correlations among PFC blood flow, metabolism, and clinical symptoms in patients with depression. More specifically, ASL and ^{18}F-FDG PET/CT were performed to assess the PFC blood flow and metabolic parameters of 17 patients with first-episode depression, which were then combined with their clinical symptoms. The results revealed a relative concordance between the glucose metabolism and blood flow alterations in the PFC of patients with depression, which were both closely associated with clinical symptoms. The left middle frontal gyrus was especially noteworthy and may be the core area of functional impairment in the PFC of patients with depression.

Functional abnormalities in the midbrain-striatum dopaminergic reward circuit may be one of the key molecular mechanisms underlying the onset of depression. Researchers at the Henan Provincial People's Hospital combined structural MRI and ^{11}C-RAC PET/CT, which were acquired using separate scanners, for the analysis of 20 patients with first-episode depression. Their results revealed significantly decreased tracer uptake in the bilateral caudate nucleus and putamen of patients with depression, while the degree of reduction was correlated with the values of factors such as clinical scores, anxiety or somatization, cognitive impairment, psychomotor retardation, and sleep disorders. This implies that abnormalities of striatal dopamine receptors may be a crucial pathogenic mechanism of depression.

Other researchers have also performed a prospective multimodal ^{11}C-RAC PET/CT and BOLD-fMRI study on patients with first-episode depression, in order to observe alterations in their striatal D2 receptor binding potential and brain functional networks. They found that patients with depression in the resting state exhibited reduced D2 receptor binding and increased brain network connectivity, signifying that changes in dopamine neurotransmission may be an important neuropathological basis for the core symptoms (emotional deficits) of depression. Furthermore, the increased network connectivity of the bilateral medial PFC in patients with depression was also shown to be negatively correlated with the D2 receptor binding potential of the ipsilateral striatum, which indicates the potential presence of abnormal regulation exerted by the PFC on the striatal dopamine circuit via the cortico-limbic pathways.

MRS and PET are generally used to detect different compounds, and it is therefore usually not possible to compare MRS and PET findings. Nevertheless, there is a common compound that can be examined using both techniques, namely, GABA, which plays a critical role in the pathophysiology of depression. Both MRS and PET findings have shown that patients with depression have lower levels of GABA compared to healthy controls, but in different brain areas. More specifically, the decreases in GABA as measured by MRS are mainly found in the occipital cortex, where those detected by PET primarily occur in the parahippocampal and temporal regions. However, to the best of our knowledge, there is only one small-sample study on the PET imaging of GABA. Although there are more MRS studies on GABA, the exact role of GABA in depression remains inconclusive, requiring further investigations and replications.

14.3.2 Research Advantages of Integrated PET/MR in Depression

Multimodal imaging involves the simultaneous acquisition of multiple parameters. The mutual complementation between the quantitative PET values of biological parameters and high-resolution MRI information will help to us gain a multi-perspective understanding of changes in the brain with respect to structure, function, and other aspects. The acquisition of multimodal imaging data from individual subjects has recently been applied to research on neurological diseases. Data analysis in studies on depression mostly involves conducting separate analyses on individual modalities before performing comparisons. However, due to the complexity and variability of neurological diseases, the results obtained through unimodal analysis may exhibit large dispersity and may not accurately reflect the covariance between different modalities. Therefore, the combination of high-sensitivity and high-resolution imaging modalities with dynamic acquisition procedures offers additional advantages that are highly appealing to clinical and research applications. On the basis of unimodal imaging, integrated PET/MR effectively addresses the limited spatial resolution of PET in order to obtain more precise PET signals, thereby achieving the further integration of multimodal information for the diagnosis of central nervous system diseases. Integrated PET/MR has recently been utilized in the detection and staging of gliomas, as well as the localization of critical functional areas adjacent to the tumor, which has crucial implications for surgical planning. PET/MR also has clinical value in detecting surgically resectable epileptic foci, as well as the identification of metabolic activity, neurotransmitter concentration, and enzymatic expression in cerebellar structures. In early- and late-stage cerebral ischemia, the co-registration of MRI with regional values of CBF, oxygen utilization, and glucose metabolism can be used to discriminate areas of irreversible damage from functionally impaired but morphologically preserved areas, thereby influencing therapeutic strategies. Additionally, longitudinal follow-up is of great significance to research on depression, while PET/MR involves a lower radiation dose compared to PET/CT, and is therefore more suitable for repeated scanning and long-term follow-up.

The research experiences above can serve as a basis for future integrated PET/MR studies on depression. Integrated PET/MR has immense potential in neuroscientific research, especially in the multiparametric analysis of complex neural network functions, the imaging of complex molecular processes in gene transfer and cellular transplantation, and the translation of novel therapeutic strategies from preclinical research to clinical applications. PET/MR has been utilized in the scientific and clinical research of neurodegenerative diseases, epilepsy, cerebrovascular disease, tumors, and other diseases. Combining the high resolution of MRI with the specific and targeted binding of biological compounds in PET imaging has had significant implications for enhancing the diagnostic accuracy and sensitivity of depression, as well as for investigating the pathophysiological mechanisms of depression. We believe that integrated PET/MR techniques will bring about more in-depth research findings on depression in the near future.

Suggested Reading

Anand A, Li Y, Wang Y, et al. Activity and connectivity of brain mood regulating circuit in depression: a functional magnetic resonance study. Biol Psychiatry. 2005;57(10):1079–88.

Baeken C, Marinazzo D, Everaert H, et al. The impact of accelerated HF-rTMS on the subgenual anterior cingulate cortex in refractory unipolar major depression: insights from ^{18}F-FDG PET brain imaging. Brain Stimul. 2015;8(4):808–15.

Boldrini M, Underwood MD, Mann J, et al. Serotonin-1A autoreceptor binding in the dorsal raphe nucleus of depressed suicides. J Psychiatr Res. 2008;42(6):433–42.

Bouckaert FM, De Winter FM, Vandenbulcke MP, et al. Grey matter volume increase following electroconvulsive therapy in patients with late life depression: a longitudinal MRI study. J Psychiatry Neurosci. 2016;41(2):105–14.

Bracht T, Linden D, Keedwell P. A review of white matter microstructure alterations of pathways of the reward circuit in depression. J Affect Disord. 2015;187:45–53.

Conway CR, Chibnall JT, Cumming P, et al. Antidepressant response to aripiprazole augmentation associated with enhanced FDOPA utilization in striatum: a preliminary PET study. Psychiatry Res. 2014;221(3):231–9.

Dou S, Fu C, Xuan A, et al. Relationship between cerebral glucose metabolism and brain functional regional homogeneity in patients with first-episode depression. Chin J Nucl Med Mol Imaging. 2015;35(1):27–31.

Esterlis I, Dellagioia N, Pietrzak RH, et al. Ketamine-induced reduction in mGluR5 availability is associated with an antidepressant response: an [^{11}C]ABP688 and PET imaging study in depression. Mol Psychiatry. 2018;23(4):824–32.

Fu C, Shi D, Gao Y, et al. Functional assessment of prefrontal lobes in patients with major depression disorder using a dual-mode technique of 3D-arterial spin labeling and 18F-fluorodeoxyglucose positron emission tomography/computed tomography. Exp Ther Med. 2017;14(2):1058–64.

Fu C, Zhang H, Shi D, et al. Changes in the resting-state glucose metabolism and perfusion of the prefrontal cortex in first-episode depression, and their correlation with clinical symptoms. Chin Med J. 2015;95(37):3017–22.

Iwabuchi SJ, Krishnadas R, Li C, et al. Localized connectivity in depression: a meta-analysis of resting state functional imaging studies. Neurosci Biobehav Rev. 2015;51:77–86.

Ji E, Guang N, Wang H, et al. Correlation of cerebral perfusion characteristics and cognitive function in patients with unipolar and bipolar depression. Chin J Behav Med Brain Sci. 2011;20(4):330–2.

Kaufman J, Sullivan GM, Yang J, et al. Quantification of the serotonin 1A receptor using PET: identification of a potential biomarker of major depression in males. Neuropsychopharmacology. 2015;40(7):1692–9.

Kreuzer PM, Lehner A, Schlee W, et al. Combined rTMS treatment targeting the anterior cingulate and the temporal cortex for the treatment of chronic tinnitus. Sci Rep. 2015;5:18028.

Lanzenberger R, Kranz GS, Haeusler D, et al. Prediction of SSRI treatment response in major depression based on serotonin transporter interplay between median raphe nucleus and projection areas. Neuroimage. 2012;63(2):874–81.

Liu Y, Du L, Li YM, et al. Antidepressant effects of electroconvulsive therapy correlate with subgenual anterior cingulate activity and connectivity in depression. Medicine. 2015;94(45):e2033.

Liu J, Fang J, Wang Z, et al. Transcutaneous vagus nerve stimulation modulates amygdala functional connectivity in patients with depression. J Affect Disord. 2016;205:319–26.

Malhi GS, Lagopoulos J, Ward PB, et al. Cognitive generation of affect in bipolar depression: an fMRI study. Eur J Neurosci. 2004;19(3):741–54.

Mcgrath CL, Kelley ME, Holtzheimer PE, et al. Toward a neuroimaging treatment selection biomarker for major depressive disorder. JAMA Psychiatry. 2013;70(8):821–9.

Meyer JH, Wilson A, Sagrati S, et al. Brain monoamine oxidase A binding in major depressive disorder: relationship to selective serotonin reuptake inhibitor treatment, recovery, and recurrence. Arch Gen Psychiatry. 2009;66(12):1304–12.

Miller JM, Hesselgrave N, Ogden RT, et al. Positron emission tomography quantification of serotonin transporter in suicide attempters with major depressive disorder. Biol Psychiatry. 2013;74(4):287–95.

Monkul ES, Silva LA, Narayana S, et al. Abnormal resting state corticolimbic blood flow in depressed unmedicated patients with major depression: a $^{15}O-H_2O$ PET study. Hum Brain Mapp. 2012;33(2):272–9.

Moriguchi S, Yamada M, Takano H, et al. Norepinephrine transporter in major depressive disorder: a PET study. Am J Psychiatry. 2017;174(1):36–41.

Murrough JW, Henry S, Hu J, et al. Reduced ventral striatal/ventral pallidal serotonin1B receptor binding potential in major depressive disorder. Psychopharmacology (Berl). 2011;213(2–3):547–53.

Ottowitz WE, Deckersbach T, Savage CR, et al. Neural correlates of strategic processes underlying episodic memory in women with major depression: a ^{15}O-PET study. J Neuropsychiatry Clin Neurosci. 2010;22(2):218–30.

Perrin JS, Merz S, Bennett DM, et al. Electroconvulsive therapy reduces frontal cortical connectivity in severe depressive disorder. Proc Natl Acad Sci USA. 2012;109(14):5464–8.

Pillai RLI, Zhang M, Yang J, et al. Will imaging individual raphe nuclei in males with major depressive disorder enhance diagnostic sensitivity and specificity? Depress Anxiety. 2018;35(5):411–20.

Redlich R, Bürger C, Dohm K, et al. Effects of electroconvulsive therapy on amygdala function in major depression-a longitudinal functional magnetic resonance imaging study. Psychol Med. 2017;47(12):2166–76.

Renner F, Derubeis R, Arntz A, et al. Exploring mechanisms of change in schema therapy for chronic depression. J Behav Ther Exp Psychiatry. 2018;58:97–105.

Savitz JB, Drevets WC. Neuroreceptor imaging in depression. Neurobiol Dis. 2013;52:49–65.

Savitz J, Nugent AC, Cannon DM, et al. Effects of arterial cannulation stress on regional cerebral blood flow in major depressive disorder. Sci Rep. 2012;2:308.

Schmaal L, Hibar DP, Sämann PG, et al. Cortical abnormalities in adults and adolescents with major depression based on brain scans from 20 cohorts worldwide in the ENIGMA Major Depressive Disorder Working Group. Mol Psychiatry. 2017;226(6):900–9.

Singh MK, Leslie SM, Bhattacharjee K, et al. Vulnerabilities in sequencing and task switching in healthy youth offspring of parents with mood disorders. J Clin Exp Neuropsychol. 2018;40(6):606–18.

Smith SM, Fox PT, Miller KL, et al. Correspondence of the brain's functional architecture during activation and rest. Proc Natl Acad Sci U S A. 2009;106(31):13040–5.

Smith GS, Workman CI, Kramer E, et al. The relationship between the acute cerebral metabolic response to citalopram and chronic citalopram treatment outcome. Am J Geriatr Psychiatry. 2011;19(1):53–63.

Sun M, Xuan A, Fu C, et al. Correlation between striatal dopamine D2 receptor non-displaceable binding potential and functional connectivity. Chin Med J. 2020;100(15):1159–63.

Sun M, Zhang H, Xuan A, et al. Non-displaceable binding potential changes of striatal dopamine D2 receptors in patients with first-episode major depressive disorder and their correlation with clinical features. Chin J Nucl Med Mol Imaging. 2017;37(9):532–7.

Szczepanik J, Nugent A, Drevets WC, et al. Amygdala response to explicit sad face stimuli at baseline predicts antidepressant treatment response to scopolamine in major depressive disorder. Psychiatry Res Neuroimaging. 2016;254:67–73.

Videbech P, Ravnkilde B, Pedersen AR, et al. The Danish PET/depression project: PET findings in patients with major depression. Psychol Med. 2001;31(7):1147–58.

Wang L, Xia M, Li K, et al. The effects of antidepressant treatment on resting-state functional brain networks in patients with major depressive disorder. Hum Brain Mapp. 2015;362(2):768–78.

Xia M, Si T, Sun X, et al. Reproducibility of functional brain alterations in major depressive disorder: evidence from a multisite resting-state functional MRI study with 1, 434 individuals. Neuroimage. 2019;189:700–14.

Xia M, Womer FY, Chang M, et al. Shared and distinct functional architectures of brain networks across psychiatric disorders. Schizophr Bull. 2019;452(2):450–63.

Zhang J, Sun M, Xuang A, et al. Multimodal imaging study of striatal dopamine D2 receptor binding potential and brain regional homogeneity in patients with first-episode major depressive disorder. Chin J Radiol. 2018;52(7):495–501.

Zhang J, Wang J, Wu Q, et al. Disrupted brain connectivity networks in drug-naive, first-episode major depressive disorder. Biol Psychiatry. 2011;704(4):334–42.

15 Research Applications of Positron Emission Tomography/Magnetic Resonance (PET/MR) Imaging in Schizophrenia

Li Sun, Zhi Wang, and Jiliang Fang

Schizophrenia is a severe, chronic mental illness, which is primarily characterized by hallucinations and delusions, a blunted affect, and cognitive difficulties. Schizophrenia has a strong genetic predisposition, and symptoms usually appear at approximately 16–30 years of age. Although its incidence in the general population is only 1%, if one in a pair of identical twins is affected, then the risk of schizophrenia for the other twin increases to 50%.

Since it was first described by Kraepelin and Bleuler, researchers have believed that schizophrenia is intimately associated with neural abnormalities, a relationship which has been explored for hundreds of years. In 1976, Johnstone et al. performed computed tomography (CT) on patients with schizophrenia and found evidence of enlargement of the lateral ventricles, thereby introducing a new direction of neuroscientific research on schizophrenia. Since that discovery, substantial progress has been made in the neuroimaging research of schizophrenia, especially with the advent and ongoing development of MRI techniques, which has opened a new chapter in the neuroscientific research on schizophrenia.

L. Sun · Z. Wang · J. Fang (✉)
Department of Radiology, Guang'anmen Hospital, China Academy of Chinese Medical Science, Beijing, China

15.1 Research Applications of MRI in Schizophrenia

The ongoing creation and improvement of advanced scan sequences and post-processing techniques have enabled researchers to utilize MRI for the non-invasive evaluation of structural, functional, and neurochemical changes in the human brain. These techniques have been extensively applied to research on the pathophysiological mechanisms of depression, dementia, and other neurological diseases and have played an especially prominent role in promoting the progress of research on the neural mechanisms of schizophrenia. Therefore, in this section, we will discuss the advances of neuroimaging techniques, such as structural MRI (sMRI), diffusion tensor imaging (DTI), functional MRI (fMRI), and magnetic resonance spectroscopy (MRS), as they apply to research in schizophrenia.

15.1.1 Neurostructural Research in Schizophrenia

A large number of cross-sectional neuroimaging studies on schizophrenia have demonstrated neurostructural changes in patients, primarily manifesting as decreased brain tissue and increased cerebrospinal fluid volumes, both of which are most prominent in the frontal lobe. Nevertheless, there is an ongoing debate regarding the

J. Lu, G. Zhao (eds.), *PET/MR: Functional and Molecular Imaging of Neurological Diseases and Neurosciences*, https://doi.org/10.1007/978-981-19-9902-4_15

neuropathological models of schizophrenia. The neurodevelopmental model posits that these structural changes in the brain are related to genetic, prenatal, and environmental factors and occur in the early stages of neurodevelopment. The post-onset progression model proposes that these changes occur after disease onset and progressively worsen with increasing disease duration. To elucidate the relationship between disease evolution and brain structure, several research teams have recently conducted longitudinal studies on the brain structure of patients with schizophrenia. These studies can be divided into the following three categories based on the various disease stages of the subjects under investigation: (1) studies on high-risk groups, primarily focusing on the neurostructural changes of high-risk groups from the pre-clinical to the initial stages of disease onset; (2) studies on first-episode patients, which encompass neurostructural changes from disease onset to disease progression; and (3) studies on chronic patients, which are longitudinal follow-up studies conducted at certain intervals on patients with non-first-episode chronic schizophrenia.

15.1.1.1 High-Risk Groups: Research from the Pre-Clinical Stage to the First Episode of Schizophrenia

1. Gray matter changes: Previous structural imaging studies of the brain involving patients with schizophrenia have demonstrated relatively consistent findings of lateral ventricular enlargement as well as volume loss in the frontal operculum and lateral temporal lobe, although there are discrepancies regarding the timing of these changes. A number of longitudinal studies on high-risk groups have found that high-risk subjects who ultimately converted to schizophrenia showed a more significant reduction in gray matter volume compared to those who did not convert and healthy controls. However, different studies showed slight variations in the regions of volume reduction, the most common of which was the prefrontal cortex (PFC); other regions included the inferior temporal gyrus, medial parietal cortex, inferior parietal lobule, left fusiform gyrus, precuneus, cingulate gyrus, and cerebellar cortex. A meta-analysis revealed that the decrease in the gray matter volumes of the superior temporal and inferior frontal gyri at baseline in high-risk groups may signify the development of schizophrenia in the future (Fig. 15.1). However, the majority of those that converted to schizophrenia in this study, as well as some of those that did not, were being treated with antipsychotic medications during the interscan interval, indicating that the researchers could not fully exclude the effects of these pharmaceutical treatments. Another multi-center, large-sample study found that high-risk individuals showed a more rapid decline in the cortical volume of the right superior frontal gyrus, middle frontal gyrus, and medial orbitofrontal cortex (OFC). Further analysis revealed that these changes in cortical and lateral ventricular volumes were not significantly associated with medication use, drug dosage, or time (Fig. 15.2) (Cannon et al. 2015). Additionally, a plasma-based aggregate index of proinflammatory cytokines was found to predict the decline in gray matter volume, and this correlation was more significant among high-risk individuals who had converted to schizophrenia.

   Taken together, the above findings indicate that patients with schizophrenia exhibit gray matter changes earlier than the onset of symptoms, which gradually worsen as the disease progresses. These gray matter changes remained significant even after excluding the influence of medications. Although preliminary investigations have been conducted on the relationship between changes in the brain volume and plasma proinflammatory cytokines, the interaction between them remains poorly understood.
2. White matter changes: Schizophrenia may be closely associated with cortico-cortical disconnection. Cross-sectional studies on high-risk groups and first-episode patients revealed that white matter volume reduction and impaired structural integrity can already be

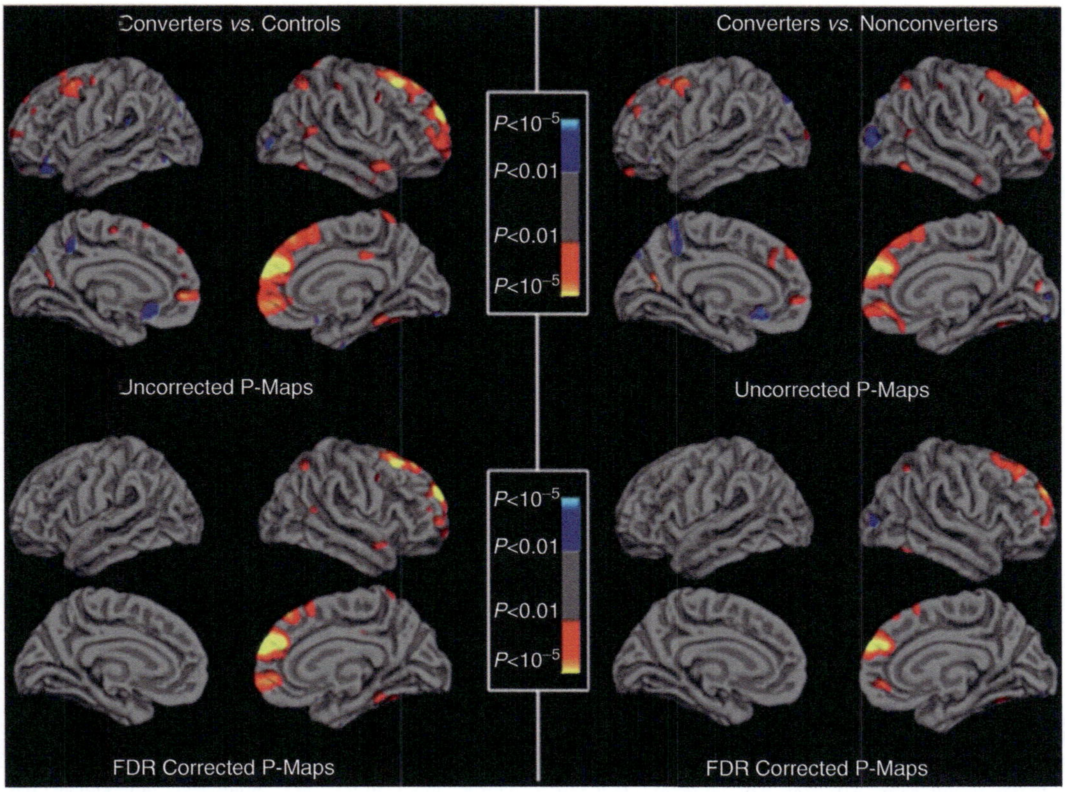

Fig. 15.1 Comparison of the rates of change in cortical thickness among high-risk subjects who converted to schizophrenia, those who did not, and healthy controls. The uncorrected results in the upper panels indicate that compared to the other two groups, high-risk individuals who converted to schizophrenia showed significant cortical thinning of the bilateral superior frontal, middle frontal, medial orbitofrontal, superior temporal, and parahippocampal gyri, as well as the right superior and inferior parietal lobules (red). The FDR-corrected results in the lower panels indicate that significant cortical thinning can only be found in the right superior frontal, middle frontal, and medial orbitofrontal gyri

observed in the early or prodromal stages of schizophrenia. At present, only one longitudinal follow-up DTI study has been performed on a population at high-risk for schizophrenia. In a comparison of fractional anisotropy (FA) values among high-risk individuals, first-episode patients, and healthy controls, it was found that first-episode patients had the lowest FA values and healthy controls had the highest, while those of high-risk individuals were somewhere between the two. Follow-up results demonstrated a progressive decline in the white matter FA values in the left frontal region among those at high-risk for converting to schizophrenia, whereas those at high-risk who did not covert did not exhibit these changes. Therefore, the results of that study confirmed that conversion to schizophrenia in high-risk groups is related to the progressive destruction of white matter integrity, particularly frontal white matter, similar to what was observed in first-episode and chronic patients.

15.1.1.2 Longitudinal Research on First-Episode Patients: Studies on Early-Stage Schizophrenia

1. Gray matter: The results of previous MRI studies on patients with first-episode schizophrenia revealed significant reductions in frontal, hypothalamic, and whole-brain gray matter volume from several to more than ten years after the first episode. Subsequent studies showed that these gray matter volume

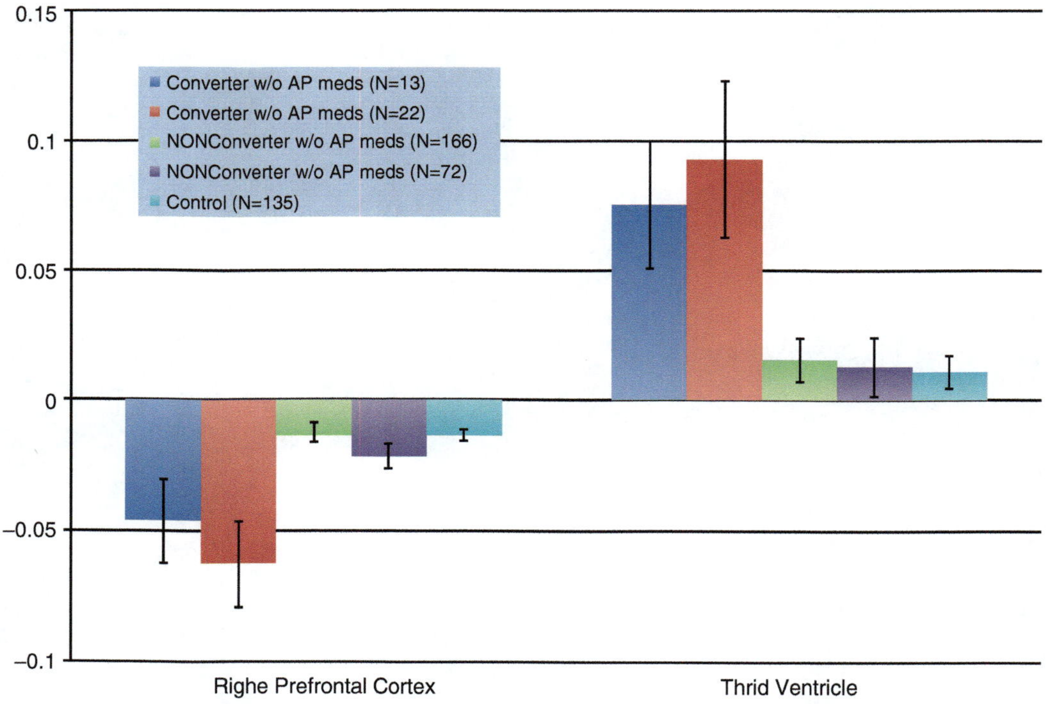

Fig. 15.2 Mean annualized rates of change in right prefrontal cortical and third ventricle volumes (Reproduced with permission from [4]). High-risk individuals that converted to schizophrenia without antipsychotic medication showed more significant changes in the right prefrontal cortex and third ventricle compared to those who didn't convert, with and without antipsychotic medication, and healthy controls, but showed no significant difference when compared to high-risk individuals who converted with antipsychotic medication. *Dark blue* high-risk individuals who converted to schizophrenia without antipsychotic medication; *red* high-risk individuals who converted to schizophrenia with antipsychotic medication; *green* high-risk individuals who did not convert to schizophrenia without antipsychotic medication; *purple* high-risk individuals who did not convert with antipsychotic medication; *light blue* healthy controls

reductions were caused by cortical thinning, rather than decreases in surface area, and these changes were most prominent in the early stages of the disease. Moreover, these gray matter changes were found to be correlated with worsening clinical presentations and cognitive decline. However, other such studies did not find significant changes in gray matter volume after the onset of the disease. These inconsistencies in research findings may be related to the differences in methodology; therefore, the question of whether patients with schizophrenia experience progressive gray matter changes remains and has not yet been definitively answered.

2. White matter: There is currently a lack of longitudinal studies on white matter changes in first-episode patients. Early volumetric studies of the brain showed that the reduction in whole-brain volume may have predominantly been due to gray matter changes, whereas no significant changes were observed in the white matter volume. In recent years, some studies have utilized DTI to perform the longitudinal tracking of microstructural changes in white matter, although the results of these studies have been inconsistent. Wang et al. showed that compared to healthy controls, previously drug-naïve patients with first-episode schizophrenia who received six weeks of drug therapy exhibited a significant decrease in the absolute FA values of white matter around the bilateral anterior cingulate cortices (ACCs) and right anterior corona radiata in the frontal lobe. Clinical symptoms improved during the treatment period, but the

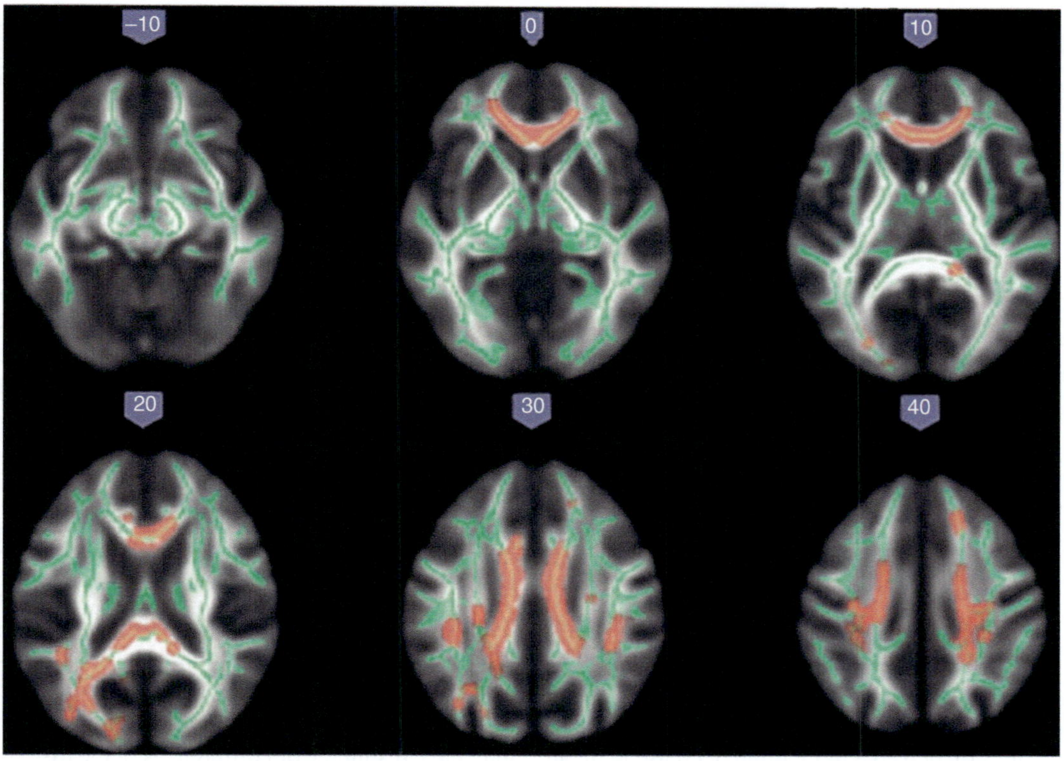

Fig. 15.3 Comparison of FA values between patients with schizophrenia and healthy controls. Green voxels represent the white matter skeleton; red and yellow voxels represent regions with lower FA values in patients with schizophrenia relative to healthy controls

changes in FA values were not correlated with changes in clinical symptoms or the dose of antipsychotic medication. In contrast to these findings, Marques et al. found increased white matter FA values in multiple regions following the use of antipsychotic medication, and these changes were positively correlated with cumulative antipsychotic dose, indicating the improvement of microstructural integrity in white matter fibers after exposure to antipsychotic medication (Fig. 15.3).

15.1.1.3 Structural Changes of the Brain in Patients with Chronic Schizophrenia

1. Gray matter: Longitudinal studies on the gray matter structure of patients with chronic schizophrenia are relatively scarce. Compared to healthy controls, patients with chronic schizophrenia exhibit more rapid cerebral gray matter atrophy, primarily in the frontotemporal region, thalamus, caudate nucleus, insula, periventricular region, putamen, and cingulate cortex. Severe cortical atrophy signifies a poor prognosis; however, not all studies have found a correlation between gray matter changes and clinical symptoms. In an almost 10-year-long follow-up study, which examined the relationship of brain volumetric changes with symptom severity, functional levels, and cognitive ability in patients with schizophrenia and healthy controls, it was found that gray matter reduction during the follow-up period was not associated with symptom severity, functional level, or cognitive decline. Some studies have found that patients with chronic schizophrenia did not exhibit any changes in the gray matter volume. Taken together, these negative findings support the hypothesis that patients with schizophrenia only exhibit gray matter

atrophy in the early stages of the disease, while gray matter changes gradually taper off and become insignificant as the disease progresses. Schnack et al. suggested that rapid changes in gray matter occurred within the first five years of disease onset, following which the gray matter volume begins to stabilize.

2. White matter: Current research on white matter in chronic schizophrenia is also relatively scarce, implying that we have a very limited understanding on the dynamic changes of the white matter microstructure and its relationship with clinical presentations among patients with chronic schizophrenia. Domen et al. utilized DTI and tract-based spatial statistics (TBSS) to study the longitudinal changes of the white matter microstructure in patients with chronic schizophrenia, non-affected siblings, and healthy controls. The results of their study indicated that at the three-year follow-up, only non-affected siblings displayed a more rapid decrease in mean FA value compared to healthy controls, while the mean FA value of patients with chronic schizophrenia was consistently lower than the baseline levels of non-affected siblings and healthy controls, although it remained relatively stable overall (Fig. 15.4). These findings are partially consistent with those of previous studies, indicating that there is persistent and stable damage to the white matter microstructure of patients with chronic schizophrenia; however, different studies have reported damage to different regions of white matter. Another study found that white matter structural damage may be associated with poor prognosis.

The results of studies on both gray and white matter suggest that structural damage to the brain in patients with schizophrenia may occur during a critical period of progression in the early stages, after which it enters a stable state. However, there are inconsistencies, or even contradictions, among some of these research findings, which may have resulted from differences in the disease subtype, follow-up duration, duration after onset

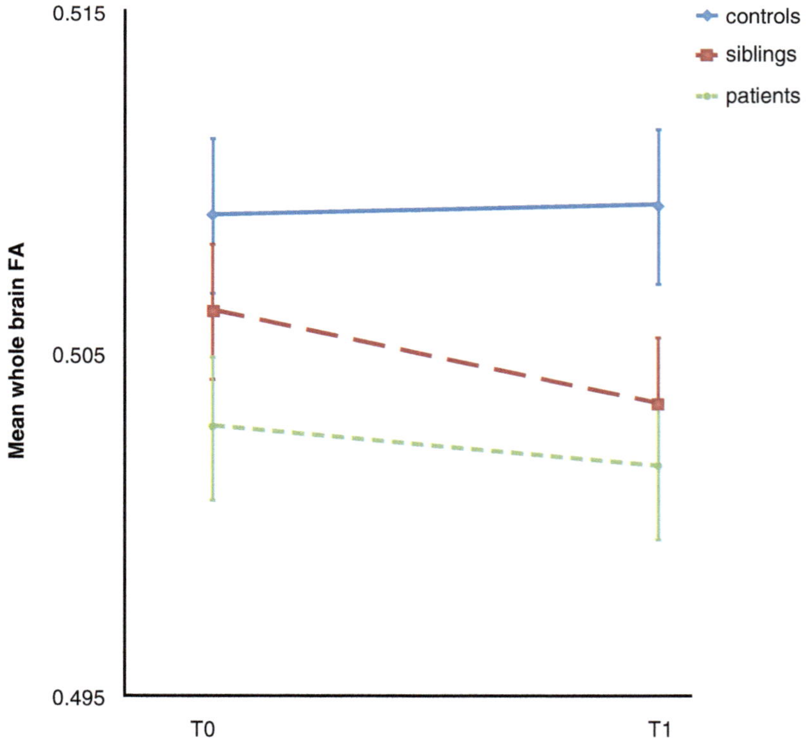

Fig. 15.4 Group comparison of changes in whole-brain FA values across the follow-up period

at the time of enrollment, and medication status of the patients enrolled in the studies. Additionally, there are also key issues in experimental methodology. For instance, the lack of consensus on the conceptual definition of first-episode patients has increased the difficulty of achieving a unified explanation and summarization of experimental results. Based on these studies, we can see that structural changes in the brains of patients with schizophrenia do not seem to occur at a uniform rate over the course of this disease. It is therefore necessary to perform more rigorous studies with larger sample sizes while gathering more unified and well-defined patient clinical information.

15.1.2 fMRI Research in Schizophrenia

Numerous studies have utilized fMRI techniques to explore the neurological changes seen in schizophrenia. These studies have observed both areas of the brain with enhanced and diminished activation, as well as both an increase in functional connectivity and a decrease in functional connectivity between different regions. Interestingly, some regions showed completely opposite results between different studies even when the same methods were used. For example, when fractional amplitude of low-frequency fluctuations (fALFF) was used to evaluate the intensity changes of spontaneous neuronal activity in the resting state among patients with schizophrenia, some researchers found that medication-naïve first-episode patients exhibited decreased fALFF in the medial PFC, whereas others found increased fALFF in the same region among medicated patients with chronic schizophrenia. In fact, many studies have demonstrated that a wide range of antipsychotic drugs can affect the resting-state or task-based fMRI signals. Studies involving medication-naïve first-episode patients with schizophrenia were able to exclude the effects of medication on brain function to the greatest possible extent and provide excellent samples for studying the neurological basis of schizophrenia. Schizophrenia is a highly hereditary disease; therefore, the study of genetically high-risk groups for schizophrenia is of crucial significance for the early detection and diagnosis of this disease. Here, we will focus on studies concerning two patient groups.

15.1.2.1 Resting-State fMRI Research

The default mode network (DMN) is a large-scale brain network which exhibits highly correlated intra-network activity that is active during the resting state. Previous studies have shown that corresponding changes occur to the DMN due to aging, as well as pathological states such as dementia and depression. Clinically, schizophrenia is primarily characterized by self-disorder and thought abnormalities, and the more closely associated these functions are to the DMN, the more marked the changes are in the DMN. To this end, the resting-state fMRI studies on schizophrenia are predominantly focused on the DMN.

In a study on first-episode, medication-naïve patients with schizophrenia, Guo et al. found that compared to healthy controls, patients with schizophrenia exhibited lower network homogeneity in the left PFC and right middle temporal gyrus, as well as increased network homogeneity in the left posterior cingulate cortex (PCC) and right cerebellum crus I. In another study, Guo et al. compared the voxel-mirrored homotopic connectivity (VMHC) intensity between 48 first-episode, medication-naïve patients with paranoid schizophrenia and 50 healthy controls. Patients with schizophrenia showed lower VMHC than healthy controls in the precuneus, precentral gyrus, superior temporal gyrus, middle occipital gyrus, fusiform gyrus, and cerebellum lobule VI, and it was found that the VMHC decrease of the precuneus and superior temporal gyrus was significantly correlated with symptom severity (Fig. 15.5). In a subsequent study, Liu et al. compared the VMHC intensity between first-episode, medication-naïve adolescent-onset patients with schizophrenia and healthy controls, which similarly revealed lower VMHC values of multiple brain regions in the patient group, primarily involving the fusiform gyrus, superior temporal gyrus/insula, precentral gyrus, and precuneus. Moreover, VMHC changes in the

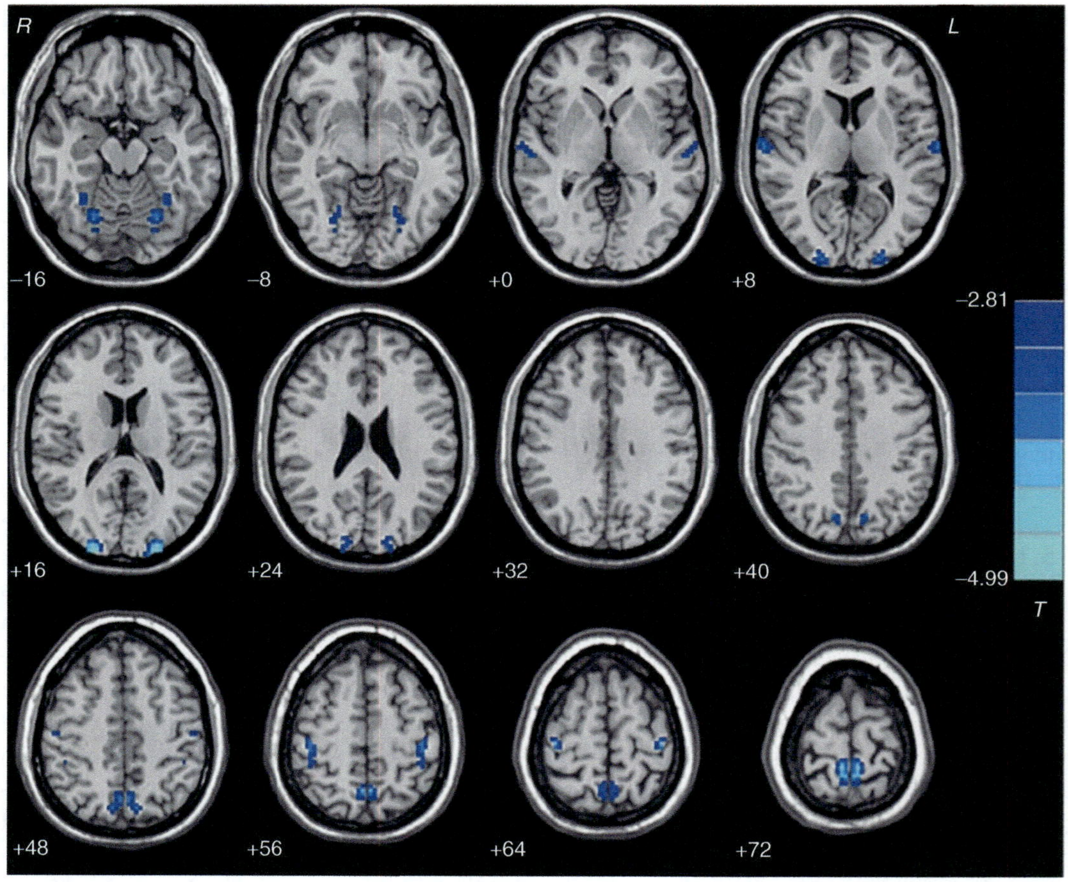

Fig. 15.5 Differences in VMHC between medication-naïve first-episode patients with paranoid schizophrenia and healthy controls (GUO W, XIAO C, LIU G, et al. Decreased resting-state interhemispheric coordination in first-episode, drug-naive paranoid schizophrenia. Prog Neuropsychopharmacol). Blue represents areas with decreased VMHC

superior temporal gyrus/insula were significantly correlated with impairments in executive function. He et al. conducted a large-sample study that included 115 medication-naïve first-episode patients with schizophrenia and 113 healthy controls. The results of their study indicated that patients had decreased fALFF values in the bilateral medial PFC and OFC and increased fALFF values in the bilateral putamen. Furthermore, patients with schizophrenia exhibited increased functional connectivity of the DMN in the left insula and bilateral dorsolateral PFC, while disease severity was associated with changes in the fALFF values of the left OFC and right putamen and functional connectivity of the DMN.

Wang et al. noted that the disrupted network connectivity patterns in patients with chronic, unmedicated schizophrenia was closely related to connection distance. More specifically, the abnormal short-range connectivity of the sensorimotor system was significantly correlated with disease duration and negative symptoms, whereas altered long-range connectivity was correlated with neurocognitive performance (Fig. 15.6). Using multimodal MRI data from 512 subjects, Xia et al. compared the common abnormalities in the functional networks of the brain across schizophrenia, bipolar disorder, and major depressive disorder. They demonstrated that in all three disorders, the brain networks exhibited a common tendency toward randomized, disrupted

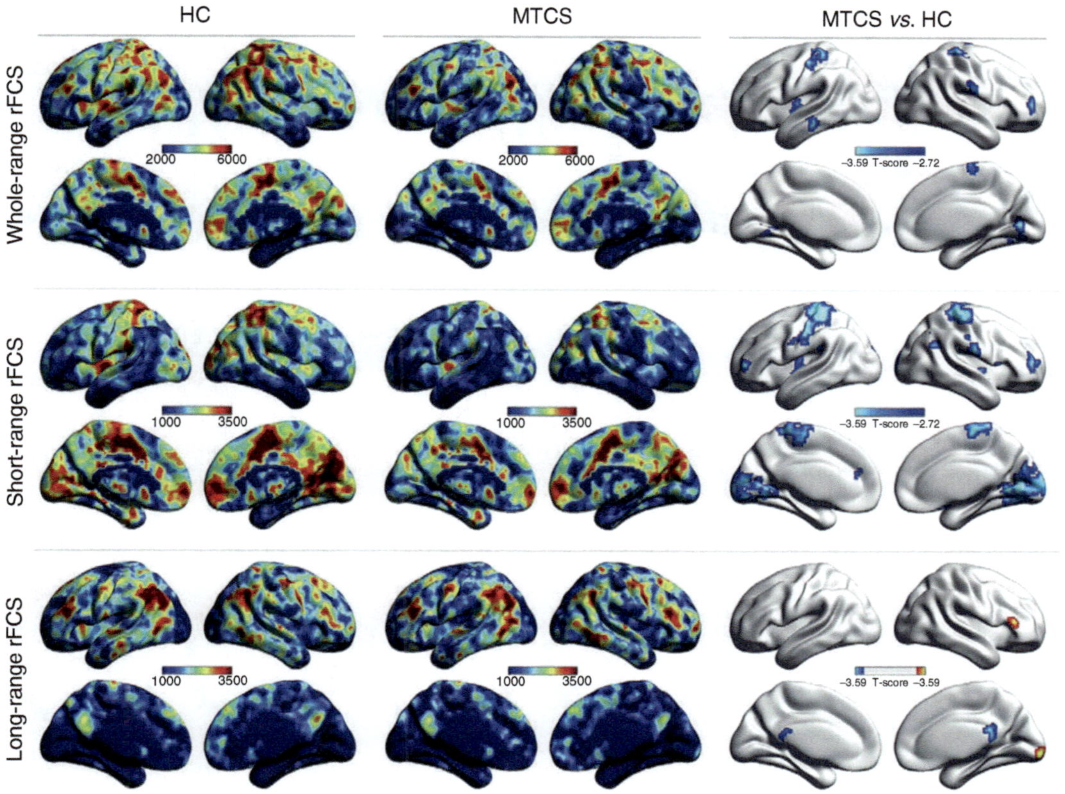

Fig. 15.6 Disrupted functional connectivity of the sensorimotor system and DMN in patients with chronic, unmedicated schizophrenia. The sensorimotor system primarily exhibited abnormalities in short-range functional connectivity, whereas the DMN primarily showed abnormalities in long-range functional connectivity. *rFCS* regional functional connectivity strength

connectivity patterns, with increased medium- to long-range connectivity in core nodes of the medial/lateral frontoparietal cortex, and decreased short-range connectivity in the primary cortices. They found that these abnormalities were most significant in patients with schizophrenia. Further investigation revealed that patients with schizophrenia had impaired modular organization in their brain networks, showing excessive inter-modular connectors, with a significant increase in the inter-modular connections of the DMN, frontoparietal network, and sensorimotor network. Furthermore, these brain network abnormalities were found to be significantly correlated with clinical symptoms (Fig. 15.7).

Relatively few studies have been conducted on individuals at high genetic risk of developing schizophrenia. Tang et al. showed that compared to healthy controls, individuals at high genetic risk showed elevated ALFF values in the striatum (including left caudate nucleus/putamen and right caudate nucleus), left medial temporal lobe (including hippocampus, parahippocampal gyrus, and fusiform gyrus), left lateral thalamus, bilateral ventral and dorsal cingulate gyri, bilateral sulcus of the corpus callosum, and precuneus, whereas regions with reduced ALFF values were primarily located in the left inferior parietal lobule/postcentral gyrus. Wang et al. found changes in the functional connectivity of the left angular gyrus and dorsolateral PFC with the insula among subjects at high genetic risk of schizophrenia. Additionally, Ma et al. compared the differences in whole-brain regional homogeneity (ReHo) and functional connectivity between 42 subjects at high genetic risk of schizophrenia and 38 healthy controls. They found that the DMN of genetic carriers showed decreased ReHo

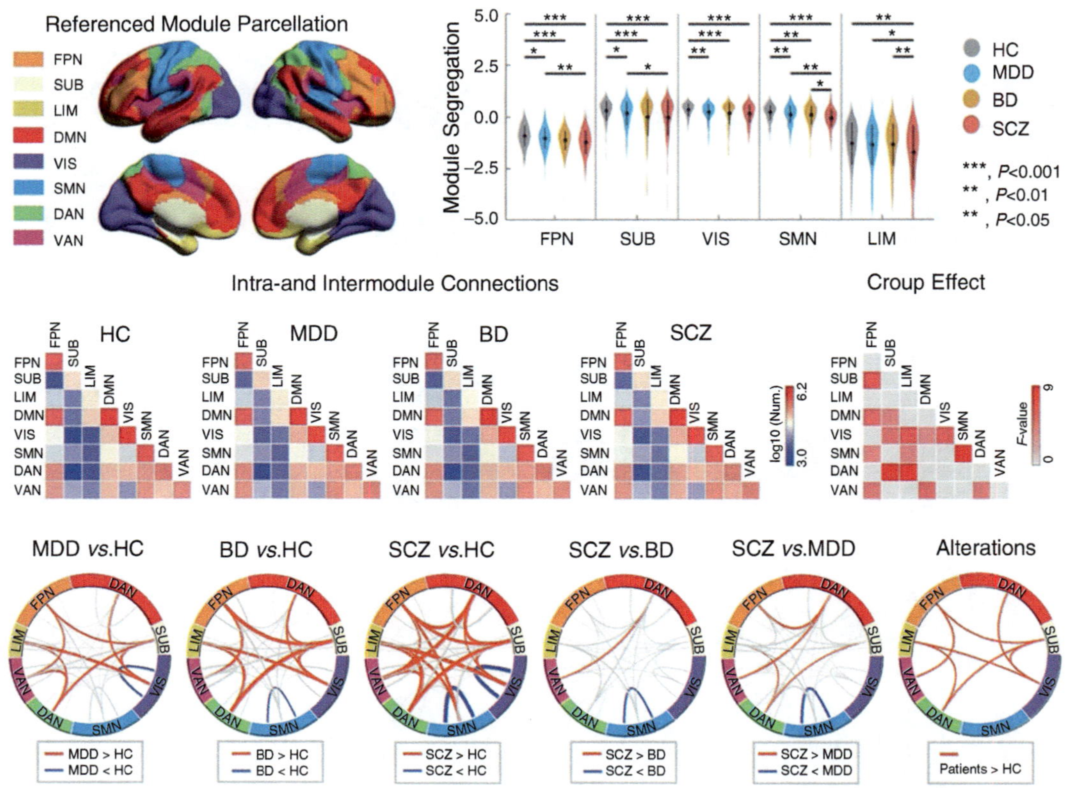

Fig. 15.7 Abnormal modular organization of functional networks of the brain in patients with schizophrenia, bipolar disorder, and major depressive disorder. Significant increases in the inter-modular connections of the DMN, frontoparietal network, and sensorimotor network, with most significant abnormalities being observed in patients with schizophrenia

values in the left ventral ACC, left caudate nucleus, bilateral middle frontal gyrus, and right superior frontal gyrus, as well as increased functional connectivity of the right superior frontal gyrus, and left OFC. Moreover, ReHo changes of the right middle frontal gyrus and right superior frontal gyrus were associated with a decline in delayed recall performance (Figs. 15.8, 15.9, and 15.10).

Therefore, both first-episode medication-naïve patients with and individuals at high genetic risk for schizophrenia exhibited widespread functional changes in the DMN. Taken together, the research findings described above indicate that the onset of schizophrenia is closely associated with impairments to the functional integrity of the DMN, and these changes may be present even before the onset of the disease. Although these studies have attempted to control for the effects of subject heterogeneity, the differences in post-processing methods, correction methods, seed selection, DMN acquisition methods, and other parameters have given rise to somewhat inconsistent conclusions across the various studies. As a whole, studies on first-episode, medication-naïve patients with schizophrenia have found that abnormal areas of the brain are primarily distributed along the prefrontal-temporal pathway, whereas individuals at high genetic risk for developing schizophrenia primarily exhibit abnormalities in the cortical-limbic-striatal system. Nevertheless, more studies are needed to determine the specific areas of the brain associated with schizophrenia.

A study by Sun et al. demonstrated the abnormal distribution of inter-subject variability in the functional connectivity of patients with schizophrenia, with significantly enhanced inter-

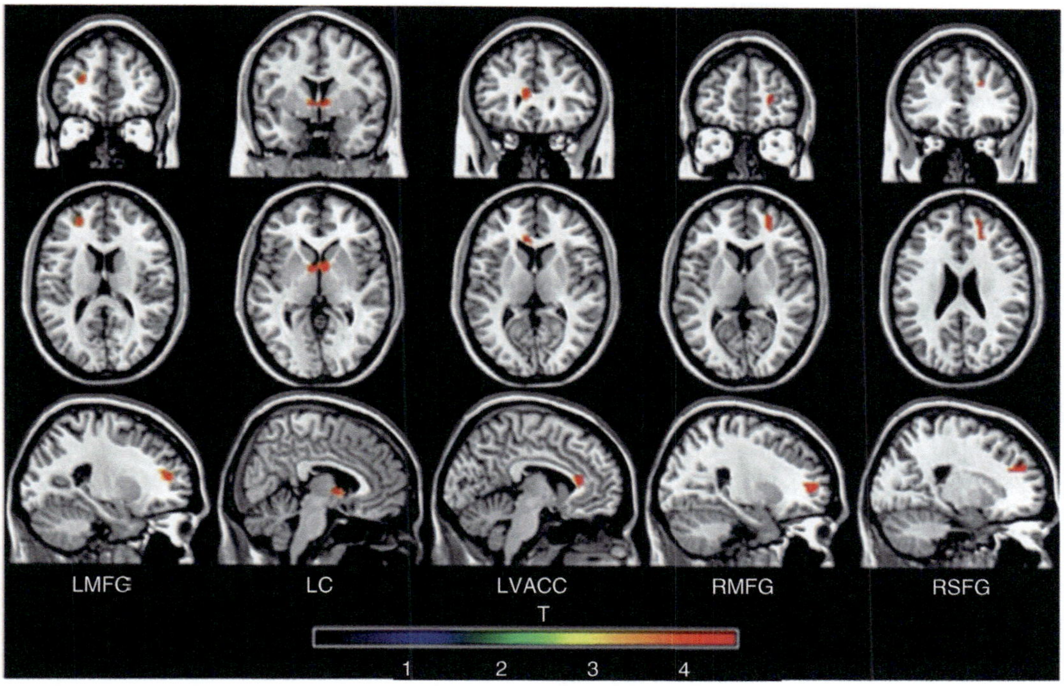

Fig. 15.8 Brain regions with significant changes in ReHo values within the DMN among individuals at high genetic risk of schizophrenia compared to healthy controls. *LMFG* left middle frontal gyrus; *LC* left caudate, *LVACC* left ventral anterior cingulate cortex; *RMFG* right middle frontal gyrus; *RSFG* right superior frontal gyrus

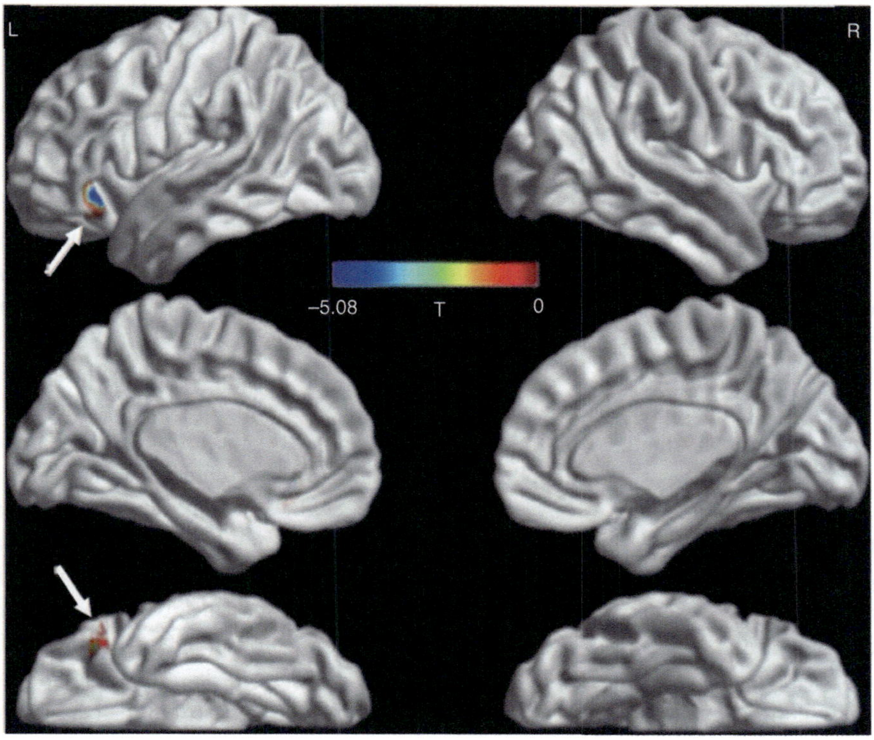

Fig. 15.9 Brain regions with significant differences in functional connectivity within the DMN among individuals at high genetic risk of schizophrenia compared to healthy controls (arrows) (Reproduced with permission from [8])

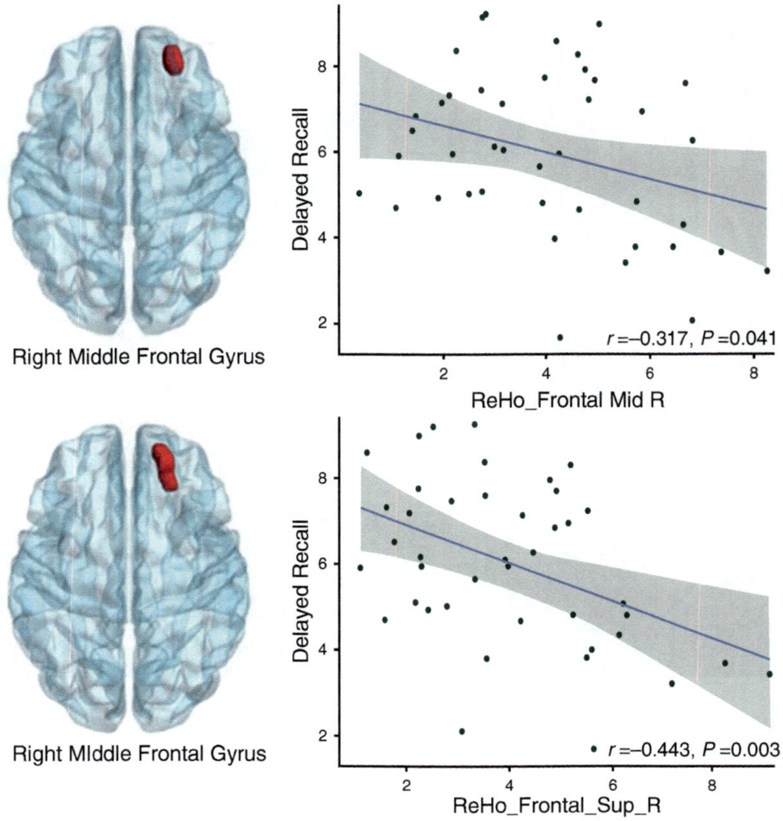

Fig. 15.10 Scatterplots showing the relationship between delayed recall performance and ReHo values in the right middle and superior frontal gyri (showing significant negative correlations) (Reproduced with permission from [8]). *Reho Frontal Mid R* Regional homogeneity of the right frontal middle gyrus; *Reho_Frontal_Sup_R* Regional homogeneity of the superior frontal gyrus

individual variation in the somatosensory, visual, auditory, and emotional integration circuitry. Furthermore, inter-individual variability was associated with age of onset, stage of disease, medication status, and severity of clinical symptoms. Therefore, we are currently still unable to rule out the possibility that the inconsistencies in the findings above are related to the patient's disease stage and its associated inclination toward certain clinical symptoms. As such, studies with more detailed classification and longer follow-up durations are needed to evaluate the relationship between these functional changes in the brain and the pathogenesis of schizophrenia. Additionally, although some studies have found that functional changes in specific areas of the brain may be associated with the clinical presentations or cognitive impairments in schizophrenia, further research is needed to clarify the relationship between these changes and specific symptoms or cognitive changes.

15.1.2.2 Task-Based fMRI Research

Task-based fMRI studies on first-episode medication-naïve patients have demonstrated task-related activation changes in multiple areas of the brain compared to healthy controls. Owing to the different types of tasks and implementation methods utilized in various studies, the resultant findings have been inconsistent regarding the activation and differential activation of various areas of the brain under different tasks, even if these studies all involved in the comparison of patients with schizophrenia and healthy controls. Nevertheless, some areas of the brain have been shown to exhibit changes in activation patterns that are widely present across different task types, the most common of which is the PFC. Hypoactivations in the PFC primarily occur in the dorsolateral PFC, OFC, and ventral PFC, which can be observed in verbal fluency tasks, eye movement tasks, the Stroop Color-Word Task, the AX-continuous performance task

(AX-CPT), explicit emotion discrimination tasks, drum beat tasks, and working memory tasks. In contrast, working memory tasks elicited stronger activation in the ventrolateral PFC. The second most common area of the brain with abnormalities is the temporal lobe. First-episode medication-naïve patients showed increased activation of the left superior temporal gyrus when performing serial reaction time (SRT) tasks but exhibited decreased activation in the superior temporal gyrus when performing verbal fluency, drumbeat, working memory, and language tasks. Furthermore, these studies have also demonstrated varying degrees of abnormal activation in the ACC, right ventral striatum, ventral premotor cortex, sensorimotor regions, thalamus, precuneus, and parietal regions.

As with the resting-state fMRI research, task-based fMRI studies on individuals at high genetic risk of schizophrenia are also relatively scarce. A study on individuals at high genetic risk showed hyperactivation of the bilateral precentral gyrus and right superior parietal lobule. The results of another study involving patients with schizophrenia, non-affected relatives at high genetic risk for developing schizophrenia, and low-risk subjects without schizophrenia-related genes indicated that when performing a visual lexical decision task, patients with schizophrenia showed significantly higher activation in the bilateral superior occipital, left superior temporal, and right inferior frontal gyri and the bilateral inferior parietal lobule, as well as significantly lower activation of the left fusiform and right parahippocampal gyri, compared to low-risk individuals. Their high-risk relatives showed significantly higher activation of the right inferior frontal gyrus, bilateral superior temporal gyrus, and right inferior parietal lobule, as well as lower activation of the right fusiform and right middle temporal gyri, compared to low-risk individuals. Therefore, the activation patterns of brain in patients with schizophrenia and their high-risk relatives were essentially the same when performing tasks, with no significant differences between the two groups. In a longitudinal study on healthy controls and individuals at high genetic risk for developing schizophrenia, it was observed that at the 18-month follow-up, those at high-risk of converting to schizophrenia showed significantly higher activation of the left middle temporal gyrus than those at high-risk who did not convert when performing the Hayling sentence completion test.

Despite the differences in task choices and activated regions of the brain across the various studies, it is still possible to identify certain common patterns of changes in task-related brain activation among first-episode medication-naïve patients with schizophrenia, that is, a higher likelihood of involvement in the prefrontal and temporal regions. This is similar to the findings of the resting-state research, indicating the presence of prefrontal-temporal pathway changes in patients with schizophrenia, particularly in the dorsolateral PFC, OFC, and left superior temporal gyrus. However, the mechanisms underlying the role of this pathway in schizophrenia are currently unclear. Research on individuals at high genetic risk of schizophrenia is relatively lacking, and there is a lack of consistent conclusions. However, both task-based and resting-state fMRI studies have together demonstrated the presence of changes in the functional networks of the brain prior to the onset of schizophrenia, as well as a certain extent of similarity and continuity between the brain network changes before and after the onset of the disease.

15.1.3 MRS Research in Schizophrenia

Over the past few decades, continued and unremitting efforts have been made to improve the abilities of MR technology to detect metabolism in the human body. Currently, MRS is the only technique available for the non-invasive in vivo detection of chemical properties in tissues. As such, it has been extensively utilized in research on metabolic dysfunction of the brain in a variety of neurodegenerative diseases and has been utilized in the detection of the biomarkers found in common mental disorders. Therefore, this technique has significant value for the identification of disease biomarkers and the prediction and evaluation of therapeutic efficacy in patients with schizophrenia.

According to previous animal studies and human post-mortem studies, schizophrenia is related to glutamatergic and GABAergic dysfunction, and MRS can be used for the non-invasive detection of glutamate and GABA metabolism in the brain. However, further validation is needed to demonstrate whether MRS can truly reflect metabolic changes in the brain of patients with schizophrenia. Here, we will focus on the glutamatergic and GABAergic systems in our discussion on the utilization of MRS in schizophrenia research and briefly introduce the research findings on other relevant metabolites.

15.1.3.1 Schizophrenia and the Glutamatergic and GABAergic Regulatory Systems

It has been hypothesized that the negative symptoms and cognitive impairment of patients with schizophrenia are related to the dopamine depletion of mesocortical neurons projecting from the ventral tegmentum to the PFC, thereby weakening the stimulation of neuronal dopamine D_1 receptors. Contrarily, the overactivation of the mesolimbic pathway (projecting to the nucleus accumbens) leading to the over-stimulation of D_2 receptors is believed to be a major factor contributing to the positive symptoms of schizophrenia. Another hypothesis posits that N-methyl-D-aspartate (NMDA) receptor hypofunction and inadequate GABAergic transmission play a major role in schizophrenia. The NMDA receptor hypofunction in patients with schizophrenia can lead to the reduced signal transduction in NMDA receptors, resulting in the disruption of excitation monitoring, in turn causing GABAergic neurons to respond as though excitatory transmission is insufficient. This diminished negative feedback from GABAergic interneurons to pyramidal neurons leads to increased glutamatergic neurotransmission and ultimately leads to excitotoxicity.

Neuroimaging studies on GABA and glutamate (Glu) are of crucial significance, due to the need for in vivo studies to verify a number of hypotheses concerning the role of GABA and Glu dysfunction in schizophrenia. Furthermore, elucidating the involvement of functional impairments of the GABAergic and glutamatergic systems in the pathophysiological process of schizophrenia in an in vivo state will facilitate the research and development of drugs that target these systems. Additionally, neuroimaging techniques that can be utilized in GABAergic and glutamatergic imaging are also useful for exploring the mechanisms of action and evaluating the therapeutic efficacy of drug treatments.

15.1.3.2 GABA ^{1}H-MRS Research in Patients with Schizophrenia

Neuroimaging techniques are able to be utilized to evaluate the GABAergic system of patients with schizophrenia. ^{1}H-MRS can be used to measure the GABA concentration of regions of interest (ROIs) and generally measures the total GABA content of all tissues (intracellular and extracellular) within each ROI. Since the measurement results also include a small number of macromolecular substances and traces of homocarnosine in addition to GABA, these measurements are usually denoted as GABA+. Based on the different ROI locations selected in various studies, we divided the following research findings into the following regions: (1) medial frontal cortex; (2) parietal/occipital cortex; (3) striatum; and (4) other regions of the brain.

The medial frontal cortex is the most studied region of the brain involving GABA ^{1}H-MRS. Approximately half of the studies have reported elevated MRS GABA levels in the medial PFC of patients with schizophrenia, whereas the other half have reported reduced levels of GABA, and a handful of studies have shown that the GABA levels of patients did not differ significantly from those of healthy controls. Egerton et al. performed a meta-analysis on the relevant findings, which revealed a marked heterogeneity across the experimental results, and no significant differences between patients with schizophrenia and healthy controls (Figs. 15.11 and 15.12).

The second most studied region of the brain is the parietal/occipital cortex, which has shown similar findings to those of the medial frontal cortex. Approximately half of the studies found that patients with schizophrenia exhibited higher MRS GABA levels than those of healthy controls, whereas the other half obtained the opposite results, and a handful of studies did not find significant between-group differences in the GABA levels of the parietal/occipital cortex. Similarly, a meta-analysis of these findings also demonstrated a marked heterogeneity across the experimental results, and no significant differences in GABA levels of the parietal/occipital cortex between patients with schizophrenia and healthy controls.

Few studies have focused on the striatum as an ROI, of which slightly more studies have found decreased GABA levels in patients with schizophrenia than those that showing increased GABA levels. However, a meta-analysis of these studies also did not reveal significant differences in MRS GABA levels between patients with schizophrenia and healthy controls. Studies on other regions of the brain include the dorsolateral PFC, hippocampus, and centrum semiovale. Due to the limited number of reports on these regions, the findings remain inconclusive.

In summary, there are significant inconsistencies in the GABA results of MRS studies on schizophrenia, which may be related to the fol-

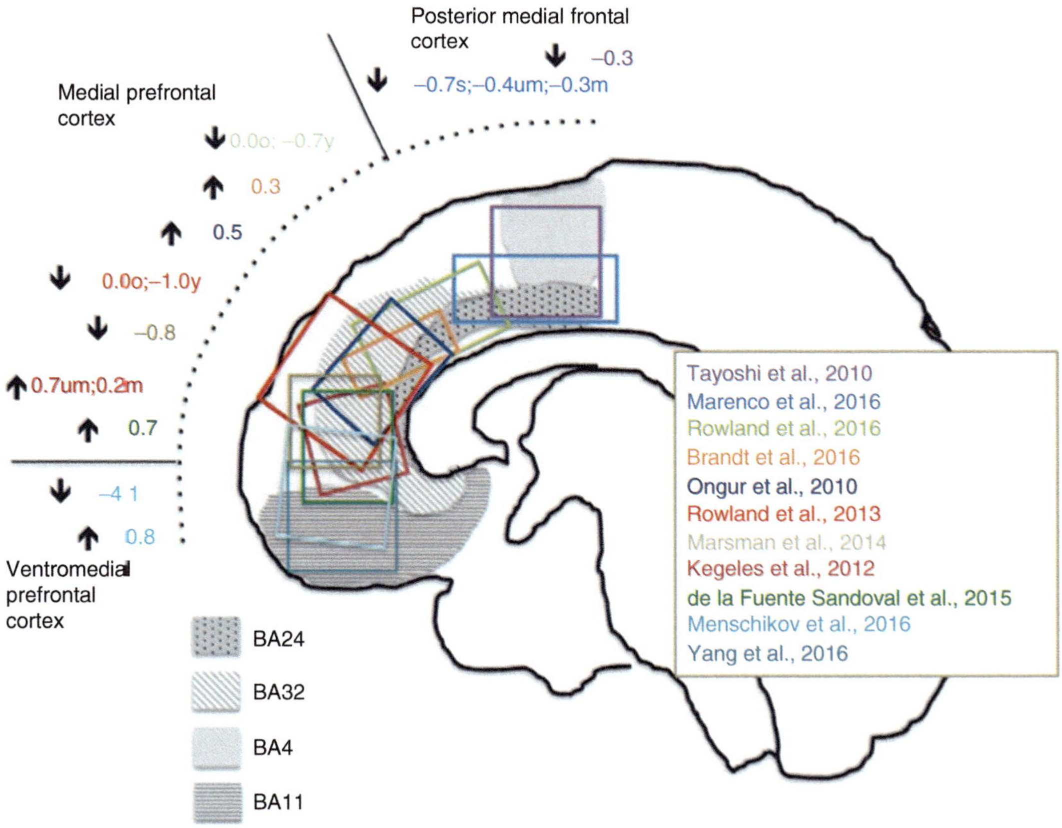

Fig. 15.11 Schematic diagram of ROI locations in the medial frontal cortex selected by different GABA ^{1}H-MRS studies. Numbers in the figure represent the effect sizes for the difference in GABA level between patients and healthy controls for each study in the meta-analysis. Negative effect sizes indicate lower GABA levels in patients compared to healthy controls

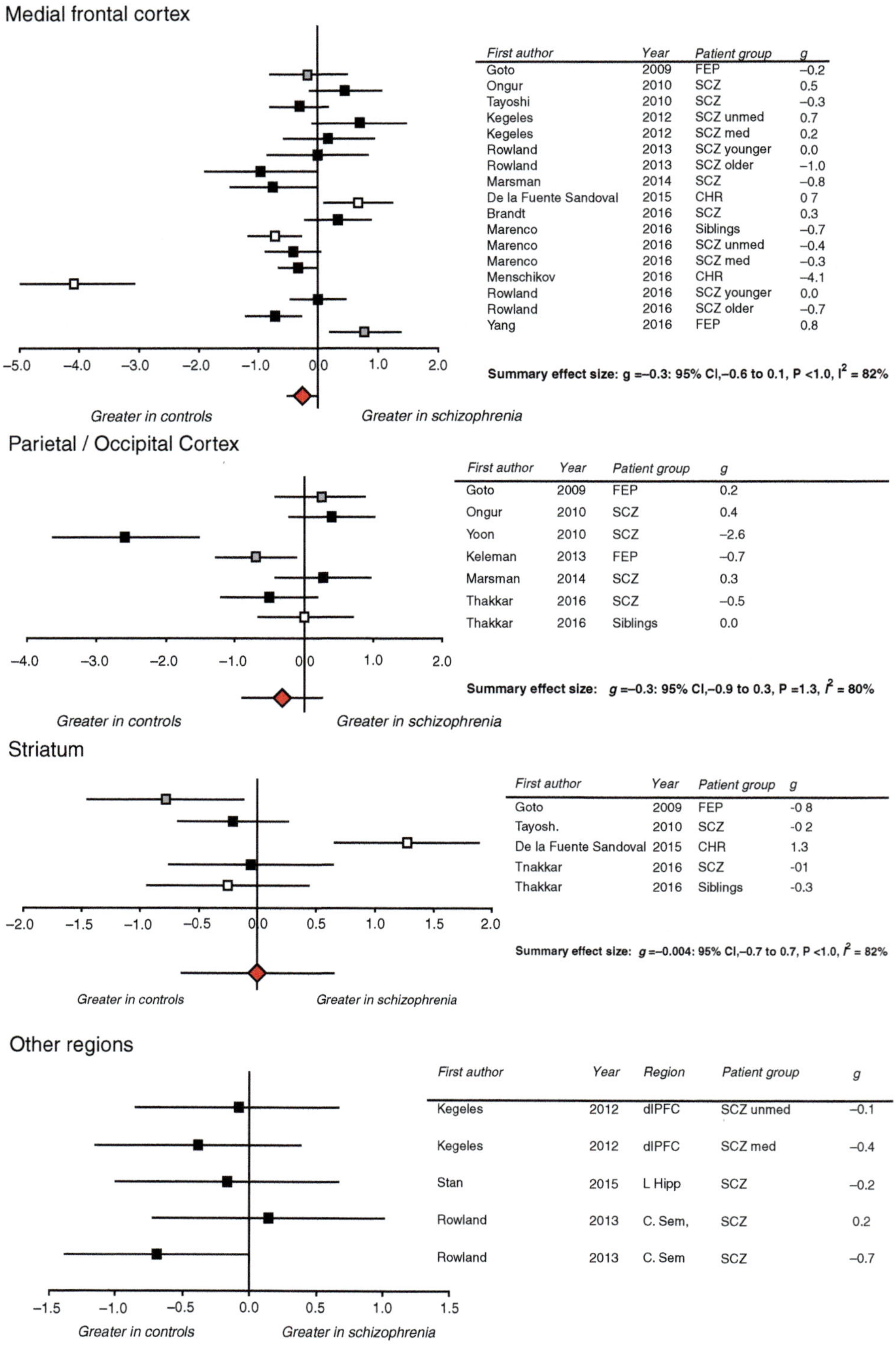

Fig. 15.12 Forest plots (Hedge's *g*) showing effect sizes of ^{1}H-MRS GABA studies comparing patients with schizophrenia and healthy controls (Reproduced with permission from [9]). Error bars represent a 95% confidence interval. Black squares indicate data from clinically confirmed cases, first-episode patients (FEP), or patients with schizophrenia (SCZ), whereas white squares indicate data from clinically high-risk (CHR) subjects or unaffected siblings. Med: currently receiving antipsychotic medication; unmed: currently not receiving antipsychotic medication

lowing: first, there are substantial variations in subject selection; second, from the perspective of experimental techniques, whole-brain acquisition cannot be achieved using MRS, which necessitates the usage of ROIs, resulting in significant variability in ROI locations and sizes across different studies; and third, with respect to the analysis of acquired data, some studies have directly utilized absolute GABA+ values, while others have opted to report relative values. Furthermore, research has also shown that using the ratios of different substances within the same subjects will give rise to differences in the significance levels of the results. Current research findings have demonstrated that there are no consistent patterns of change in GABA concentrations in patients with schizophrenia, as measured by ^{1}H-MRS. Moreover, most studies have small sample sizes and highly heterogeneous data. In the future, studies with larger sample sizes and greater homogeneity may help to produce more valuable conclusions, while studies that directly compare patient subgroups may also prove useful. Additionally, based on the results of postmortem studies, future research should also focus on the dorsolateral PFC, ACC, and hippocampus.

15.1.3.3 ^{1}H-MRS Research on Glu and Glutamine (Gln) in Patients with Schizophrenia

According to numerous reports on Glu and Gln changes in the nervous systems of patients with schizophrenia, changes in the concentration of glutamatergic metabolites in the brain occur in a time-dependent manner. Some studies have found that medication-naïve patients in the early stage exhibited an increase in Glu and Gln levels and/or the Gln/Glu ratio, whereas patients with chronic schizophrenia often showed a decrease in the level of these amino acids. A recent meta-analysis revealed that Glu and Gln levels decreased with increasing age and disease duration.

^{1}H-MRS is able to measure neurochemical information in the resting state, while task-related ^{1}H-MRS, i.e., functional MRS (fMRS), can be used to obtain specific measurements of dynamic changes in glutamatergic and energy metabolism during neural activation. fMRS studies require MRS methods with high sensitivity and high stability. A 7 Tesla (T) fMRS study found that compared with healthy controls, patients with schizophrenia showed a delayed increase in Glu levels during cognitive tasks, signifying the degeneration of neurons involved in glutamatergic transmission and oxidative metabolism.

15.1.3.4 N-Acetylaspartate (NAA) ^{1}H-MRS Research in Patients with Schizophrenia

NAA is widely recognized as a marker for neuronal integrity and is the most abundant metabolite detected in the ^{1}H-MR spectrum of the adult mammalian central nervous system. More intuitive results can be obtained through the in vivo ^{1}H-MRS measurements of NAA, and therefore, more consistent findings have been observed among the NAA measurements of patients with schizophrenia. According to previous studies, patients with schizophrenia exhibited lower NAA levels in various brain areas (e.g., frontal lobe, hippocampus, and thalamus) compared to healthy controls, while the extent of the decrease of NAA in patients with chronic schizophrenia was more significant than that of first-episode patients. Nevertheless, other studies have also observed elevated NAA levels in the hippocampus of patients with chronic schizophrenia and the PFC of high-risk adolescents. Bustillo et al. demonstrated that with increasing age, the NAA level of gray matter increased while that of white matter decreased in the cerebral cortex of patients with schizophrenia. A meta-analysis revealed that the cerebral concentration of NAA in patients with schizophrenia decreased with increasing age and disease duration, which may reflect the persisting damage inflicted on the neuronal metabolic integrity of patients over time.

15.1.3.5 Glutathione ^{1}H-MRS Research in Patients with Schizophrenia

Glutathione is an important cellular redox regulator that has antioxidative effects and can protect cells from damage induced by reactive oxygen species. Decreased glutathione levels have been observed in the cerebrospinal fluid and medial PFC of patients with chronic schizophrenia, and this decrease was found to be directly proportional to the severity of negative symptoms. Research has shown that subjects carrying polymorphisms in the glutamate-cysteine ligase catalytic subunit (*Gclc*) gene were at a higher risk for schizophrenia and exhibited lower glutathione concentration in the medial PFC compared to low-risk individuals. Patients with schizophrenia with a low genetic risk had lower levels of Glu in the PFC, indicating that glutamatergic impairments may be a major pathogenic factor among patients with a low-risk *Gclc* genotype. Nevertheless, other studies have also found no significant difference in the glutathione levels in the brain between patients and healthy controls. This may have been due to the differences in the distribution of *Gclc* polymorphisms between the study populations, and/or the fact that measurements were primarily performed in the resting state, as the resting-state changes may be less significant than changes measured under specific conditions, such as under stressful mental states. Further validation is needed for stress-induced glutathione changes in patients or subjects at risk for schizophrenia. Additionally, other studies have found that glutathione was associated with white matter integrity and the resting-state functional connectivity of the cingulate fasciculus, whereas the relationship between glutathione and functional connectivity may be disrupted in the early stages of psychosis.

15.1.3.6 ^{31}P-MRS Research on Nicotinamide Adenine Dinucleotide (NAD)+/NADH in Patients with Schizophrenia

The balance between the oxidized (NAD+) and reduced (NADH) forms of NAD plays a key role in a number of biological processes, including energy metabolism, antioxidation, and calcium homeostasis. The ratio between NAD+ and NADH is a reflection of cellular redox state, and the low concentration and limited spectral resolution of these two compounds have substantially increased the challenge involved in their in vivo measurement. A strong magnetic field can significantly enhance sensitivity and spectral dispersion, which can in turn improve spectral fitting. There have been recent studies reporting on utilization of ^{31}P-MRS for the in vivo measurement of NAD+ and NADH in the human brain. One of these studies demonstrated that early-stage and chronic patients with psychosis exhibited significant reductions in the NAD+/NADH ratio. These findings are the first to directly support the redox imbalance of NAD+/NADH in patients with schizophrenia, and such alterations may be related to mitochondrial dysfunction and impaired energy metabolism.

15.1.3.7 ^{31}P-MRS Research on Mitochondrial Dysfunction in Patients with Schizophrenia

Patients with schizophrenia may also display abnormalities in mitochondrial function and energy metabolism. Although current ^{31}P-MRS studies have shown inconsistent changes of adenosine triphosphate (ATP), phosphocreatine, and inorganic phosphate (Pi) in the frontal, temporal, and subcortical regions of the brain, ^{31}P-MRS magnetization transfer experiments have demonstrated that the reaction rate of creatine kinase, which catalyzes the conversion of phosphocreatine from ATP, was reduced in the ACC of patients with schizophrenia. Apart from methodological differences, potential compensatory mechanisms in the resting state may also contribute partially to the changes detected. In contrast, dynamic changes can still be observed, even when the total resting-state level remains unchanged. Furthermore, the accumulation of lactate (Lac) has been observed in the medial PFC and cerebrospinal fluid of patients with schizophrenia, suggesting the shift of energy production toward a greater dependence on glycolysis, which may lead to lactic acidosis, as seen by a ^{31}P-MRS study which found that patients with schizophrenia had relatively low brain pH values.

In summary, despite the numerous confounding factors involved (e.g., MRI methods, disease stage, geographical differences, differences in patient grouping, and different medication effects, among others), it has still been possible to detect the presence of glutamatergic, redox, and mitochondrial dysfunction in the brains of patients with schizophrenia using MRS. It is worth noting that the compensatory mechanisms in the resting state may mask changes in metabolite concentrations. In contrast, measurements based on dynamic MRS are more reliable, indicating that more information can be obtained by performing fMRS studies and magnetization experiments on patients.

Another point worth considering is that at present, only a small proportion of the Glu and GABA measured is involved in neurotransmission. Therefore, ^{13}C-MRS studies will need to be conducted in the future to directly investigate the abnormal neurotransmission and energy metabolic pathways of Glu and GABA, which will hopefully provide new insights on the pathophysiology of schizophrenia.

15.2 Research Applications of PET Imaging in Schizophrenia

PET allows for the non-invasive, in vivo functional imaging of the brain and can evaluate characteristics such as cerebral blood flow (CBF), glucose metabolism, and neurotransmission. PET neurotransmitter imaging can provide a wide range of information on neurotransmitters, including pre- and post-synaptic function and anatomical location. Therefore, this technique has been applied to the pathophysiological research of various mental illnesses, including schizophrenia, as well as the mechanisms of action underlying psychiatric medications. In particular, PET probes that can bind to monoamine receptors and transporters have been extensively utilized in the study of neurotransmission mediated by monoamine neurotransmitters, such as dopamine, serotonin (5-HT), and norepinephrine. These neurotransmitters are involved in a wide range of cognitive processes, including memory and executive function, and are also the primary targets of antipsychotics and antidepressants. Therefore, PET studies conducted using such probes can not only elucidate the pathological mechanisms of various mental illnesses (including schizophrenia) but can also further clarify the mechanisms of action underlying antipsychotic medications. In this section, the PET probes were categorized according to the type of receptor(s) to which they bind, in order to briefly describe the research findings obtained through the use of monoamine neurotransmitter imaging to explore the relationship between neurotransmission and cognitive function in healthy controls and patients with schizophrenia, as well as the effect of drugs on cognitive performance and their mechanisms of action.

15.2.1 Dopamine

Dopamine is a major neurotransmitter that is intimately associated with the pathophysiology and treatment of schizophrenia. A variety of PET tracers are able to display the dopamine pathway, and as such, also reveal the various abnormalities of dopaminergic transmission in schizophrenia.

15.2.1.1 D_1 Receptors

D_1 receptors are uniformly distributed across cortical regions, but are concentrated primarily in the striatum. Evidence from animal and human clinical studies have demonstrated the presence of PFC dysfunction in patients with schizophrenia, while D_1 receptors in this region play a key role in a number of frontal lobe functions.

A PET imaging study using the ^{11}C-SCH23390 tracer found that patients with schizophrenia had a lower D_1 receptor occupancy in the PFC; the activity of D_1 receptors in the PFC was negatively correlated with the severity of negative symptoms and was also associated with the decline of frontal lobe functions, such as executive function. Another imaging study using the ^{11}C-NNC112 tracer found that the D_1 receptor activity in the dorsolateral PFC of medication-naïve patients with schizophrenia was higher than that of healthy controls and that the increase in activity was associated with their performance in a working memory task (n-back task). The results

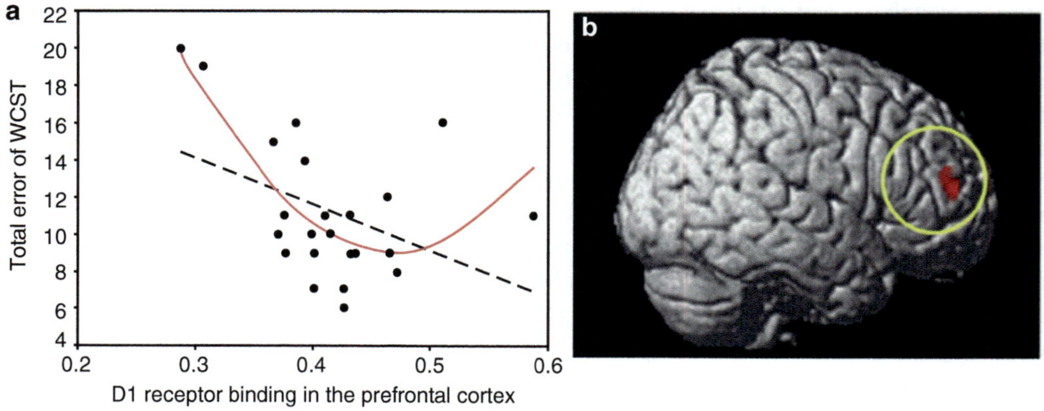

Fig. 15.13 Relationship between D_1 receptor binding in the PFC and WCST performance. ROI analysis shows an inverted U-shaped relationship between D_1 receptor binding in the PFC and total error of WCST. Red solid line: quadratic regression; black broken line: linear regression (**a**). SPM analysis also shows a quadratic regression between prefrontal D_1 receptor binding and total error of WCST. *Red region* area of D_1 receptor binding in the PFC; *yellow circle* delineated ROI for analysis (**b**)

by Takashi et al. may provide a possible explanation for this group difference: using the ^{11}C-SCH23390 tracer, they found that the D_1 receptor activity of healthy subjects showed a U-shaped relationship with performance in the Wisconsin Card Sorting Test (WCST) (Fig. 15.13), indicating that both the under- and over-stimulation of D_1 receptors will hinder working memory and set-shifting performance. This hypothesis has also been verified through animal studies. Nevertheless, we cannot rule out the possibility that the differences in these results may be attributable to the differences in the patients' basic characteristics (age, sex, and previous use of antipsychotic medication) and radiotracers utilized.

15.2.1.2 D_2/D_3 Receptors

Dopaminergic neurons are densely distributed in the striatum, and PET imaging is usually performed using probes with moderate affinity, such as ^{11}C-raclopride (^{11}C-RAC). In contrast, fewer D_2/D_3 receptors are found in extra-striatal regions (including the cerebral cortex, limbic regions, and thalamus); therefore, high-affinity PET probes (e.g., ^{11}C-FLB457 and ^{18}F-fallypride) are often selected for scanning. These tracers are all benzamide derivatives that are antagonistic to D_2 and D_3 receptors.

D_2 and D_3 receptors are currently the primary targets of antipsychotic drugs. According to previous reviews and meta-analyses, medication-naïve patients with schizophrenia showed no difference or only a small increase in striatal D_2/D_3 receptor activity in the resting state compared to healthy controls. However, the majority of these studies were focused on psychopathology, especially the positive symptoms, and only a handful assessed the subjects' cognitive function. Therefore, the relationship between striatal dopamine D_2 receptors and cognitive impairment in patients with schizophrenia remains inconclusive. In a ^{11}C-RAC PET study on six monozygotic and five dizygotic unaffected co-twins of patients with schizophrenia, as well as four monozygotic and four dizygotic healthy control twin pairs, it was found that dopamine D_2 receptor activity was upregulated in the caudate nucleus of monozygotic unaffected co-twins of patients with schizophrenia. Moreover, this upregulation was associated with poor performance in cognitive tasks (e.g., subtests of the Wechsler Memory Scale and California Verbal Learning Test).

Significant differences were also demonstrated in extra-striatal D_2/D_3 receptors between patients with schizophrenia and healthy controls, especially in the thalamus. A meta-analysis

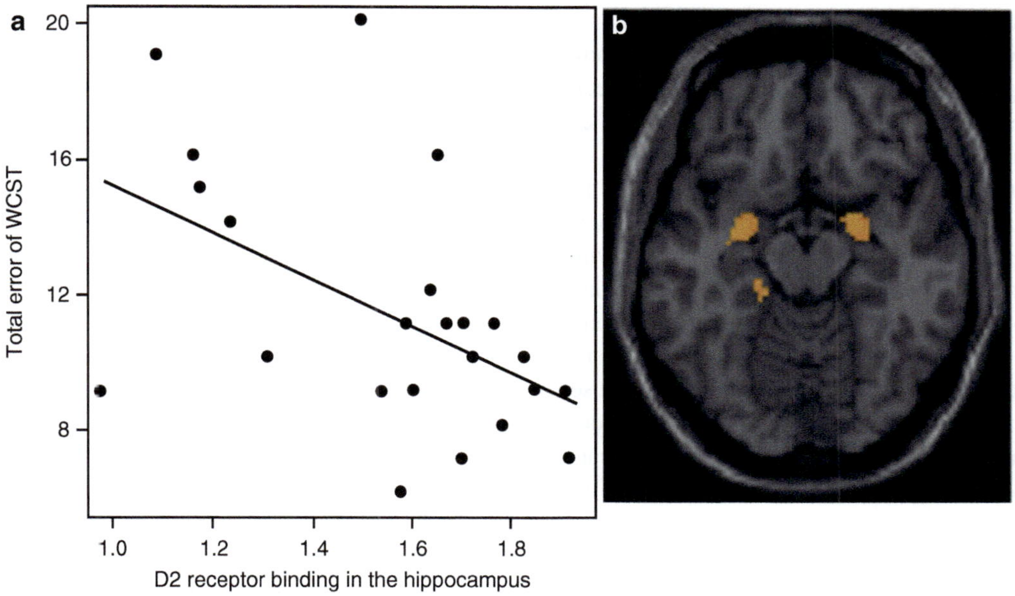

Fig. 15.14 Linear relationship between D_2 receptor binding in the hippocampus and WCST performance (Reproduced with permission from [10]). ROI analysis of the hippocampus shows a positive linear correlation between D_2 receptor binding in the hippocampus and total error of WCST (**a**). SPM analysis also shows a linear correlation between hippocampal D_2 receptor binding and total error of WCST (**b**)

revealed that the summary effect size of thalamic D_2/D_3 receptor availability between patients and healthy controls was d = −0.32, but was not statistically significant. ^{18}F-fallypride was utilized to assess the executive dysfunction and memory impairment of patients with schizophrenia, which revealed a negative or low correlation between D_2/D_3 receptor activity and WCST performance in patients, whereas healthy controls exhibited a positive correlation between the two, i.e., a higher D_2/D_3 receptor activity was associated with better performance. This disparity was especially prominent in the thalamus. Similarly, patients showed a negative or extremely low correlation between frontal-striatal-thalamic D_2/D_3 receptor activity and performance in the California Verbal Learning Test, whereas healthy controls showed a positive correlation between the two (Fig. 15.14).

15.2.1.3 Dopamine Transporter (DAT)

The majority of molecular imaging studies on striatal DAT activity did not find significant differences between healthy controls and treatment-naïve patients with schizophrenia. This finding is supported by a recent meta-analysis that included PET and single photon emission computed tomography (SPECT) studies. Another study demonstrated that the DAT activity in patients with schizophrenia with tardive dyskinesia was lower than that of patients without this symptom. Furthermore, striatal DAT activity was correlated with the severity of negative symptoms, as well as the cognitive and anxiety/depression scores on the Positive and Negative Syndrome Scale (PANSS). However, the majority of patients in this study were medicated; hence, the effects of medication must be considered. Moreover, none of the patients underwent MRI scans, and some patients did not have PANSS scores.

15.2.1.4 Levodopa (L-DOPA) Uptake (Dopamine Synthesis Capacity)

6-^{18}F-L-DOPA and L-β-^{11}C-DOPA, both of which are radioactive analogues of the dopamine precursor L-DOPA that can detect the dopamine synthesis capacity of the presynaptic terminal, are commonly used to determine the synthesis rate of endogenous dopamine. Compared to healthy controls, patients with schizophrenia have been shown to have a stronger capacity for dopamine synthesis, a finding that has been further validated by a recent meta-analysis. In a study on medication-naïve patients with schizophrenia involving ^{18}F-DOPA and ^{15}O-H_2O as PET imaging probes, patients with schizophrenia were found to exhibit higher dopamine synthesis capacity in the striatum compared to healthy controls, suggesting that patients had enhanced striatal presynaptic dopamine function. Furthermore, patients with schizophrenia exhibited a close correlation between increased CBF in the dorsolateral PFC and striatal dopamine synthesis capacity when performing the WCST, whereas this relationship was not found among healthy controls. PET imaging studies of the brain performed using ^{18}F-DOPA revealed that the dopamine synthesis capacity of the dorsal ACC in medicated patients with schizophrenia was correlated with their performance on the Stroop Color-Word Test; that patients with prodromal symptoms of schizophrenia showed an elevated dopamine synthesis capacity in the striatum; and that subjects at high risk for psychosis showed a negative correlation between striatal dopamine synthesis capacity and performance on a semantic verbal fluency tasks, such that a higher synthesis was associated with a lower accuracy rate and a lower verbal fluency.

15.2.2 5-HT

The 5-HTergic system in the human brain consists of 14 different receptor subtypes and transporters. Extensive research has been conducted on the 5-HT_1A and 5-HT_2A receptors and the 5-HT transporter (5-HTT), which are also major targets of many psychiatric medications. However, there is a lack of PET studies on the 5-HTergic system in schizophrenia.

15.2.2.1 5-HT_1A Receptor

5-HT_1A receptors are widely distributed in the hippocampus, insula, neocortex, and dorsal raphe nucleus. Additionally, 5-HT_1A receptors can regulate the entire 5-HTergic system and are therefore one of the most important subtypes of 5-HT receptors. According to animal and pharmacological studies, the 5-HT_1A receptor plays an important role in cognitive function and is a potential target for controlling the cognitive and emotional symptoms in a variety of neuropsychiatric diseases.

At present, four studies have been conducted using the PET tracer ^{11}C-WAY100635 to detect the activity of 5-HT_1A receptors in patients with schizophrenia. One study found that patients with schizophrenia exhibited increased 5-HT_1A activity in the medial temporal cortex, whereas another study found reduced 5-HT_1A activity in the amygdala. The remaining two studies demonstrated no difference in 5-HT_1A activity between patients with schizophrenia and healthy controls. A meta-analysis on post-mortem studies revealed that patients with schizophrenia had increased prefrontal 5-HT_1A receptors.

In a study on healthy subjects, Yasuno et al. found that hippocampal memory function was negatively correlated with 5-HT_1A receptor activity. However, other PET studies using ^{11}C-WAY100635 found that 5-HT_1A receptor activity in the raphe nucleus, hippocampus, and neocortical regions was not correlated with performance in any cognitive domain. As of yet, no PET studies have been conducted on cognitive function and 5-HT_1A receptor activity in patients with schizophrenia.

15.2.2.2 5-HT_2A Receptor

A large number of post-mortem and pharmacological studies have demonstrated that the 5-HT_2A receptor plays a crucial role in schizophrenia and cognitive function. A meta-analysis on post-mortem studies showed a decrease in prefrontal 5-HT_2A receptors among patients with schizophrenia. A few researchers have conducted 5-HT_2A receptor PET imaging studies on first-episode medication-naïve patients with schizophrenia, but their results lack consistency. In a recent study, PET imaging was performed on 30 patients with schizophrenia and matched healthy controls using ^{18}F-altanserin, which is a highly selective tracer for 5-HT_2A receptors. The results of that study revealed that patients with schizophrenia had lower 5-HT_2A activity in the PFC compared to healthy controls. However, 5-HT_2A activity was not correlated with cognitive function (e.g., working memory, attention, and executive function), implying that at least in the early stages of schizophrenia, 5-HT_2A receptors are not associated with cognitive dysfunction.

15.2.2.3 5-HTT

Previous PET studies using the 5-HTT-selective tracer ^{11}C-DASB showed no significant difference in 5-HTT activity between patients with schizophrenia and healthy controls, while 5-HTT activity was not correlated with schizophrenia symptoms. In contrast, ^{11}C-DASB PET studies on healthy subjects found that 5-HTT activity in the frontostriatal region was correlated with performance in executive function and logical reasoning. As of yet, however, no PET studies have been conducted on the relationship between 5-HTT activity and cognitive function in patients with schizophrenia.

15.2.2.4 Other Components of the 5-HTergic System

PET probes targeting 5-HT_1B, 5HT4, 5-HT6, and 5-HT have been successfully utilized in human brain imaging. However, at present, there have been no clinical studies involving the application of these probes to the neuroimaging of patients with schizophrenia.

15.2.3 Norepinephrine

The central norepinephrinergic system plays a critical role in wakefulness and attentional focus, while the norepinephrine transporter is a target of drug therapy for depression and attentional deficit hyperactivity disorder. Despite its importance, however, PET probes are rarely utilized in the imaging of norepinephrine transporters. There are currently no reports on the PET imaging of norepinephrine transporters in patients with schizophrenia.

PET imaging provides a direct approach to study the neurotransmitters and neurophysiology involved in schizophrenia. A large number of PET studies have demonstrated the presence of differences between the brains of patients with schizophrenia and healthy controls, while the relationship between these changes in the brain and scores on symptom scales signifies that these changes constitute the pathophysiological basis of these diseases. However, as mentioned above, only a small number of PET studies have directly examined the relationship between schizophrenia and cognitive impairment and elucidated the link between neurotransmitters and cognitive function. Current findings indicate that impaired striatal dopamine synthesis and prefrontal D_1 and D_2/D_3 receptor activity may be related to cognitive impairment in patients with schizophrenia. However, currently available studies are not only limited in quantity, but also lack uniformity in methodology. For instance, the differences in radiotracers used, quantification methods, neurocognitive tests, and patient characteristics (e.g., disease stage, duration of antipsychotic use, age, and sex) may lead to contradictory results between different studies. It is thought that these deficiencies can be addressed in the future by conducting large-sample, standardized, uniform studies that can provide new theories concerning the neurobiology of cognitive impairment in schizophrenia.

15.3 Research Applications of PET/MR in Schizophrenia

Schizophrenia involves the impairment of perception, thinking, emotion, and behavior, as well as the incoherence of mental activities. A wide range of cognitive and behavioral impairments have been demonstrated in patients with schizophrenia through neuropsychological and clinical studies. Over the past few decades, functional neuroimaging techniques have gradually taken their place as the primary methods used in schizophrenia research. Of these, MRI and PET imaging have enabled us to understand the underlying functional characteristics of the brain in patients with schizophrenia at the level of the nervous system, bringing together the fields of genetics, behavioral studies, and psychology. Integrated

PET/MR allows the simultaneous acquisition of PET and MRI information, which avoids the interference of external stimuli and spatial variability caused by imaging at different time points, thereby greatly enhancing the accuracy of image co-registration. With the continued advancement of technology and broadening of clinical applications, integrated PET/MR has demonstrated its usefulness in investigating the pathogenesis, diagnosis, and differential diagnosis of mental illnesses. However, there are currently no reports on the use of PET/MR in the field of schizophrenia. As the most advanced technique at the cutting-edge of functional and molecular imaging technology, the integration of PET and MRI will maximize the combination of function and structure and enable the exploration of neurophysiological changes in schizophrenia in a multimodal manner.

15.3.1 Research Advances of Neuroimaging in Schizophrenia

Schizophrenia is a condition caused by neurodevelopmental aberrations, presenting with non-specific prodromal symptoms. The evaluation criteria for high-risk individuals with prodromal symptoms primarily involve the combination of genetic factors and presentation of prodromal syndrome. Neuroimaging research revealed that abnormal changes in brain structure and function were already present in high-risk populations. Therefore, performing the clinical diagnosis and evaluation of high-risk populations, as well as exploring the pathological mechanisms involved, in accordance with these abnormalities is of crucial significance to the early identification of ultra-high-risk individuals, reducing the incidence of schizophrenia, improving patient prognosis, and alleviating the treatment burden of the disease.

Prior to onset, patients with schizophrenia often present with mild, early-stage clinical abnormalities, and this high-risk syndrome is known as clinical high risk (CHR). By utilizing different imaging techniques, researchers have found that high-risk patients exhibited structural abnormalities in various brain regions, including the frontal lobe, medial temporal lobe, ACC, and superior temporal gyrus. Furthermore, these abnormalities were compatible with those of first-episode or chronic patients, indicating that these structural abnormalities were present prior to the onset of schizophrenia and were markers of disease progression. Structure is the carrier of function. Research findings on gray matter structure have confirmed the presence of asymmetric gray matter abnormalities in patients with schizophrenia, which were significantly associated with sex and family history.

Investigations based on fMRI techniques have been conducted on the changes of neurological function in schizophrenia. The results indicate that first-episode medication-naïve patients with schizophrenia showed gray matter abnormalities and that local gray matter abnormalities were associated with clinical symptoms. Patients with familial schizophrenia and their parents showed more significant reductions in thalamic gray matter density compared to patients with sporadic schizophrenia and their parents. Therefore, it has been suggested that alterations in thalamic gray matter may be genetically related and can serve as a potential imaging marker for the evaluation of clinical symptoms and prognosis of patients with familial and sporadic schizophrenia. Some researchers have also examined whether there are changes in the functional connectivity of brain areas with structural abnormalities, and whether these changes are correlated with clinical symptoms. A study on brain areas with gray matter abnormalities in patients with schizophrenia revealed no changes in the resting-state functional connectivity. Given that the mechanisms underlying the drug treatment of schizophrenia remain poorly understood, and the adverse reactions are significant, fMRI has also been utilized to study the effects of drug treatment on brain function in schizophrenia. These studies revealed that antipsychotics exerted extensive effects on the brain structure and function of patients with schizophrenia within a short period of time, manifesting as reduced functional connectivity in various brain areas, and these functional changes were correlated with clinical symptoms. However, the relationship of these structural and functional changes with the evaluation of therapeutic efficacy remains inconclusive, requiring further verification through multimodal imaging data. Furthermore, the longitudinal follow-up studies are also needed to determine the long-term effects of drug treatment.

MRS is the only technique available for the non-invasive in vivo detection of chemical properties in tissues. As such, it has been extensively applied to research on metabolic dysfunction of the brain in a variety of neurodegenerative diseases and has been utilized in the detection of biomarkers in mental illnesses. Therefore, this technique has significant potential for the identification of disease biomarkers, and the prediction and evaluation of therapeutic efficacy in patients with schizophrenia. Previous animal and human post-mortem studies have demonstrated schizophrenia is related to glutamatergic and GABAergic dysfunction, while MRS can be used to perform the non-invasive detection of their metabolic status in the brain. However, further verification is needed to demonstrate whether MRS detection can truly reflect metabolic changes of the brain in patients with schizophrenia.

PET enables the non-invasive evaluation of brain metabolic activity and blood flow, as well as the determination of the distribution of key neurotransmitters in the human brain. Unlike traditional imaging techniques, different tracers can be used in PET imaging for the qualitative and quantitative analysis of brain glucose metabolism, blood flow, dopamine, and 5-HT neurotransmission, and changes in receptor affinity, distribution, and activity. Therefore, this technique has been extensively utilized in research on the neurochemical and pathophysiological mechanisms of schizophrenia and is a direct approach for studying the neurotransmitters and neurobiology involved in this condition. Previous PET studies have shown that there are differences between the brains of patients with schizophrenia and healthy controls, while the relationship between these differential changes and scores on symptom scales signifies that these changes constitute the pathophysiological basis of this disease. However, as mentioned in Sect. 15.2 above, only a small number of PET studies have directly examined the relationship between schizophrenia and cognitive impairment and elucidated the link between neurotransmitters and cognitive function. Current findings indicate that impaired striatal dopamine synthesis and prefrontal D_1 and D_2/D_3 receptor activity may be related to cognitive impairment in patients with schizophrenia.

15.3.2 Advantages of Multimodal Imaging in Schizophrenia Research

Multimodal imaging can help us to understand the human brain from multiple perspectives, such as changes in gray matter volume, structural and functional connectivity of the brain, and neurotransmission function. In recent years, the acquisition of multimodal imaging data from individual subjects has been applied to research on neurological diseases, such as schizophrenia and depression. However, these studies mostly involve conducting separate analyses for individual modalities before performing comparisons across modalities, and therefore do not fully utilize the shared information between multimodal data. However, due to the complexity and variability of neurological diseases, the results obtained through unimodal analysis may exhibit large dispersity and may not accurately reflect the covariance between different modalities. Therefore, multimodal data analysis has begun to garner growing interest in the academic community. MRI is currently the main imaging method utilized in the diagnosis of most neurological diseases, while PET can provide information on brain metabolism, receptors, and hemodynamics and is therefore also widely used in clinical practice. Built on the basis of unimodal imaging, integrated PET/MR can effectively address the limited spatial resolution of PET in order to obtain more precise PET signals, thereby achieving the further integration of multimodal information for the diagnosis of central nervous system diseases. By analyzing the ^{18}F-FDG PET,

^{11}C-FMZ PET, and fMRI data of eight healthy subjects, researchers were able to determine their whole-brain glucose metabolism, GABA metabolism, and fMRI metrics (ALFF, ReHo, and whole-brain connectivity). Their results revealed that glucose metabolism was significantly positively correlated to ALFF, ReHo, and GABA metabolism, while GABA metabolism was also significantly positively correlated to ALFF. However, there are currently no multimodal imaging studies on patients with schizophrenia. Previous studies have reported that structural and functional alterations were already present in individuals at high risk of schizophrenia. Furthermore, brain structure and function generally undergo a process of dynamic change in patients with schizophrenia. Therefore, longitudinal follow-up studies are of crucial significance to research on schizophrenia. The combination of PET and MRI can provide more functional and structural information and either modality alone. Moreover, the absence of ionizing radiation in MRI makes it more suitable for repeated scanning and long-term follow-up.

Additional longitudinal, multimodal imaging data are needed for the evaluation of drug treatments in schizophrenia, as their underlying mechanisms are still poorly understood, and previous unimodal studies have demonstrated the presence of short- and long-term effects of drug treatment on schizophrenia. Owing to the high complexity of functional and structural alterations of the brain in patients with schizophrenia, integrated PET/MR can enable the acquisition of metabolic and functional information of the brain under the same normal physiological and pathological states, thereby organically combining metabolic, functional, and structural imaging. In addition to providing more accurate structural information, fMRI can also complement PET metabolic imaging. Furthermore, through the use of different tracers, PET can be utilized for the in vivo imaging of neurotransmitter metabolic processes. There are currently no reports on whether neurotransmitter changes are related to fMRI abnormalities or to clinical characteristics. Therefore, the utilization of multimodal imaging techniques to gain a more complete picture of alterations in the brain of patients with schizophrenia will help to promote our understanding of a neurophysiological basis for the onset and development of symptoms in patients with schizophrenia.

PET/MR offers one-stop multimodal imaging of the brain with simultaneous acquisition and automatic image registration, fundamentally avoiding possible biases in subsequent image co-registration. It also ensures that structural, perfusion, functional metabolic, and other information can be acquired under the same physiological and pathological states. Therefore, it offers unique advantages for research on the pathogenic mechanisms of schizophrenia. Furthermore, PET/MR can overcome the drawbacks and deficiencies of unimodal imaging techniques, in order to implement multimodal investigations on the pathogenic mechanisms of diseases, thereby providing a better understanding on the complex pathological changes of neurological conditions. We expect that the application and promotion of PET/MR scanners in clinical practice will further drive the progress of research on schizophrenia.

Suggested Reading

González-Vivas C, Soldevila-Matías P, Sparano O, et al. Longitudinal studies of functional magnetic resonance imaging in first-episode psychosis: a systematic review. Eur Psychiatry. 2019;59:60–9.

Dietsche B, Kircher T, Falkenberg I. Structural brain changes in schizophrenia at different stages of the illness: a selective review of longitudinal magnetic resonance imaging studies. Aust N Z J Psychiatry. 2017;51(5):500–8.

Gutiérrez-Galve L, Chu EM, Leeson VC, et al. A longitudinal study of cortical changes and their cognitive correlates in patients followed up after first-episode psychosis. Psychol Med. 2015;45(1):205–16.

Cannon TD, Chung Y, He G, et al. (2015) progressive reduction in cortical thickness as psychosis develops: a multisite longitudinal neuroimaging study of youth at elevated clinical risk. Biol Psychiatry. 2015;77(2):147–57.

Van Haren NEM, Schnack HG, Koevoets MGJC, et al. Trajectories of subcortical volume change in schizophrenia: a 5-year follow-up. Schizophrenia Res. 2016;173(3):140–5.

Domen P, Peeters S, Michielse S, et al. Differential time course of microstructural white matter in patients with psychotic disorder and individuals at risk: a 3-year follow-up study. Schizophr Bull. 2017;43(1):160–70.

Liu Y, Guo W, Zhang Y, et al. Decreased resting-state interhemispheric functional connectivity correlated with neurocognitive deficits in drug-naive first-episode adolescent-onset schizophrenia. Int J Neuropsychopharmacol. 2018;21(1):33–41.

Ma X, Zheng W, Li C, et al. Decreased regional homogeneity and increased functional connectivity of default network correlated with neurocognitive deficits in subjects with genetic high-risk for schizophrenia: a resting-state fMRI study. Psychiatry Res. 2019;281:112603.

Egerton A, Modinos G, Ferrera D, et al. Neuroimaging studies of GABA in schizophrenia: a systematic review with meta-analysis. Transl Psychiatry. 2017;7(6) e1147.

Takahashi H. PET neuroimaging of extrastriatal dopamine receptors and prefrontal cortex functions. J Physiol Paris. 2013;107:503–9.

Yuksel C, Tegin C, O'connor L, et al. Phosphorus magnetic resonance spectroscopy studies in schizophrenia. J Psychiatr Res. 2015;68:157–66.

Bustillo JR, Jones T, Chen H, et al. Glutamatergic and neuronal dysfunction in gray and white matter: a spectroscopic imaging study in a large schizophrenia sample. Schizophr Bull. 2017;43(3):611–9.

Wijtenburg SA, Wright SN, Korenic SA, et al. Altered glutamate and regional cerebral blood flow levels in schizophrenia: a ^{1}H-MRS and pCASL study. Neuropsychopharmacology. 2017;42(2):562–71.

Sonnay S, Gruetter R, Duarte JMN. How energy metabolism supports cerebral function: insights from ^{13}C magnetic resonance studies in vivo. Front Neurosci. 2017;11:288.

Zhu X, Lu M, Lee BY, et al. In vivo NAD assay reveals the intracellular NAD contents and redox state in healthy human brain and their age dependences. Proc Natl Acad Sci U S A. 2015;112(9):2876–81.

Rowland LM, Krause BW, Wijtenburg SA, et al. Medial frontal GABA is lower in older schizophrenia: a MEGA-PRESS with macromolecule suppression study. Mol Psychiatry. 2016;21(2):198–204.

Weinstein J, Chohan MO, Slifstein M, et al. Pathway-specific dopamine abnormalities in schizophrenia. Biol Psychiatry. 2017;81(1):31–42.

Howes OD, Kambeitz J, Kim E, et al. The nature of dopamine dysfunction in schizophrenia and what this means for treatment. Arch Gen Psychiatry. 2012;69(8):776–86.

Hirvonen J, Van Erp TG, Huttunen J, et al. Increased caudate dopamine D2 receptor availability as a genetic marker for schizophrenia. Arch Gen Psychiatry. 2005;62(4):371–8.

Vyas NS, Buchsbaum MS, Lehrer DS, et al. D2/D3 dopamine receptor binding with [18F]fallypride correlates of executive function in medication-naive patients with schizophrenia. Schizophr Res. 2017;192:442–56.

Nozaki S, Kato M, Takano H, et al. Regional dopamine synthesis in patients with schizophrenia using L-[beta-11C]DOPA PET. Schizophr Res. 2009;108(1–3):78–84.

Vernaleken I, Buchholz HG, Kumakura Y, et al. Prefrontal cognitive performance of healthy subjects positively correlates with cerebral FDOPA influx: an exploratory [^{18}F]-fluoro-L-DOPA-PET investigation. Hum Brain Mapp. 2007;28(10):931–9.

Paterson LM, Kornum BR, Nutt DJ, et al. 5-HT radioligands for human brain imaging with PET and SPECT. Med Res Rev. 2013;33(1):54–111.

Yasuno F, Suhara T, Ichimiya T, et al. Decreased 5-HT$_1$A receptor binding in amygdala of schizophrenia. Biol Psychiatry. 2004;55(5):439–44.

Penttila J, Hirvonen J, Tuominen L, et al. Verbal memory and 5-HT$_1$A receptors in healthy volunteers-a PET study with [carbonyl-(11)C]WAY-100635. Eur Neuropsychopharmacol. 2016;26(3):570–7.

Rasmussen H, Erritzoe D, Andersen R, et al. Decreased frontal serotonin2A receptor binding in antipsychotic-naïve patients with first-episode schizophrenia. Arch Gen Psychiatry. 2010;67(1):9–16.

Paterson LM, Tyacke RJ, Nutt DJ, et al. Measuring endogenous 5-HT release by emission tomography: promises and pitfalls. J Cereb Blood Flow Metab. 2010;30(10):1682–706.

Mizrahi R, Addington J, Rusjan PM, et al. Increased stress-induced dopamine release in psychosis. Biol Psychiatry. 2012;71(6):561–7.

Moriguchi S, Yamada M, Takano H, et al. Norepinephrine transporter in major depressive disorder: a PET study. Am J Psychiatry. 2017;174(1):36–41.

Kahn RS, Sommer IE. The neurobiology and treatment of first-episode schizophrenia. Mol Psychiatry. 2015;20(1):84–7.

Wang Q, Cheung C, Deng W, et al. White-matter microstructure in previously drug-naive patients with schizophrenia after 6 weeks of treatment. Psychol Med. 2013;43(11):2301–9.

Marques TR, Taylor H, Chaddock C, et al. White matter integrity as a predictor of response to treatment in first episode psychosis. Brain. 2014;137(pt1):172–82.

Schnack HG, Van Haren NE, Nieuwenhuis M, et al. Accelerated brain aging in schizophrenia: a longitudinal pattern recognition study. Am J Psychiatry. 2016;173(6):607–16.

Tang Y, Chen K, Zhou Y, et al. Neural activity changes in unaffected children of patients with schizophrenia: a resting-state fMRI study. Schizophr Res. 2015;168(1–2):360–5.

Takahashi H, Kato M, Hayashi M, et al. Memory and frontal lobe functions; possible relations with dopamine D2 receptors in the hippocampus. NeuroImage. 2007;34(4):1643–9.

Nugent AC, Martinez A, D'alfonso A, et al. The relationship between glucose metabolism, resting-state fMRI BOLD signal, and GABAA-binding potential: a preliminary study in healthy subjects and those with temporal lobe epilepsy. J Cereb Blood Flow Metab. 2015;35(4):583–91.

Research Applications of Positron Emission Tomography/Magnetic Resonance (PET/MR) Imaging in Other Neurological Diseases

16

Jing Huang, Qianwen Li, and Jie Lu

16.1 Research Applications of PET/MR in Multiple Sclerosis (MS)

MS is the most common inflammatory demyelinating disease of the central nervous system (CNS) and primarily involves the brain, optic nerves, and spinal cord. This disease frequently occurs in young and middle-aged adults, affecting more than 2.5 million patients worldwide, and is one of the major causes of disability among younger patients. The incidence of MS varies by population, as evidenced by a meta-analysis that included 59 countries which revealed that the incidence of MS increased significantly with increasing geographic latitude. The exact etiology and pathological mechanisms of MS are not fully understood. It is currently believed that the onset of this disease is jointly determined by genetic and environmental factors, with autoimmunity and neurodegeneration playing a dominant role in its pathological processes. The pathological features of MS are primarily characterized by inflammation, demyelination, axonal injury, and gliosis, and when axonal injury exceeds a specific threshold, MS clinically manifests as a progressive phase. MS can be classified based on its disease course into relapsing-remitting multiple sclerosis (RRMS) and progressive multiple sclerosis (PMS), while the latter can be further subdivided into primary progressive multiple sclerosis (PPMS) and secondary progressive multiple sclerosis (SPMS).

MS involves a wide variety of clinical signs and symptoms. At present, the clinical diagnosis of MS is primarily based on the dissemination of lesions in time and space. MRI not only enables the visualization of the location, number, size, and distribution of MS lesions, but also allows the dynamic observation of lesion evolution over time. Therefore, it is helpful for the differential diagnosis of MS, the evaluation of therapeutic efficacy, and the determination of patient prognosis, particularly in evaluating the natural course of this disease. However, conventional T_1-weighted imaging (T_1WI) and T_2-weighted imaging (T_2WI) sequences lack the specificity needed to obtain this detailed information. In recent years, novel MRI techniques have been utilized in the quantitative assessment of MS-related structural and functional changes of the brain, helping us to understand the pathogenic mechanisms of this disease. In particular, these techniques can be used to observe functional changes in brain tissues in order to explore the pathophysiological mechanisms of MS.

J. Huang · Q. Li · J. Lu (✉)
Department of Radiology and Nuclear Medicine, Xuanwu Hospital, Capital Medical University, Beijing, China

J. Lu, G. Zhao (eds.), *PET/MR: Functional and Molecular Imaging of Neurological Diseases and Neurosciences*, https://doi.org/10.1007/978-981-19-9902-4_16

16.1.1 Research Applications of MRI in MS

16.1.1.1 Research Applications of Voxel-Based Morphometry (VBM) in MS

In the past, MS was regarded as a demyelinating disease that only affected white matter. However, recent VBM studies have detected the presence of progressive gray matter atrophy in various MS subtypes. Reductions in gray matter volume can occur throughout the brain, but occur most prominently in the deep gray matter nuclei and the limbic lobe. Gray matter atrophy in MS is primarily attributed to the following pathological mechanisms: (1) demyelinating lesions of brain white matter leading to progressive axonal degeneration; (2) focal inflammatory lesions of the gray matter itself and diffuse leptomeningeal lesions; (3) 60% loss of glial cells; and (4) impaired axonal iron export, resulting in abnormal iron deposition. The gray matter involvement of MS has garnered increasing attention, with a growing body of evidence suggesting that gray matter atrophy is closely related to clinical function scores, including motor, sensory, cognitive, and other functions. Striatal volume and the cortical thickness of the middle frontal gyrus are positively correlated with cognitive function, whereas thalamic volume is negatively correlated with disease duration and the Expanded Disability Status Scale. VBM was performed to analyze the status of brain atrophy in MS and neuromyelitis optica (NMO), and to compare between the two conditions. The results of that study revealed that brain atrophy was extensively distributed in MS and was most prominent in the bilateral thalamus and caudate nucleus, whereas brain atrophy was relatively mild and restricted in NMO, primarily found in the cortical regions, with no significant atrophy of deep gray matter. Brain regions with significant differences in gray matter volume between the two diseases included the bilateral thalamus, caudate nucleus, parahippocampal gyrus, and left insula (Fig. 16.1).

16.1.1.2 Research Applications of Diffusion Tensor Imaging (DTI) in MS

MS lesions cause changes in the structure and/or permeability of barriers to water molecule diffusion in the CNS, while axonal injuries reduce the restricted diffusion in the vertical direction of nerve fibers. These changes are primarily characterized by a decrease in fractional anisotropy (FA) and an increase in axial diffusivity (AD), the latter of which is related to myelin damage, as well as elevated apparent diffusion coefficient (ADC) and mean diffusivity (MD) values. In the early stages of MS, i.e., the clinically isolated syndrome (CIS) phase, DTI can be used to detect abnormal changes in white matter tracts, which occur less frequently than in patients with more advanced MS (Fig. 16.2). Studies have shown that the abnormal diffusion of water molecules in the corpus callosum can be detected during the CIS phase of MS, which can serve as an important indicator for predicting CIS conversion. Approximately 91% of cases converted to MS within 3 years in patients with abnormal diffusion in more than three white matter tracts (e.g., corticospinal tract, corpus callosum, optic radiation, etc.) during the CIS phase. DTI can also be used to observe microscopic changes in perilesional areas, where structural abnormalities cannot be detected using conventional MRI. Typical DTI abnormalities in MS include elevated MD and reduced FA, which are generally more significant than those of normal white matter regions. Furthermore, MS lesions in gray matter exhibit higher FA values than normal gray matter, which may reflect the axonal loss, neuronal injury, and microglial activation in gray matter lesions.

In recent years, tract-based spatial statistics (TBSS) has been utilized in research on inflammatory demyelinating diseases of the CNS. TBSS is a method of analysis based on DTI data that implements a "skeletonized" data processing approach in order to objectively reflect the integrity of white matter tracts. It has a higher accu-

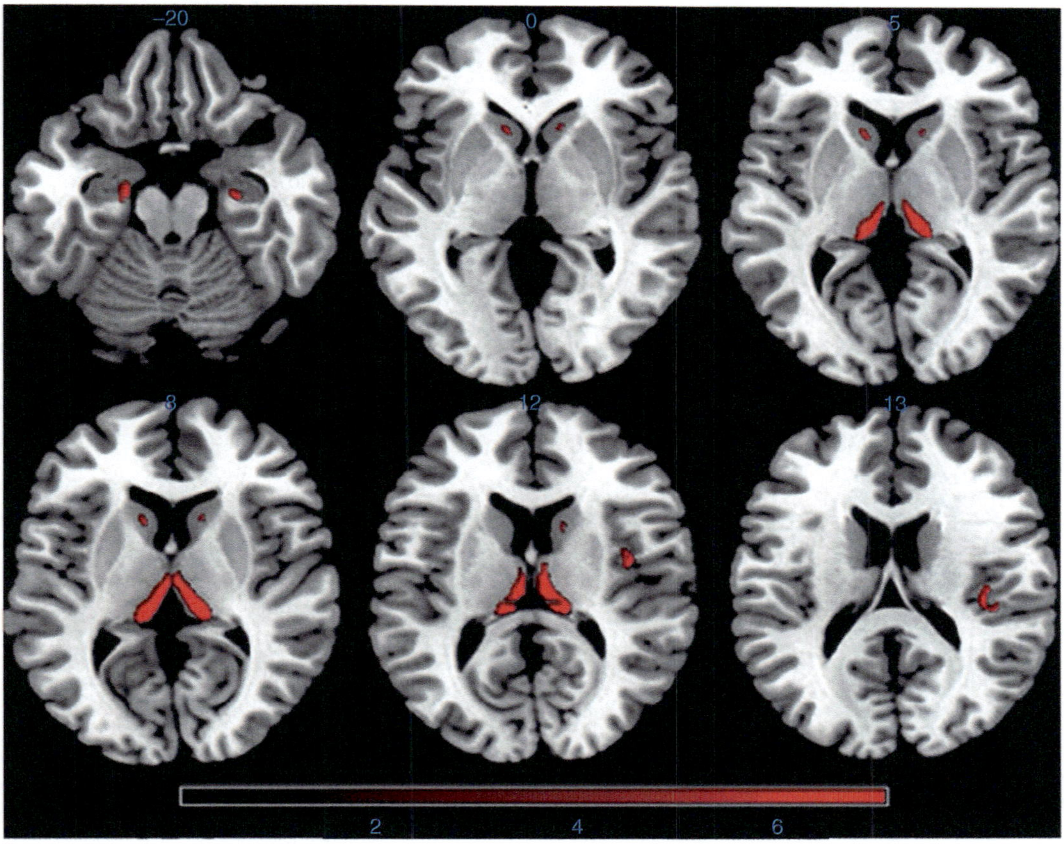

Fig. 16.1 VBM comparison of whole-brain gray matter volume between MS and NMO. Compared to brain atrophy in NMO, patients with MS showed significantly lower gray matter volume (red) in regions that included the bilateral thalamus, caudate nucleus, parahippocampal gyrus, and right insula

racy than conventional DTI and can help reduce the occurrence of false positive results. Using TBSS, patients with RRMS were found to have more extensive involvement of white matter tracts, including the commissural, association, and projection fibers, as well as the those in the brainstem. Of these, the commissural and association fibers were most significantly affected, although all white matter tracts showed varying decreases in FA values. Compared to patients with MS, patients with CIS exhibited milder and more restricted involvement of white matter tracts, as well as a smaller decrease in FA values. Furthermore, unlike the involvement of movement, sensation, and cognition-related white matter tracts in patients with MS, CIS mainly affected cognition-related tracts, such as the corpus callosum. The TBSS comparison of areas of the brain with significant differences between the two conditions is shown in Fig. 16.3.

Diffusion tensor tractography (DTT) can be used to trace specific white matter tracts, such as the corticospinal tract, corpus callosum, and optic radiation. DTT studies demonstrated that patients with MS had higher MD and lower FA values in white matter tracts compared to healthy controls. One drawback of DTT studies is that the appearance of focal and diffuse changes in brain tissues over the course of the disease can lead to a decrease in white matter anisotropy, which then increases the uncertainty of major eigenvectors in DTT.

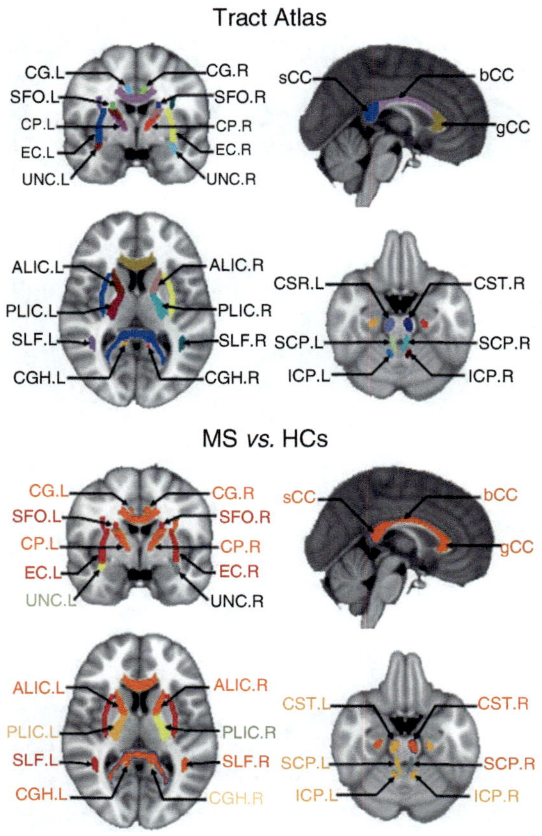

Fig. 16.2 Differences in DTI metrics in atlas-based tract analysis among CIS, MS, and healthy control groups. Gray represents normal diffusion metrics; yellow represents abnormalities in one diffusion metric; light orange represents abnormalities in two diffusion metrics; dark orange represents abnormalities in three diffusion metrics; and red represents abnormalities in all diffusion metrics. *CG* cingulate gyrus; *SFO* superior fronto-occipital fasciculus; *CP* cerebral peduncle; *EC* external capsule; *UNC* uncinate fasciculus; *sCC* splenium of corpus callosum; *bCC* body of corpus callosum; *gCC* genu of corpus callosum; *ALIC* anterior limb of internal capsule; *PLIC* posterior limb of internal capsule; *SLF* superior longitudinal fasciculus; *CGH* cingulum at hippocampus; *CST* corticospinal tract; *SCP* superior cerebellar peduncle

16.1.1.3 Research Applications of fMRI in MS

(1) Task-based fMRI
   (a) Motor tasks: A wide range of task paradigms have been utilized to explore the functions of the brain related to the motor system, the most common of which are finger flexion-extension tasks. However, despite the differences in motor tasks, similar patterns of change have been elicited in functional areas. Patients in all stages of MS (e.g., CIS and RRMS, or SPMS and PPMS) all exhibited more extensive cortical activation than healthy controls, often involving the motor-related areas of the bilateral cerebral hemispheres. Patients in full remission after relapse also displayed a wider extent of activation in motor areas compared to healthy controls, involving the entire affected cerebral hemisphere. These findings, therefore, provide a new understanding of functional reorganization following acute brain injury. Nevertheless, different patterns of motor activation can be exhibited throughout the various stages of MS. CIS is generally characterized by unilateral motor activation, RRM by bilateral activation, and SPMS by more extensive activation, even affect-

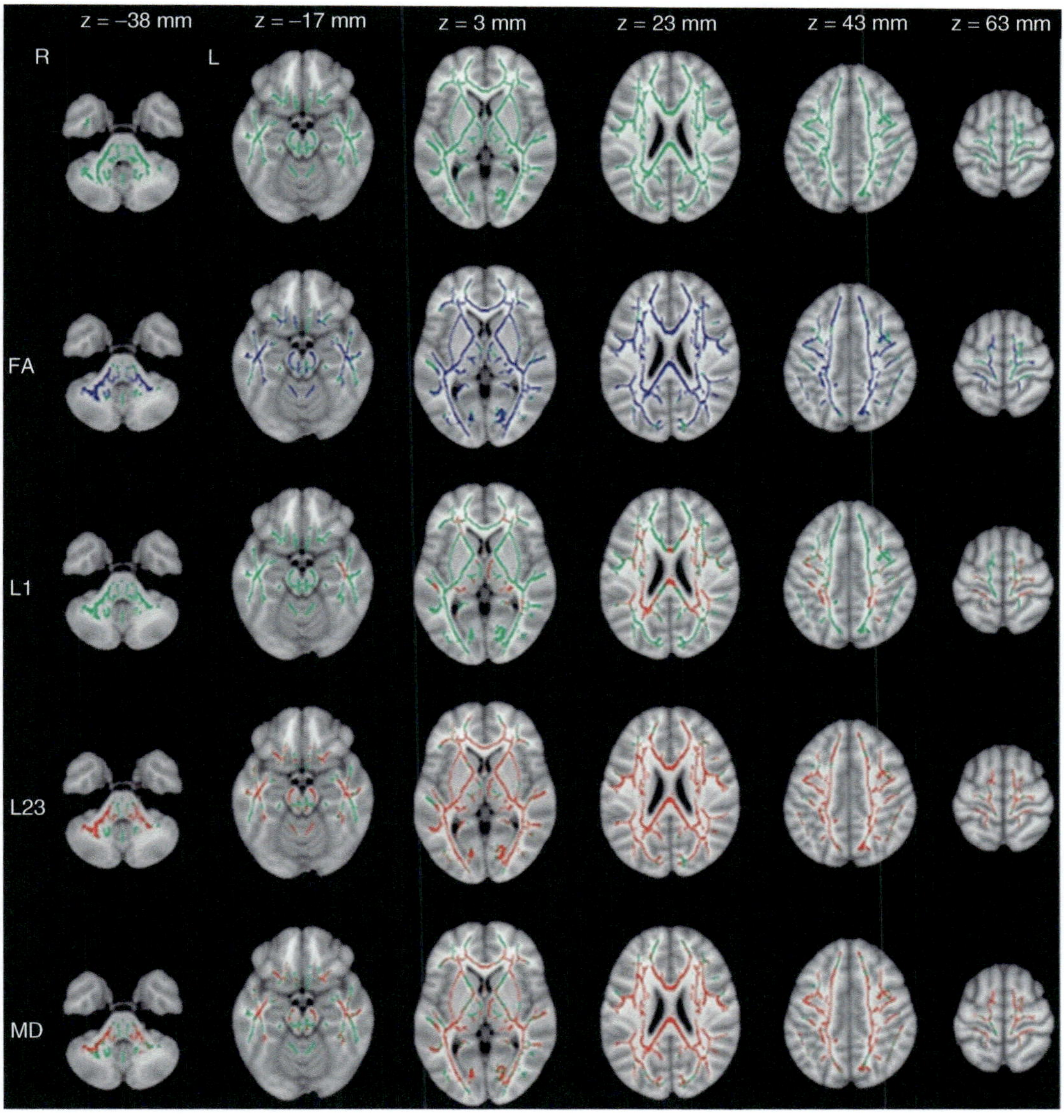

Fig. 16.3 TBSS comparison of CIS and MS. Blue represents white matter areas with decreased FA values (first row), while red represents white matter tracts with increased λ_1 (second row), λ_{23} values (third row), and MD (fourth row) ($P < 0.05$, family-wise error corrected)

ing regions beyond the motor system. Combining fMRI with structural MRI enables us to examine the correlation between functional and structural changes, as structural data can be used to assess the injury load, while DTI can be used to evaluate the integrity of white matter structures and for the quantitative analysis of white matter injuries. In general, the increase in sensorimotor activation is correlated to the severity of tissue damage, especially in specific white matter regions, such as the corticospinal tract.

(b) Cognitive tasks: The majority of studies have reported that compared to healthy controls, MS patients without or with mild cognitive impairment exhibited more extensive activation of the cerebral cortex when performing cognitive tasks. During memory and attention tasks, MS patients with higher cognitive ability showed increased activation of the cerebral cortex, whereas those with lower cognitive ability did not show a significant increase. When performing memory tasks, MS patients with cognitive impairment showed a lower activation of the hippocampal neural network compared to those without cognitive impairment. Furthermore, attention tasks of varying complexity elicited additional activation in patients with MS. However, additional activation was not observed in the prefrontal cortex (PFC) or motor cortex of patients with severe MS, suggesting that compensatory mechanisms may have been depleted in that group. Moreover, patients with RRMS showed more widespread cortical activation with increasing task difficulty than patients with CIS. In contrast, patients with SPMS only showed a slight increase in cortical activation with increasing task difficulty, suggesting that their functional reserve was limited. These abnormally activated areas of the brain were also correlated with structural damage in the brain, such as lesion load, loss of white matter integrity as measured by DTI, or brain atrophy.

Longitudinal task-based fMRI studies are relatively scarce. A study found that at the 12-month follow-up, the prolonged activation of the PFC was significantly correlated with improvements in the cognitive function of patients with MS. This implies that the improvement of cognitive performance in patients with MS over time is related to the increased activation of relevant cortical regions.

(2) Resting-state fMRI (RS-fMRI): There is currently a plethora of RS-fMRI studies on patients with MS. Commonly used functional metrics include amplitude of low-frequency fluctuation (ALFF) and functional connectivity (FC), while commonly used methods of analysis include independent component analysis (ICA) and graph theory methods. RS-fMRI studies have shown that the ALFF of patients with MS was lower than that of healthy controls after their first demyelinating event, while patients with CIS also showed significant reductions in the ALFF values for the anterior cingulate cortex (ACC), caudate nucleus, and cuneus (Fig. 16.4). These findings indicate that resting-state functional changes can be detected even in the earliest stages of MS, and that these changes can evolve over the course of the disease. Furthermore, other studies have found that patients with MS showed increased ALFF in the thalamus and some cortical regions, and indicated that these changes were related to the degree of dysfunction.

Within the six resting-state networks extracted by ICA, patients with CIS showed a higher level of synchronization than healthy controls and patients with MS, including in the default mode

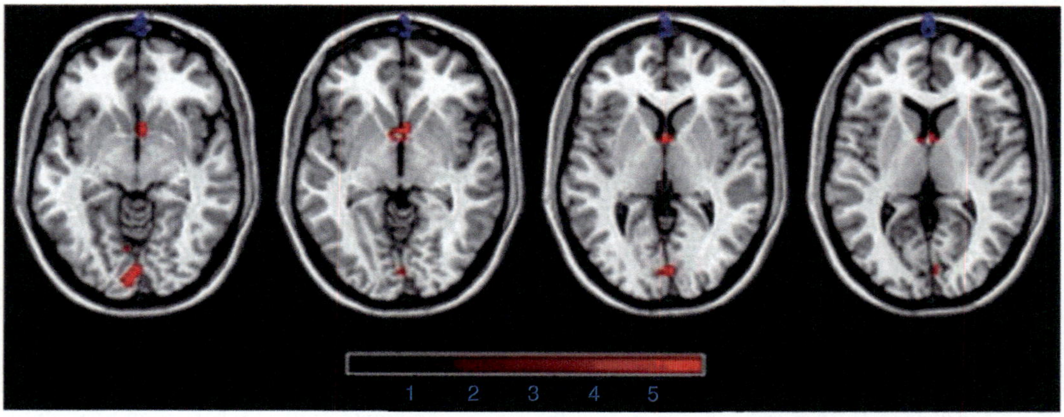

Fig. 16.4 ALFF of levels in patients with CIS. Brain areas with significant reductions include the anterior cingulate cortex, caudate nucleus, and cuneus

network (DMN) and sensorimotor network, whereas patients with MS did not show significant functional differences compared to healthy controls. Additionally, patients with MS exhibited gradual decreases in the FC of the memory and executive function networks, which were correlated with greater injury. This implies that the cortical functional reorganization of the resting-state networks is a phenomenon that occurs in the early stages of MS and gradually declines with disease progression and greater injury accumulation. Some studies have suggested that the enhanced FC of the dorsal frontoparietal, right ventral frontoparietal, and prefronto-insular networks was negatively correlated with Multiple Sclerosis Functional Composite Score. Additionally, functional changes of the DMN were found to be correlated with fatigue and clinical disability indicators. Compared to healthy controls, patients with MS showed a progressive decline in anterior DMN activity, and these changes were more prominent in MS patients with cognitive impairment. These findings may be related to the DTI changes in the corpus callosum and cingulate gyrus. Compared to MS patients without fatigue, MS patients with fatigue showed increased FC in the posterior DMN and primary motor cortex, as well as decreased FC in the anterior DMN and supplementary motor cortex. MS patients exhibited lower FC in the bilateral peristriatal visual cortex than healthy controls, whereas patients with visual symptoms showed higher FC in the extrastriate cortex and right middle occipital gyrus. These differences were correlated with the number of visual symptom episodes in patients with MS, but not with regional gray matter atrophy. Compared to healthy controls, CIS patients without brain lesions exhibited decreased FC in the visual areas and increased FC in the left thalamus and visual areas (Fig. 16.5).

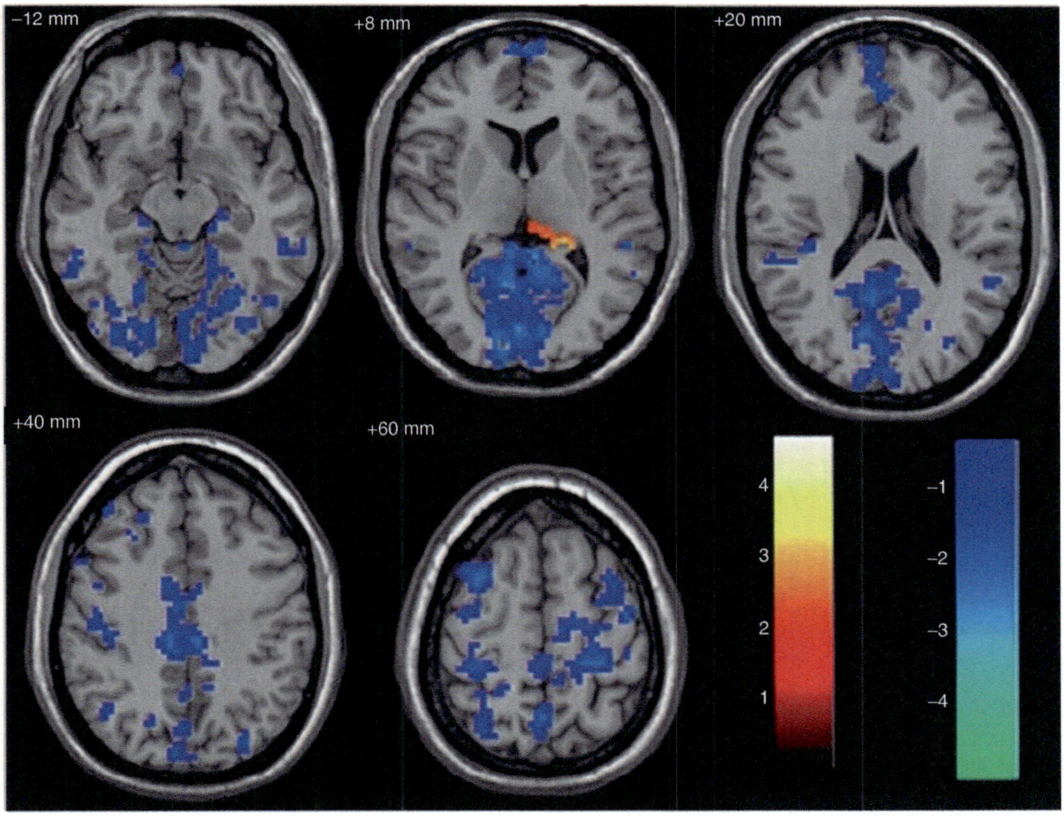

Fig. 16.5 Whole-brain functional connectivity of the primary visual cortex in CIS patients without brain lesions. Blue represents regions with decreased functional connectivity, primarily found in the visual cortices; red represents regions with increased functional connectivity, primarily found in the left thalamus

Current studies have utilized seed-based methods to explore the FC of the thalamus. Compared to healthy controls, patients with MS showed coexisting regions of increased and decreased FC in the thalamus (Fig. 16.6). Interestingly, thalamic FC was negatively correlated with cognitive function, suggesting that a closer connectivity between the thalamus and certain brain areas is associated with more severe cognitive impairment. Additionally, patients with MS were reported to have decreased FC between the thalamus and several brain regions, including the right middle frontal gyrus, parahippocampal gyrus, and left inferior parietal lobule, while increased intra- and inter-thalamic FC was negatively correlated with disease duration. In another seed-based RS-fMRI study that evaluated the relationship between sensorimotor network FC and upper limb motor deficits, motor-preserved patients with MS showed stronger FC in visual information processing areas than motor-impaired patients with MS, whereas motor-impaired patients showed weaker FC in the sensorimotor and somatosensory association cortices. These findings suggest that more severe structural damage can be observed throughout the brain of motor-impaired patients.

At present, longitudinal RS-fMRI studies are relatively scarce. After the initial onset of acute demyelination injuries, functional reorganization may lead to changes in injury-related networks, but without changes in the chronic phase. In another study, patients with MS who were within 24 h of the acute phase showed stronger long- and short-range FC than healthy controls, while at the 2-year follow-up, the FC decreases of those patients were correlated with disability progression. Therefore, the decrease in connectivity signified the depletion of functional compensation. By performing graph theory analysis on the brain networks of a large cohort of patients with MS, researchers revealed the presence of abnormalities in global network features, which may serve as a potential method for differentiating between patients with MS and healthy controls.

Over the years, fMRI, which can be used to detect functional changes related to clinical improvements and has shown that certain brain areas may play a critical role in recovery, has provided important evidence for the plasticity and functional reorganization of MS injuries. More longitudinal studies on MS involving larger samples sizes are needed, however, to verify these results.

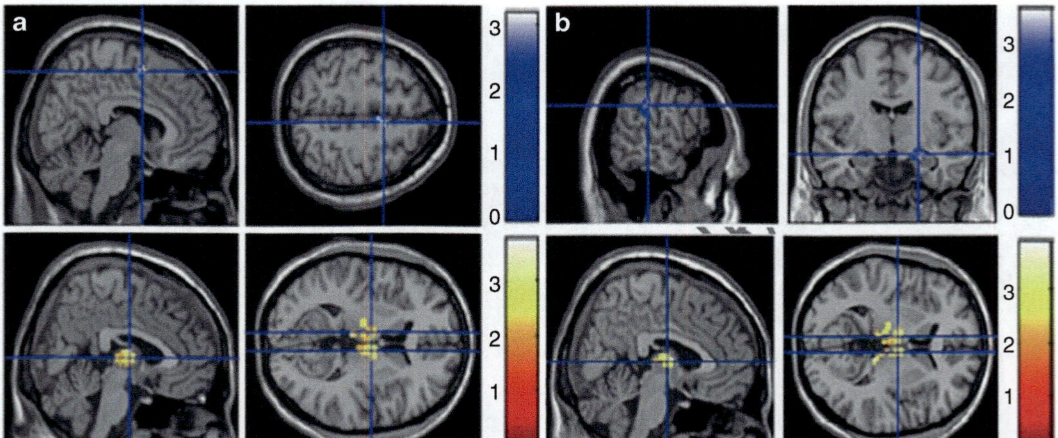

Fig. 16.6 Whole-brain functional connectivity changes of the left (**a**) and right thalamus (**b**) in patients with MS. Decreased functional connectivity in the right middle frontal gyrus (top row) and increased functional connectivity in the bilateral thalamus (bottom row) (**a**). Decreased functional connectivity in the right parahippocampal gyrus (top row) and increased functional connectivity in the bilateral thalamus (bottom row) (**b**). The color scale represents *t* values

16.1.1.4 Research Applications of Magnetic Resonance Spectroscopy (MRS) in MS

^{1}H-MRS can be utilized to elucidate the pathogenesis of MS from a metabolic perspective. A substantial decrease in N-acetylaspartate (NAA) can be observed in acute demyelinating diseases, and since NAA can only be detected in neurons and their axons, the decrease in NAA can be attributed to axonal injury. An increase in glutamate (Glu) suggests that there is an association between axonal injury in active lesions and Glu excitotoxicity. Furthermore, elevated choline (Cho) and lactate (Lac) peaks can also be observed. Changes in Cho peak are predominantly caused by the increase in membrane phospholipids released during the active degradation of myelin sheaths. The increase in Lac peak may reflect the metabolism of inflammatory cells. In large acute demyelinating lesions, a decrease in creatine (Cr) peak and increases in lipid and myo-inositol (mI) peaks can be observed.

Following the acute phase, the Lac peak of injured tissues gradually decreases to normal levels over the subsequent several days, several weeks, the Cr peak returns to normal within a few days, while mI levels increase slightly, which may be related to gliosis. The Cho and lipid peaks return to normal levels after a few months. The NAA peak may continue to decline or recover partially soon after the acute phase and persist for several months. The recovery of NAA may be related to the subsidence of edema, increase in axonal diameter, and reversible metabolic changes in neurons. MRS can also be used to visualize abnormal metabolic alterations in white matter regions. A smaller decrease in the NAA peak is observed with increasing distance from the center of the lesion. Regions with gliosis exhibit higher Cr and mI peaks, as well as an elevated Glu peak, which signifies excitotoxic effects. NAA/Cr is highly correlated with clinical disability in patients with CIS and RRMS. Moreover, the decrease in white matter NAA/Cr is also strongly correlated with the likelihood of clinical disability, while this correlation is stronger in patients with early-stage RRMS, and is decreased in patients with SPMS. In addition to NAA and Cr, Cho and lipid levels can also reflect the severity of acute inflammation, whereas mI can reflect the degree of brain gliosis in MS and may be associated with the likelihood of clinical disability.

An MRS study demonstrated that NAA was reduced in occult lesions in patients with MS, whereas patients with NMO did not exhibit a decrease in NAA, indicating the presence of axonal or neuronal injury in MS. In contrast, patients with NMO exhibited a slight increase in Cho in occult lesions, suggesting that only subtle metabolic changes had occurred in NMO (Fig. 16.7).

16.1.2 Research Applications of PET Imaging in MS

PET imaging can be utilized in the research of the pathological basis for neuroinflammation, neurological dysfunction, demyelination, and remyelination in MS, thereby supplementing the findings of MRI studies to achieve the accurate diagnosis of, monitoring of clinical progression, and formulation of treatment plans for MS.

16.1.2.1 Research Applications of ^{18}F-Fluorodeoxyglucose (^{18}F-FDG) PET in MS

^{18}F-FDG was one of the first tracers utilized in the imaging of inflammation due to the increased uptake of the radiotracer as a result of the increased glucose utilization rate of inflammatory cells. In MS, ^{18}F-FDG can not only serve as a marker of inflammation, but also as a marker of neurodegeneration due to the higher metabolic rate of activated immune cells. Research has shown that deep white matter lesions exhibited higher ^{18}F-FDG uptake than bilateral paraventricular lesions, suggesting that lesions at different locations are subjected to different extents of infiltration by inflammatory cells. Lesions in the acute and remission phases exhibit different patterns of ^{18}F-FDG uptake, which may be related to the degree of inflammatory response in the lesions,

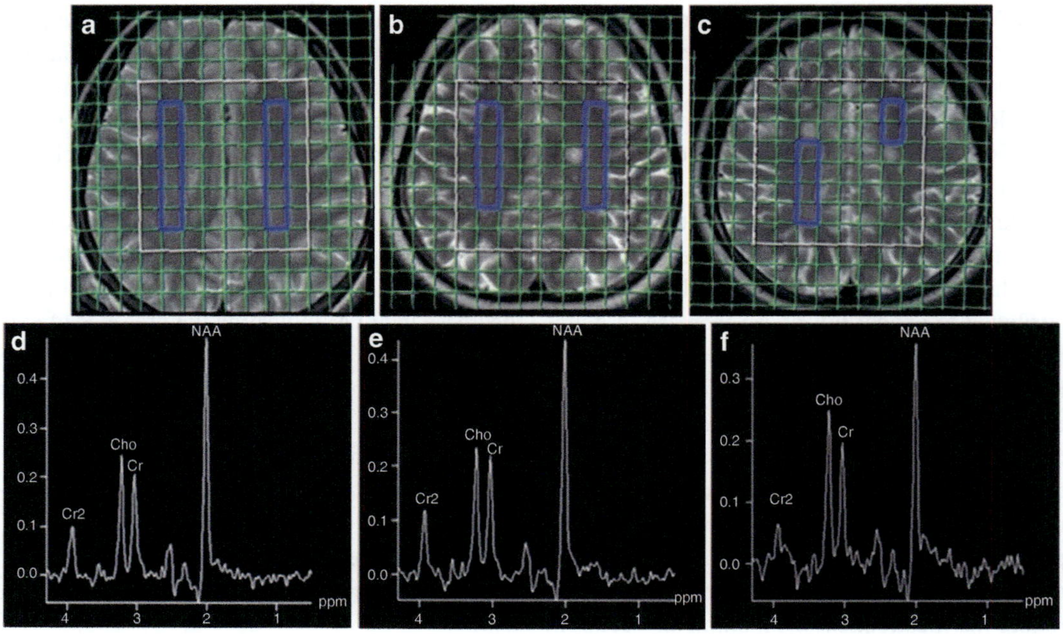

Fig. 16.7 Voxel placement and MR spectra. Selected voxel positions of normal-appearing white matter in conventional MRI among healthy controls (**a**), patients with NMO (**b**), and patients with MS (**c**). Corresponding MR spectra (**d–f**)

and can therefore be used to evaluate the status of disease. Most lesions in patients at various stages of MS exhibit high ^{18}F-FDG uptake, suggesting the presence of active inflammation, while lesions appear as hypo- or isometabolic in the remission and acute phases. Some researchers believe that ^{18}F-FDG can be used to classify white matter lesions according to regional glucose metabolism into acute (hypometabolic) and chronic (hypometabolic or isometabolic) lesions. Furthermore, in addition to changes in lesional glucose metabolism, patients with MS also exhibited alterations in cortical glucose metabolism, which could be attributed to the decline in cerebral cortical function induced by axonal injury, thereby giving rise to clinically relevant cognitive impairments. A longitudinal follow-up PET study revealed that cortical glucose uptake decreased with increasing disease duration and was most significant in the frontoparietal cortex. Moreover, a decline in glucose metabolism occurred at a faster rate than the progression of the clinical symptoms.

16.1.2.2 Neuroinflammation and Activated Microglia

Microglia account for 10% of the total number of brain cells and are involved in the immune defense of the CNS. Following CNS injury, microglia become activated and can be identified based on their morphological and immunophenotype changes, which allow them to be differentiated from their phenotype in the quiescent state. The participation of activated microglia in acute inflammation is generally beneficial. Conversely, chronic inflammation and sustained microglial activation can produce adverse effects in chronic neuroinflammatory diseases such as MS. However, the exact role of sustained microglial activation in such diseases is still poorly understood.

Microglial activation can upregulate the expression of translocator protein (TSPO), which is a protein involved in the release of pro-inflammatory cytokines during inflammation and is found at extremely low levels in the CNS of healthy subjects. Currently, the most widely used tracer is the first-generation PET tracer, ^{11}C-

PK11195, which is also the most classic TSPO-targeting radioligand. However, owing to the short half-life of ^{11}C, ^{11}C-PK11195 has relatively low bioavailability in brain tissue and high levels of non-specific binding with normal tissue, causing a low signal-to-noise ratio, therefore restricting its application in clinical practice. These defects have prompted the development of second-generation radioligands, the most important of which is ^{11}C-PBR28. ^{11}C-PBR28 and the ^{18}F-labelled TSPO ligand, ^{18}F-PBR06, can display the sites of inflammation (Fig. 16.8), and enable the dynamic monitoring of macrophage changes during the inflammatory process, thereby reflecting the course of inflammatory responses, and monitoring the progression and severity of neuroinflammation.

Activated microglia play a critical role in the pathological processes of MS. The lesions revealed by MRI exhibit an increased expression of TSPO in PET. ^{11}C-PBR28 PET imaging has shown that focal hypermetabolism in the brains of MR patients occurs earlier than MRI abnormalities. In activated MS plaques, TSPO expression is significantly elevated in microglia or macrophages, whereas in chronic MS plaques, the increase is more pronounced in reactive astrocytes. This indicates that the pathological mechanism of TSPO elevation during the inflammatory phase of MS may differ from that of the chronic phase, with increased ^{11}C-PK11195 uptake observed not only within white matter lesions, but also in normal gray and white matter. The increased TSPO expression of cerebral gray matter in MS (Fig. 16.9) was found to be correlated with the level of clinical neurological dysfunction. In addition, TSPO PET imaging can also be utilized to evaluate the efficacy of MS treatments. Patients with MS who were treated with glatiramer acetate showed significantly reduced cerebral ^{11}C-PK11195 uptake, suggesting that the extent of microglial activation is diminished following MS treatment.

16.1.2.3 Myelin Imaging

Although the spontaneous myelin repair that occurs during the pathological process of MS is incomplete, it can mitigate focal and diffuse white matter injury. Pathological evidence from post-mortem examinations have shown that after undergoing MS-related demyelination, remyelination can be observed in the lesions and white matter of all MS subtypes. Moreover, in patients with MS, more active remyelination was detected in new lesions.

The application of PET imaging in the study of myelin dynamics has been garnering growing interest in recent years. In 2006, the first myelin PET tracer, ^{11}C-1, 4-bis (p-aminostyryl)-2-methoxybenzene (^{11}C-BMB), was evaluated in baboons. The tracer demonstrated a high affinity for white matter, but poor gray/white matter contrast and a long acquisition time, which prevented the further development of this tracer given the

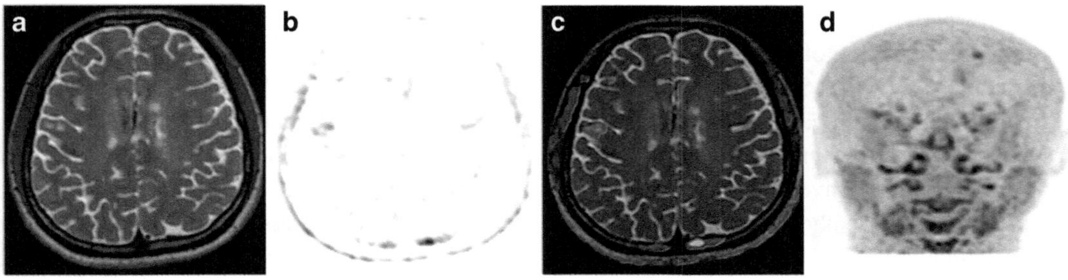

Fig. 16.8 Sites of inflammation revealed by the TSPO ligand ^{18}F-PBR06. A 49-year-old female patient who suffered from SPMS for 17 years. Transverse MR T_2-weighted imaging shows multiple bilateral cingulate gyrus and right fronto-subcortical white matter hyperintensities (**a**). Transverse ^{18}F-PBR06 PET (**b**), integrated ^{18}F-PBR06 PET/MR (**c**), and coronal ^{18}F-PBR06 PET (**d**) show corresponding increases in the ^{18}F-PBR06 uptake of right fronto-subcortical lesions, indicating that the lesions are active inflammatory lesions

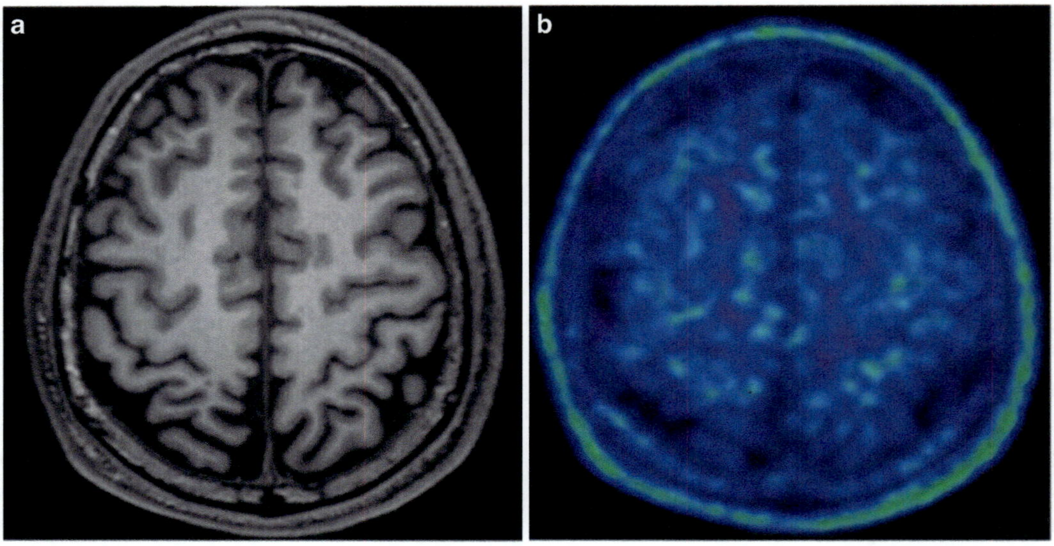

Fig. 16.9 Elevated TSPO expression of cerebral gray matter in MS. A 35-year-old male patient who suffered from RRMS for 3 years. Transverse MR T_1-weighted imaging (**a**) and integrated ^{18}F-PBR28 TSPO PET/MR (**b**) show significantly elevated TSPO in the gray matter of the frontal and parietal lobes

short half-life of ^{11}C. ^{11}C-Case Imaging Compound (^{11}C-CIC), which has a similar structure to ^{11}C-BMB, has also been tested for the evaluation of myelin dynamics in preclinical studies. However, the ability of ^{11}C-CIC to detect remyelination could not be confirmed by ex vivo data in preclinical models. In contrast, ^{11}C-N-methyl-4,4′-diaminostilbene (^{11}C-MeDAS) has exhibited pharmacokinetics, tissue binding, and blood-brain barrier penetration characteristics that are more conducive to imaging. ^{11}C-MeDAS can bind selectively to white matter regions in the brain and spinal cord and has shown a very high sensitivity and specificity to myelin content in experimental models of MS. In autoimmune encephalitis, ^{11}C-MeDAS uptake was found to decrease during inflammatory demyelination and gradually increased over the course of subsequent spontaneous remyelination, which is consistent with histopathological findings and clinical symptoms.

^{11}C-Pittsburgh compound B (^{11}C-PiB), a PET tracer for visualizing amyloid deposition in patients with dementia, has now been utilized in MS research. In a mouse model of demyelination, ^{11}C-PiB was able to clearly distinguish between demyelinated and remyelinated lesions. The standardized uptake value (SUV) of ^{11}C-PiB did not differ significantly between patients with MS and healthy controls, but there was a progressive decrease in ^{11}C-PiB binding from whole-brain normal-appearing white matter (NAWM) to MS lesions, which reflected the decrease in myelin content.

16.1.3 Research Applications of PET/MR in MS

Although substantial progress has been achieved in MRI techniques for the evaluation of MS (i.e., DTI, fMRI, ^{23}Na MRI, magnetization transfer imaging), these techniques cannot be utilized to fully detect the pathophysiological processes in the early stages of the disease. PET, on the other hand, is ideal for detecting microglial activation (using TSPO tracers) or myelin changes (using amyloid tracers), although it has a very limited spatial resolution, which can reduce the accuracy of quantification, especially in small lesions. Integrated PET/MR combines the two techniques to overcome the limitations of unimodal imaging, so as to comprehensively display the structural, functional, and metabolic changes in MS, which will facilitate our future clinical understanding on the pathogenesis of MS. Although only a handful of integrated PET/MR studies have been conducted thus far, their number is constantly increasing.

An ^{18}F-FDG PET/MR study involving 17 patients with RRMS revealed that the mutually complementary PET (glucose metabolic rate of the basal ganglia) and MRI (reduced gray matter density of the frontal, parietal, and temporal regions) findings provided a better explanation for fatigue-related areas of the brain (fatigue affects up to 80% of patients with MS). Integrated PET/MR can also be used to observe the correlation between two inflammatory markers in patients with MS. For example, the simultaneous acquisition of mI MRS and TSPO PET can help to reveal the different stages or subtypes of inflammation. Furthermore, multimodal imaging that combines PET with MRI can elucidate different characteristics of demyelinating diseases within the same imaging environment; therefore, furthering our understanding on the pathological processes, such as neuroinflammation and remyelination, of MS. Longitudinal studies based on TSPO PET/MR can simultaneously assess glial activation in white matter lesions, as well as T_2 lesion volume and NAWM magnetization transfer ratio, which explained 90% of the variance in enlarging T_2 lesion volume and brain atrophy in patients with MS at a 1-year follow-up. The use of integrated PET/MR can further improve patient compliance and enhance spatial resolution and registration accuracy. Additionally, the simultaneous acquisition of PET and MRI allows for the motion correction of PET data, which minimizes ambiguity in quantification, and is especially important when processing subtle changes in longitudinal studies. There is enormous potential for the application of PET/MR in MS, offering considerable advantages for both spatial and temporal synchronization when studying inflammation and neuronal activity in MS.

16.2 Research Applications of PET/MR in Encephalitis

Encephalitis refers to inflammatory lesions of the brain, which can manifest as a series of clinical symptoms, primarily including altered mental status, memory loss, epileptic seizures, and disorders of sleep and consciousness, among others. There are numerous causes for encephalitis, which can be grouped into two major types: autoimmune and infectious encephalitis. Autoimmune encephalitis is an inflammatory disease caused by abnormal immune responses produced by the body's immune system against neuronal antigenic components. Histopathologically, it is chiefly characterized by the infiltration of inflammatory cells into the brain parenchyma, and the formation of "sleeve-like" structures around blood vessels, with no evidence of specific infection in brain tissue and cerebrospinal fluid. Infectious encephalitis is generally the result of infection by viruses, bacteria, or other pathogens. In addition to neurological symptoms, patients may also present with fever and other symptoms and signs of systemic infection.

16.2.1 Research Applications of MRI in Encephalitis

16.2.1.1 Research Applications of Conventional MRI in Encephalitis

Conventional MRI is the preferred method of imaging for patients with suspected encephalitis. Abnormal structural alterations can be detected in 50–70% of patients with autoimmune encephalitis, and the affected areas have been shown to be associated with neuronal antibodies and clinical syndrome. Limbic encephalitis is characterized by abnormal MRI signals in the medial temporal lobe (MTL), and patients with bilateral MTL involvement (accompanied by cerebrospinal fluid or electroencephalography abnormalities) can be diagnosed as having limbic encephalitis independently of antibody tests. Owing to the differences in the course of the disease, lesions may exhibit hypo- or isointense signals on T_1WI (predominantly hypointensities), slightly hyperintense or hyperintense signals on T_2WI, and slightly hyper- or isointense signals on diffusion-weighted imaging (DWI). All lesions show hyperintense signals on the fluid attenuated inversion recovery (FLAIR) sequence, as this sequence suppresses the hyperintense signals of free water, but not those of lesions, thereby effectively highlighting the latter. The FLAIR sequence has a high sensitivity and is highly valuable for detecting lesions and determining the extent of lesions. Abnormal signals can usually be detected in the bilateral MTL, manifesting as T_1 hypointensities and T_2 and FLAIR hyperintensities in the majority of limbic encephalitis cases related to anti-γ- aminobutyric acid β receptor (GABABR), anti-α-amino-3-hydroxy--5-methyl-4-isoxazoleproprionic acid receptor (AMPAR), and leucine-rich glioma-inactivated 1 (LGI1) antibodies. Anti-GABABR encephalitis may also exhibit multi-focal lesions involving the cortical and subcortical regions, as well as T_2 and FLAIR hyperintensities, which are primarily found in the frontal and temporal lobes, and less commonly in the cerebellum and basal ganglia. These lesions do not exhibit restricted diffusion or enhancement. Approximately 50% of patients with anti-N-methyl-D-aspartate receptor (NMDAR) encephalitis show brain MRI abnormalities with no specific manifestations. Lesions can involve a number of brain areas, including the cortex, white matter, hippocampus, cerebellum, and basal ganglia, as well as exhibit T_1 hypointensities and T_2 and FLAIR hyperintensities. Some researchers have classified the head MRI findings of patients with anti-NMDAR encephalitis into the following four types: (1) Type I, normal; (2) Type II, hippocampal involvement; (3) Type III, extra-hippocampal involvement; and (4) Type IV, involvement of hippocampus and other areas. The hippocampus is the most commonly affected area and is associated with poor prognosis (Fig. 16.10). The presence of non-specific white matter lesions indicates that the patient should be screened for demyelination-related antibodies (e.g., aquaporin 4 or oligodendrocyte glycoprotein).

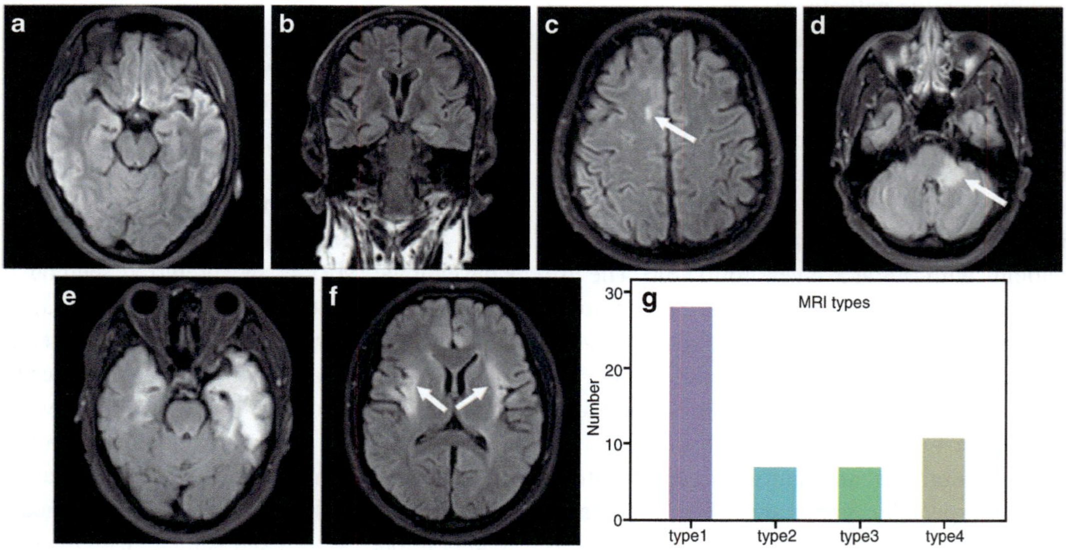

Fig. 16.10 MRI findings and difference analysis of patients with anti-NMDAR encephalitis. Type I, a 23-year-old male patient with anti-NMDAR encephalitis showing a normal brain MRI (**a**). Type II, a 29-year-old female patient showing lesions in the left hippocampus and a mild reduction in bilateral hippocampal volume (**b**). Type III (**c**, **d**), a 28-year-old male patient with lesions in the right frontal lobe (arrow in Fig. **c**) and left brachium pontis (arrow in Fig. **d**). Type IV (**e**, **f**), a 25-year-old male patient with lesions in the bilateral frontal lobes, temporal lobes, insula (arrows in Figs. **e**, **f**), hippocampus, and cingulate gyrus, and a reduction in left hippocampal volume. Histogram showing the four types of brain MRI findings (**g**)

16.2.1.2 Research Applications of DTI in Encephalitis

Although DTI has been widely utilized in a wide range of neurological diseases, it is rarely applied to infectious diseases. Using the region-of-interest (ROI) method, researchers analyzed the DTI changes in regions of the brain with abnormal T_2WI signals in patients with herpes simplex encephalitis. The results of that study indicated that in the early stages of inflammation, patients showed a slight decrease in MD and an increase in FA, whereas on or after the 14th day of inflammation, patients showed an increased MD and decreased FA, which were consistent with changes associated with inflammatory vasogenic edema. In another controlled study, DTI and fMRI were performed on 55 healthy controls and 11 pediatric patients with serologically confirmed tick-borne encephalitis (TBE) showing CNS involvement. No significant differences were found in the DTI findings between the two groups, whereas fMRI revealed differential activation of cortical areas related to working memory in patients, suggesting that functional changes preceded structural alterations.

16.2.1.3 Research Applications of MRS in Encephalitis

^{1}H-MRS allows the pathogenic mechanisms of encephalitis to be explored from a metabolic perspective. In patients with glutamate receptor encephalitis, the lower NAA peak found in cortical hyperintense lesions on FLAIR sequences signifies the presence of neuronal injuries. A longitudinal ^{1}H-MRS study of patients with Rasmussen encephalitis revealed that the metabolites underwent dynamic changes over the course of disease progression. More specifically, the early stages were chiefly characterized by a decreased NAA peak in the lesion area, whereas the later stages were characterized by increased lactic acid and glutamine/glutamate peaks. These findings suggest that Rasmussen encephalitis involves progressive brain damage, as well as the occurrence of neuronal injury and repair. In TBE patients, decreased NAA/Cr and increased Cho/Cr were observed in the bilateral thalamus, indicating that neuronal injury and metabolic abnormalities are present in TBE. Therefore, MRS can serve as a sensitive tool for evaluating brain metabolite changes in TBE patients.

16.2.1.4 Research Applications of fMRI in Encephalitis

fMRI has been extensively utilized in research on neurological and psychiatric diseases. Nevertheless, fMRI studies on encephalitis are relatively scarce, with only a handful of studies conducted in China and abroad, most of which are focused on autoimmune encephalitis.

Anti-NMDAR encephalitis is the most common form of autoimmune encephalitis. This disease generally occurs in young women, and 40–60% of cases in female patients are associated with ovarian teratoma. Typical clinical symptoms include low-grade fever, headache, and fatigue during the prodromal phase, later followed by psychiatric symptoms including anxiety, psychosis, delusions, and hallucinations. As the disease progresses further, patients may present with abnormal movements such as orofacial dyskinesia, dystonia, dysautonomia, epileptic seizures, and impaired consciousness. Some patients may also exhibit persistent cognitive deficits, including memory and impairments in executive function.

Reports have suggested that only 23–50% of patients with anti-NMDAR encephalitis exhibit structural abnormalities in brain MRI involving the frontal lobe, parietal lobe, and MTL, while the involvement of the cingulate gyrus, thalamus, cerebellum, and brainstem has also been reported. A long-term follow-up MRI study revealed that severe disease can lead to hippocampal atrophy and mild whole-brain atrophy, which was partially reversible at the 5- and 7-year follow-up. Patients in the acute phase showed impaired microstructural integrity in the hippocampus, while hippocampal volume and microstructural integrity were correlated with memory performance, disease severity, and disease duration.

According to fMRI studies, functional changes in the brain are associated with cognitive impairment following anti-NMDAR encephalitis. An fMRI analysis of anti-NMDAR encephalitis patients after the acute phase revealed that the FC between the DMN (including the medial PFC, ACC, part of the posterior cingulate cortex, and part of the MTL) and bilateral anterior hippocampus decreased, and that this FC decrease was also correlated with patient's memory impairment. Patients with acute anti-NMDAR encephalitis exhibited a disconnect between the MTL and DMN, impaired frontotemporal FC, and decreased hippocampal FC. In addition to the DMN, patients with anti-NMDAR encephalitis also showed functional impairments in other brain networks. For example, schizophrenia-like symptoms (e.g., hallucinations, delusions, and mutism) were correlated with impaired FC in the frontoparietal network. Animal models of anti-NMDAR encephalitis have been established based on these clinical and imaging findings. Pathological analysis showed that widespread labelling of anti-NMDAR antibodies could be observed in the hippocampus, and this region also exhibited reduced total and synaptic NMDAR cluster densities and total NMDAR protein concentration. These findings suggest that abnormal hippocampal function is associated with antibody-related damage, thereby forging a link between hippocampal dysfunction and cognitive impairment in immune-mediated neuroinflammatory diseases. These experiments have also provided a theoretical basis for treatments that seek to reduce anti-NMDAR antibodies and immunocompetent cells.

Patients with anti-LGI1 encephalitis present with subacute memory deficit, along with various neuropsychiatric symptoms, such as disorientation, impaired consciousness, temporal lobe epileptic seizures, and behavioral abnormalities. Patients are generally over 40 years of age, and men are more susceptible than women. Anti-LGI1 encephalitis is rarely associated with systemic tumors and initiating immunotherapy in the early stages will result in a good overall prognosis. Limbic LGI1 encephalitis is often accompanied by faciobrachial dystonic seizures (FBDS), which are brief, convulsive, high-frequency dystonic attacks that usually affect the upper limb and face unilaterally on the affected side. fMRI performed after the acute phase on patients with anti-LGI1 encephalitis revealed that the areas of the brain affected by this disease extended beyond the limbic system, and chiefly manifested as increased FC of the dorsal and ventral DMN, as well as decreased FC of the salience network, which were correlated with memory and cognition. Therefore, it was speculated that FC changes may be secondary or compensatory changes resulting from focal hippocampal injuries. Taken together, the functional studies above support the view that anti-LGI1 encephalitis can cause extensive brain dysfunction and functional reorganization.

Voltage-gated potassium channel (VGKC) antibodies can be detected among patients with limbic encephalitis, neuromyotonia, and Morvan's syndrome. These antibodies do not act directly on VGKCs, but on target proteins related to the VGKC complex, i.e., LGI1 and contactin-associated protein-like 2 (CASPR2). Patients with this form of autoimmune anti-VGKC antibody (VGKCC-Ab)-associated encephalitis exhibit varying degrees of MTL atrophy, accompanied by cognitive impairment. During the follow-up period, nearly 50% of patients developed hippocampal sclerosis. fMRI studies conducted on patients with anti-VGKCC-Ab encephalitis revealed that brain network FC changes were correlated with memory, but not with hippocampal volume. Therefore, FC impairments may serve as a better imaging marker of cognitive function in patients with VGKCC-Ab encephalitis. However, the majority of fMRI studies on encephalitis are cross-sectional; therefore, it is necessary to perform longitudinal research to explore the evolutionary patterns of brain activation and brain network activity over time.

16.2.2 Research Applications of PET Imaging in Encephalitis

Patients with encephalitis often present with negative findings on conventional MRI, and increasing attention has been paid to neuroimaging research on the early diagnosis of encephalitis.

PET allows us to observe the abnormal changes in brain tissues from a metabolic perspective. Studies have reported that the diagnostic sensitivity of PET (78%) for autoimmune encephalitis is higher than that of conventional MRI (63%). The utilization of PET has enabled the more detailed study of the pathogenesis and pathophysiological mechanisms of encephalitis, and the most common finding in autoimmune encephalitis is high ^{18}F-FDG uptake in the MTL. ^{18}F-FDG PET can display extra-lesional areas of the brain with increased glucose metabolism, such as the brainstem, cerebellum, or cerebral cortex, and the increase is more closely associated with clinical symptoms compared to MRI findings.

An ^{18}F-FDG PET study on patients with herpes simplex encephalitis demonstrated that high ^{18}F-FDG uptake could be observed in the hippocampus, temporal lobe, and striatum during the acute phase, as well as in the cerebral cortex (except the temporal lobe). During the recovery phase (after 3–6 months), the hippocampus and temporal lobe showed low ^{18}F-FDG uptake, which may have been related to gliosis and brain atrophy.

^{18}F-FDG PET imaging of patients with anti-NMDAR encephalitis revealed hypermetabolism in the frontotemporal lobe and hypometabolism in the parieto-occipital lobe, whereas the opposite trend was observed during the recovery process. Moreover, the increase in glucose metabolism between the frontotemporal lobe and occipital lobe was positively correlated with disease severity. In another PET study, patients with anti-NMDAR encephalitis showed whole-brain abnormalities in glucose metabolism compared to classic limbic encephalitis. Furthermore, a longitudinal PET study found that abnormalities in cerebral glucose metabolism improved with disease remission, with the cerebral cortex exhibiting diffuse hypometabolism during the early recovery phase, which returned to normal in the late recovery phase. Conversely, patients with worsening clinical symptoms showed further increases in regional glucose metabolism of the brain.

In anti-LGI1 encephalitis, approximately 70% of patients with T_2WI hyperintensities in the basal ganglia showed hypermetabolism on PET, whereas the PET findings of patients without abnormal signals in the basal ganglia revealed striatal hypermetabolism. Additionally, glucose hypermetabolism was observed in the cerebellum, glucose hypometabolism in the cingulate gyrus, occipital lobe, and precentral gyrus, and no significant changes were observed in the glucose metabolism of the MTL. These changes might be related to the disease duration, but longitudinal follow-up PET studies are needed to verify this claim. Changes in temporal glucose metabolism were better correlated with disease duration, such that limbic encephalitis patients with normal temporal glucose metabolism had better clinical prognosis.

PET imaging of patients with VGKCC-Ab encephalitis revealed that regions with temporal hypermetabolism agreed with MRI findings of hippocampal swelling and T_2WI hyperintensities. Only the unilateral temporal lobe and hippocampus were affected in the initial stages, but hypometabolism occurred in the bilateral lobes at the 2-year follow-up. Anti-AMPAR encephalitis is common among female patients, and 70% of patients have various types of tumors. The typical presentations of anti-AMPAR encephalitis include limbic encephalitis, accompanied by epileptic seizures, memory impairment, and psychiatric symptoms. Lesions are most commonly located in the MTL. PET can be used to display the increased glucose metabolism of the hippocampus, which remains in a hypermetabolic state even after the swelling has subsided. After anti-epileptic treatment of persistent temporal lobe seizures, patients experienced an improvement in memory symptoms, and a decrease in hippocampal hypermetabolism, showing a trend toward normal levels. In anti-GABABR encephalitis, GABABR is expressed throughout the brain, especially in the hippocampus, thalamus, and cerebellum. Anti-GABABR encephalitis typically manifests as limbic encephalitis, with 50% of cases associated with small cell lung cancer or neuroendocrine tumors. PET studies have shown that the majority of patients exhibited glucose hypermetabolism in the MTL, while some patients with anti-GABABR encephalitis presented with diffuse hypometabolism of the cerebral cortex. PET imaging of patients positive for anti-Ma2 antibodies revealed that glucose metabolism in the MTL increased with increasing anti-Ma2 antibody titer.

PET can contribute significantly to the diagnosis of autoimmune encephalitis. Encephalitis lesions may present with hypermetabolic or hypometabolic changes on PET, but the pattern of their metabolic changes remain inconclusive, and the predictive value of these changes for the prognosis of encephalitis is still unclear.

16.2.3 Research Applications of PET/MR in Encephalitis

The glucose hypermetabolism detected by PET is closely associated with the inflammatory process of encephalitis, whereas glucose hypometabolism may be caused by widespread neuronal injury in the chronic phase, but the mechanisms underlying this hypometabolism is still poorly understood. Multimodal imaging that combines PET and MRI provides a comprehensive understanding on the pathological mechanisms of encephalitis from the metabolic, structural, and functional perspectives. This provides important information for the clinical evaluation of the pathogenesis and the evaluation of therapeutic efficacy of encephalitis (Fig. 16.11).

16.3 Research Applications of PET/MR in Migraine

Migraine is a common chronic neurovascular disease, generally presenting as a recurrent pulsatile headache that is most often unilateral, but can also be bilateral, sometimes accompanied by symptoms such as nausea, vomiting, phonophobia, and photophobia. The most common type of migraine is migraine without aura (MwoA), which accounts for approximately 80% of migraine cases. A minority of cases are preceded by sensory and motor disturbances, which are known as an aura. Such cases are known as migraine with aura (MwA), or classic migraine, and account for 10% of all migraine cases. The global prevalence of migraine is about 10%, and its lifetime prevalence is about 14%. Among adults, the male-to-female ratio of migraine prevalence is 1:3 vs. 1:2, whereas among prepubescent children, there is no significant gender difference in prevalence. Studies on the family history of migraine suggest that it exhibits significant familial clustering, with 50–80% of patients reporting a positive family history.

Migraine attacks are associated with physical and chemical factors, psychological factors, and changes in hormone levels and are frequently induced by triggers. A study found that approximately 85% of patients were able to report their triggers, which often involved multiple factors. A classic migraine attack consists of the aura phase, attack phase, and interictal phase. Thus far, a theoretical consensus has yet to be achieved

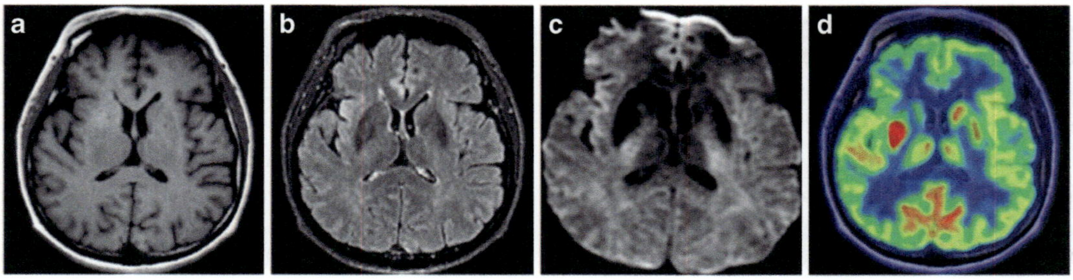

Fig. 16.11 Autoimmune encephalitis. A 46-year-old female patient. Transverse MR T_1WI shows slight hypointense signals in the right basal ganglia (**a**); transverse FLAIR (**b**) and DWI (**c**) show no abnormal signals; transverse ^{18}F-FDG PET (**d**) shows significantly increased glucose metabolism in the right caudate nucleus and putamen, with a maximum SUV of approximately 19.80

regarding the pathogenesis of migraine, but the following theories are currently widely accepted: (1) the vasogenic theory, (2) the theory of cortical spreading depression (CSD), and (3) the trigemino-vascular theory. It is generally believed that different types of migraine involve different pathogenic mechanisms. The clinical diagnosis of migraine is based primarily on the physician's subjective judgement with reference to the diagnostic criteria published by the International Headache Society (IHS), i.e., the International Classification of Headache Disorders Third Edition-Beta (ICHD-IIIβ), relevant scales, and relevant symptoms reported by the patient. It was previously believed that patients with migraine did not exhibit abnormal changes in brain imaging, and the goal of imaging examinations was to exclude organic diseases. However, with the advancement of new imaging techniques, researchers began detecting structural and functional changes in the brains of migraine patients, which may reflect the pathophysiological mechanisms underlying the neuronal alterations and brain functional abnormalities caused by recurrent migraine attacks.

16.3.1 Research Applications of MRI in Migraine

16.3.1.1 Research Applications of Conventional MRI in Migraine

1. Research applications of VBM in migraine: VBM-based comparisons of gray matter densities between migraine patients and healthy controls revealed that migraine patients had significantly lower gray matter densities in the bilateral insula, motor and premotor areas, PFC, cingulate gyrus, and right posterior parietal cortex, which were negatively correlated with disease duration and overall frequency of migraine attacks. These results suggest that recurrent migraine attacks led to selective changes in the areas of the brain involved in central pain regulation. Migraine patients also had lower gray matter densities in the temporal and frontal lobes, which were correlated with age and disease duration, as well as higher density in periaqueductal gray matter (PAG). Furthermore, the gray matter densities of the PAG and dorsolateral pons were higher among MwA than MwoA patients.
2. Research applications of DTI in migraine: DTI studies have demonstrated that the brainstem plays a crucial role in the pathogenesis of migraines. Early DTI studies found that MwoA and MwA patients showed lower FA values in white matter compared to the control group. DTI abnormalities, however, occurred in various locations across different studies in patients with migraine compared to healthy controls. After receiving drug treatment, MwoA patients showed improvements in clinical symptoms, as well as significantly increased FA values in affected areas, such as the corpus callosum. This implies that effective treatment can lead to the reversal of microstructural damage in the nerve fibers of the corpus callosum.

16.3.1.2 Research Applications of fMRI in Migraine

1. Research applications of fMRI in the aura phase of migraine: fMRI studies on the aura phase in MwA patients showed that CSD propagated at a velocity of 3.5 mm/min to the adjacent occipital cortex, then gradually spread to the entire cerebral cortex. This led to an initial decrease, followed by an increase, in glial and neuronal activities, as well as an initial hypoperfusion, followed by hyperperfusion, in corresponding areas of the brain. The propagation velocity of aura symptoms was similar to the velocity of cerebral blood flow (CBF) changes in experimental CSD. These findings have demonstrated the occurrence of CSD during the aura phase, suggesting that CSD is involved, to some extent, in the pathological changes during this phase.
2. Research applications of fMRI during the attack phase
   (a) Research applications of fMRI in spontaneous migraine attacks: A major limitation of performing fMRI studies during spontaneous migraine attacks is the

unpredictability and relatively short duration of migraine attacks. To address this issue, researchers have utilized event-related fMRI, by using pain, visual, olfactory, and other stimuli to induce migraine attacks, in order to perform functional imaging during the stimulation process. The purpose of this is to study the perceptual and affective abnormalities in the pain processing network of migraine patients.

(b) Research applications of fMRI during pain stimulation: Trigeminal nerve stimulation has been widely utilized to examine the pathophysiological mechanisms of migraine during the attack and interictal phases. Although the brainstem is considered to be highly associated with migraine attacks, these attacks are not solely related to a single area of the brain, but also involve the hypothalamus and cerebellum. Standard trigeminal nerve stimulation studies have demonstrated that the posterior thalamus is a critical structure for acute pain response, whereas the inferior part of the anterior thalamus may be key site implicated during migraine attacks. During specific stages of the migraine cycle, different functional changes can be observed in each subregion of the hypothalamus. Schultze and May performed a comprehensive study on the correlation between the migraine cycle and trigeminal nerve stimulation. Their results showed that hypothalamic activity, as a response to trigeminal nerve stimulation, increased over the period toward the next migraine attack. Furthermore, the hypothalamus showed altered FC values of the spinal trigeminal nuclei and dorsal thalamus, which was correlated to the prodromal and attack phases.

(c) Research applications of fMRI during visual stimulation: Aura in MwA patients is often a visual symptom; therefore, visual stimuli are frequently utilized in studies. Photophobia is a clinical sign of migraine during the attack and interictal phases. Migraine with visual aura is associated with the CSD of neuronal activity in the primary motor cortex, and the hyperexcitability of the visual cortex may be related to the integration mechanisms between the cortical regions and trigeminal nerve pathway. The primary visual and motor cortices and lateral geniculate nucleus of migraine patients showed greater responses to visual stimuli, which implies that cortical hyperresponsiveness is associated with migraine auras. Cortical hyperresponsiveness is not only found in the primary visual cortex, but also in higher-order visual cortices (inferior parietal lobule and frontal gyrus).

(d) Research applications of fMRI during olfactory stimulation: Although not mentioned in the classification criteria of the IHS, migraine patients may exhibit osmophobia during the attack and interictal phases, and certain odors can trigger migraine attacks. Relevant studies have found that migraine patients showed increased activation of the limbic system (amygdala and insula) and dorsal medulla oblongata during the attack phase, but there was no difference between patients and healthy controls during the interictal phase. This suggests that olfactory stimuli may induce functional changes, thereby demonstrating that the significant physiological connections between olfaction and the trigeminal nociceptive pathway are involved in the onset of migraine, and that odor-induced activation of the dorsal medulla oblongata may be the mechanism which odors trigger migraine attacks.

3. Research applications of fMRI during the interictal phase: Studies on the interictal phase of migraine attacks primarily involve utilizing RS-fMRI to study functional changes of the brain in patients, as well as the correlation of such changes with attack frequency and disease duration. Patients with MwoA and MwA showed decreased FC in the PFC and tempo-

ral regions of the DMN, as well as the frontoparietal region of the executive network (middle frontal gyrus and ACC). These functional abnormalities and structural changes may not be associated with clinical symptoms. Instead, FC changes in the DMN and PFC may be related to corresponding stimulus-induced responses or may be characteristic of migraine patients. Other RS-fMRI studies on migraine patients found that FC abnormalities were primarily located at the level of pain processing networks. For example, in the pain and somatosensory processing pathways, increased FC was observed between the PAG and cerebral regions. At present, relatively similar conclusions have been obtained across studies conducted in China and abroad. More specifically, migraine patients showed significantly lower FC values in brain regions such as the middle frontal gyrus and ACC, as well as the frontal and temporal lobes in the DMN. Based on these findings, it can be concluded that the widespread attenuation of FC in migraine patients are adaptive changes to pain stimuli, and long-term pain stimulation can lead to diminished responses and sensitivity to pain in the brains of patients with migraine.

4. Research applications of perfusion imaging in migraine
   (a) Research applications of perfusion-weighted imaging (PWI) in migraine: PWI studies have reported that during migraine attacks, patients may exhibit local aura- or headache-related perfusion abnormalities, but current findings are inconsistent, or even contradictory. Early studies revealed that patients with chronic or persistent aura exhibited both hyper- and hypoperfusion. Subsequent studies later found that in migraine with visual aura, patients exhibited hypoperfusion of the occipital cortex contralateral to the visual field defect, which showed decreased CBF and cerebral blood volume.
   (b) Research applications of arterial spin labelling (ASL) in migraine: As with the research findings of PWI in migraine, ASL has also yielded inconsistent results in migraine patients, which include the following: (1) no significant differences in whole-brain or regional cerebral perfusion; (2) hyper- and hypoperfused regions observed in MwA patients during the attack phase, which are reversible in some patients; and (3) positive correlation between CBF changes and attack frequency. These findings could be attributed to the regional functional remodeling of areas of the brain in patients with migraine.

   In a study on the efficacy evaluation of drug treatment using ASL, ASL imaging was performed in a single 32-year-old migraine patient 1 h after the attack, the results of which revealed hypoperfusion in the bilateral medial thalamus and hypothalamus, as well as hyperperfusion of the bilateral frontal cortex. ASL imaging was repeated 1 h after the oral administration of rizatriptan, which indicated improvements in the perfusion of the bilateral medial thalamus and hypothalamus. These findings also suggest that the hypothalamus and adjacent areas are involved in the onset of migraine attacks.

5. Research applications of DWI and susceptibility-weighted imaging (SWI) in migraine: During migraine attacks, regions of the brain related to aura or headache may exhibit regional restricted diffusion, hypoperfusion, vascular changes, and other manifestations. Altinok et al. reported that during the aura phase of one patient with migraine, PWI revealed hypoperfusion in the cerebral hemisphere contralateral to aura symptoms, DWI revealed regional restricted diffusion in the parietal lobe of the same side, while SWI showed significantly dilated cortical veins in the same cerebral hemisphere. These abnormalities had returned to normal during follow-up after 2 days.
6. Research applications of MRS in migraine: In a study by Sarchielli et al., MwA patients exhibited increased lactic acid levels and decreased NAA levels following visual stimu-

lation, whereas these changes were not observed in MwoA patients. Therefore, these findings indicate that migraine is not entirely a functional disease but may also have microstructural alterations. Compared to healthy controls, MwoA patients showed increased GABA concentrations in the brain. It was therefore speculated that the imbalance in the "excitation-inhibition" homeostasis between GABA in inhibitory neurons and glutamate in excitatory neurons may lead to migraine attacks. Furthermore, migraine patients treated with levetiracetam showed decreased GABA levels in the cingulate cortex, suggesting that GABA could serve as a biomarker for evaluating therapeutic efficacy in migraine.

16.3.2 Research Applications of PET Imaging in Migraine

Common radiotracers utilized in PET studies include ^{18}F-FDG and ^{15}O-H_2O. According to PET studies comparing the differences in cerebral glucose metabolism between migraine patients and healthy controls, migraine patients showed significant decreases in the glucose metabolism of areas of the brain known to be associated with central pain processing, such as the bilateral insula, bilateral ACC and posterior cingulate cortex, and PFC. Metabolism in the insula and ACC was found to be negatively correlated with disease duration and lifetime headache frequency.

Owing to the unpredictability of migraine attacks and the relatively stringent requirements of experimental conditions, very few studies have been conducted on spontaneous migraine attacks. Weiller et al., who pioneered the functional imaging of spontaneous migraine attacks, demonstrated using ^{15}O-H_2O PET that the CBF of the dorsal pons was significantly elevated during these attacks and remained at an elevated level even after treatment with sumatriptan for pain relief. Based on these findings, they proposed the theory of the "brainstem migraine generator." Thereafter, ^{15}O-H_2O PET studies on migraine observed significantly elevated CBF in the midbrain, pons, and hypothalamus, and these activated areas also persisted even after treatment with sumatriptan. Taken together, these findings indicate that in addition to the brainstem, the hypothalamus also plays a critical role in the pathophysiology of migraine attacks. A recent PET study on patients with spontaneous prodromal vestibular migraine revealed that patients had increased glucose metabolism in the vestibulo-thalamo-cortical pathway, and decreased glucose metabolism in the visual cortex, which may be attributed to the mutual inhibition between the visual and vestibular systems. PET studies involving the imaging of 5-hydroxytryptamine (5-HT) receptors showed increased 5-HT synthesis during the migraine attack phase and increased 5-HT receptor availability in the pons during the early stage of migraine attacks. In a recent study involving a selective radiotracer for L-type opioid receptors, it was found that during migraine attacks, PFC μ opioid receptors (which are involved in pain regulation) were activated and correlated with the availability of μ opioid receptors. These findings have elucidated the mechanisms of the central L-type opioid system underlying allodynia during spontaneous migraine attacks. Another study showed that the level of μ opioid receptors is reduced in the endogenous opioid system involved in pain regulation. Therefore, it was speculated that these receptors may have been occupied, which could be an antagonistic response to persistent pain and injury.

A variety of imaging techniques have been utilized to study the structural and functional changes of the brain in patients with migraine. The mutual complementation of these techniques has provided new insights on the pathogenic mechanisms of migraine. There are also contradictions or controversies among current research results, which may be related to the heterogeneity of subjects enrolled and differences in imaging methods across different studies. Nevertheless, the combination of different imaging techniques and further investigations on their interrelationships will be of crucial significance. In future, these imaging techniques will serve as new indicators for evaluating the onset and development of migraine, as well as new methods and targets for the evaluation and treatment of migraine in a more objective and visible manner.

Suggested Reading

Antonio C, Beniamino G, George D, et al. [18F] Florbetapir PET/MR imaging to assess demyelination in multiple sclerosis. Eur J Nucl Med Mol Imaging. 2020;47(2):366–78.

Bolcaen J, Acou M, Mertens K, et al. Structural and metabolic features of two different variants of multiple sclerosis: a PET/MRI study. J Neuroimaging. 2013;23(3):431–6.

Burns R, de Malherbe M, Chadenat ML, et al. Arterial spin labeled MR imaging detecting biphasic neurovascular changes in migraine with persistent aura. Headache. 2017;57(10):1627–8.

Cecchin D, Palombit A, Castellaro M, et al. Brain PET and functional MRI: why simultaneously using hybrid PET/MR systems? QJ Nucl Med Mol Imaging. 2017;61(4):345–59.

Coppola G, Di Renzo A, Tinelli E, et al. Resting state connectivity between default mode network and insula encodes acute migraine headache. Cephalalgia. 2018;32(5):846–54.

Datta G, Colasanti A, Kalk N, et al. 11C-PBR28 and 18F-PBR111 detect white matter inflammatory heterogeneity in multiple sclerosis. J Nucl Med. 2017;58(9):1477–82.

Datta G, Colasanti A, Rabiner EA, et al. Neuroinflammation and its relationship to changes in brain volume and white matter lesions in multiple sclerosis. Brain. 2017;140(11):2927–38.

Datta G, Violante IR, Scott G, et al. Translocator positron-emission tomography and magnetic resonance spectroscopic imaging of brain glial cell activation in multiple sclerosis. Mult Scler. 2017;23(11):1469–78.

Denuelle M, Fabre N, Payoux P, et al. Hypothalamic activation in spontaneous migraine attacks. Headache. 2007;47(10):1418–26.

Dodich A, Cerami C, Iannaccone S, et al. Neuropsychological and FDG-PET profiles in VGKC autoimmune limbic encephalitis. Brain Cogn. 2016;103(10):81–7.

Fillippi M, Rocca MA. M R imaging of multiple sclerosis. Radiology. 2011;259(3):659–81.

Gil-Gouveia R, Pinto J, Figueiredo P, et al. An arterial spin labeling MRI perfusion study of migraine without aura attacks. Front Neurol. 2017;8:280.

Graus F, Titulaer MJ, Balu R, et al. A clinical approach to diagnosis of autoimmune encephalitis. Lancet Neurol. 2016;15(4):391–404.

Kara B, Kiyat Atamer A, Onat L, et al. DTI findings during spontaneous migraine attacks. Clin Neuroradiol. 2013;23(1):31–6.

Kreisl WC, Jenko KJ, Hines CS, et al. A genetic polymorphism for translocator protein 18 kDa affects both in vitro and in vivo radioligand binding in human brain to this putative biomarker of neuroinflammation. J Cereb Blood Flow Metab. 2013;33(1):53–8.

Law-Ye B, Fargeot G, Leclercq D. Arterial spin labeling hypoperfusion in migraine aura. Headache. 2017;57(6):935–6.

Li Q, Chen CHF, Gong T, et al. High-field MRS study of GABA+ in patients with migraine: response to levetiracetam treatment. Neuroreport. 2018;29(12):1007–10.

Louapre C, Perlbarg V, Garcia-Lorenzo D, et al. Brain networks disconnection in early multiple sclerosis cognitive deficits: an anatomofunctional study. Hum Brain Mapp. 2014;35(9):4706–17.

Maleki N, Becerra L, Upadhyay J, et al. Direct optic nerve Pulvinar connections defined by diffusion MR tractography in humans: implications for photophobia. Hum Brain Mapp. 2012;33(1):75–88.

Maniyar FH, Sprenger T, Monteith T, et al. Brain activations in the premonitory phase of nitroglycerin-triggered migraine attacks. Brain. 2014;137(Pt 1):232–41.

Matteo B, Selene C, Stefano R, et al. Molecular imaging of multiple sclerosis: from the clinical demand to novel radiotracers. EJNMMI Radiopharm Chem. 2019;4(1):6.

May A. Understanding migraine as a cycling brain syndrome: reviewing the evidence from functional imaging. Neurol Sci. 2017;38(Suppl 1):125–30.

Moccia M, De Stefano N, Barkhof F. Imaging outcome measures for progressive multiple sclerosis trials. Mult Scler. 2017;23(12):1614–26.

Navarro V, Kas A, Apartis E, et al. Collaborators motor cortex and hippocampus are the two main cortical targets in LGI1-antibody encephalitis. Brain. 2016;139(Pt 4):1079–93.

Neeb L, Bastian K, Villringer K, et al. No microstructural white matter alterations in chronic and episodic migraineurs: a case-control diffusion tensor magnetic resonance imaging study. Headache. 2015;55(2):241–51.

Pagani M, Giuliani A, Öberg J, et al. Progressive disintegration of brain networking from Normal aging to Alzheimer disease: analysis of independent components of ^{18}F-FDG PET data. J Nucl Med. 2017;58(7):1132–9.

Politis M, Giannetti P, Su P, et al. Increased PK11195 PET binding in the cortex of patients with MS correlates with disability. Neurology. 2012;79(6):523–30.

Probasco JC, Solnes L, Nalluri A, et al. Decreased occipital lobe metabolism by FDG-PET/CT: an anti-NMDA receptor encephalitis biomarker. Neurol Neuroimmunol Neuroinflamm. 2017;5(1):e413.

Rom S, Persidsky Y. Cannabinoid receptor 2: potential role in immunomodulation and neuroinflammation. J Neuroimmune Pharmacol. 2013;8(3):608–20.

Schulte LH, Allers A, May A. Hypothalamus as a mediator of chronic migraine: evidence from high-resolution fMRI. Neurology. 2017;88(21):2011–6.

Schulte LH, May A. The migraine generator revisited: continuous scanning of the migraine cycle over 30 days and three spontaneous attacks. Brain. 2016;139(Pt 7):1987–93.

Sijbesma JW, Dierckx RA, Buchpiguel CA, et al. PET imaging of demyelination and remyelination in the cuprizone mouse model for multiple sclerosis: a comparison between [11C] CIC and [11C] MeDAS. NeuroImage. 2014;87(2):395–402.

Singhal T, O'connor K, Dubey S, et al. 18F-PBR06 versus 11C-PBR28 PET for assessing white matter translocator protein binding in multiple sclerosis. Clin Nucl Med. 2018;43(9):e289–95.

Spatola M, Petit-Pedrol M, Simabukuro M, et al. Investigations in GABAA receptor antibody-associated encephalitis. Neurology. 2017;88(11):1012–20.

Stankewitz A, May A. Increased limbic and brainstem activity during migraine attacks following olfactory stimulation. Neurology. 2011;77(5):476–82.

Szots M, Blaabjerg M, Orsi G, et al. Global brain atrophy and metabolic dysfunction in LGI1 encephalitis: a prospective multimodal MRI study. J Neurol Sci. 2017;376(15):159–65.

Van Sonderen A, Thijs RD, Coenders EC, et al. Anti-LGI1 encephalitis: clinical syndrome and long-term follow-up. Neurology. 2016;87(14):1449–56.

Venneti S, Lopresti BJ, Wiley CA. Molecular imaging of microglia-macrophages in the brain. Glia. 2013;61(1):10–23.

Weiller C, May A, Limmroth V, et al. Brain stem activation in spontaneous human migraine attacks. Nat Med. 1995;1(7):658–60.

Yuan J, Guan H, Zhou X, et al. Changing brain metabolism patterns in patients with ANMDARE: serial 18F-FDG PET/CT findings. Clin Nucl Med. 2016;41(5):366–70.

GPSR Compliance

The European Union's (EU) General Product Safety Regulation (GPSR) is a set of rules that requires consumer products to be safe and our obligations to ensure this.

If you have any concerns about our products, you can contact us on ProductSafety@springernature.com

In case Publisher is established outside the EU, the EU authorized representative is:

Springer Nature Customer Service Center GmbH
Europaplatz 3
69115 Heidelberg, Germany

Batch number: 10731383

Printed by Printforce, the Netherlands